D1128232

Adolescent Psychiatry
in Clinical Practice

Adolescent Psychiatry in Clinical Practice

Edited by

Simon G. Gowers FRCPsych MPhil

Professor of Adolescent Psychiatry, University of Liverpool and Honorary Consultant in
Adolescent Psychiatry, Mersey Regional Young People's Centre, Chester, UK

A member of the Hodder Headline Group
LONDON
Co-published in the USA by
Oxford University Press, Inc., New York

First published in Great Britain in 2001 by
Arnold, a member of the Hodder Headline Group,
338 Euston Road, London NW1 3BH

http://www.arnoldpublishers.com

Co-published in the USA by
Oxford University Press Inc.,
198 Madison Avenue, New York, NY10016
Oxford is a registered trademark of Oxford University Press

© 2001 Arnold

All rights reserved. No part of this publication may be reproduced or
transmitted in any form or by any means, electronically or mechanically,
including photocopying, recording or any information storage or retrieval
system, without either prior permission in writing from the publisher or a
licence permitting restricted copying. In the United Kingdom such licences
are issued by the Copyright Licensing Agency: 90 Tottenham Court Road,
London W1P 0LP.

Whilst the advice and information in this book are believed to be true and
accurate at the date of going to press, neither the authors nor the publisher
can accept any legal responsibility or liability for any errors or omissions
that may be made. In particular (but without limiting the generality of the
preceding disclaimer) every effort has been made to check drug dosages;
however, it is still possible that errors have been missed. Furthermore,
dosage schedules are constantly being revised and new side-effects
recognized. For these reasons the reader is strongly urged to consult the
drug companies' printed instructions before administering any of the drugs
recommended in this book.

British Library Cataloguing in Publication Data
A catalogue record for this book is available from the British Library

Library of Congress Cataloging-in-Publication Data
A catalog record for this book is available from the Library of Congress

ISBN 0 340 76231 4

1 2 3 4 5 6 7 8 9 10

Typeset in 10/13 pt Sabon by Genesis Typesetting, Rochester, Kent
Printed and bound in Great Britain by MPG Books Ltd, Bodmin, Cornwall

What do you think about this book? Or any other Arnold title?
Please send your comments to feedback.arnold@hodder.co.uk

CONTENTS

PREFACE

Despite growing concern about high levels of psychiatric morbidity in teenagers and the pleas of two reports from the Health Advisory Service, adolescent psychiatry remains a small, underdeveloped sub-speciality in the UK. A succession of reports, including the recent Audit Commission and Young Minds reviews of CAMHS, have pointed to the contrast between the growing morbidity of adolescents and the lack of provision of services for them, particularly at the older end of the age span.

Child and adolescent psychiatry has benefited from a significant increase in the number of academic posts over the past decade, many of which have contributed notably to clinical and research knowledge in the adolescent age group. However, given the high rates of disorder in adolescence and the increasing risk of mental illness at this stage of development, one gets an impression of a mismatch between morbidity and academic development.

When the University of Liverpool generously offered me the first chair dedicated to adolescent psychiatry in the UK, I felt a bit like Groucho Marx, who was memorably disinclined to join a club who would have him as a member. On the one hand I felt ill-equipped to be its academic standard-bearer and, on the other hand, disappointed by the small size of the club!

I was aware, however, that there existed a significant body of experienced clinicians with a wealth of clinical expertise, up-to-date research literature at their fingertips and time on their hands to put this knowledge to paper!

This book was conceived, therefore, with the aim of drawing together the expertise of a number of adolescent psychiatrists. Many have gained their clinical experience as consultants to Regional Adolescent Services, supplemented by others with specialist knowledge in such areas as the law, drug and alcohol misuse, liaison psychiatry and forensic services, to provide a comprehensive account of current best clinical practice. All the chapters aim to reflect the current evidence-base underlying their clinical guidance. They are readable and practical with appropriate clinical examples, but also, hopefully, scholarly.

Although all but one of the contributors are psychiatrists, this book is intended for all members of multidisciplinary child and adolescent mental health teams working with adolescents. Equally importantly, I hope that those who often fill the gaps in service provision, paediatricians and clinicians in adult services, for example, will find it helps them in liaising with CAMHS and feeling better equipped to manage complex cases themselves.

Simon G. Gowers

ACKNOWLEDGEMENT

I am grateful to Arthur Crisp and David Taylor for encouraging me to develop an academic career in adolescent psychiatry, and to the multidisciplinary teams at Colwood, Prestwich and Chester YPC who contributed to my understanding.

I would like to thank the young people at Chester YPC and M for contributing the illustrations, and Gill, Imogen and Christy for tolerating my conduct/emotional/eating disorder and periodic regression to adolescence at times of stress.

Finally, special thanks to Linda Rhodes for her tireless help in collating the manuscript and liaising with the authors and publishers.

FOREWORD

Contemporary western societies are preoccupied with the issue of troubled adolescents. Indeed, during recent years there has been a tremendous growth of research into both adolescent development and adolescent psychopathology. We now know a great deal about the epidemiology of mental disorders in adolescence. Knowledge is also accumulating about how best to treat these disorders. For example, during the past five years the results of randomised trials of treatment for several important adolescent problems have been published, including major depression, anxiety, and conduct disorders.

This rapid growth in research has not been matched by the development of a separate clinical speciality of adolescent psychiatry. In many countries adolescent psychiatry is still practised by general child psychiatrists. Nevertheless, as this book shows, clinical practice in the field has advanced considerably. The principal objective of this volume is to provide practical guidelines for the health professional who deals with troubled adolescents. The authors are experienced clinicians and their feel for the clinical needs of adolescent patients comes through in every chapter. The book begins with helpful reviews of normal development, influences on the development of psychopathology, and the classification and epidemiology of adolescent disorders. Each of the major disorders is then considered in turn. Treatments are then discussed in chapters that deal with all of the major therapies, including cognitive approaches, medication, family therapy and individual therapy.

Clinicians are likely to enjoy reading *Adolescent Psychiatry in Clinical Practice* from cover to cover. The approach taken is broad ranging and authoritative. It provides a comprehensive account of current clinical practice and introduces new approaches for understanding psychopathology in this age group.

Richard Harrington

LIST OF CONTRIBUTORS

Dr Sue Bailey
Consultant Adolescent Forensic Psychiatrist
Adolescent Forensic Service, Research and Development Unit, Mental Health
Services of Salford, Bury New Road, Prestwich, Manchester, M25 3BL

Dr Rachel M. Calam
Senior Lecturer in Clinical Psychology
University Department of Clinical Psychology, Research and Teaching Unit,
Withington Hospital, West Didsbury, Manchester, M20 8LR

Dr Paul Cawthron
Consultant in Child and Adolescent Psychiatry
Nottingham Healthcare NHS Trust, Thorneywood Adolescent Unit, Porchester
Road, Nottingham, NG3 6LF

Dr Andrew Clark
Senior Lecturer/Consultant in Child and Adolescent Psychiatry
Adolescent Psychiatry Service, Mental Health Services of Salford
Bury New Road, Prestwich Manchester, M25 3BL

Dr Andrew J. Cotgrove
Consultant in Adolescent Psychiatry
Young People's Centre, Pine Lodge, 79 Liverpool Road, Chester, CH2 1AW

Dr Rachel Davis
Consultant in Child and Adolescent Psychiatry
Craigavon and Banbridge Health Trust, Child and Family Clinic, Bocombra
Lodge, 2 Old Lurgan Road, Portadown, Northern Ireland, BT63 5SQ

Dr Mary Eminson
Consultant Child and Adolescent Psychiatrist
Child and Family Services, Bolton Hospitals NHS Trust, Royal Bolton
Hospital, Minerva Road, Farnworth, Bolton, BL4 OJR

Dr David M. Foreman
Consultant/Senior Lecturer in Child and Adolescent Psychiatry
Department of Psychiatry, Keele University, Thornburrow Drive, Hartshill,
Stoke-on-Trent, ST4 7QB

Dr Robin Glaze
Consultant in Adolescent Psychiatry
Young People's Unit, Royal Edinburgh Hospital, Tipperlin Road, Edinburgh,
EH10 5HF

Dr Michael Göpfert
Consultant Psychotherapist
Webb House Democratic Therapeutic Community, Victoria Avenue, Crewe,
CW2 7QS

Professor Simon G. Gowers
Professor of Adolescent Psychiatry
University of Liverpool, Academic Unit, Young People's Centre, Pine Lodge,
79 Liverpool Road, Chester, CH2 1AW

Professor Jonathan Hill
Professor of Child and Developmental Psychiatry
University of Liverpool, University Child Mental Health, 1st Floor, Mulberry
House, Alder Hey Children's Hospital, Eaton Road, Liverpool, L12 2AP

Dr John Merrill
Consultant in Drug Dependence
Drugs North West, Kenyon House, Mental Health Services of Salford, Bury
New Road, Prestwich, Manchester, M25 3BL

Dr Julia Nelki
Consultant Child and Adolescent Psychiatrist
Seymour House, 41–43 Seymour Terrace, Liverpool, L3 5TE

Dr Clive North
Consultant Child and Adolescent Psychiatrist
North Essex Child and Family Consultation Service, 25 West Avenue,
Clacton-on-Sea, Essex, CO15 1EN

Dr Lesley Peters
Clinicial Research Fellow
Drugs North West, Kenyon House, Mental Health Services of Salford, Bury
New Road, Prestwich, Manchester, M25 3BL

Dr Tania Stanway
Consultant in Adolescent Psychiatry
16–19 Service, Tarvin Ward, West Cheshire Hospital, Countess of Chester
Health Park, Liverpool Road, Chester, CH2 1UL

Dr Andrew Weaver
Consultant Child and Adolescent Psychiatrist
East Cheshire NHS Trust, Child and Adolescent Mental Health, Alderley
Building, Macclesfield General Hospital, Victoria Road, Macclesfield,
SK10 3BL

Dr Alison J. Wood
Consultant Child Psychiatrist
Child and Adolescent Psychiatry, South Manchester University Hospitals NHS
Trust, Carol Kendrick Unit, Withington Hospital, Nell Lane, West Didsbury,
Manchester, M20 2LR

Dr Michael Venables
Consultant in Child and Adolescent Psychiatry
Child and Adolescent Mental Health Services (CAMHS), The Annexe
Horsham Hospital, Hurst Road, Horsham, RH12 2DR

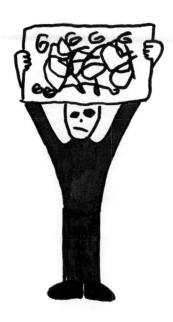

Chapter 1

NORMAL DEVELOPMENT
IN ADOLESCENCE

Rachel M. Calam

INTRODUCTION

Hall (1904), who characterised adolescence with the phrase 'sturm und drang' (storm and stress), indicated the complexity of understanding adolescent development in the title of his paper 'Adolescence: its psychology and its relation to physiology, anthropology, sociology, sex, crime, religion and education'.

Adolescence is a time of substantial change. At present, we lack a unified theory of development in adolescence (Durkin, 1995), but the complexity of the stage may make it difficult to arrive at a single model. Many studies reflect a preoccupation with the problems that may present in adolescence, rather than the normal course of development (Hill, 1993). The literature on normal development suggests rather a different picture, with only 5–15% of adolescents showing severe psychological disturbance (Kazdin, 1990; Offer *et al.*, 1988). Of these, a high percentage will have had difficulties in childhood (Rutter, 1976). In this chapter, the literature on the normal development of the adolescent will be reviewed with an emphasis on the importance of context. Substantial physical, cognitive and psychological developments take place during adolescence, and this chapter will also consider these in turn, together with the changes in relationships that they contribute to.

The role of the major contexts for development, the family, the school and the peer group, will be considered. It is clear that each of these will have an influence on development, but that there are interactions between the ways in which adolescents experience each of these contexts and the contribution that the adolescent brings to relationships in each of these settings. Family relationships predict adjustment to school and the quality of peer relationships, while peer relationships and behaviour in school relate to academic performance. Successful adjustment in school will influence access to the world of work, which is considered in the final section of the chapter.

THE DEFINITION OF ADOLESCENCE

One of the difficulties in describing adolescence lies in the lack of any clearly defined start or finishing point. Physical, pubertal maturation, often taken as a marker for entry into adolescence, may occur at very different ages. The end of adolescence is even more difficult to define; economic independence will be affected by socioeconomic factors and other markers may be highly culturally defined. In the West, our definitions of adolescence have changed markedly since the Industrial Revolution, and each of the post war decades has seen shifts in society's perception of the adolescent.

'. . . we like to believe that we know one when we see one, but *adolescent* is an inherently fuzzy concept. It labels a diversity of young people, and covers a lengthy developmental span.' (Durkin, 1995, p. 508).

THE DEVELOPMENTAL TASKS OF ADOLESCENCE

Adolescence presents the youngster and family with a number of tasks, the successful accomplishment of which will be more or less essential to good mental health. The tasks change over time, and there are clear cultural and gender differences which may become more marked with increasing age. It is becoming increasingly clear from the work on attachment theory that the way in which transitions are negotiated will reflect prior experience within the network of relationships in the family and broader social context. Prior experience will influence current behaviour as the adolescent encounters new settings and experiences.

The major tasks of this time involve the movement from small, familiar settings to larger and more impersonal ones, e.g. secondary schools, and the exploration of new possibilities in relationships, leisure and, later, work settings. In all these changes, the peer group is of importance. Underlying all of this is the relationship to the family. The wider cultural context and prevailing socioeconomic conditions will also have an important impact on development. All of these are areas to which we will return.

ADOLESCENT DEVELOPMENT IN THE CONTEXT OF THE LIFESPAN

Coleman and Hendry (1999) summarise some of the main principles of lifespan developmental psychology which are of clear relevance to the understanding of adolescent development. They emphasise the human ecology of development, and the geographical, historical, social and political context of the family. A further important concept is that of the reciprocal influence of individuals and families on one-another.

Rutter and Rutter (1992) set out a number of principles and concepts central to the consideration of development across the lifespan. They note the importance of *genetic and biological factors*. The adolescent makes the change from child to adult, undergoing change in the bodily configuration and a range of different changes arising as a result in changes in hormonal activity that precede and continue through puberty. In this chapter, sociobiological concepts will be referred to, giving examples of adolescent behaviour which may have their origins in reproductively advantageous strategies. These changes lay the foundations for the establishment of adult sexual relationships. *Timing* is a further important factor in changes; this chapter will present examples of the influence of timing of, for example, pubertal maturity on behaviour. Rutter and Rutter emphasise the degree to which people are *active*, rather than passive participants in their own development, shaping their own world through their interactions and negotiations with others. The way that adolescents will feel, think and act in given circumstances will vary. The meaning of *transitions* and their interpretation is also important. Again, the chapter will give examples of the experiences and development of adolescents from families with different ideologies and ways of interacting, and from different socioeconomic and ethnic groups. *Protective factors* which enhance development in adolescence will be a focus. A final area highlighted by Rutter and Rutter is the existence of *chain and strand effects*, in which there is carry-over from childhood into adolescence and then into adulthood.

ATTACHMENT IN ADOLESCENCE

One central, unifying theory in understanding development is that of attachment theory (Ainsworth *et al.*, 1978; Bowlby, 1969). In studies of infants and caregivers, three types of attachment were identified by Ainsworth *et al.*: *secure*, *anxious-avoidant* and *anxious-resistant*. Research shows that prior attachment status at age 12–18 months is predictive of later behaviour in other settings. It has become clear that secure attachment is beneficial to development across the lifespan. A small number of studies (e.g. Erikson *et al.*, 1985) have tracked the same individuals over time and have shown that insecure attachment is associated with poor peer relationships in childhood, which, as is known from other studies, are likely to be associated with poor social competence in adolescence. Central to attachment theory is the concept of the *internal working model*, the model of interpersonal relationships which has been developed from within the context of these early attachments. The nature of the internal working model is thought to have a profound influence on the way in which new relationships will be approached and formed, and would thus be likely to have an influence throughout the lifespan. The quality of close relationships plays an important role in adjustment throughout the lifespan and 'human beings at any age are most well-adjusted when they have confidence in the accessibility and responsiveness of a trusted other' (Armsden and Greenberg, 1987, p. 428).

Some studies have attempted to measure the nature of the current attachment relationship between the adolescent and parent or have asked for a description of the earlier relationship (Armsden and Greenberg, 1987). These studies show that secure attachment in adolescence, or self-report of having had a secure attachment, is associated with greater social competence and adjustment, and with lower anxiety, hostility and greater ego resiliency. Secure attachment is also likely to be associated with acceptance of conventional norms of behaviour and hence reduce the risk of antisocial behaviour. The ability to establish and maintain social relations will have its roots in attachment relationships. At all stages in the life cycle, it is important to be able to establish and maintain relationships and a network of supportive ties which, although changing over time, provide resources for individual well-being. Hence, quality of attachment relationships, rather than family structure, was found to be important in preventing delinquent behaviour (Sokol-Katz et al., 1997), with secure attachment being associated with law-abiding beliefs and behaviour. Attachment relationships are, therefore, of considerable importance and we will return to the subject of family relationships later in the chapter.

DEVELOPMENT IN ADOLESCENCE

PHYSICAL AND BIOLOGICAL DEVELOPMENT IN ADOLESCENCE

Puberty is a time of change and development in a range of bodily functions. In addition to the changes in the reproductive system and secondary sex characteristics, there are changes in the functioning of the neuroendocrine system, heart, cardiovascular system, lungs and musculature. The growth spurt may begin in boys between 10 and 16, and in girls, at 7, 8 or 12–14, although for boys it tends to be around 13 and around 11 for girls. There is a marked increase in strength and endurance, particularly for boys. Coleman and Hendry (1999) provide a clear summary of changes at this time. Figure 1.1 illustrates the main changes. The rapid change in physical state has a profound effect on the individual, leading to much preoccupation with the self, and there may be a period of clumsiness as adaptation occurs. For males and females, the physical developments may have different, culturally determined meanings, and may lead to differences in self-perception. Differences in timing of these events, early or late relative to peers, may also be related to behaviour and self-concept.

(a) Females

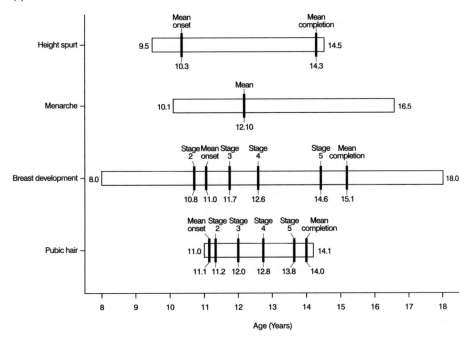

(b) Males

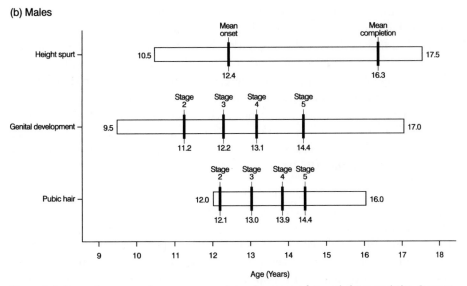

Figure 1.1 Normal range and average age of development of sexual characteristics. Source: Tanner, J. M. (1978) *Foetus into Man*. London: Open Books

GIRLS

In the West, menarche generally occurs between the ages of 10 and 16. In less affluent societies, menarche is later, e.g. in Papua New Guinea, where it may occur between 18 and 20. Age of puberty tends to follow dietary, workload and morbidity patterns, with age decreasing as these improve. Over the past century, in industrialised societies, the age of menarche has dropped considerably. Baker and Bellis (1995) summarise these findings. Within a society, diet and physical activity levels are an important influence (Bullough, 1981). Even in the biological sphere, the influence of family and social context is important, to the extent that Belsky *et al.* (1991) suggest that onset of menstruation be seen as a dependent, rather than independent variable in development. Girls who grow up in households where there is family conflict and father absence show early menarche (Aro and Taipale, 1987). These girls started dating, drinking and smoking earlier, so that biological and behavioural developments were closely linked. These behaviours might, in turn, lead to further conflict within the family. These rule-breaking behaviours were more likely to be seen in girls in mixed sex schools, showing an influence of peer group on behaviour.

There appear to be important influences on the ways in which girls perceive menstruation. While some girls are positive, others are negative or ambivalent. The perception of the physical changes associated with puberty and timing of onset of menstruation relative to other girls are important. Girls with particularly negative expectations, pre-menarche, also describe the most negative experiences after menarche (Brooks-Gunn and Reiter, 1990). Early pubertal onset is associated with greater psychological distress, perhaps because girls have less time to prepare for the event and because girls who mature early have to confront new expectations, stressors or environments before they are psychologically ready to deal with them (Ge *et al.*, 1996). Here, a dynamic relationship can be seen between the individual's physical and emotional state and family, peer group and other environmental factors. Late menarche appears to carry far less risk of associated disturbance. Girls tend to begin to diet around puberty and it appears that it is their attitude to weight gain, rather than puberty itself, which lies behind this (Rutter and Rutter 1992).

BOYS

The sequence of sexual maturation of boys occurs approximately 18–24 months later than it does for girls. There seems to be a strong association between physical maturation and peer group status. Boys who mature early are perceived more positively by peers and develop better self-image (Rutter and Rutter, 1993). Psychobiological explanations suggest that strong, athletic physique associated with early development is a marker for reproductive effectiveness (Weisfield *et al.*, 1987).

There are probably considerable differences in the ways in which parents talk to boys and girls about puberty and communicate expectations about changes at this time. While girls generally have some discussion of menstruation with their mothers or another confidante, boys generally have no discussion of spermarche with their fathers (Durkin, 1995).

SEXUAL BEHAVIOUR

The development of sexual awareness is an important aspect of adolescence. This comes at a time of concurrent developments in self-awareness and self-esteem, leading to increased vulnerability. Ninety-five percent of boys and 60% of girls masturbate. In early to mid adolescence, Western adolescents begin to engage in sexual activity with others (Katchadourian, 1990). Recent figures for the UK collected by the Brook Advisory Service (1998) show that 20% of young people have intercourse before their 16th birthday, with most having their first experience at 17. The figures across Europe are relatively consistent with this. Timing of first intercourse in boys is related to early physical maturity, parental transitions, e.g. having new partners, and with antisocial behaviour and substance use (Capaldi et al., 1996). It may be that the direct experience of having a parent introduce a new partner into the household heightens the adolescent's awareness of sexuality. It may also be associated with reduced monitoring of the adolescent's activities.

The rate of teenage pregnancy has dropped since the introduction of freely available contraception in 1975. Low educational attainment, poverty, emotional difficulties and being a child of a teenage mother are all associated with teen pregnancy. The rates of abortion for pregnant teenagers are related to socioeconomic status, with girls from deprived areas being more likely to continue with a pregnancy (Brook Advisory Service, 1998).

At the turn of the millennium, parents remain more concerned over the emerging sexuality of their daughters rather than sons. While the value of female chastity varies markedly across cultures, the role of the male as predator is widespread. Sociobiologists have plausible explanations of this, which can be explored in Baker and Bellis (1995). In evolutionary terms, the most successful male will be the one who fertilises the most females; for the female, allowing eggs to be fertilised by a sub-optimal male will reduce her reproductive success.

Whatever the underlying reasons, males and females have different scripts for sexual activity. First intercourse for the male is a highly regarded event (Zani, 1991), while reports given by females have been described as more anxious (Gordon and Gilgun, 1987). As Durkin (1995) points out, however, prevailing attitudes and behaviour may change; while more male than female adolescents report sexual activity, the gap has narrowed over time (Gordon and Gilgun, 1987).

BISEXUAL AND HOMOSEXUAL ACTIVITY

Homosexuality is one area which may cause parents great concern. It is also an area where there are tremendous differences between societies and cultures, and between generations. Studies by Ford and Beach (1952) suggested that on some islands in the South West Pacific, homosexual activity between men was fairly universal. In 40% of the countries they surveyed, including the UK, homosexual activity was more rare and subject to social taboo. For males, homosexual activity is more common in the young and pre-reproductive, and is associated with having more partners. A recent study estimated that 30–40% of men will have had some sort of homosexual experience; the majority of these take place in adolescence and around 1–3% of men describe themselves as having a stable homosexual identity. A further 1–3% of men continue in bisexual activity, although predominantly heterosexual (McKnight, 1997). A high percentage of young lesbian women do not report a consistent pattern of same-sex attraction through adolescence; in one study, 40% said that they had undergone a change in attraction over time and a quarter said that their strongest prior attraction had been to a man (Diamond, 1998). This would suggest different causes for males and females, and for different individuals.

Again, Baker and Bellis (1995) provide fascinating data and draw comparisons across species, indicating the homosexual activity is relatively common and may confer reproductive advantage. They suggest that homosexual behaviour may be adaptive; in primates, early attempts at copulation are often incomplete and biological preparedness for adolescent homosexual practice may increase reproductive efficiency. In humans, cultural sanctions against early conception may mean that girls are less willing to allow boys the opportunity to experiment and practice copulatory skills. While these sociobiological arguments are outside the scope of this chapter, it may be important for parents and adolescents to know that homosexual behaviour is far more common in adolescence than in adulthood and that there may be a range of positive, biological reasons for its existence.

The majority of adolescents who try out homosexual behaviour do not become committed homosexuals. For those who do, a critical factor in mental health appears to be the anticipated responses of others (Rotheram-Borus *et al.*, 1991). Fear of rejection, ridicule and physical assault are important. Positive self-image is associated with refusal to accept the negative views of others, and finding coping resources (Savin-Williams, 1990). Parental acceptance, particularly by the mother, appears to be of particular importance.

COGNITIVE AND SOCIAL DEVELOPMENT

COGNITIVE DEVELOPMENT

The most influential work on cognitive development is that of Piaget (1972). His theory explained the formation and modification of schemas, the basic actions of knowing. In the infant, these include repertoires of physical actions associated with particular objects, people or contexts. Later, in childhood, schemes are mental actions such as classifying and comparing, developing in adolescence into processes of deductive analysis or systematic reasoning. Schemes are modified and adapted through *assimilation*, where new experiences are taken in and incorporated into existing schemes, often with some modification of the incoming information, and *accommodation*, where existing schemes are modified to fit new experiences or create new schemes when new information cannot be made to fit.

Piaget described a series of stages through which the search for, and integration of information about the self and the outside world could be observed and explained. Piaget drew attention to the clear differences between the thinking of young children and adolescents. Between the ages of 7 and 11, the child develops the ability to formulate hypotheses and explanations of concrete events. The child develops rules or strategies which Piaget termed *concrete operations*. These operations include addition, subtraction, reversibility, ordering and conservation. Of all these, Piaget considered reversibility to be the most critical. A demonstration of this is seen in the classic conservation experiments; the child becomes able to recognise that a ball of clay can be rolled into a sausage, then back into a ball, without there being a change in the amount of clay. In this way, the child learns to overcome the purely perceptual aspects of a task and think more logically about a process. Bee (1994) provides a clear overview of this work.

In adolescence, Piaget described the development of *formal operations*, with *abstract reasoning* a feature of the stage. This abstract reasoning allows the adolescent to entertain and consider a range of possibilities, and to reflect upon these, providing a range of possible solutions to the questions that arise at this time. There are examples of the ways in which the shift from concrete to formal operations may be seen in the abstract problems that adolescents are able to solve in mathematics and science.

Subsequent research has suggested that only 50–60% of 18–20 year olds use formal operations (Keating, 1990). It may be that this reflects the types of tasks used to measure formal operations, or that formal operations can only be applied with information or tasks which are already familiar to the adolescent. It may also be that many everyday contexts do not require their use. It is thought that, while adolescents have the capacity to develop formal operations, the right environmental demands may be essential for this development to take place (Bee 1994).

The ability to think in hypothetical terms and consider a range of possibilities helps in the formulation of arguments and counter-arguments (Steinberg, 1993). This is an aspect of adolescence that parents will recognise! This ability also helps in the development of perspective-taking skills. The ability to think in abstract concepts also means that adolescents are able to use more advanced reasoning and logical processes to think about, for example, morality, friendships, responsibility and ideology.

A further important aspect of thinking is that of *metacognition*, the ability to think about thinking. While young children show the beginnings of under-standing metacognition, this shows further development through adolescence and adolescents are better able to describe the thought processes that they are using. There is also likely to be increased self-consciousness and introspection. These permit the sorts of self-examination and exploration that contribute to the development of a coherent sense of identity. Here, as in other aspects of development, the attainment of new cognitive skills may also lead to disturbance; greater awareness gives more scope for anxiety and depression, as subsequent chapters will show. Again, the family context and the child's history of relationships may influence the development of metacognitive abilities.

One feature of this stage of cognitive development is a degree of preoccupation with the self which has been termed *egocentrism*. Piaget (1972) described this phenomenon in much younger children, suggesting that the child has difficulty in seeing that other people may have a perspective different to their own. Vygotsky (1962) suggested that egocentrism might, in young children, be functional in developing an understanding of the world, aiding the control of action, the internalisation of the views of other people and the understanding of other people's perspectives. For the adolescent, the exposure to new ideas and challenges may lead to an increase in self-absorption, or apparent egocentrism, and it is presumably within the context of this preoccupation with the self that there is the opportunity for further cognitive development in the understanding of yet wider perspectives.

Elkind (1985) suggested that preoccupation with the self might be associated with the sense of an 'imaginary audience', a sense of being on show. In the company of this imaginary, private audience, the adolescent can conduct private experiments in anticipation of eliciting a more predictable response from others in the outside world. As with many other form of play, the rehearsal functions to allow the adolescent a greater self-awareness and degree of control over the environment.

The ability to think *multidimensionally* is a further change in thinking seen in adolescence. This is the kind of thinking required to try to understand, for example, complex historical events, for instance how England were knocked out of the 1998 football World Cup. (A unidimensional explanation would simply blame David Beckham, who was sent off for retaliation, a singularly adolescent example of self-destructiveness.) The ability to understand sarcasm, for example, has been documented as a late development; this requires the combination of information from a number of different sources (Steinberg 1993). At the same time, adolescent thinking shows a shift from the concrete, black and white thinking of childhood to the ability to see things as relative, to question assertions and refuse to accept 'facts'. *Adolescent relativism* may lead considerable scepticism and doubt (Chandler, 1987), and it has been suggested that this, too, contributes to the development of more sophisticated understanding of complexity.

INFORMATION PROCESSING

The literature indicates that development occurs on a number of fronts which foster abstract, multidimensional thinking (Steinberg, 1993). Adolescents become more skilled in the use of both selective and divided attention; short-term and long-term memory improve, and organisational strategies for the control of thinking also undergo development. With the development of metacognition, the adolescent enjoys access to a powerful set of mental tools.

One particularly interesting finding to have emerged questions the old wisdom that boys and girls show differences in their patterns of ability. While it used to be the case that girls showed superior verbal IQ, and boys, greater mathematical and spatial ability, many of these differences have now disappeared (Jacklin, 1989); the only difference remaining is in spatial ability. There is therefore clear evidence that abilities can be influenced by social and environmental pressures.

SOCIAL COGNITION

While the study of thinking and reasoning shows how children are able to develop into adolescents capable of a wider range of mental tasks, the greatest challenges to parents, peers and teachers often lie in the ways in which the adolescent understands him or herself, and relates to others. At the core of good peer relations lies *social cognition*, the ability to think about people, social relationships and social institutions (Lapsley, 1989). Adolescents show a range of developments that constitute this ability.

Role-taking ability continues to develop through adolescence and, in addition to being able to understand the perspective of another person, they are able to appreciate that other person's perspective of their point of view (Selman, 1980). This contributes to the ability to argue effectively.

Conceptions of morality and social convention are also more fully appreciated. There is a shift from the acceptance of rules as 'given', to a more reasoned understanding of the reasons for their existence. The moral principles of fairness, justice and equality begin to be considered in more abstract ways (Kohlberg, 1976). Through the development of these principles, adolescents reach a point where they see that social conventions serve a functional purpose in regulating and coordinating actions between people (Steinberg, 1993). Adolescents who show higher levels of development of these social cognitive abilities appear better able to behave in more socially competent ways (Ford, 1982).

UNDERSTANDING OF THE SELF

It takes time for children and adolescents to form a unified, consistent representation of themselves. Even at 14 and 15, children will endorse mutually self-contradictory self-descriptions (Harter, 1986); with further development, however, these become more consistent. Here, too, the influence of peers, family and school environment is seen. Again, reflection on experience leads to development and the degree of challenge experienced will be important.

SELF-ESTEEM

There has been a considerable amount of research on self-esteem in adolescence, probably due to its importance to overall well-being. Adolescents compare themselves to others in order to ascertain their level of worth, a process which begins around 6 or 7 and intensifies in adolescence (for summary, see Coleman and Hendry, 1999). It appears that self-esteem is most closely tied to valued domains of skills and activities (Harter, 1983). Some studies show that self-esteem appears to drop in early adolescence (Simmons and Blyth, 1987), but then to recover later. There is some evidence that self-esteem in early adolescence is higher in those who are physically more mature, particularly boys. Overall, studies appear to show an increase from early to late adolescence. This may reflect the range of challenges presented by change of school, increasing parental and scholastic expectations, coupled with an increase in self-awareness and reflection, and mastery of a range of domains with increasing age. Most adolescents show variation in their estimation of their self-worth across different contexts, with validation support in a particular context being a significant contributor to self-perception. The ways in which adolescents evaluate themselves in different contexts is critical to their overall sense of worth as a person (Harter *et al.*, 1998). If adolescents are comfortable in some domains, it may make lack of success in others more tolerable and lessen the impact on global self-esteem (Coleman and Hendry, 1999).

IDENTITY

Erikson (1959) discussed the concept of an 'identity crisis' in adolescence, as the young person struggled to decide who he or she is and wants to become. Identity development continues through adolescence and is a life-long process. Marcia (1966) investigated the notion of development of identity, suggesting four types of identity status:

(1) *Identity diffusion*, with an avoidance of commitment and decision making.
(2) *Identity foreclosure*, with the tentative acceptance of the views of others, e.g. parents.
(3) *Moratorium*, a state of crisis with active attention to major decisions and exploration of possibilities but no firmly resolved commitments.
(4) *Identity achievement*, where crisis is resolved and firm commitments are made to ideals and plans.

There are indications that identity achievers may be more likely to be better adjusted in a range of social situations. Marcia's four categories are of particular interest in relation to work on the family. A review by Adams *et al.* (1994) indicates that family style is associated with different types of development. Diffusion appears to be associated with rejecting and detached families, foreclosure, with child-centred and conformist families, while moratorium and identity achievement are associated with warmth and support, and encouragement of initiative and independence. It is probable that some of these styles of relating to children will also be linked to patterns of attachment relationships.

Class differences and educational opportunity may have an important influence; higher education may extend the moratorium period (Munro and Adams, 1977). Durkin (1995) summarises studies which have shown that ethnic and cultural context are important, with ethnic minority youngsters being later to achieve advanced identity status. There is a suggestion, however, that certain cultural factors may protect the adolescent against identity confusion; the Muslim culture, for example, provides a strong sense of place within the extended family, community and within Islam, which may lead to a clear sense of identity. Again, the social context of the adolescence and their relationship to networks outside the immediate family are likely to be of considerable importance.

AUTONOMY

Closely tied in with the notion of identity is that of autonomy, although there is a range of different definitions of this. Steinberg and Silverberg (1986) suggested that development occurs in three domains, (1) emotional autonomy, (2) resistance to peer pressure and (3) subjective sense of self-reliance. It is noteworthy that girls tend to score more highly on all measures. Ryan and Lynch (1989) suggested that attachment theory is an important basis for the understanding of the development of emotional autonomy; the emotional support and acceptance of the parent allows individuation for the securely attached adolescent. Without this sense of support, adolescents become more reliant on peers. This peer influence may, of course, foster good adjustment, but may also lead to antisocial behaviours.

LONELINESS

To what extent is loneliness a normal part of adolescence? While transient loneliness may act as a spur for to seek out companionship, prolonged loneliness may make it more difficult to break out of a solitary pattern. 'Existential loneliness' may appear as the adolescent realises that they are separate from everyone else. Larson (1997) suggests that time alone becomes more voluntary through the teenage years and that, by late adolescence, solitary time has positive after-effects. Adolescents who spend an intermediate amount of time alone appear better adjusted than those who spend little or a great deal of time alone. Adolescent solitude may, therefore, be more normal and less worrying than parents may perceive it to be, and have a constructive role in allowing time for reflection.

ADOLESCENT DEVELOPMENT IN THE CONTEXT OF THE FAMILY

A popular notion in the common sense view of adolescence is that of the generation gap. Again, the research literature does not support this view (Brown, 1990). Rather, it would appear that parents and adolescents generally communicate and get on well. While there are likely to be numerous disagreements, particularly over limit-setting, families are able to come to mutual agreement on such issues, and adolescents generally accept parental values. In a Dutch study, 96% of adolescents were satisfied with the situation at home (Du Bois-Reymond, 1989). There appears to be considerable agreement between parents and children on moral, political and social beliefs and attitudes (Adams *et al.*, 1994).

CONFLICT

In parallel with these findings, several studies show that there is an increase in parent–child conflict in adolescence (Paikoff and Brooks-Gunn, 1991). Given the many changes and developments that the young person is undergoing, it is perhaps unsurprising that this should be so. Parents will not be surprised to know that one study suggests that adolescents report an average of seven disagreements daily (Laursen and Collins, 1994). Most conflicts involve mothers, followed by siblings, friends, romantic partners, fathers, other peers and adults. Adolescents argue with parents over autonomy, authority and responsibility. With siblings they also argue over the latter two, but also about interpersonal concerns. With peers, interpersonal behaviour and relational difficulties form the focus. Cognitive developments such as enhanced hypothetical reasoning may lead to arguments (Laursen and Collins, 1994). Sociobiologists see conflict as an adaptive strategy, leading to greater autonomy and peer contact (Steinberg, 1993). Smetana (1993) points out the value of conflict in the resolution of different social cognitive perspectives. These conflicts help to prepare the young person for a life independent from the parent and for the necessary separation which this entails. Furthermore, as Durkin points out, conflict occurs in all close relationships, whatever the age of the participants, and, statistically, is much more frequent in families with very young children. Shantz and Hartup (1992) provide a good review of the literature and set adolescent conflict in context, suggesting: '*Conflicts*, defined as oppositional interactions, are seen as natural interpersonal sequelae of shifts in role expectations associated with age-graded transitions and maturational changes' (Shantz and Hartup, 1992, p. 216).

Their review suggests that adolescent sense of identity and social cognition is linked to responsiveness in the relationship with the parent, and that supportive but challenging discussion of issues is associated with more advanced reasoning. However elegant the developmental purpose, the majority of conflicts end in stand-off or power assertion, rather than disengagement. With age, the ability to bring conflict to resolution develops, and conflict becomes better managed.

ADOLESCENT DEVELOPMENT AND THE FAMILY LIFE CYCLE

In considering the relationship between adolescent development and the family, it is important to look at this stage of the life cycle from a broader perspective and to see what other family members may be experiencing. The parents of adolescents are typically aged 35–45, although this is likely to change as mothers have their children at increasingly later ages. There is evidence that middle adulthood can be a time of difficulty for adults (Farrell and Rosenberg, 1981); anxieties over changes in physical state and attractiveness coincide; mothers may be experiencing the menopause, and fathers, a loss of potency. Perceptions of time and the future change, and, at the point where the adolescent is beginning to explore the possibilities of the future, the parent may feel increasingly trapped in a particular pathway or set of circumstances (Steinberg, 1993). Parents may also have concerns about their own ageing parents, and thus be carrying a range of roles and responsibilities which may be perceived to be burdensome.

There are some indications that parents may be adversely affected by their child's development into adolescence. Mothers of girls and fathers of boys show more psychological distress and less satisfaction with marriage as their children mature and distance themselves emotionally. Parental characteristics, such as self-esteem, are associated with the ability to grant autonomy to the child (Small, 1988).

PARENTING STYLES

There are a number of approaches to the study of parenting and its relationship to adolescent development. In one influential set of studies, Baumrind (1987) suggested that two relatively independent aspects of parenting were of considerable importance; parental responsiveness and parental demandingness. This led to a four-way classification of parenting into indulgent (high responsiveness, low demand), authoritative (high responsiveness, high demand), authoritarian (low responsiveness, high demand) and indifferent (low responsiveness, low demand).

Subsequent studies have shown these styles of parenting to be associated with different adolescent outcomes.

- *Authoritative* parents, who are warm and firm, have realistic expectations of their children which they help the child to meet. They value autonomy, but are prepared to take ultimate responsibility. These families are characterised by rational discussion of issues, including discipline. Adolescents growing up in this context tend to be more responsible, self-assured, adaptive, creative, curious and socially skilled. They are also more successful in school.
- *Authoritarian* parents value obedience and conformity, and tend to be more punitive in their approach and more absolute in their demands. The child is expected to accept rules without question and autonomy is restricted. Adolescents in this kind of family tend to be more dependent and passive, less socially skilled and assured, and less curious.
- *Indulgent* parents are accepting and benign, placing little demand on the child. They are more likely to believe that the imposition of rules or control is an infringement of the child's rights and may have a negative effect on development. These parents are more likely to see themselves as available resources for the child to use. In this context, adolescents are often more irresponsible and less mature, and less able to take on a leadership role.
- *Indifferent* parents arrange family life in a way which minimises the demands of the child on themselves and may, in extreme cases, be neglectful. They may show little interest in the child's school work, other activities or whereabouts and structure home life around their own needs. Adolescents in this context are more likely to be impulsive, engage in delinquent behaviour and precocious experimentation with drugs, sex and alcohol.

These patterns have been seen in a number of studies of children in different ethnic and socioeconomic groups (Steinberg *et al.*, 1991).

It is not difficult to see why the authoritative position is likely to promote good developmental outcomes. The adolescent is protected by the rules which have been clearly set out, and which provide a secure and predictable base. The flexibility of the parent is valuable to the family as a whole in allowing successful adaptation to changing needs of family members at different stages of the life cycle and they can moderate their parenting to suit the current needs of the adolescent.

Discussion of rules and social responsibilities and the willingness of parents to negotiate helps the adolescent's sense of autonomy and self-efficacy, and also helps directly in the development of negotiation skills. Intellectual development and reasoning is promoted in this way, as is moral development and empathy. The warmth of the relationship promotes identification with the parent's values and approaches. The child themselves may be an active participant in promoting and continuing authoritative parenting through warmth and responsivity.

ADOLESCENT RELATIONSHIPS WITH SIBLINGS

The sibling relationship is a distinct one, different to that with parents or peers, yet is relatively little studied. Adolescents rate sibling relationships like those with parents for companionship and importance, but more like those with peers for power, assistance and satisfaction with the relationship. What distinguishes the sibling relationship is the degree of conflict; adolescents do indeed argue a good deal more with siblings than they do with anyone else! It may be that the closeness of the shared environment provides more opportunity for both positive and negative interaction (Steinberg, 1993). While sharing the same macro-environment of the family, each sibling lives in a micro-environment of unique relationships. Siblings experience the family context in different ways, and there is very little correlation between sibling scores on personality traits. Siblings give very different accounts of their experiences of the family. The best adjusted adolescents are more likely to report a close relationship with their mother, that they are involved in family decision making and that they are given high levels of responsibility around the house (Daniels *et al.*, 1985).

PEER RELATIONSHIPS

Peer relationships become increasingly important in adolescence, as the young person pursues a range of activities outside the parental home (Brown, 1990). Peer-orientated activities become more important (Adams *et al.*, 1994), as does identification with a peer group as a means of becoming more competent in the extra-familial environment. Peer group membership is associated with the development of autonomy and skills in maintaining relationships, and lack of a peer group is far more risky in development (Kirchler *et al.*, 1991).

It will come as no surprise to parents that adolescents spend twice as much time with peers than anyone else (Brown, 1990) and adolescents moods are more positive in this setting. The post-war 'baby boom' led to a bulge in the adolescent population during the late 1960s and early 1970s, which led to cultural shifts in the ways in which adolescent behaviour, and particularly peer group behaviour, was represented and studied (Steinberg, 1993). Social identity theory (Tajfel, 1978) described processes of social categorisation, social comparison and psychological group distinctiveness. Self-categorisation describes the way in which people form opinions which concur with those of people who are important to them, which are then the focus of social comparison, where the value of the group is considered in relation to the value of other groups. Such categorisation and comparison contributes to social identity through the formation of ingroups and outgroups. Research on adolescents shows support for these processes, with strong identification with a group being associated with positive views of self and others (Palmonari *et al.*, 1990). Social identity may also, however, restrict options for the adolescent; 'oppositional social identity' arising from, for example, racism, may lead to rebellion against the school system and consequent under-achievement (Clark, 1991).

The peer group provides a network of significant others from outside the family. A characteristic of these groups in adolescence is the extent to which, in common with the peer groups of children, they continue to be sex segregated. The groups tend to be larger than the small groups of three or four friends characteristic of childhood (Steinberg, 1993). It is helpful to think of two kinds of peer groups; cliques and crowds. *Cliques* are made up of two to 12 individuals, generally of the same sex and age. The members feel they know each other well and appreciate each other. *Crowds* are larger, reputation-based structures; the nerds, gothics or druggies. Adolescents use these larger structures to locate themselves in the social context. The adolescent continues to learn social skills within the clique and to feel secure within the wider setting of, for example, school, while the crowd provides a sense of identity and self-concept. Social support buffers adolescents against stress at school (Hauser and Bowlds, 1990).

Adolescents tend to form cliques with other young people of the same age, social class and race as themselves, with these differences becoming more marked as they get older. Clique formation appears to be influenced by shared interests, orientation towards school and towards the teen culture (Steinberg, 1993).

Conformity to culturally valued norms is a characteristic of peer group relationships. While conformity to prosocial pressure is greatest at 11–12 years, conformity to antisocial suggestions peaks at 14–15, probably reflecting the struggle for autonomy from parents. The peer group offers the possibility for creation of a shared culture (Lightfoot, 1992) and thus offers an important context for mastery across a number of areas of development with people who are at an equivalent stage. Social comparison with other groups allows for increasing cohesion and sense of self-worth.

Identification with the peer group and the family are not mutually exclusive; adolescents who feel strongly identified with their peer group also are strongly committed to their family (Kirchler *et al.*, 1991). Parenting style is associated with adolescent social behaviour and choices, and the kinds of peer groups selected. A consistent finding is that while peers are rated as increasingly significant with age, family members are rated as the most significant people in their lives and remain an important source of advice on major decisions (Durkin, 1995).

During late adolescence, there is a weakening of the peer group, which is replaced by loosely associated pairs of couples. The experience of the peer group has laid the foundation for this, facilitating the development of skills in the maintenance of close relationships outside the family context, and providing a context for experimentation with and discussion of intimate relationships.

PEER ACCEPTANCE, POPULARITY AND REJECTION

Acceptance by the peer group is of considerable importance. Popular adolescents are friendly, good natured, humorous and intelligent. Popularity may not necessarily be associated with leadership; leaders appear to be chosen on the basis of their likelihood of getting things done.

Social rejection is associated with poor social skills; the adolescent may be tactless or aggressive or may show behaviour that leads to unpopularity, e.g. drawing attention to themselves excessively (Steinberg, 1993). Children neglected by their peers may be withdrawn, shy or unenthusiastic. Where children have a poor view of themselves and judge themselves to be low in competence with peers, there is an increased risk of victimisation, which can create a vicious cycle of bullying (Egan and Perry, 1998). Rejected adolescents are more lonely and more likely to develop disturbance (Parker and Asher, 1987), and lack of acceptance is associated with low achievement, school dropout, delinquency, and with emotional and mental health problems in adulthood (Savin-Williams and Berndt, 1990).

YOUTH ORGANISATIONS

There are many organisations where adolescents enter into adult-led activities. Where these are well run, they offer the adolescent to explore new opportunities and develop their abilities. They offer opportunities to learn understanding of organisations, roles and social rules. Where adolescents attend organised activities, they are more likely to see unrelated adults as significant influences, offering opportunities for modelling, personal growth and development. Some studies indicate that these kinds of unrelated adults are not seen as resources when there is a problem; parents or teachers are more likely to be sought out. Youth leaders do, however, offer an important resource and may be described as role models by the adolescent (Hendry *et al.*, 1992). They have the benefits of being more distant from peer and family network and conflicts, able to see the young person independently of their family history, and can offer an adult view and interpretation of experiences. In sports, group leaders may have a particularly salient mentoring role and their attention may be much prized by the adolescent (Gottlieb, 1991).

SCHOOL

THE SCHOOL ENVIRONMENT

Adolescents make active choices in the degree to which they fit in with the demands of school and quality of the school environment is an important factor in this. Adolescents value being treated as intelligent, responsive individuals, and their motivation to work needs careful management and understanding by the teachers and school system. The extent to which goals are meaningful and relevant will influence the extent to which the adolescent will engage with the system. Semmens (1990, p. 28) suggests that as a key social environment for the young person, it is a source of a 'redemptive pathway' towards adulthood. A good school can, therefore, help to provide a supportive environment in which positive development can be fostered. Such an environment needs to provide resources for young people to work on particular needs, e.g. social relationships, which will be based on an understanding of adolescent development and peer networks. Good schools will work towards making school structures small, adults accessible, promote healthy peer relations, and allow authentic experiences of success and self-responsibility (Gregory, 1995).

EDUCATIONAL ATTAINMENT AND THE FAMILY

The family and school environments both contribute to academic attainment; as might be expected, a stable, affluent, stimulating home with parents who are aware of the value of education is associated with better outcome (Bo, 1994). Congruence with the values of the school is also important (Steinberg, 1993). Higher levels of aspiration are associated with higher socioeconomic status (Entwhistle, 1990). There are considerable differences across children from different ethnic backgrounds; in a study of children in the UK, Scarr et al. (1983) found West Indian children to have lower attainment than peers of English or Asian background, and that this gap widened in adolescence.

SCHOOL, ATTAINMENT AND SOCIAL RELATIONSHIPS

The extent to which children are able to establish friendships and acceptance by their peer group is related to their academic success. It appears that prosocial behaviour in the adolescent is particularly important in this process (Wentzel and Caldwell, 1997). There are clearly relationships between social and academic competence, and this is likely, in turn, to be related to family factors. Bagwell et al. (1998), in a longitudinal study of friendship and adjustment, suggest that poor peer relationships may be a marker for other underlying difficulties, e.g. in the family, and that the additional stress of peer rejection may interact with existing vulnerabilities to create disturbance. On the other hand, good peer relationships may foster resilience, and moderate the risk of difficulties in adjustment.

FROM EDUCATION TO EMPLOYMENT

Educational attainment is, in turn, directly linked to attainment in the occupational sphere and here the chain effects described by Rutter and Rutter

(1992) referred to earlier are very apparent. One of the clearest demonstrations of this comes from the work of Caspi *et al.* (1987), who observed links from childhood behaviour though to educational attainment, occupational status, and success in marriage and parenting at ages 30 and 40. Clearly, children whose attainment declines in adolescence can be disadvantaged across the lifespan. Adolescents who emerge from school at times of economic recession and high unemployment are likely to be particularly disadvantaged.

MOVING TOWARDS ADULTHOOD

WHAT MAKES FOR A SUCCESSFUL TRANSITION INTO ADULT LIFE?

Active planning for the future can be protective of mental health (Clausen, 1991). Adolescents who show a *future time perspective* are aware of the structure of the future and the relationship between their current activities and later outcomes. This, in turn, is associated with the family; where parents express interest and provide input, adolescents develop clearer and more positive plans (Pullikinen, 1990). Current relationships with peers are also important in this respect; with increasing age, adolescents come to share a view of the future and their part in it, and develop shared norms which influence the direction that is taken (Greene, 1990).

RELATIONSHIP FORMATION AND MATE SELECTION

The formation of a long-term relationship and, traditionally, marriage, are features of young adulthood. We have seen how adolescents are biologically motivated to prepare for this stage, and how changes in the experience and structure of the peer group help to pave the way. Within the UK at the turn of the millennium, we have a range of different views of marriage. Parents of adolescents born in the 1980s who grew up in a culture where marriage was expected of them by their parents may see their own children living together or delaying the establishment of long-term relationships. In many cases, parental divorce may have been a factor in this. Across the ethnic minority groups, there are differences in the attitudes and expectations concerning marriage, ranging from the traditional, arranged marriages of some cultures to an amalgam of traditional and new attitudes. The range of possible outcomes has never been so varied as it has been for the millennial adolescent.

Mates tend to be selected from within the same socioeconomic, educational and occupational strata (Eshelman, 1985), and a number of important principles come into play in mate selection. Physical attractiveness appears to be highly salient (Jackson, 1992). In traditional African and Asian countries, home-keeping potential and the desire for a home and children are valued, whereas in European cultures, love, character and maturity are more prized (Buss *et al.*, 1990). The value of chastity also varies markedly across cultures.

The tendency for males to seek younger females and females to seek older partners is consistent across most cultures. Adolescent boys, however, have a wider range of acceptability, including older partners, a finding that has been suggested to relate to fertility and reproductive advantage (Kenrick *et al.*, 1996), although it may be governed by perceived willingness to participate in sexual activity.

WORK AND UNEMPLOYMENT

Super (1985) developed a theory of vocational self-concept within a lifespan perspective. He described *crystallisation*, a time when vocational options are narrowed down, and then *specification*, in the late teens and early 20s at which stage a specific choice is made. Given changing economic conditions and high levels of unemployment, however, the picture is more complex. The quality of adolescence is affected by economic circumstances; a large, international study by Offer *et al.* (1988) showed that the more wealthy the country, the better the mood of the adolescents living there. Durkin (1995) summarises the different experiences of adolescents leaving school, looking at those going into work full time or being under-employed or unemployed.

For those in work, access to money is highly valued, and young adults in full employment regard themselves as more grown up and self-confident. This appears to be particularly the case for males. Males are more likely to be offered training than females. Young women remain more focused on marriage and rate children as important. In some Western countries, a relatively small percentage of school leavers can expect to find work. As Durkin points out, this is likely to influence the extent to which young people feel that they have 'grown up' and are able to develop self-reliance as adults. These young people may also be living in households already hit by economic disadvantage; this influences both family dynamics and vulnerability to antisocial behaviour.

Employment status and the way that it is perceived by the young person have an impact on mental health. Boring, low-level jobs are associated with disturbance, including depression (O'Brien, 1990) and there may be no benefit of low-status, unskilled jobs over unemployment (Winefield and Winefield, 1992). A longitudinal study of young people on the Isle of Sheppey, an area of the UK with exceptionally high unemployment, showed that young people moving into the workforce found work less enjoyable than they had expected and half had experienced feeling 'really desperate' in low-paid, unskilled jobs (Wallace, 1989).

The way in which youth unemployment is perceived is likely to influence the way in which it is experienced. Psychological distress is associated more with subjective financial strain than actual income (Ullah, 1990). Relative deprivation theory (Sabini, 1995) suggests that people compare themselves with others around them and if others seem to be having an equally difficult time, may adapt. While newly unemployed young people may protest, with time they adapt, losing the sense that they could bring about change in their circumstances (O'Brien, 1990), an adaptation which can be seen as learned helplessness.

SUMMARY

Adolescence is characterised by the movement from the family into the wider world, a time when the young person matures rapidly and undergoes a number of transformations in their physical state, thinking and behaviour which are a preparation for adult life. The course of development in adolescence can be influenced a great deal by family, peers and the wider social context, while the adolescent as an individual makes a substantial contribution to the course of their own development and relationships.

Adolescents will try out their developing mental powers, and will question and debate. As their peer group becomes more important, they will spend a great deal of time with friends and will be happier in their company than with anyone else. As adolescence progresses, there will be experimentation with the formation of couple relationships. Movement into the worlds of work and unemployment reflect individual characteristics and attainments, but also contextual factors. Parents may experience these changes as challenging and wonder about their own role, but the family remains a significant influence throughout development into early adulthood.

REFERENCES

Adams, G. R., Gullotta, T. P. and Markstrom-Adams, C. (1994) *Adolescent Life Experiences*, 3rd edn, Pacific Grove, CA: Brooks/Cole

Ainsworth, M. D. S., Blehar, M., Waters, E. and Wall, E. (1978) *Patterns of Attachment*. Hillsdale, NJ: Erlbaum.

Armsden, G. and Greenberg, M. (1987) The inventory of parent and peer attachment: individual differences and their relationship to psychological well-being in adolescence. *Journal of Youth and Adolescence*, **16**, 427–453.

Aro, H. and Taipale, V. (1987) The impact of timing of puberty on psychosomatic symptoms among 14 to 16 year old Finnish Girls. *Child Development*, **58**, 261–268.

Bagwell, C. L., Newcomb, A. F. and Bukowski, W. M. (1998) Preadolescent friendship and peer rejection aas predictors of adult adjustment. *Child Development*, **69**, 146–153.

Baker, R. R. and Bellis, M. A. (1995) *Human Sperm Competition: Copulation, Masturbation and Infidelity*. London: Chapman & Hall.

Baumrind, D. (1987) Parental disciplinary patterns and social competence in children. *Youth and Society*, **9**, 239–276.

Bee, H. (1994) *Lifespan Development*. New York: Harper Collins.

Belsky, J., Steinberg, L. and Draper, P. (1991) Childhood experience, interpersonal development and reproductive strategy: an evolutionary theory of socialisation. *Child Development*, **62**, 647–670.

Bo, I. (1994) The socio-cultural environment as a source of support. In F. Nestemann and R. Hurrelmann (eds), *Social Networks and Social Support in Childhood*. Berlin: de Gruyter.

Bowlby, J. (1969) *Attachment and Loss, Vol 1: Attachment*. London: Hogarth.

Brook Advisory Service (1998) *Teenagers and Sex: A Briefing Paper*. London: Brook Advisory Centres.

Brooks-Gunn, J. and Reiter, E. O. (1990) The role of pubertal processes. In S. S. Feldman and G. R. Elliott (eds), *At the Threshold: The Developing Adolescent*. Cambridge: Cambridge University Press.

Brown, B. B. (1990) Peer groups and peer cultures. In S. S. Feldman and G. R. Elliott (eds), *At the Threshold: The Developing Adolescent*. Cambridge: Cambridge University Press.

Bullough, V. (1981) Age at menarche: a misunderstanding. *Science*, **213**, 365–366.

Buss, D. M. and associates (1990) International preferences in selecting mates: a study of 37 cultures. *Journal of Cross-Cultural Psychology*, **21**, 5–47.

Capaldi, D. M., Crosby, L. and Stoolmiller, M. (1996) Predicting the timing of first sexual intercourse for at-risk adolescent males. *Child Development*, **67**, 344–359.

Caspi, A., Elder, G. H., Jr and Bem, D. J. (1987) Moving against the world: the life course patterns of explosive children. *Developmental Psychology*, **23**, 308–313.

Chandler, M. (1987) The Othello effect; essay on the emergence and eclipse of skeptical doubt. *Human Development*, **30**, 137–159.

Clark, M. L. (1991) Social identity, peer relations and academic competence of African-American adolescents. *Education and Urban Society*, **24**, 41–52.

Clausen, J. S. (1991) Adolescent competence and the shaping of the life course. *American Journal of Sociology*, **96**, 805–842.

Coleman, J. C. and Hendry, L. (1999) *The Nature of Adolescence*, 3rd edn. London: Routledge.

Daniels, D., Dunn, J., Furstenberg, F., Jr and Plomin, R. (1985) Environmental differences within the family and adjustment differences within pairs of adolescent siblings. *Child Development*, **56**, 764–774.

Diamond, L. M. (1998) Development of sexual orientation among adolescent and young adult women. *Developmental Psychology*, **34**, 1085–1095.

Du Bois-Reymond, M. (1989) School and family in the lifeworld of youngsters. In F. Nestemann and R. Hurrelmann (eds), *Social Networks and Social Support in Childhood*. Berlin: de Gruyter.

Durkin, K. (1995) *Developmental Social Psychology: From Infancy to Old Age.* Oxford: Blackwell.

Egan, S. K. and Perry, D. G. (1998) does low self regard invite victimisation? *Developmental Psychology*, **34**, 299–309.

Elkind, D. (1985) Egocentrism redux. *Developmental Review*, **5**, 218–226.

Entwhistle, D. R. (1990) Schools and the adolescent. In S. S. Feldman and G. R. Elliott (eds), *At the Threshold: The Developing Adolescent*. Cambridge: Cambridge University Press.

Erikson, E. (1959) Identity and the life cycle. *Psychological Issues*, **1**, 1–171.

Erikson, M. F., Sroufe, L. A. and Egeland, B. (1985) The relationship between quality of attachment and behaviour problems in preschool in a high-risk sample. *Growing Points of Attachment Theory and Research: Monographs of the Society for Research in Child Development*, **50**, 147–193.

Eshelman, J. R. (1985) One should marry a person of the same religion, race, ethnicity and social class. In H. Feldman and M. Feldman (eds), *Current Controversies in Marriage and the Family*. Newbury Park, CA: Sage.

Farrell, M. P. and Rosenberg, S. D. (1981) *Men at Midlife*. Boston, MA: Auburn House.

Ford, C. S. and Beach, F. A. (1952) *Patterns of Sexual Behaviour*. London: Eyre & Spottiswode.

Ford, M. (1982) Social cognition and social competence in adolescence. *Developmental Psychology*, **18**, 323–340.

Ge, X., Conger, R. D. and Elder, G. H. (1996) Coming of age too early: pubertal influences on girls' vulnerability to psychological distress. *Child Development*, **67**, 3386–3400.

Greene, A. L. (1990) Great Expectations: constructions of the life course during adolescence. *Journal of Youth and Adolescence*, **19**, 289–306.

Gordon, S. and Gilgun, J. F. (1987) Adolescent sexuality. In V. B. van Hasselt and M. Hersen (eds), *Handbook of Adolescent Psychology*. New York: Pergamon.

Gottlieb, B. H. (1991) Social supports in adolescence. In M. E. Colten and S. Gore (eds), *Adolescent Stress: Causes and Consequences* New York: McGraw Hill, pp. 281–306.

Gregory, L. W. (1995) The 'turnaround' process: factors influencing the school success of urban youth. *Journal of Adolescent Research*, **10**, 135–164.

Hall, G. S. (1904) *Adolescence: Its Psychology and its Relation to Physiology, Anthropology, Sociology, Sex, Crime, Religion and Education*. New York: Appleton, 2 vols.

Harter, S. (1983) Developmental perspectives on the self-system. In E. M. Hetherington (ed.), *Handbook of Child Psychology, Vol. 4. Socialisation, Personality and Social Development*. New York: Wiley.

Harter, S. (1986) Cognitive developmental processes in the integration of concepts about emotions and the self. *Social Cognition*, **4**, 119–151.

Harter, S, Waters, P. and Whitesell, N. R. (1998) Relational self-worth: differences in perceived worth as a person across interpersonal contexts among adolescents. *Child Development*, **69**, 756–766.

Hauser, S. T. and Bowlds, M. K. (1990) Stress, coping and adaptation. In S. S. Feldman and G. R. Elliott (eds), *At the Threshold: The Developing Adolescent.* Cambridge: Cambridge University Press

Hendry, L. B., Roberts, W., Glendinning, A. and Coleman, J. C. (1992) Adolescents' perceptions of significant individuals in their lives. *Journal of Adolescence*, **15**, 255–270.

Hill, P. (1993) Recent advances in selected areas of adolescent development. *Journal of Child Psychology and Psychiatry*, **34**, 69–99.

Jacklin, C. (1989) Female and male: issues of gender. *American Psychologist*, **44**, 127–133.

Jackson, L. A. (1992) *Physical Appearance and Gender; Sociobiological and Sociocultural Perspectives.* Albany, NY: State University of New York Press.

Katchadourian, H. (1990) Sexuality. In S. S. Feldman and G. R. Elliott (eds), *At the Threshold: The Developing Adolescent.* Cambridge: Cambridge University Press.

Kazdin, A. E. (1990) Psychotherapy for children and adolescents. *Annual Review of Psychology*, **41**, 21–54.

Keating, D. P. (1990) Adolescent thinking. In S. S. Feldman and G. R. Elliott (eds), *At the Threshold: The Developing Adolescent.* Cambridge: Cambridge University Press.

Kenrick, D. T., Keefe, R. C., Gabrielidis, C. and Cornelius, J. S. (1996) Adolescents' age preferences for dating partners: support for an evolutionary model of life-history strategies. *Child Development*, **67**, 1499–1511.

Kirchler, E., Pombeni, M. L. and Palomnari, A. (1991) Sweet sixteen . . . adolescent's problems and the peer group as a source of support. *European Journal of Psychology of Education*, **6**, 393–410.

Kohlberg, L. (1976) Moral stages and moralisation: the cognitive-development approach. In T. Lickona (ed.), *Moral Development and Behaviour.* New York: Holt, Rinehart & Winston.

Lapsley, D. (1989) Continuity and discontinuity in adolescent social development. In R. Montemayor, G. Adams and T. Gullota (eds), *Advances in Adolescence Research.* Beverley Hills, CA: Sage, Vol. 2.

Larson, R. W. (1997) The emergence of solitude as a constructive domain of experience in early adolescence. *Child Development*, **68**, 80–93.

Laursen, B. and Collins, W. A. (1994) Interpersonal conflict during adolescence. *Psychological Bulletin*, **115**, 197–209.

Lightfoot, C. (1992) Constructing self peer and culture: a narrative perspective on risk taking. In L. T. Winegar and J. Valsiner (eds), *Children's Development within Social Context, Vol. 2. Research and Methodology.* Hillsdale, NJ: Erlbaum.

McKnight, J. (1997) *Straight Science? Homosexuality, Evolution and Adaptation*. Routledge: London.

Marcia, J. (1966) Development and validation of ego-identity status. *Journal of Personality and Social Psychology*, **3**, 551–558.

Munro, G. and Adams, G. R. (1977) Ego-identity formation in college students and working youth. *Developmental Psychology*, **13**, 523–524.

O'Brien, G. E. (1990) Youth unemployment and employment. In P. C. L. Heaven and V. J. Callan (eds), *Adolescence: An Australian perspective*. Sydney: Harcourt Brace Jovanovitch.

Offer, D., Ostrov, E., Howard, K. I. and Atkinson, R. (1988) *The Teenage World: Adolescents' Self Image in Ten Countries*. New York: Plenum.

Paikoff, R. L. and Brooks-Gunn, J. (1991) Do parent-child relationships change during puberty? *Psychological Bulletin*, **110**, 47–66.

Palmonari, A., Pombeni, M. L. and Kirchler, E. (1990) Adolescents and their peer groups: a study on the significance of peers, social categorisation processes and coping with developmental tasks. *Social Behaviour*, **5**, 33–48.

Parker, J. G. and Asher, S. R. (1987) Peer relations and later personal adjustment: are low-accepted children at risk? *Psychological Bulletin*, **102**, 357–389.

Piaget, J. (1972) *The Principles of Genetic Epistemology*. London: Routledge & Kegan Paul.

Pullikinen, L. (1990) Home atmosphere and adolescent future orientation. *European Journal of Psychology of Education*, **5**, 33–43.

Rotheram-Borus, M. J., Rosario, M. and Koopman, C. (1991) Minority youths at high risk: gay males and runaways. In M. E. Colten and S. Gore (eds), *Adolescent Stress: Causes and Consequences*. New York: Aldine de Gruyter.

Rutter, M. (1976) Family, area and school influences in the genesis of conduct disorders. In L. Hersov, M. Berger and D. Shaffer (eds), *Aggression and Antisocial Behaviour in Childhood and Adolescence. Journal of Child Psychology and Psychiatry Book Series No. 1*. Oxford: Pergamon.

Rutter, M. and Rutter, M. (1992) *Developing Minds: Challenge and Continuity across the Lifespan*. Harmondsworth: Penguin.

Ryan, R. M. and Lynch, J. H. (1989) Emotional detachment versus autonomy: revisiting the vicissitudes of adolescence and young adulthood. *Child Development*, **60**, 340–356.

Sabini, J. (1995) *Social Psychology*, 2nd edn. New York: Norton.

Savin-Williams, R. C. (1990) *Gay and Lesbian Youth: Expressions of Identity*. New York: Hemisphere.

Savin-Williams, R. C. and Berndt, T. J. (1990) Friendship and peer relations. In S. S. Feldman and G. R. Elliott (eds), *At the Threshold: The Developing Adolescent*. Cambridge: Cambridge University Press.

Scarr, S., Caparulo, B. K., Ferdman, B. M., Tower, R. B. and Caplan, J. (1983) Developmental status and school achievements of minority and non-minority children from birth to 18 years in a British Midlands town. *British Journal of Developmental Psychology*, **1**, 31–48.

Selman, R. (1980) *The Growth of Interpersonal Understanding: Developmental and Clinical Analyses.* New York: Academic Press.

Shantz, C. U. and Hartup, W. W. (1992) *Conflict in Child and Adolescent Development.* Cambridge: Cambridge University Press.

Simmons, R. G. and Blyth, D. A. (1987) *Moving into Adolescence: The Impact of Physical Change and School Context.* New York: Aldine de Gruyter.

Small, S. (1988) Parental self-esteem and its relationship to childrearing practices, parent-adolescent interaction and adolescent behaviour. *Journal of Marriage and the Family*, **50**, 1063–1072.

Smetana, J. G. (1993) Understanding of social rules. In M. Bennett (ed.), *The Child and Psychologist: An Introduction to the Development of Social Cognition.* New York: Harvester Wheatsheaf.

Sokol-Katz, J., Dunham, R. and Zimmerman, R. (1997) Family structure versus parentqal attachment in controlling deviant adolescent behaviour: a social control model. *Adolescence*, **32**, 199–215.

Steinberg, L. (1993) *Adolescence*, 3rd edn. New York: McGraw Hill.

Steinberg, L. and Silverberg, S. (1986) The vicissitudes of autonomy in early adolescence. *Child Development*, **57**, 841–851.

Steinberg, L., Mounts, N., Lambourn, S. and Dornbusch, S. (1991) Authoritative parenting and adolescent adjustment across various ecological niches. *Journal of Research on Adolescence*, **1**, 19–36.

Super, D. E. (1985) Coming of age in Middletown: careers in the making. *American Psychologist*, **40**, 405–414.

Tajfel, H. (1978) Social categorisation, social identity and social comparison. In H. Tajfel (ed.), *Differentiation between Social Groups.* London: Academic Press, pp. 61–76.

Ullah, P. (1990) the association between income, financial strain and psychological well-being among unemployed youths. *Journal of Occupational Psychology*, **63**, 317–330.

Vygotsky, L. S. (1962) *Thought and Language.* New York: Wiley.

Wallace, C. (1989) Social reproduction and school leavers: a longitudinal perspective. In K. Hurrelmann and U. Engel (eds), *The Social World of Adolescents: International Perspectives.* Berlin: de Gruyter.

Weisfield, G. E., Muczenski, D. M., Weisfield, C. C. and Omakr, D. R. (1987) Stability of boys social success among peers over an eleven year period. In J. A. Meacham (ed.), *Interpersonal Relations: Family, Peers, Friends.* Basel: Karger.

Wentzel, K. R. and Caldwell, K. (1997) Friendships, peer acceptance and group membership: relations to academic achievement in middle school. *Child Development*, **68**, 1198–1209.

Winefield, H. and Winefield, A. (1992) Psychological development in adolescence and youth: education, employment and vocational identity. In P. C. L. Heaven (ed.), *Life Span Development*. Sydney: Harcourt Brace Jovanovitch.

Zani, B. (1991) Male and female patterns in the discovery of sexuality during adolescence. *Journal of Adolescence*, **14**, 163–178.

Chapter 2

INFLUENCES ON THE DEVELOPMENT OF PSYCHOPATHOLOGY IN ADOLESCENCE

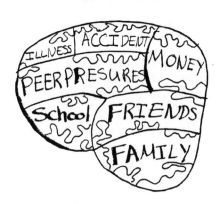

Rachel Davis

INTRODUCTION

The preceding chapter has shown that adolescence is a period of rapid physiological, social and cognitive change. Fortunately, the majority of adolescents are able to cope with these normative changes without developing any psychological difficulties and develop a healthy sense of themselves by the time they reach adulthood. In addition to these normative developmental changes, adolescents can also experience non-normative changes like parental divorce or bereavement in this period. Again, most young people cope effectively with these adversities. In a minority of adolescents, however, this period can so difficult for some teenagers to negotiate successfully, that it can result in the development of mental health problems.

Coleman's focal theory (1978) suggests that developmental tasks are managed more effectively if they occur in a sequence rather than simultaneously. Thus too many changes occurring at once are more likely to lead to stress, which in turn increases the likelihood of psychopathology developing in that young person. If one considers the number of changes that occur in adolescence in comparison to other developmental periods, it is not surprising that an increase in psychological disturbance during adolescence compared to earlier childhood has been found (Lewinsohn *et al.*, 1994). Some disorders, e.g. mood disorders of mild to moderate severity, suicide and alcohol abuse or dependence, have also been reported in adolescence as both increasing in prevalence and presenting at a younger age over the latter part of the 20th century (Lewinsohn *et al.*, 1993). In addition, behavioural and emotional problems co-occur at remarkably high rates in adolescents (Feehan *et al.*, 1994; Fleming and Offord, 1990).

When it comes to trying to understand the individual contributions of different factors to the development of adolescent psychopathology, whereas previously the nature–nuture controversy was hotly contested, most experts now hold the view that both individual and environmental factors are constantly changing and interacting together, and both contribute to adolescent psychopathology.

For the remainder of this chapter, various factors, both normative and non-normative in origin, which have been shown to influence the development of psychopathology in adolescence will be discussed. These will include biological, environmental and individual factors. However, as I have mentioned above, it is often impossible to identify the individual contribution of each factor to the development of psychopathology as they frequently co-exist and interact together. The impact of puberty on adolescent mental health will be described initially.

PUBERTY

Dramatic biological changes occur in adolescence, and the associated physical and sexual changes vary between adolescents with regard to their age of onset and rate of progression (Crockett and Petersen, 1993; Tanner, 1972). Puberty in females has a range of onset from 8.5 to 13 years (Marshall and Tanner, 1969) and in males from 9.5 to 13.5 years (Marshall and Tanner, 1970). Puberty lasts on average 4 years but again can range from 1.5 to 6 years.

IMPACT OF PUBERTY

During and following puberty, adolescents compare themselves to other individuals on many different levels, including their appearance, intellect and social skills. How an adolescent perceives their own physical attractiveness and body image has been shown to be related to their self-evaluation and self-esteem (Thornton and Ryckman, 1991). The overall time span and pace of puberty can therefore exert a significant influence upon a young persons' body image and self-esteem. For example, adolescents who have thought themselves too short or too fat compared to their peers are more likely to have a poorer self-concept (Hogan and McWilliams, 1978). Low self-esteem in adolescence has previously been shown to be associated with depression and suicidal ideation (Crockett and Petersen, 1993; Rutter, 1986), anxiety disorders (Greenberg *et al.*, 1992), eating disorders (Button, 1990), and other problems like delinquency and substance misuse (Reardon and Griffing, 1983).

Changes brought about by puberty have been thought to be experienced more negatively by girls in comparison to boys. Puberty bestows the advantage of increased size and strength on males. In contrast, girls perceive their bodies as getting heavier and body fat is significantly increased (Richards *et al.*, 1990). In Western societies there has been a shift in the appreciation of the hour glass figure to the 'leaner look'. Consequently girls can react negatively to these natural alterations of their figure, which are markedly dissimilar to our current Western ideal female stereotype. This in turn can affect a teenager's self-image and self-esteem. Overall, body image and self-esteem have been reported as declining initially in early adolescence and then increasing later, but with lower levels for females compared to males (Petersen *et al.*, 1994).

The timing of puberty itself can significantly affect the development of psychopathology in adolescence, and again its impact differs between males and females. In the original studies on pubertal timing, early maturation in males was reported as having positive effects with an almost linear relationship between the timing of puberty and positive feelings about oneself (Crockett and Petersen, 1987). Usually boys who matured early were thought to be at an advantage physically in comparison to their peers. They were seen as being more likely to be treated in a more mature way, to have a more positive body image, self-esteem and mood, and to form relationships with the opposite sex more quickly. In comparison, late maturing boys showed an initial decline in body image, but this improved substantially over subsequent years (Petersen *et al.*, 1994). Others have found that unusually early or late pubertal development in males was related to risk behaviours, like alcohol and drug use.

Early maturing females have been reported as being more at risk of having a variety of psychological difficulties, including internalising symptoms (Hayward *et al.*, 1997), dissatisfaction with or a disturbed body image (Alsaker, 1992), eating disorders (Attie and Brooks-Gunn, 1989; Graber *et al.*, 1994), scholastic underachievement (Alasker, 1992), conduct or delinquent problems (Alasker, 1992) and high-risk behaviours, e.g. excessive drinking (Magnusson *et al.*, 1985). These difficulties were found to decrease over time and the higher levels of delinquency did not persist into adulthood. In contrast, females who experience a delay in the starting up of this maturational process have been described as being less concerned with their body image, more popular with peers, achieving more academically and exhibiting fewer behaviour problems (Petersen, 1988).

HORMONAL CHANGES

The changes in hormones which occur during puberty have been thought to account for behaviour changes and depressed feelings in adolescence. Earlier animal studies revealed a link between aggressive behaviour and androgen levels in male animals and less consistently in female animals (Bouissou, 1983). In adolescents, Olweus *et al.* (1980) found that testosterone levels did not have an effect on male adolescent aggressive and antisocial behaviour, but higher levels of testosterone were related to higher levels of provoked aggressive behaviour in these boys. He subsequently suggested that testosterone levels exerted an indirect causal influence on provoked aggression with low frustration tolerance acting as a mediating variable (Olweus, 1986). Other researchers have looked at the relationship between the combination of particular gonadal and adrenal hormones and behaviour. Susman et al. (1987) found that the combination of lower gonadal steroid levels and relatively high adrenal androgen levels were related to adjustment problems and rebellious behaviour in some boys. This was particularly true of those males with this hormonal combination and who were of a relatively higher chronological age (late maturers). This led to the hypothesis that asynchrony of hormone levels and age may be related to adjustment difficulties in adolescence. These findings were, however, less consistent for girls (Nottelmann et al., 1987).

Focusing on girls, Brooks-Gunn and Warren (1989) found that rising levels of reproductive hormones influenced the emergence of depressive symptomatology in adolescent females. Specifically, girls who had the most rapidly increasing hormone levels had the highest reports of depressed affect in comparison to girls who had either significantly lower levels or who had adult levels of these hormones. Although Warren and Brooks-Gunn (1989) did not find an interactive effect between oestrogen levels and negative life events, Buchanan et al. (1992) suggested that an increasing hormonal activity may cause heightened reactivity or mood lability following stressors. In the wider context, however, Buchanan et al. (1992) found that other factors such as an individual's physical health, life events or environmental influences played a more significant role in an adolescents emotions and adjustment than did hormonal changes associated with puberty.

ADVERSITY

Adversities or stressors are usually divided into two types. An acute stressor is typically one of sudden rapid onset, severe in intensity and usually of short duration, e.g. a natural disaster. A chronic stressor in contrast is characterised by having a more gradual onset, being less severe in intensity and occurring over a prolonged period, e.g. long-standing parental mental or physical illness, or family discord. Stressful life events do not typically result in the development of a specific type of disorder in children and adolescents although adolescents can develop post-traumatic stress disorder in response to particularly severe trauma.

Negative discrete life events or stressors themselves have been shown to be associated with emotional disorders like depression (Williamson et al., 1995), anxiety (Bernstein and Hoberman, 1989) and behavioural problems (Swearingen and Cohen, 1985) in adolescents. Chronic adversities are thought to impact more negatively on an adolescents mental health or psychological functioning compared to discrete events (Compas et al., 1989). Different adversities can also occur simultaneously and not surprisingly the higher the number of these present, the more likely an adolescent's self-esteem is to be compromised (Youngs et al., 1990) and the greater the risk of mental health problems developing (Rutter, 1984).

Despite the significant impact that both acute and chronic stressors can have on a person's mental health, not all young people exposed to adversity develop psychological difficulties. This is because we all have our own individual resources to help us cope with stresses in our lives. These resources operate together to create what is termed one's 'resilience'. This is made up of both personal and environmental factors which can protect or lessen the impact of a particular stressor (Rutter, 1987). Personal factors in an adolescent can include characteristics like having a high intellect, high self-esteem, an internal locus of control and having problem-focused coping skills. Environmental factors include being a member in a cohesive family with warm caring supportive parents and having close friendships or good social support from others. As expected, the more of these protective factors a young person has, the better able one is to cope with adversity.

Throughout this chapter different types of adversities will be discussed further in relation to adolescent psychopathology. It is important to bear in mind that even though these adversities are associated with an increase in psychopathology, their presence does not necessarily result in psychological difficulties, particularly if a young person's resilience is able to withstand them.

CHRONIC PHYSICAL ILLNESS

The impact of a chronic medical illness during the sensitive stage of adolescence has been studied in two main ways. Some studies have selected groups of teenagers with a specific chronic condition whilst others have chosen to study adolescents with chronic illnesses irrespective of their nature. In the latter non-categorical approach different chronic illnesses are viewed as impacting on a young person's life in similar ways, regardless of the idiosyncratic nature of each condition. Studies have provided conflicting results regarding the prevalence of psychopathology in these children and adolescents, and this may be due to a variety of reasons, such as different types of chronic conditions being studied, the illnesses having different degrees of severity or associated disability, different participant groups being used (clinic sample versus community sample), or different data collection methods (parent versus adolescent report).

Those studies that have found an increased level of psychopathology and adjustment problems suggest that the rate of psychological problems is approximately double that found in healthy adolescents (Gortmaker et al., 1990) with affective and anxiety disorders particularly being increased (Suris et al., 1996). Some studies have found females to be more affected (Suris et al., 1996), whilst others have shown that this is the case for males (Pless et al., 1993). In some instances particular psychiatric disorders have been reported as occurring more commonly with certain chronic illnesses, e.g. Pumariega *et al.* (1986) found that adolescents with cystic fibrosis were at an increased risk of developing an eating disorder.

Certain factors associated with a chronic medical illness have been suggested as potentially influencing the rate of psychopathology and are discussed below. The age of onset of a chronic illness is thought to be important as it can have a more negative impact on an adolescent compared to a younger child as it occurs at a time when one's identity, self-esteem and self-image is developing, and peer relationships are very important. Having a chronic illness can get in the way of a teenager getting involved in the usual adolescent activities like playing sports, dating and learning to drive. A young person can end up feeling resentful, unaccepting of the illness, uncooperative with treatment and unwilling to take responsibility for treatment. Psychological difficulties are also more likely to occur in adolescents with poorly controlled illnesses (Liss *et al.*, 1998) or more severe forms of an illness (Garralda *et al.*, 1988). One would also expect that an illness with an associated disability or disfigurement would be more likely to pose difficulties for an adolescent to handle compared to a younger child, as it may impact upon the development of a young person's self-esteem, self-image and relationship with others. However, research in this area has provided conflicting results (Wolman *et al.*, 1994). Chronic illnesses which affect the central nervous system, e.g. epilepsy, have higher rates of emotional and behavioural problems than chronic physical conditions which do not (Rutter *et al.*, 1970). The types of psychiatric disorders in adolescents with chronic illnesses affecting the central nervous system, however, are generally not different from those in adolescents with chronic illnesses not affecting it. Specific psychoses, however, have been reported in children and adolescents with particular types of epilepsy (Taylor, 1975).

INTELLECTUAL IMPAIRMENT

Rutter *et al.* (1970) found that behaviour problems, both mild and severe, in mentally retarded children and adolescents were three to four times more common than in randomly selected children of a corresponding age group. Gillberg *et al.* (1986) found that more than half of mentally retarded children aged between 13 and 17 years had additional psychiatric symptoms. Sixty-four percent of severely retarded teenagers and 57% of the mildly retarded teenagers had a handicapping psychiatric condition. Autism-like 'psychotic behaviour' was reported as being common in the severely retarded group, with 0.2% of the total group having a combination of mental retardation and psychotic symptoms. Gillberg and colleagues also found that puberty sometimes aggravated problems, especially in the group with psychotic behaviour, but only rarely caused them.

FAMILY INFLUENCES

In the last 50 years there have been significant social changes in the developed world including increased urbanisation, a greater number of both working mothers and single parent families, and a higher divorce rate. Obviously these changes will in turn influence what is meant by the term 'family life'. So, for example, the experience of being an adolescent now is quite different to that of a teenager 50 years ago. Certain aspects of current family life which can play a part in the development of adolescent psychopathology will be discussed below.

WORKING FAMILIES

Overall little difference has been found in the children and adolescents with one wage earning parent compared with those with two wage earners, although some studies have reported lower school performance and an increase in aggressive behaviour in sons but not daughters in middle class families with full-time working mothers (Hoffman, 1980; Montemayor and Clayton, 1983). Studies looking at 'latchkey' adolescents likewise have not reported differences in these children's feelings about themselves, their academic achievement or their peer relations compared to their counterparts (Vandell and Ramanan, 1991). For these children and adolescents what seems to be important is the quality of care that young person receives from his or her parents, where he or she stays after school and whether parental supervision is present even if this occurs at a distance (Lerner and Galambos, 1991).

PARENTING STYLES

Parenting is affected by a variety of factors including the relationship between a parent and their teenage son or daughter, their marital relationship, family functioning, extended family support, and the community where the family resides. Many studies of parenting during adolescence have examined the relations between parenting characteristics and child and adolescent outcomes (Ge et al., 1996). Most often parenting style is usually conceptualised along two dimensions – parental demandingness (control) and parental responsiveness (warmth) which can be combined to form four categories of parenting. Studies have found that adolescents with parents who were authoritative in their parenting style (highly demanding and highly responsive parents) had the best outcome behaviourally and academically in school (Baumrind, 1991; Steinberg et al., 1989). Permissive-indulgent (undemanding and highly responsive parents) parents were more likely to have offspring with a mixture of positive and negative features. Although they were more psychologically well adjusted than the latter two groups described below, they were also more likely to engage in moderate levels of deviant behaviour

(Lamborn *et al.*, 1991). Authoritarian parenting (highly demanding and unresponsive parents) was associated with lack of social competence with peers, a tendency to withdraw instead of taking the initiative, low self-esteem, an external locus of control and also academic difficulties up to the age of 17 years (Baumrind, 1991). Permissive-indifferent or neglecting (unresponsive and undemanding) parents were found to have the least well-adjusted adolescents. These children were the least competent academically and socially and had the highest levels of behaviour problems and internalising symptoms.

Harsh and inconsistent parenting has been reported as being associated with antisocial behaviour in children and adolescents (Farrington, 1991). Adolescents in families where physical punishment is used have also been found to have higher levels of psychiatric symptoms and a lower sense of well-being (Bachar *et al.*, 1997), and with some modelling their parents aggressive behaviour (Johnson and O'Leasry, 1987).

FAMILY FUNCTIONING

Family functioning has been measured in different ways and has been shown to influence adolescent depressive symptomatology (Martin *et al.*, 1995), suicidal behaviours (Martin *et al.*, 1995), suicide rates (McKenry *et al.*, 1982) and substance abuse (McKay *et al.*, 1991).

Children and adolescents living in families with high levels of conflict or discord are more likely to have both internalising and externalising problems, immaturity, low self-esteem, and academic difficulties compared with controls (Fendrich *et al.*, 1990). Forehand *et al.* (1991a) reported that as parental conflict increased, adolescent functioning deteriorated. Conger *et al.* (1991) found a relationship between spousal conflict and early alcohol use in their offspring. In families where children and adolescents witness violence between parents, an increased rate of internalising and externalising symptomatology has been reported with some developing symptoms of post-traumatic stress disorder (Masten *et al.*, 1990).

Although there are clear associations between family dysfunction and increased levels of psychopathology in the offspring living within these families, it is difficult, particularly retrospectively, to determine whether the presence of a disturbed adolescent in a family results in the problematic communication or vice versa. Overall it is thought to be more likely that a vulnerable adolescent is at greater risk of becoming disturbed or relapsing in the presence of problematic communication within the family.

PARENTAL PSYCHOPATHOLOGY

The association between parental psychiatric illness and emotional or behavioural difficulties in children and adolescents has been shown to hold for parents with alcohol problems (Hill and Muka, 1996), substance abuse (Stephenson *et al.*, 1996), depression (Downey and Coyne, 1990), anxiety disorders and obsessive-compulsive disorders (Turner *et al.*, 1987). Many reasons have been hypothesised regarding the transmission of psychopathology from one generation to the next. These include genetic transmission of the disorder itself or the presence of environmental factors like family discord or dysfunction. Living in a stressful environment, poor parenting practices or particular types of interactions between the parent and child can result from having an ill parent (Downey and Coyne, 1990; Rutter, 1990).

Much information on the inheritance of psychopathology has come from twin, adoption and family studies, segregation analysis, and more recently from molecular genetic studies. Research so far has found that most aspects of childhood and adolescent psychopathology are moderately genetically influenced (Lombroso *et al.*, 1994). Most psychiatric disorders are also thought to be due to the expression of more than one gene. Lombroso *et al.* (1994), in a review, identified that genetic factors played an important role in the aetiology of attention deficit hyperactivity disorder, autism, affective disorders, obsessive-compulsive disorder, Gilles de la Tourette's syndrome and specific reading disability.

Environmental influences also play an important role in the development of psychopathology. These are divided into shared environmental factors (i.e. those shared by siblings reared in the same family) and non-shared ones (those which are not shared by siblings in a family). In behavioural genetic studies shared environmental factors are thought to have a minimal influence on sibling psychological similarity (Tellegen *et al.*, 1988) whilst non-shared influences play a more major role (Plomin and Daniels, 1987). Although there are exceptions, e.g. several adoption studies have found that being reared in an alcoholic family does increase a person's chances of becoming an alcoholic (McGue, 1993), overall most of the environmental influence appears to be of the non-shared variety.

Pike and Plomin (1996), in their review, reported that shared environmental influences account for little if any variation (with the possible exception of juvenile delinquency where shared environmental factors contribute more than in other disorders) while non-shared environmental influences account for much of the variation. They reported this to be the case for autism, hyperactivity, anorexia nervosa, Tourette's syndrome and depressive symptoms. Other studies found that there was a larger genetic contribution to depressive symptomatology in adolescence compared to younger children, although this was not replicated by Pike and Plomin (1996).

Genetic and environmental influences can interact together in a variety of ways. For example, they can have an additive effect; genetically determined character-istics may influence the exposure or sensitivity to environmental risks or genetic influences can lead indirectly to psychopathology through related genetically influenced characteristics such as personality (Kendler and Eaves, 1986). Changes in the environment may also impact on the strength of the genetic effect. Developmentally the magnitude of the genetic and environmental contribution to psychopathology can vary over time as seen in twin studies of temperamental dimensions (McCartney *et al.*, 1990).

PARENTAL DEVIANCE

Numerous studies have shown an association between criminality and antisocial behaviour in parents and delinquency and conduct disorders in their offspring (Phares and Compas, 1992). Loeber and Stouthamer-Loeber (1986) described particular features within these families that could contribute to this association which included parental insensitivity to the child's needs, a lack of parental supervision and involvement with their children, a high incidence of condoning abnormal behaviour in the children, and also significant family discord. These factors were more important for younger children, whereas factors like economic deprivation, poor school functioning and having deviant friends were found to be more important contributors for adolescents.

DIVORCE AND SINGLE PARENT FAMILIES

Divorce can impact on a teenager in many ways and its effects can depend on a variety of factors, e.g. relationships within the family prior and following the divorce, the reasons for the divorce, problematic court proceedings, the decisions made by the court with regard to custody and access, a sudden drop in income, and the changes in parenting subsequently experienced by an adolescent. The overall effects of divorce on adolescent functioning are similar to those seen in children (Forehand *et al.*, 1991b). Adolescents from disrupted families have been shown to be more likely to engage in behaviours that could damage health, e.g. cannabis use or alcohol consumption, to have conduct problems (Allison and Furstenberg, 1989), to develop emotional problems (Zill *et al.*, 1993) and to exhibit academic difficulty or drop out of high school (Hetherington *et al.*, 1982), compared to adolescents in intact families. These problems have been correlated with inept parenting by the custodial parent, e.g. a lower level of monitoring and control over the teenagers activities (Hetherington, 1982). The negative effects of divorce have also been reported to be particularly associated with the absence of the father, economic disadvantage and continuing parental conflict (Amato and Keith, 1991). Residing with a parenting figure of the same sex after divorce has also been shown to be of some protective importance (Peterson and Zill, 1986). To put this all in perspective, however, although most children and adolescents exhibit short-term developmental disruptions, emotional distress and behaviour problems, most usually adapt to their new set of circumstances within the first 2 years after the divorce (Hetherington *et al.*, 1982), unless there are additional stressors. Differences between the adjustment of children in divorced and intact families are therefore not large (Amato and Keith, 1991), and in some families adolescents psychological well-being improves after their parents' divorce (Bilge and Kaufman, 1983).

REMARRIAGE AND STEPFAMILIES

Most reconstituted families manage to adjust and build adequate step-parent and stepchild relationships; however, the adjustment of an adolescent particularly in early adolescence to remarriage and the presence of a step-parent seems to be more problematic than for younger children (Hetherington, 1989). Hetherington and Clingempeel (1986) found both girls and boys aged between 9 and 15 years at the time of remarriage to often have marked behaviour problems and difficulties in the parent–child relationship which did not improve greatly over the following 2 years. Zimiles and Lee (1991) found that academic achievement was lower and school drop-out was higher in adolescents in reconstituted families than in intact families. Stepfather and adolescent stepdaughter relationships have been reported as being particularly problematic (Hetherington and Clingempeel, 1992).

CHROMOSOMAL DISORDERS

In this section I want to briefly comment on some of the findings regarding the mental health or psychological well-being of adolescents with particular chromosomal disorders which either occur more commonly or which are more likely to have an impact in the adolescent period will be discussed. They are classified according to whether the defect affects a sex chromosome or autosomal chromosome.

SEX CHROMOSOME ABNORMALITIES

The main sex chromosome disorders include Klinefelter's syndrome, XYY syndrome, Turner's syndrome and Fragile X. As the process of puberty involves sexual development and adolescence is a time of increased self-consciousness when young people are likely to compare themselves to others, any interference in the initiation or progress of puberty is more likely to result in psychological problems for that individual than in a young person whose puberty progresses normally. As the sex chromosomes are involved in these disorders, the process of puberty can be affected in these young people. For example, in Turner's syndrome, most affected females are of short stature and have gonadal dysgenesis, and usually lack a spontaneous puberty. Alternatively puberty is usually delayed by 6 months in XYY males.

In addition to this, one would expect an adolescent whose physical features or intellectual capacities are obviously different from his or her peers, to be more likely to have psychological difficulties than his or her unaffected counterparts. Adolescent boys with Klinefelter's syndrome or Fragile X have typical physical stigmata which often become more pronounced with the onset of puberty. They have intellectual impairment of varying degrees and are at increased risk of being bullied or stigmatised, and consequently of developing psychological difficulties compared to their unaffected peers.

A variety of studies have specifically tried to determine the prevalence of mental health problems in individuals with sex chromosome disorders. Some studies have reported a higher rate of mental health problems in adolescents with Turner's syndrome compared to controls (Cunniff et al., 1995); however, the majority of studies seem to suggest that although females with Turner's syndrome are at increased risk for subtle behaviour problems, they have a lower rate of mental illness than expected (McCawley et al., 1995). In the case of Fragile X, a spectrum of possible involvement has been recognised ranging from unaffected carriers to those with the full associated phenotype, significant learning disability and higher prevalence of psychopathology. A variety of behavioural and emotional disorders has been described in association with this syndrome, primarily in adult cases (Hagerman and Sobesky, 1989), including an increased frequency of schizotypal features and chronic affective disorder (Reiss and Freund, 1990), although their relationship to the fragile X chromosome is unclear. In one study of obligate female carriers, the degree of fragility was found to be a potentially important predictor of psychopathology among female carriers with normal IQ (Freund et al., 1992). Males with Klinefelter's syndrome and XXY males have been described as being unpopular with their peers, introverted and prone to temper outbursts. Additional studies have reported an increased incidence of psychological consultations in males with Klinefelter's syndrome (Sorensen, 1992) and of mental health problems in XXY males (Nielsen et al., 1980).

AUTOSOME CHROMOSOMAL ABNORMALITIES

These include disorders like Down's syndrome, Prader–Willi syndrome, Wilson's disease (hepatolenticular degeneration) and Huntington's disease. As some of these disorders have associated physical stigmata and impaired intellectual development, one would expect individuals with these disorders, particularly during adolescence, to be more at risk of psychological problems. In Down's syndrome there is also an increased incidence of other medical problems, e.g. congenital cardiac abnormalities, sensory impairment and leukaemia. Again in view of this one would anticipate adolescents with this disorder to have a higher prevalence of psychiatric disorder. Some studies have shown this to be the case (Myers and Pueschel, 1991); however, overall, Down's syndrome has not been found to be associated with a higher rate of mental health problems compared to other causes of mental retardation.

Children and adolescents with Prader–Willi syndrome have a variable phenotypic profile including short stature, delayed onset of puberty, varying degrees of intellectual impairment and childhood onset of hyperphagia, which often leads on to severe food-related difficulties including food foraging and life threatening obesity. They have also been described as having a variety of emotional and behavioural difficulties (Dykens and Cassidy, 1995). The obesity often becomes more of a problem in adolescence as it becomes even more difficult to control the child's food intake. In one study over 50% of adolescents with Prader–Willi syndrome fulfilled the criteria for a definite or probable DSM-III diagnosis with a high preponderance of reported neurotic disorders, primarily compulsive and anxious types (Whitman and Accardo, 1987), but matched controls were not used.

Wilson's disease is an uncommon inborn error of metabolism affecting copper excretion. Although it usually presents in the second and third decade of life with neurological or psychiatric signs and symptoms, it can appear in childhood or adolescence (Akil and Schwartz, 1991). Scheinberg and Sternlieb (1984) reported that most patients with clinically evident Wilson's disease developed psychiatric symptoms of some kind and that in general 10–25% of cases can present initially with psychiatric symptoms. Psychiatric symptoms reported in the past include affective disorders, anxiety, affective or schizophrenic psychoses, emotional lability or incongruity, changes in personality, or non-specific behavioural or emotional problems.

Huntington's disease is an autosomal dominant inherited disorder with an onset before 14 years, in 5%. It can first present in a child or teenager in a variety of ways with neurological symptoms, intellectual deterioration, disturbed or withdrawn behaviour, or a loss of interest in school work.

SCHOOL

The transition to secondary or middle school can result in increased anxiety and also reduced self-esteem in adolescents (Cotterell, 1992), although overall adolescents have been found to be more positive about their new school after the transition (Berndt and Mekos, 1995). Factors like school size and teachers expectations have also been shown to influence a student's behaviour (Gabarino, 1980). Children and adolescents who have a low IQ or a specific learning difficulty and do poorly at school are at increased risk for psychiatric disorders. These disorders include conduct disorder (Rutter et al., 1970), delinquency (West and Farrington, 1973), hyperactivity (Hinshaw, 1992), depressive symptoms (Fleming et al., 1989) and anxiety symptoms (Williams et al., 1989).

Teenagers can truant or drop-out of school for many reasons. Those who do are more likely than those who remain in school to be emotionally troubled, lack confidence in their self-worth, have low esteem, and have higher rates of drug use, delinquency and depression (Dryfoos, 1991). The exact mechanism by which poor school performance leads to increased rates of psychiatric disorder has not been fully determined as yet.

PEERS

In adolescence young people like to conform more with peer values, current peer culture and spend less time with parents. Peer group interaction, acceptance by peers and the development of an intimate sexual relationship become increasingly more important in the process of developing an identity.

Friendships can impact in both positive and negative ways on an adolescents psychological well-being. Young people who have more intimate friends have been described as being less hostile, less anxious, less depressed, more sociable and having a higher self-esteem than adolescents with less intimate friendships (Buhrmester, 1990). On the other hand, participation in the peer culture can also result in a young person engaging in dangerous behaviors, e.g. drug experimentation. When peer groups assume an unusually dominant role in the lives of adolescents, this is just as likely to be a consequence of inadequate parental attention as it is to do with the attractiveness of the peer group (Galambos and Silbereisen, 1987).

Being rejected or bullied by ones peers affects ones self-esteem and has been shown to result in serious problems like delinquency, drug abuse or depression (Parkhurst, 1992). In a review, Parker and Asher (1987) reported a positive correlation between rejection by peers in childhood and later problems, including neurotic and psychotic illnesses, conduct disorders, delinquency, disturbances in sexual behaviour, and school maladjustment. On recognising these associations, however, it is difficult to determine the direction of causality.

WORK

Deciding on ones chosen career and taking steps to achieve that goal is one of the major developmental tasks of adolescence. Studies looking at the impact of part-time work in adolescents still attending school have shown that this can have positive psychological benefits when conditions are good. However, when the job involved working long hours, was felt to be stressful or when it interfered with school work then it impacted negatively on that particular young person's psychological well-being (Mortimer et al., 1992). As in the adult population, unemployment or job loss after leaving school can result in significant psychological distress for a person with increased anxiety, depression or psychosomatic complaints. Feehan et al. (1995) found that after adjusting for mental disorder at age 15 years, unemployment remained an independent predictor of mental disorder at age 18 years for both sexes.

ADOLESCENT PREGNANCY

Pregnancy in adolescence, whether it results in subsequent marriage or not, is associated with many difficulties. Many are still in the process of growing up, are still in need of parenting themselves and are not adequately prepared for motherhood (Osofsky, 1990). Not only is the teenager trying to cope with the developmental tasks that need to be negotiated in adolescence and being a mother to her baby, but she is also often struggling to finish school or to find a job. Pregnant adolescents are also more likely than their non-pregnant peers to live in socially disadvantaged circumstances, be unemployed or if employed to have lower paying occupations (Brooks-Gunn and Chase-Lansdale, 1995). All these factors affect the emotional, social, physical and economic well-being of the parent and child. In one study, 59% of adolescent mothers of 1–3 year olds met the criteria for adult depression (Colletta, 1983).

ENVIRONMENT

SOCIOECONOMIC DISADVANTAGE

There is a strong and consistent relationship between socioeconomic disadvantage and adolescent psychiatric disorder (Offord, 1990). This relationship is stronger in younger children compared with adolescents (Rutter, 1981). It is thought to be mediated by parental and family characteristics like family dysfunction or marital discord, or attributes of the children associated with economic disadvantage, e.g. low intellect, rather than economic disadvantage itself (Rutter and Giller, 1983). Studies have shown that economic hardship can have a direct negative effect on marital happiness and the parent–offspring relationship (Ho et al., 1995), and also that the marital relationship can mediate the effect of economic hardship on child and adolescent outcomes by disturbing the parent–offspring relationship (Fauber et al., 1990). Studies concentrating on economically disadvantaged parents have found them to more frequently display inconsistent discipline (Lempers et al., 1989), rejecting behaviour (Conger et al., 1984), less nurturance (Lempers et al., 1989), less support (Flanagan, 1990) and to be more autocratic (Flanagan, 1990). Conger et al. (1993) also demonstrated that socioeconomic disadvantage has an effect on adolescent adjustment by increasing parental depression which in turn is associated with less involved parenting.

COMMUNITY

A growing body of research has shown that social support is positively associated with parenting behaviour (Taylor and Roberts, 1995). Abuse and neglect occur less frequently in families with strong social support (Garbarino, 1989). Taylor and Roberts (1995) demonstrated a positive association between kinship social support and adolescent adjustment. Social support has been shown by others to be negatively associated with adolescent anxiety (McLoyd et al., 1994) and problem behaviour (Taylor and Roberts, 1995). They have suggested that the positive effects of social support on adolescent adjustment may be mediated by the association of kinship support with more adequate parenting. Thus social support may enhance parent child-rearing practices, which in turn may enhance adolescent functioning. Aneshensel and Sucoff (1996) also found that the perception of ones neighbourhood as being dangerous has been shown to influence adolescent mental health. The more threatening a neighbourhood is perceived, the more common are symptoms of depression, anxiety, oppositional defiant disorder and conduct disorder.

CULTURE

Most of the research in adolescence so far has typically been carried out with white middle class subjects and it is not always appropriate to generalise findings from this group to those adolescents in minority groups, particularly as there is evidence from several community studies that emotional and behavioural problems vary by race or ethnic minority. Cultural factors like child-rearing practices, social standards, religious beliefs, coping strategies used and educational provision all affect the prevalence of disorders. Different expectations and restrictions are also placed on adolescents depending on the particular culture in which they grow up.

A variety of studies have looked at the prevalence of mental health problems in different cultures in the UK in the younger age groups. For example, Rutter et al. (1974) found that 10-year-old children from West Indian immigrant families had higher rates of antisocial symptoms, restlessness and impaired concentration reported by teachers compared with non-immigrant families. This increased rate of disorder was associated with an increased rate of educational retardation in this group (Yule et al., 1975), and also other factors including family disruption and dysfunction. In contrast, children of Asian origin living in the UK appear to have comparable or slightly reduced rates of psychiatric disorder compared to white children (Cochrane, 1979). In North America, American Indian children have been reported as having higher rates of emotional and behavioural disorders compared to their counterparts (Beiser and Attneave, 1982), with adolescent girls being particularly at risk (Offord, 1990). Also in the US, young black people have been found to have higher rates of behavioural problems, especially serious offences (Rutter and Giller, 1983), and also depressive symptoms compared to their white counterparts (Garrison *et al.*, 1985).

For minority groups, the beliefs and practices of child-rearing will also be affected by acculturation of the minority group to the culture of the dominant group (Sodowsky *et al.*, 1991). Discord and stress typically arises between parents and adolescents over dating, marriages and career choices because of antagonism caused by conflict between the old and new cultural values (Nguygen and Williams, 1989).

In addition to this, minority groups like African-American adolescents are more likely to experience additional stressors or negative life events like higher rates of unemployment and teenage pregnancy (Rogers and Lee, 1992), lower income, discrimination and increased exposure to violent crime (Wright *et al.*, 1996) compared to their white counterparts. Adolescents in minority groups are also more likely to perform poorly at school and experience family adversity (Offord, 1990). All these factors play a part in the higher rate of mental health problems in minority adolescents.

RESIDENTIAL CARE, FOSTER PLACEMENT AND ADOPTION

In comparison to younger children, adolescents tend to be admitted into local authority care for longer periods and this is often associated with severe behaviour problems, chronic social difficulties, neglect or abuse (Triseliotis and Hill, 1990). Overall, children and adolescents admitted to residential care have a much higher rate of psychiatric disorder than other children (Wolkind and Rutter, 1973). In particular, adolescents admitted to residential care fare worse than children admitted at an earlier age (Garnett, 1990). This high level of disorder is thought to be due to other life experiences, e.g. longer exposure to adverse family factors, rather than being a result of being in residential care (Wolkind and Rutter, 1973).

Similarly, children and adolescents in permanent foster care placements had a higher level of difficulties compared to controls (Parker, 1966). Those settled in these placements at an older age have been described as faring worse with higher rate of placement breakdown (Parker, 1966).

Interracial adoption, intercountry adoption and the adoption of hard to place youngsters has increased over the years. The adoption of older children, particularly adolescents and those with special needs, has increased (Barth and Berry, 1988). Adopted children are thought to be at higher risk for problems for a number of reasons, including exposure to early negative experiences like inadequate care, separation from mother, institutional care, increased genetic vulnerability and problems concerning their personal identity. Transracially adopted children may also be vulnerable to feeling excluded because of their different appearance.

Overall, adoptees have been shown to be at a slightly greater risk of psychiatric disorder in clinic populations and non-clinic samples (Maughan and Pickles, 1990). Studies have suggested that those adopted at an earlier age have a better outcome than older adoptees (Triseliotis and Russell, 1984). Adoptees at the age of approximately 11 years have been noted to be most maladjusted and this is thought to be related to possible concerns over identity (Maughan and Pickles, 1990). In two subsequent studies, Verhulst *et al.* (1992) and Verhulst and Versluis-Bieman (1995) demonstrated that the age at placement of individuals did not contribute to the prediction of later maladjustment independent of the influence of early adversities. Secondly, he postulated that although adverse environmental pre-adoption experiences are associated with higher levels of problem behaviour which may make adoptees vulnerable to later maladjustment, other factors pertaining to adolescent development may also interact negatively with adoption-specific factors. These are then likely to render individuals vulnerable to deviation from the normal developmental pathway. Follow-up studies of adoptees in adulthood have found them to have a stronger sense of self, and a higher level of functioning on a personal, social and economic level compared to adults who had previously been fostered (Triseliotis and Hill, 1990). These authors suggested that adoption had a greater capacity to reverse earlier adverse experiences and encouraged a stronger sense of belonging and permanence than those in foster or residential care.

ABUSE

Physical, emotional or sexual abuse, like other adversities, can be either acute or chronic in origin. Garbarino (1989) reported that the incidence of adolescent maltreatment equalled or exceeded the incidence of maltreatment of younger children. Psychological and sexual abuse predominated. Females are more likely to be abused in adolescence than at any other time; however, some studies have found that adolescent boys develop more problems following sexual abuse than girls (Garnefski and Diekstra, 1997).

The effects of abuse are often studied in children and adolescents over wide age ranges, and different types of abuse often co-occur and are studied simultaneously. The consequences of any form of abuse on adolescent adjustment can be severe, chronic and multiproblematic (Garnefski and Diekstra, 1997). These can include emotional disturbances including depressive, anxiety or post-traumatic symptoms (Kiser *et al.*, 1991), deliberate self-harm or suicide (Wagner, 1997), somatic complaints, negative self-image (Hjorth and Ostrov, 1982), behavioural problems including conduct disorders, aggression, substance use (Garbarino and

Plantz, 1986), academic delay or difficulties (Kurtz *et al.*, 1993) and, in the case of sexual abuse, additional effects on an adolescent's sexuality.

CONCLUSION

Adolescence is a time when many new challenges appear on the way to reaching adulthood. In addition to these new challenges some youngsters enter adolescence with adversities dating back to earlier in their childhood, for example, chronic illness. Others meet new stressors during this period. Adversities interact together in complex ways and are moderated by an adolescent's resilience.

If an adolescent's resilient qualities are unable to withstand the impact of these adversities, mental health problems can occur. For some these problems can even continue into adulthood. To further understand how adversities and resilient factors interact together and can sometimes result in mental health problems, more prospective studies need to be carried out in these areas.

REFERENCES

Akil, M. and Schwartz, J. A. (1991) The psychiatric presentations of Wilson's disease. *Journal of Neuropsychiatry and Clinical Neurosciences*, **3**, 377–382.

Allison, P. D. and Furstenburg, F. F. (1989) How marital dissolution affects children: variations by age and sex. *Developmental Psychology*, **25**, 540–549.

Alsaker, F. D. (1992) Pubertal timing, overweight, and psychological adjustment. *Journal of Early Adolescence*, **12**, 396–419.

Amato, P. R. and Keith, B. (1991) Consequences of parental divorce for the well-being of children: a meta-analysis. *Psychological Bulletin*, **110**, 26–46.

Aneshensel, C. and Sucoff, C. (1996) The neighbourhood context of adolescent mental health. *Journal of Health and Social Behaviour*, **37**, 293–310.

Attie, I. and Brooks-Gunn, J. (1989) Development of eating problems in adolescent girls: a longitudinal study. *Developmental Psychology*, **25**, 70–79.

Bachar, E., Canetti, L., Bonne, O., Kaplan DeNour, A. and Shalev, A. Y. (1997) Physical punishment and signs of mental distress in normal adolescents. *Adolescence*, **32**, 945–958.

Barth, R. P. and Berry, M. (1988) *Adoption and Disruption. Rates, Risks and Responses.* New York: Aldine De Gruyter.

Baumrind, D. (1991) Effective parenting during the early adolescent transition. *Advances in Family Research*, **2**, 111–163.

Beiser, M. and Attneave, C. L. (1982) Mental disorder among Native American children: rates and risk periods for entering treatment. *American Journal Psychiatry*, **139**, 193–198.

Berndt, T. J. and Mekos, D. (1995) Adolescents' perceptions of the stressful and desirable aspects of the transition to junior high school. *Journal of Research on Adolescence*, 5, 123–142.

Bernstein, G. A. and Hoberman, H. M. (1989) Self-reported anxiety in adolescents. *American Journal of Psychiatry*, **146**, 384–386.

Bilge, B. and Kaufman, G. (1983) Children of divorce and one-parent families: cross-cultural perspectives. *Family Relations*, **32**, 59–71.

Bouissou, M. F. (1983) Andogens, aggressive behaviour and social relationships in higher mammals. *Hormone Research*, **18**, 43–61.

Brooks-Gunn, J. and Chase-Lansdale, P. L. (1995) Adolescent parenthood and parenting: development in context. In M. H. Bornstein (ed.), *Handbook of Parenting: Vol. 3. Status and Social Conditions of Parenting*. Hillsdale, NJ: Erlbaum.

Brooks-Gunn, J. and Warren, M. P. (1989) Biological and social contributions to negative affect in young adolescent girls. *Child Development*, **62**, 40–55.

Buchanan, C. M., Eccles, J. S. and Becker, J. B. (1992) Are adolescents the victims of raging hormones? Evidence for activational effects of hormones on moods and behaviour at adolescence . *Psychological Bulletin*, **111**, 62–107.

Buhrmester, D. (1990) Intimacy of friendship, interpersonal competence, and adjustment during preadolesence and adolescence. *Child Development*, **61**, 1101–1111.

Button, E. (1990) Self-esteem in girls aged 11–12: baseline findings from a planned prospective study of vulnerability to eating disorders. *Journal of Adolescence*, **13**, 407–413.

Cochrane, R. (1979) Psychological and behavioural disturbances in West Indians, Indians and Pakistanis in Britain: a comparison of rates among children and adults. *British Journal of Psychiatry*, **134**, 201.

Coleman, J. (1978) Current contradictions in adolescent theory. *Journal of Youth and Adolescence*, **6**, 139–154.

Colletta, N. D. (1983) At risk for depression: a study of young mothers. *Journal of Genetic Psychology*, **142**, 301–310.

Compas, B. E., Howell, D. C., Phares, V., Williams, R. A. and Giunta, C. T. (1989) Risk factors for emotional/behavioural problems in young adolescents: a prospective analysis of adolescent and parental stress and symptoms. *Journal of Consulting and Clinical Psychology*, **57**, 732–740.

Conger, R. D., McCarty, J. A., Young, R. K., Lahey B. B. and Kropp, J. P. (1984) Perception of child, child-rearing values, and emotional distress as mediating links between environmental stressors and observed maternal behaviour. *Child Development*, **54**, 2234–2247.

Conger, R. D. Lorenz, F. O., Elder, G. H., Melby, J. N., Simons, R. L. and Conger, K. J. (1991) A process model of family economic pressure and early adolescent alcohol use. *Journal of Early Adolescence*, **11**, 430–449.

Conger, R. D., Conger, K. J. Elder, G. H., Lorenz, F. O., Simons, R. L. and Whitebeck, L. B. (1993) Family economic stress and adjustment of early adolescent girls. *Developmental Psychology*, 29, 206–219.

Cotterell, J. L. (1992) School size as a factor in adolescents' adjustment to the transition to secondary school. *Journal of Early Adolescence*, 12, 28–45.

Crockett, L. J. and Petersen, A. C. (1987) Pubertal status and psychosocial development : Findings from the early adolescent study. In R. M. Lerner and T. T. Roch (eds), *Biological and Social Interactions in Early Adolescence: A Life-span Perspective*. Hillsdale, NJ: Erlbaum, pp. 173–188.

Crockett, L. J. and Petersen, A. C. (1993) Adolescent development: health risks and opportunities for health promotion. In S. G. Millstein, A. C. Petersen and E. O. Nightingale (eds), *Promoting the Health of Adolescents: New Directions for the Twenty-First Century*. New York: Oxford University Press, pp. 13–37.

Cunniff, C., Hassed, S. J., Hendon, A. E. and Rickert, V. I. (1995) Health care utilisation and perceptions of health among adolescents and adults with Turner's syndrome. *Clinical Genetics*, 48, 17–22.

Downey, G. and Coyne, J. C. (1990) Children of depressed parents: an integrative review. *Psychological Bulletin*, 108, 50–76.

Dryfoos, J. G. (1991) Adolescents at risk: a summation of work in the field: programs and policies. *Journal of Adolescent Health*, 12, 620–637.

Dykens, E. M. and Cassidy, S. B. (1995) Correlates of maladaptive in children and adults with Prader–Willi syndrome. *American Journal of Medical Genetics*, 60, 546–549.

Farrington, D. P. (1991) Childhood aggression and adult violence: early precursors and later life outcomes. In D. J. Pepler and K. H. Rubin (eds), *The Development And Treatment of Childhood Aggression*. Hillsdale, NJ: Erlbaum, pp. 5–29.

Fauber, R., Forehand, R., McCombs Thomas, A. and Wierson, M. (1990) A mediational model of the impact of marital conflict on adolescent adjustment in intact and divorced families: the role of disrupted parenting. *Child Development*, 61, 1112–1123.

Feehan, M., McGee, R., Nada-Raja, S. and Williams, S. M. (1994) DSM-III-R disorders in New Zealand 18 -year-olds. *Australian and New Zealand Journal of Psychiatry*, 28, 87–99.

Feehan, M., McGee, R., Williams, S. M. and Nada-Raja, S. (1995) Models of adolescent psychopathology: childhood risk and transition to adulthood. *Journal of the American Academy of Child and Adolescent Psychiatry*, 34, 670–679.

Fendrich, M., Warner, V. and Weissman, M. M. (1990) Family risk factors, parental depression, and psychopathology in offspring. *Developmental Psychology*, 26, 40–50.

Flanagan, C. A. (1990) Change in family work status: effects on parent–adolescent decision making. *Child Development*, **61**, 163–177.

Fleming, J. E., Offord, D. R. and Boyle, M. H. (1989) Prevalence of childhood and adolescent depression in the community: Ontario Child Health Study. *British Journal of Psychiatry*, **155**, 647–654.

Fleming, J. E. and Offord, D. R. (1990) Epidemiology of childhood depressive disorder: a critical review. *Journal of the American Academy of Child and Adolescent Psychiatry*, **29**, 571–580.

Forehand, R., Wierson, M., McCombs Thomas, A., Armistead, L., Kempton, T. and Neighbors, B. (1991a) The role of family stressors and parent relationships on adolescent functioning. *Journal of American Academy of Child and Adolescent Psychiatry*, **30**, 316–322.

Forehand, R., Wierson, M., Thomas, A. M., Fauber, R., Armistead, L., Kempton, T. and Long, N. (1991b) A short-term longitudinal examination of young adolescent functioning following divorce: the role of family factors. *Journal of Abnormal Child Psychology*, **18**, 323–340.

Freund, L. S., Reiss, A. L., Hagerman, R. and Vinogradov, S. (1992) Chromosome fragility and psychopathology in obligate female carriers of the fragile X chromosome. *Archives of General Psychiatry*, **49**, 54–60.

Galambos, N. L. and Silbereisen, R. K. (1987) Influence of income change and parental acceptance on adolescent transgression proneness and peer relations. *European Journal of Psychology of Education*, **1**, 17–28.

Garbarino, J. (1980) Some thoughts on school size and its effects on adolescent development. *Journal of Youth and Adolescence*, **9**, 19–31.

Garbarino J. (1989) Troubled youth, troubled families: the dynamics of adolescent maltreatment. In D. Cicchetti and V. Carlson (eds), *Child Maltreatment. Theory and Research on the Causes and Consequences of Child Abuse and Neglect*. New York: Cambrige University Press, pp. 685–706.

Garbarino, J. and Plantz, M. C (1986) Child abuse and juvenile delinquency: what are the links? In Garbarino, C. J. Schellenbach and J. M. Sebes (eds), *Troubled Youth, Troubled Families*. New York: Aldine de Gruyter, pp. 41–54.

Garnefski, N. and Diekstra, R. F. W. (1997) Child sexual abuse and emotional and behavioural problems in adolescence: Gender differences. *Journal of the American Academy of Child Psychiatry*, **36**, 323–329.

Garnett, L. (1990) *Leaving Care for Independence: A Follow-up Study to the Placement Outcomes Project*. Report to the Department of Health. Quoted in the Department of Health, *1991 Patterns and Outcomes in Child Placement*. London: HMSO.

Garralda, M. E., Jameson, R. A., Reynolds, J. M. and Postlethwaite, R. J. (1988) Psychiatric adjustment in children with chronic renal failure. *Journal of Child Psychology and Psychiatry*, **29**, 79–90.

Garrison, C. Z., Schoenbach, V. J. and Kaplan, B. H. (1985) Depressive symptoms in early adolescence. In A. Dean (ed.), *Depression in a Multidisciplinary Perspective*. New York: Brunner-Mazel.

Ge, X., Best, K. M., Conger, R. D and Simons, R. L. (1996) Parenting behaviours and the occurrence and co-occurrence of adolescent depressive symptoms and conduct problems. *Developmental Psychology*, **32**, 717–731.

Gillberg, C., Persson, M., Grufman, M. and Themner, U. (1986) Psychiatric disorders in mildly and severely mentally retarded urban children and adolescents: epidemiological aspects. *British Journal of Psychiatry*, **149**, 68–74.

Gortmaker, S. L., Walker, D. K., Weitzman, M. and Sobol, A. M. (1990) Chronic conditions, socioeconomic risks, and behavioural problems in children and adolescents. *Pediatrics*, **85**, 267–276.

Graber, J. A., Brooks-Gunn J., Paikoff, R. L. and Warren M. P. (1994) Prediction of eating problems: an eight year study of adolescent girls. *Developmental Psychology*, **30**, 823–834.

Greenberg, J., Pyszczynski, T., Burling, J., Simon, L., Solomon, S., Rosenblatt, A. *et al.*, (1992) Why do people need self-esteem? Converging evidence that self-esteem serves an anxiety buffering function. *Journal of Personality and Social Psychology*, **63**, 913–922.

Hagerman, R. J. and Sobesky, W. E. (1989) Psychopathology in Fragile X syndrome. *American Journal of Orthopsychiatry*, **59**, 142–152.

Hayward, C., Killen, J. D., Wilson, D. M., Hammer, L. D., Litt, I. F., Kraemer, H. C., Haydel, F., Varady, A. and Barr Taylor, C. (1997) Psychiatric risk associated with early puberty in adolescent girls. *Journal of American Academy of Child and Adolescent Psychiatry*, **36**, 255–262.

Hetherington, E. M. (1989) Coping with family transitions: winners, losers, and survivors. Meetings of the Society for Research in Child Development, 1987, Baltimore, Maryland. *Child Development*, **60**, 1–14.

Hetherington, E. M. and Clingempeel, G. W (1986) The adjustment of parents and children to divorce and remarriage. Symposium presented at the *Southeastern Regional Meeting of the Society for Research in Child Development*, Nashville, TN.

Hetherington, E. M., Cox, M. and Cox, R. (1982) Effects of divorce on parents and children. In M. E. Lamb (ed.), *Nontraditional Families: Parenting and Child Development*. Hillsdale, NJ: Erlbaum, pp. 233–288.

Hetherington, E. M., Clingempeel, G. W., Anderson, E. R., Deal, J. E., Hagan, M. S., Hollire, E. A. and Lidner, M. S. (1992) Coping with marital transitions: a family systems perspectives. *Monographs of the Society for Research in Child Development*, **57** (2–3), serial no. 227.

Hill, S. Y. and Muka, D. (1996) Childhood psychopathology in children from families of alcoholic female probands. *Journal of American Academy of Child and Adolescent Psychiatry*, **35**, 725–733.

Hinshaw, S. P. (1992) Externalising behaviour problems and academic under-achievement in childhood and adolescence: causal relationships and under-lying mechanisms. *Psychological Bulletin*, 111, 127–155.

Hjorth, C. W. and Ostrov, E. (1982) The self-image of physically abused adolescents. *Journal of Youth and Adolescence*, 11, 71–76.

Ho, C. S., Lempers, J. D. and Clark-Lempers, S. (1995) Effects of economic hardship on adolescent self-esteem: a family mediation model. *Adolescence*, 30, 118–131.

Hoffman, L. W. (1980) The effects of maternal employment on the academic attitudes and the performance of school-aged children. *School Psychology Review*, 4, 319–336.

Hogan, H. W. and McWilliams, J. M. (1978) Factors related to self-actualization. *Journal of Psychology*, 100, 117–122.

Johnson, P. L. and O'Leasry, D. (1987) Parental behavior patterns and conduct disorders in girls. *Journal of Abnormal Child Psychology*, 15, 573–581.

Kendler, K. S. and Eaves, L. J. (1986) Models for the joint effect of genotype and environment on liability to psychiatric illness. *American Journal of Psychiatry*, 143, 279–289.

Kiser, L. J., Heston, J., Millsap, P. A. and Pruitt, D. B. (1991) Physical and sexual abuse in childhood: relationship with post-traumatic stress disorder. *Journal of the American Academy of Child Psychiatry*, 30, 776–783.

Kurtz, P. D. Gardin, J. M. Wodarski, J. S. and Howing, P. T. (1993) Maltreatment and the school-aged child: school performance consequences. *Journal of Child Abuse and Neglect*, 17, 581–589.

Lamborn, S. D., Mounts, N. S., Steinberg, L. and Dornbusch, S. M. (1991) Patterns of adjustment and competence among adolescents from author-itative, authoritarian, indulgent and neglectful families. *Child Development*, 61, 1049–1065.

Lempers, J. D., Clark-Lempers, D. and Simons, R. L. (1989) Economic hardship, parenting and distress in adolescence. *Child Development*, 60, 25–39.

Lerner, J. V. and Galambos, N. L. (eds) (1991) *Employed Mothers and their Children*. New York: Garland.

Lewinsohn, P. M., Rohde, P., Seeley, J. R. and Fischer, S. A. (1993) Age-cohort changes in the lifetime occurrence of depression and other mental disorders. *Journal of Abnormal Psychology*, 102, 110–120.

Lewinsohn, P. M., Clarke, G. N., Seeley, J. R. and Rohde, P. (1994) Major depression in community adolescents. Age at onset, episode duration, and time to recurrence. *Journal of the American Academy of Child and Adolescent Psychiatry*, 33, 809–818.

Liss, D. S., Waller, D., Kennard, B., McIntire, D., Capra, P. and Stephens, J. (1998) Psychiatric illness and family support in children and adolescents with diabetic ketoacidosis: a controlled study. *Journal of the American Academy of Child and Adolescent Psychiatry*, 37, 536–544.

Loeber, R. and Stouthamer-Loeber, M. (1986) Family factors as correlates and predictors of juvenile conduct problems and delinquency. In M. Toury and M. Morris (eds), *Crime and Justice*. Chicago, IL: University of Chicago Press, vol. 7, pp. 29–149.

Lombroso, P. J., Pauls, D. L. and Leckman, J. F. (1994) Genetic mechanisms in childhood psychiatric disorders. *Journal of American Academy of Child and Adolescent Psychiatry*, 33, 921–938

Magnusson, D., Stattin, H. and Allen, V. (1985) Biological maturation and social development: a longitudinal study of some adjustment processes from mid-adolescence to adulthood. *Journal of Youth and Adolescence*, 14, 267–283.

Marshall, W. A. and Tanner, J. M. (1970) Variations in the pattern of pubertal changes in boys. *Archives of Disease in Childhood*, 45, 13–23.

Martin, G., Rozanes, P., Pearce, C. and Allison, S. (1995) Adolescent suicide, depression and family dysfunction. *Acta Psychiatrica Scandinavia*, 92, 336–344.

Masten, A. S., Best, K. M. and Garmezy, N. (1990) Resilience and development: contributions from the study of children who overcame adversity. *Development and Psychopathology*, 2, 425–444.

Maughan, B. and Pickles, A. (1990) Adopted and illegitimate children growing up. In L. N. Robins and M. Rutter (eds), *Straight and Devious Pathways from Childhood to Adulthood*. Cambridge: Cambridge University Press, pp. 36–61.

McCartney, K., Harris, M. J. and Bernieri, F. (1990) Growing up and growing apart: a meta-analysis of twin studies. *Psychological Bulletin*, 107, 226–237.

McCawley, E., Ross, J. L., Kushner, H. and Cutler, G. (1995) Self esteem and behaviour in girls with Turners syndrome. *Developmental and Behavioral Pediatrics*, 16, 82–88.

McGue, M. (1993) From proteins to cognitions: the behavioural genetics of alcoholism. In R. Plomin and G. E. McClearn (eds), *Nature, Nuture and Psychology*. Washington, DC: American Psychological Association, pp. 245–268.

McKay, J. R., Murphy R. T., Rivinus, T. R. and Maisto, S. A. (1991) Family dysfunction and alcohol and drug use in adolescent psychiatric inpatients. *Journal of the American Academy of Child and Adolescent Psychiatry*, 30, 967–972.

McKenry, P. C., Tishler, C. L. and Kelley, C. (1982) Adolescent suicide: a comparison of attempters and nonattempters in an emergency room population. *Clinical Pediatrics*, 21, 266–270.

McLoyd, V. C., Jayaratne, T. E., Ceballo, R. and Borquez, J. (1994) Unemployment and work interruption among African American single mothers: effects on parenting and adolescent socioemotional functioning. *Child Development*, 65, 562–589.

Montemayor, R. and Clayton, M. D. (1983) Maternal employment and adolescent development. *Theory Practice*, **22**, 112–118.

Mortimer, J. T., Finch, M., Shanahan, M. and Ryu, S. (1992) Work experience, mental health, and behavioral adjustment in adolescence. *Journal of Research on Adolescence*, **2**, 25–57.

Myers B. A. and Pueschel S. M. (1991) Psychiatric disorders in persons with Down syndrome. *Journal of Nervous and Mental Disease*, **179**, 609–613.

Nguyen, N. and Williams, H. (1989) Transition from east to west: Vietnamese adolescents and their parents. *Journal of the American Academy of Child and Adolescent Psychiatry*, **28**, 505–515.

Nielsen, J., Johnsen, G. and Sorensen, K. (1980) Follow-up 10 years later of 34 Klinefelter males with karyotype 47, XXY and 16 hypogonadal males with karyotype 46, XY. *Psychological Medicine*, **10**, 345–352.

Nottelmann, E. D., Susman, E. J., Inoff-Germain, G., Cutler, G. B., Jr, Loriaux, D. L. and Chrousos, G. P. (1987) Developmental processes in early adolescence: relations between adolescent adjustment problems and chronological age, pubertal stage and puberty-related serum hormone levels. *Journal of Pediatrics*, **110**, 473– 480.

Offord, D. R. (1990) Social factors in the aetiology of childhood disorders. In B. Tonge, G. Burrows and J. Werry (eds), *Handbook of Studies on Child Psychiatry*. Amsterdam: Elsevier, pp. 55–68.

Olweus, D. (1986) Aggression and hormones: behavioural relationships with testosterone and adrenaline. In D. Olweus, J. Block, and M. Radke-Yarrow (eds), *Development of Antisocial and Prosocial Behaviour: Research Theories and Issues*. Orlando, FL: Academic Press, pp. 51–72.

Olweus, D., Mattson, A., Schelling, D. and Low, H. (1980) Testerone aggression physical and personality dimensions in normal adolescent males. *Psychosomatic Medicine*, **42**, 253– 269.

Osofsky, J. D. (1990) Risk and protective factors for teenage mothers and their infants. *Society for Research in Child Development Newsletter*, Winter, 1–2.

Parker, R. (1966) *Decision in Child Care: A Study of Prediction in Fostering*. London: Allen & Unwin.

Parker, J. G. and Asher, S. R. (1987) Peer relation and later adjustment: are low-accepted children 'at risk'? *Psychology Bulletin*, **102**, 357–389.

Parkhurst, J. T. (1992) Peer rejection in middle school: subgroup differences in behavior, loneliness, and interpersonal concerns. *Developmental Psychology*, **28**, 231–241.

Petersen, A. C. (1988) Adolescent development. *Annual Review of Psychology*, **39**, 583–608.

Petersen, A. C., Leffert, N., Graham, B., Ding, S. and Overbey, T. (1994) Depression and body image disorders in adolescence. *Women's Health Issues*, **4**, 98–108

Peterson, J. L. and Zill, N. (1986) Marital disruption, parent–child relationships, and behaviour problems in children. *Journal of Marriage and the Family*, **48**, 295–307.

Phares, V. and Compas, B. E. (1992) The role of fathers in child and adolescent psychopathology: make room for daddy. *Psychological Bulletin*, **111**, 387–412.

Pike, A. and Plomin, R. (1996) Importance of nonshared environmental factors for childhood and adolescent psychopathology. *Journal of the American Academy of Child Psychiatry*, **35**, 560–570.

Pless, I. B., Power, C. and Peckham, C. S. (1993) Long-term psychosocial sequelae of chronic physical disorders in childhood. *Pediatrics*, **91**, 1131–1136

Plomin, R. and Daniels, D. (1987) Why are children in the same family so different from one another? *Behavioural and Brain Sciences*, **10**, 1–16.

Pumariega, A. J., Pursell, J., Spock, A. and Jones, J. D. (1986) Eating disorders in adolescents with cystic fibrosis. *Journal of the American Academy of Child and Adolescent Psychiatry*, **25**, 269– 275.

Reardon, B. and Griffing, P. (1983) Factors related to the self-concept of institutionalized, white, male, adolescent drug abusers. *Adolescence*, **18**, 29–41.

Reiss, A. L. and Freund, L. (1990) Review: Fragile X syndrome. *Biological Psychiatry*, **27**, 223–240.

Richards, M. H., Petersen, A. C., Boxer, A. M. and Albrecht, R. (1990) Relation of weight to body image in pubertal girls and boys from two communities. *Developmental Psychology*, **26**, 313–321.

Rogers, E. and Lee, S. H. (1992) A comparison of the perceptions of the mother–daughter relationship of black pregnant and nonpregnant teenagers. *Adolescence*, **27**, 555–564.

Rutter, M. (1981) The city and the child. *American Journal of Orthopsychiatry*, **51**, 610–625

Rutter, M. (1984) Psychopathology and development. I. Childhood antecedents of adult psychiatric disorder. *Australian and New Zealand Journal of Psychiatry*, **18**, 225–234.

Rutter, M. (1986) The developmental psychopathology of depression: issues and perspectives. In M. Rutter, C. Izard and P. Read (eds), *Depression in Young People: Developmental and Clinical Perspectives*. New York: Guilford Press, pp. 3–30.

Rutter, M. (1987) Psychosocial resilience and protective mechanisms. *American Journal of Orthopsychiatry*, **57**, 316–331.

Rutter, M. (1990) Commentary: some focus and process considerations regarding the effect of parental depression on childhood. *Developmental Psychology*, **26**, 60–67.

Rutter, M, and Giller, H. (1983) *Juvenile Delinquency: Trends and Perspectives*. New York: Guilford Press.

Rutter M., Tizard, J. J. and Whitmore, K. (eds) (1970) *Education, Health and Behaviour*. London: Longmans.

Rutter, M., Yule, W., Berger, M., Yule, B., Morton, J. and Bagley, C. (1974) Children of West Indian immigrants. I: Rates of behavioural deviance and psychiatric disorder. *Journal of Child Psychology and Psychiatry*, **15**, 241–262.

Scheinberg, I. H. and Sternlieb, I. (1984) Wilson's Disease. In L. H. Smith (ed.), *Major problems in Internal Medicine*. Philadelphia, PA: W. B. Saunders, vol. 23, pp. 76–89.

Sodowsky, G. R., Lai, E. W. M. and Plake, B. S. (1991) Moderating effects of sociocultural variables on acculturation attitudes of Hispanics and Asian Americans. *Journal of Counselling and Development*, **70**, 194–204.

Sorensen, K. (1992) Physical and mental development of adolescent males with Klinefelter syndrome. *Hormone Research*, **37** (Suppl. 3), 55–61.

Steinberg, L., Elmen, J. D. and Mounts, N. S. (1989) Authoritative parenting, psychosocial maturity, and academic success among adolescents. *Child Development*, **60**, 1424–1436.

Stephenson, A. L., Henry, C. S. and Robinson, L. C. (1996) Family characteristics and adolescent substance use. *Adolescence*, **31**, 59–77.

Susman, E. J., Inoff-Germain, G., Nottlemann, E. D., Loriaux, D. L., Cutler, G. B. and Chrousos, G. P. (1987) Hormones, emotional dispositions and aggressive attributes in young adolescents. *Child Development*, **58**, 1114–1134.

Suris, J.-C., Papera, N. and Puig, C. (1996) Chronic illness and emotional distress in adolescence. *Journal of Adolescent Health*, **19**, 153–156.

Swearingen, E. M. and Cohen, L. H. (1985) Life events and psychological distress: a prospective study of young adolescents. *Developmental Psychology*, **21**, 1045–1054.

Tanner, J. M. (1972) Sequence, tempo and individual variation in growth and development of boys and girls aged twelve to sixteen. In J. Kagan and R. Coles (eds), *Twelve to Sixteen: Early Adolescence*. New York: Norton, pp. 1–24.

Taylor, D. C. (1975) Factors influencing the occurrence of schizophrenia like psychoses in patients with temporal lobe epilepsy. *Psychiatric Medicine*, **5**, 249.

Taylor, R. D. and Roberts, D. (1995) Kinship support and maternal and adolescent well-being in economically disadvantaged African-American families. *Child Development*, **66**, 1585–1597.

Tellegen, A., Lykken, D. T., Bouchard, T. J., Jr, Wilcox, K. J., Segal, N. L. and Rich, S. (1988) Personality similarity in twins reared apart and together. *Journal of Personality and Social Psychology*, **54**, 1031–1039.

Thornton, B. and Ryckman, R. M. (1991) Relationship between physical effectiveness and self-esteem: a cross-sectional analysis among adolescents. *Journal of Adolescence*, **14**, 85–98.

Triseliotis, J. and Hill, M. (1990) Contrasting adoption, fostercare, and residential rearing. In D. M. Brodzinsky and M. D. Schecter (eds), *The Psychology of Adoption*. New York: Oxford University Press, pp. 107–120.,

Triseliotis J. and Russell J. (1984) *Hard to Place: The Outcome of Adoption and Residential Care*. London: Heinemann Educational.

Turner, S. M., Beidel, D. C. and Costello, A. (1987) Psychopathology in the offspring of anxiety disorder patients. *Journal of Consulting and Clinical Psychology*, **55**, 229–235.

Vandell, D. L. and Ramanan, J. (1991) Children of the National Longitudinal Survey of Youth: choices in after-school care and child development. *Developmental Psychology*, **27**, 637–643.

Verhulst, F. C., Althaus, M. and Versluis-Den Bieman, H. J. M. (1992) Damaging backgrounds: later adjustment of international adoptees. *Journal of the American Academy of Child and Adolescent Psychiatry*, **3**, 518–524.

Verhulst, F. C. and Versluis-Den Bieman, H. J. M. (1995) Developmental course of problem behaviours in adolescent adoptees. *Journal of the American Academy of Child and Adolescent Psychiatry*, **34**, 151–159.

Wagner, B. M. (1997) Family risk factors for child and adolescent suicidal behaviour. *Psychological Bulletin*, **121**, 246–298.

Warren, M. P. and Brooks-Gunn, J. (1989) Mood and behaviour at adolescence: evidence for hormonal factors. *Journal of Clinical Endocrinology and Metabolism*, **51**, 1150–1157.

West, D. J. and Farrington, D. (1973) *Who Becomes Delinquent?* London: Heinemann Educational.

Whitman, B. Y. and Accardo, P. (1987) Emotional symptoms in Prader–Willi syndrome adolescents. *American Journal of Medical Genetics*, **28**, 897–905.

Williams, S., McGee, R. O. and Anderson, J. (1989) The structure and correlates of self reported symptoms in 11-year old children. *Journal of Abnormal Child Psychology*, **17**, 55.

Williamson, D. E., Birmaher, B., Anderson, B. P., Al-Shabbout, M. and Ryan N. D. (1995) Stressful life events in depressed adolescents: the role of dependent events during the depressive episode. *Journal of the American Academy of Child and Adolescent Psychiatry*, **34**, 591–598.

Wolkind, S. and Rutter, M. (1973) Children who have been 'in care': an epidemiological study. *Journal of Child Psychology and Psychiatry*, **14**, 97–105.

Wolman, C., Resnick, M. D., Harris, L. J. and Blum, R. W. (1994) Emotional well-being among adolescents with and without chronic conditions. *Journal of Adolescent Health*, **15**, 199–204.

Wright Berton, M. and Stabb, S. D. (1996) Exposure to violence and post-traumatic stress disorder in urban adolescents. *Adolescence*, **31**, 489–498

Youngs, G. A., Jr, Rathge, R., Mullis, R. and Mullis, A. (1990) Adolescent stress and self esteem. *Adolescence*, **25**, 333–341.

Yule, W., Berger, M., Rutter, M. and Yule, B. (1975) Children of West Indian immigrants. II: Intellectual performance and reading attainment. *Journal Child Psychology and Psychiatry*, **16**, 1–17.

Zill, N., Morrison, D. R. and Corio, M. J. (1993) Long-term effects of parental divorce on parent–child relationships, adjustment, and achievement in young adulthood. *Journal of Family Psychology*, **7**, 91–103.

Zimiles, H. and Lee, V. E. (1991) Adolescent family structure and educational progress. *Development Psychology*, **27**, 314–320.

Chapter 3

CLASSIFICATION AND EPIDEMIOLOGY

Robin Glaze

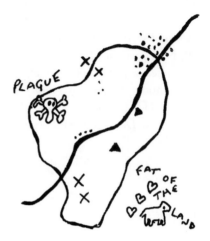

INTRODUCTION

It is possible to work in everyday clinical practice with neither a knowledge of detailed epidemiology nor an internalised framework for childhood psychiatric disorder, but to do so is to deny the richness and complexity of these fascinating disorders, to risk missing the increasingly recognised co-morbid disorders and to condemn your patients and their families to limited and partial interventions. This chapter gives an overview of the main classificatory systems, their history and usage. In the second part, an up-to-date table of the prevalence rates of adolescent disorders is presented. Finally, gender differences, racial issues, urban–rural differences and trends over time are tabled and discussed, alongside the difficulties inherent in this type of research.

DEFINITIONS

This chapter focuses on the naming, categorisation, ordering and incidence of psychiatric diseases within adolescence. *The Shorter Oxford English Dictionary* states that classification is 'The result of classifying; a systematic distribution or arrangement in a class or classes'. Likewise epidemiology is 'The branch of medicine that deals with the incidence and transmission of disease in populations-...with the aim of controlling it; the aspects of disease relating to its incidence and transmission'. Classification and epidemiology are central to the study of adolescent psychiatry because they provide a means of not only grouping and ordering psychological disturbances, personality characteristics and diseases in a way that facilitates communication between professionals, but also because the patterns of occurrence of these findings point the way to further studies into aetiology and course.

Medical classifications were first developed in order to group causes of death (Rutter *et al.*, 1975). Clearly, psychiatric classifications attempt much more than this and are hampered by the fact that there is no underlying, or natural, scheme waiting to be discovered by doing the correct research (Jaspers, 1962). This is why the standard schemes of classification are multi-axial and attempt classification of the patterns of psychological disturbance, e.g. following trauma, psychosocial background, personality characteristics and measures of adaptive functioning in addition to the illnesses themselves.

HISTORY OF ADOLESCENT PSYCHIATRIC CLASSIFICATIONS

Anna Freud's developmental profile (1965) and the categorisation of the Group for the Advancement of Psychiatry (1966) were the first significant attempts at diagnostic schemes for children and adolescents. Both were extensively based on psychoanalytic concepts. Rutter *et al.*'s (1969) proposal for a tri-axial classification, the work of the Washington University group (Feighner *et al.*, 1972) and the findings from the field trials for the International Classification of Mental and Behavioural Disorders (ICD-9) by the World Health Organization (1978) that there was good agreement between psychiatrists on disorders defined phenomenologically, but little agreement on those defined theoretically, pointed the way to classifications based on patterns of symptoms rather than theoretical constructs that lacked empirical validation.

THE ARGUMENT FOR A MULTI-AXIAL CLASSIFICATION

Approaches to modern classificatory systems are either categorical as in ICD-10 and the Diagnostic and Statistical Manual of Mental Disorders (DSM)-IV or dimensional, e.g. as found in Achenbach and Edelbrock (1978). As the names suggest, categorical systems involve making a selection from a list of diagnoses where the symptoms and symptom timings have been specified, whereas dimensional systems look to see if behavioural symptoms cluster together statistically to form groups or characteristic patterns. In the dimensional approach multivariate statistical methods like factor analysis are used to uncover the tendency of specific types of behaviour to cluster in patterns (as the dimensions of illness). Further statistical examination of the dimensions using principal component analysis or cluster analysis can then assign individual symptoms to mutually exclusive diagnostic groups.

Dimensional approaches may give different results according to the precise statistical analysis used and the results are not always clinically meaningful. As yet there is no agreement on the best dimensions to use for classification purposes, and despite the fact that they increase reliability and communicate more clinical information (such as symptoms that would be beneath threshold in a categorical system), they are much less familiar than the regular categorical names for disorders in common usage. Categorical approaches work best when the members of a diagnostic class are homogeneous and where the classes themselves have clear boundaries, whilst also being mutually exclusive.

Being based on diagnosis, neither approach comes close to describing the full complexity of an individual child's difficulties. The most widely used schemes (ICD-10 worldwide, and DSM-IV in the US, Canada and Australia) have thus developed a five-axis categorisation to broaden the descriptive power for any individual child. The usage of these axes is handled very differently between the two manuals.

The broad categories are:

- Clinical disorders and other conditions
- Personality disorders and mental retardation
- General medical conditions
- Psychosocial and environmental problems
- Global assessment of functioning

Routine use of a multi-axial system provides for more comprehensive attention to these areas, in a convenient format for both recording and conveying clinical information. In addition, the complexity and heterogeneity of the individual is more easily described, and a biopsychosocial model is emphasised.

THE DSM-IV AND ICD-10 SYSTEMS

HISTORICAL BACKGROUND

The need to collect census information in the US acted as an initial driver for the development of some form of classificatory system. The frequency of 'idiocy/insanity' was collected for the 1840 census and by 1880 seven categories of mental illness were included (mania, melancholia, monomania, paresis, dementia, dipsomania and epilepsy). In 1917 the Committee on Statistics of the American Medico-Psychological Association, along with the National Commission on

Mental Hygiene, set about helping the Bureau of the Census to gather statistics on disorders across mental hospitals. The American Medico-Psychological Association became the American Psychiatric Association in 1921, and subsequently worked with the New York Academy of Medicine to produce the first national psychiatric nomenclature for diagnosing inpatients with severe psychiatric and neurological disorders. This classification was subsequently incorporated into the first edition of the American Medical Association's *Standard Classified Nomenclature of Disease.*

The need to better understand the outpatient presentations of World War II servicemen and veterans led to a broader system being developed by the US Army, and modified by the Veterans Administration. This included 10 categories for psychoses, nine for neuroses, and a further seven for problems of character, behaviour and intelligence. DSM-I was published in 1952 by the American Psychiatric Association Committee on Nomenclature and Statistics as a variant of the ICD-6. It was the first official manual to focus on clinical utility.

The first edition of the International Classification of Disease to include a section on mental disorders was ICD-6. Neither ICD-6 nor ICD-7 gained widespread acceptance, which led the World Health Organisation to commission a comprehensive review of diagnostic issues by Stengel. In the early 1960s, the World Health Organisation had a series of multinational, multidisciplinary, multischool of thought meetings. This in turn stimulated research on classification and diagnostic reliability, whilst at the same time creating a vast network of individuals and centres prepared to work on issues surrounding psychiatric classification. Extensive consultation led to the production of ICD-8. International collaborative studies, new treatments and close links with the American Psychiatric Association continued. ICD-9 was published in 1975, DSM-III in 1980. DSM-III featured diagnostic criteria and a multi-axial classification for the first time, whereas the ICD-9's purpose of allowing international collection of basic health statistics made this of lesser importance. The ICD-9 was, however, later modified for use in the US (ICD-9-CM) by the addition of clinical diagnostic criteria.

A number of inconsistencies and lack of clarity led to a revision work group and the publication of DSM-III-R in 1987. The vast expansion of research into diagnosis that followed the publication of DSM-III and DSM-III-R greatly facilitated the DSM-IV work groups that conducted comprehensive reviews of this material, re-analysed existing data and conducted extensive field trials. Twelve field trials, involving more than 70 test sites and 6000 subjects, compared DSM-III, DSM-III-R, ICD-10 and the proposed DSM-IV criteria sets.

DSM-IV

DSM-IV is available as a book, as a desk or quick reference to the diagnostic criteria, and as a set of classification sheets containing Axes I and II categories and codes, in a brochure format. DSM-IV is also available in several electronic formats, audio and video formats, and there are even several primary care versions, including a book on the classification of child and adolescent mental illness diagnosis in primary care, published by the American Academy of Pediatrics.

DSM-IV disorders are grouped into 16 major diagnostic classes (e.g. Disorders usually first diagnosed in infancy, childhood or adolescence, Mood disorders, Schizophrenia and other psychotic disorders, etc.). There is one further class, 'Other conditions that may be a focus of clinical attention'. The class of disorders usually first diagnosed in infancy, childhood and adolescence is a useful convenience, but is not intended to imply that young people can have only those disorders. All diagnostic classes may be used in this age group. The 'other conditions' class is divided into six categories with a rich variety of subtypes:

- Psychological factors affecting medical condition
- Medication-induced movement disorder
- Other medication-induced disorder
- Relational problems
- Problems related to abuse or neglect
- Additional conditions that may be a focus of clinical attention

The manual's introduction includes extensive historical information, a definition of mental disorder and a discussion of usage with respect to the limitations of using a categorical approach, usage of clinical judgement, use in forensic settings, ethnic and cultural issues, treatment planning, and the distinction between mental and general medical conditions. It is made clear that diagnostic categories, criteria and textual descriptions should only be used by people with appropriate clinical training and experience in diagnosis. Particularly, the specific diagnostic criteria are intended to represent guidelines to clinical judgement and not as a sort of scientific recipe.

The same definition of mental disorder persists from DSM-III and includes the following features:

- Clinically significant behavioural, or psychological syndrome, or pattern occurring in an individual
- Associated with present distress, or disability, or with a significantly increased risk of death, pain, disability or an important loss of freedom
- The syndrome or pattern must not be merely an expectable and culturally sanctioned response to a particular event, e.g. in the death of a loved one
- Whatever the original cause, the disorder must currently represent a manifestation of behavioural, psychological or biological dysfunction
- Political, religious or sexually deviant behaviour, and conflicts between the individual and society shall not be seen as mental disorders unless they fulfil the above criteria

DSM-IV diagnostic codes are numeric codes of up to five digits (3 + 2) separated by a decimal point. The general disorder type is specified by the first three digits, e.g. developmental disorders of learning, motor skills and communication are 315. The fourth, and sometimes fifth, digits are used to specify subtype, thus reading disorder is 315.00, mathematics disorder is 315.1 and mixed receptive-expressive language disorder is 315.32.

DSM-IV diagnoses are usually used to denote current illness, but facility exists within the severity and course specifiers to record extra detail if necessary or useful. The following specifiers may be used:

- Mild (few if any symptoms extra, minor impairment in social, educational or occupational functioning)
- Moderate (symptoms and functional impairment between mild and severe)
- Severe (many extra symptoms, or several especially severe symptoms, with marked impairment in social, educational or occupational functioning)
- In partial remission (some residual symptoms)
- In full remission (no residual symptoms)
- Prior history (perhaps of the same or related illness)

Some diagnoses have specific criteria for mild, moderate and severe illness, e.g. conduct, manic episode, major depressive episode and mixed episode disorders. Others have specific criteria for partial remission. Finally, the issue of recurrence is considered. In clinical practice it is often the case that individuals re-present with a partial set of symptoms of a previous disorder. In these cases clinicians have the following options:

- To code the disorder as current or provisional
- The 'not otherwise specified' category
- The 'prior history' category

Epidemiological data shows that the co-occurrence of two or more separate child psychiatric conditions (co-morbidity) often occurs (Caron and Rutter, 1991). DSM-IV copes with this by coding a principal diagnosis or reason for visit, along with as many other diagnoses required to account for the full range of presenting symptoms. Multiple diagnoses may be listed in order, both multi-axially or non-axially. Where a multi-axial scheme is used, the principal diagnosis is assumed to be the first diagnosis on axis one. If the principal diagnosis is on Axis II, the qualifying phrase 'principal diagnosis' is used next to it. There is also a 'provisional diagnosis' specifier for those situations where only partial history is present, but there is strong reason to suspect that full criteria will eventually be met.

In recognition of the diversity of clinical presentations, some of which do not meet explicit criteria for disorder, DSM-IV includes the 'not otherwise specified' category. There are four situations in which it may be used:

- Atypical or mixed presentations where criteria for a specific disorder are not met, but the general criteria for the diagnostic class are
- Where clinical distress is being caused by a symptom pattern not included
- Where there is uncertainty about the aetiology
- Where complete data cannot be gathered

Although DSM-IV encourages multiple diagnoses it discourages unnecessary coding of co-morbidity, by setting rules for the formulation of a diagnostic hierarchy, and setting criteria to exclude other diagnoses and suggest a differential diagnosis for some disorders. This assists in the following situations:

- Where mental disorder is induced by a general medical condition, or is substance induced, this diagnosis pre-empts the primary diagnosis for the same symptoms
- When a more pervasive disorder (e.g. schizophrenia) includes the defining symptoms of the identified disorder, the less pervasive disorder includes an exclusion criteria set showing that only the schizophrenia is diagnosed

In situations where the boundaries between conditions are hard to call, the phrase 'not better accounted for by. . .' is used. In some situations both diagnoses would be better coded.

ICD-10

ICD-10 is available in two main forms, the traditional *Clinical Descriptions and Diagnostic Guidelines* and the *Diagnostic Criteria for Research*, although there is also a primary care version (*Diagnostic and Management Guidelines for Mental Disorders in Primary Care*). Mental and behavioural disorders are listed as a shortened glossary in Chapter V(F) of the ICD-10 itself and is not recommended for mental health clinicians to use. The following description refers to the Clinical Descriptions and Diagnostic Guidelines version of ICD-10 only.

ICD-10 has 10 specific categories of mental illness and one residual category for unspecified mental disorder:

- Organic, including symptomatic, mental disorders
- Mental and behavioural disorders due to psychoactive substance use
- Schizophrenia, schizotypal and delusional disorders
- Mood disorders
- Neurotic, stress-related and somatoform disorders
- Behavioural syndromes associated with physiological disturbances and physical factors
- Disorders of adult personality and behaviour
- Mental retardation
- Disorders of psychological development
- Behavioural and emotional disorders occurring in childhood and adolescence
- Unspecified mental disorder

ICD-10 uses an alphanumeric code rather than the simple numeric code of DSM-IV. The initial character is a letter indicating the chapter of ICD-10 in use, the following characters are numeric with a two-digit category code (e.g. F80, Specific Developmental Disorders of Speech and Language), followed by an additional digit after the decimal point to denote a specific disorder and a possible fifth digit to further define the individual disorder. In other words, each category of disorder has up to 10 subcategories (e.g. F10–F19), and within the subcategories up to 10 discrete disorders, and within that up to 10 further specifications for those discrete disorders. In total it is thus technically possible to have up to 100 disorders in each category, though none of them are actually full. The fourth and fifth character codes can be seen in action in F32.1 (Moderate depressive disorder) and F32.11 (Moderate depressive disorder with somatic syndrome).

ICD-10 uses a similar definition of disorder to that found in DSM-IV:

- Implies the existence of a clinically recognisable set of symptoms or behaviour
- Associated with distress and interference in personal functioning
- Social deviance or conflict alone, without personal dysfunction, is not included

Similarly, the ICD-10 encourages the recording of as many diagnoses as are necessary to cover the clinical picture. Again it is suggested that a main diagnosis is coded, where possible, most suited to the task in hand. In the clinical setting this will be the diagnosis causing outpatient consultation, or day or inpatient care. In other settings the lifetime diagnosis (e.g. schizophrenia) may have primary importance. Where there is uncertainty for the diagnostician, it is suggested that the list of disorders is based on the numeric order of the codes as presented in ICD-10.

Again, disorders from any category may present in adolescence, although the final three categories have particular relevance to the child and adolescent psychiatrist:

- Mental retardation (F70–F79)
- Disorders with onset specific to childhood (F80–F89)
- Behavioural and emotional disorders with onset usually occurring in childhood and adolescence (F90–F98)

Examples of disorders occurring in other groups include mood, schizophrenia, gender identity and eating disorders.

COMPARISON OF MULTI-AXIAL ASSESSMENT IN DSM-IV AND ICD-10

There are numerous coarse and fine detail differences between the two classifications (Table 3.1). ICD-10 allows coding of deliberate self-harm and

Table 3.1 Comparison of multi-axial assessment in DSM-IV and ICD-10

Axis no.	ICD-10	DSM-IV
I	Clinical psychiatric syndrome (F codes)	Clinical syndromes and other conditions that may be a focus of clinical attention
II	Developmental disorders (F80–F89)	Developmental disorders, personality disorders and mental retardation
III	Intellectual level (F70)	General medical conditions
IV	Other conditions from ICD-10 often associated with mental and behavioural disorders (A50–S06)	Psychosocial and environmental problems
V	Psychosocial stressors (Z00–Z99)	Global assessment of functioning
Self-harm	External causes of morbidity and mortality (X60–X84)	No equivalent
Assault	External causes of morbidity and mortality (X93–Y07)	No equivalent

physical assault, whereas DSM-IV does not. DSM-IV has several scales for global assessment of functioning, whereas ICD-10 has none.

Clinical psychiatric syndromes

Both systems use a categorical system, based on an atheoretical approach, using specific diagnostic criteria arising from both the phenomenology of the case and the timing of the disorders' development, and its relationship to precipitating trauma. A comparison of the clinical groupings can be found below.

Developmental disorders

Both language and learning disorders are frequently associated with impaired social skills, peer relationships and self-esteem (Cantwell and Baker, 1988). Axis I disorders are also frequently associated with developmental disorders.

Intellectual functioning

Both ICD-10 and DSM-IV divide mental retardation into the four categories of mild, moderate, severe and profound according to IQ derived from standardized tests (Table 3.2). Both ICD-10 and DSM-IV include a 'severity unspecified' category (F79 and 319, respectively) for use where there is a strong presumption of mental retardation, but where the person is untestable by standard tests. ICD-10 also has a category (F78) 'other mental retardation' for use where associated sensory deficits (e.g. blindness or deafness) make them difficult to test.

Table 3.2 Categories of mental retardation

	ICD-10	DSM-IV
Mild	50–69	50–55 to 70
Moderate	35–49	35–40 to 50–55
Severe	20–34	20–25 to 35–40
Profound	<20	<20 or 25

Associated medical conditions

DSM-IV uses the ICD-9-CM codes for selected general medical conditions. These codes are presented in two parts: (1) codes for general medical conditions over 18 separate categories and (2) codes for medication induced disorders (Table 3.3).

ICD-10 has a similar list of conditions frequently associated with mental illness as an annex (the A to S codes), though there is nothing to stop you using any of the physical codes found in the complete ICD-10 listings, indeed this is strongly

Table 3.3 Associated medical conditions

General medical conditions	Medication-induced disorders
Nervous system	Analgesics and antipyretics
Circulatory system	Anticonvulsants
Respiratory system	Antiparkinsonian medications
Neoplasms	Neuroleptic medications
Endocrine diseases	Sedatives, hypnotics and anxiolytics
Nutritional diseases	Other psychotropic medications
Metabolic diseases	Cardiovascular medications
Diseases of the digestive system	Primarily systemic agents
Genitourinary diseases	Medications acting on muscles and the respiratory system
Haematological diseases	Hormones and synthetic substitutes
Diseases of the eye	Diuretics and mineral and uric acid metabolism drugs
Diseases of the ear, nose and throat	
Musculoskeletal diseases	
Diseases of the skin	
Congenital malformations, deformations and chromosome abnormalities	
Diseases of pregnancy, childbirth and the puerperium	
Infectious diseases	
Overdose	

recommended. Sixteen categories are provided with the following differences to DSM-IV:

- No separate categories for nutritional or metabolic diseases
- Symptoms, signs, and abnormal clinical and laboratory findings absent in DSM-IV
- Injury, poisoning and certain other consequences of external causes in addition to the 'overdoses' category in DSM-IV.

Psychosocial stressors

In ICD-10 psychosocial stressors are expressed within factors influencing health status and contact with health services (Z codes). There are 27 categories including 91 subcodes. The ICD-10 field trials showed poor inter-clinician agreement, which is reflected in the minimal instructions for usage. In the author's experience, there are two schools of thought on the usage of Z codes: (1) to take an exhaustive approach in which every code applicable is used, and (2) to take a minimalist approach whereby only a few codes are used, and each code recorded is seen as 'using up' the clinical circumstances and thereby excluding further similar codes.

In DSM-IV a psychosocial problem is defined as a negative life event, or an environmental difficulty or deficiency, a familial or other interpersonal stress, an inadequacy of social support or personal resources, or any other problem defining the context of the development of the persons difficulties. Additionally, positive life experiences may also represent stressors and can therefore be coded in situations where the person is having difficulty coping with the transition. As many codes as necessary may be used though, unless there is clear relevance to the noted psychopathology, only those present in the year previous to the presentation should be used. The DSM-IV categories are shown below:

I.   Problems with primary support group
II.   Problems related to the social environment
III. Educational problems
IV.   Occupational problems
V.   Housing problems
VI.   Economic problems
VII. Problems with access to health care services
VIII. Problems related to interaction with the legal system/crime
IX.   Other psychosocial and environmental problems

Global assessment of functioning

DSM-IV uses the Global Assessment of Functioning (GAF) scale. The GAF is a derivation of the Global Assessment Scale (GAS) (Endicott et al., 1976), itself a derivation of the Health-Sickness Rating Scale (Luborsky, 1962). The observer-rated scale gives a score between 1 and 100, with lower scores equating to more disabled.

ICD-10 does not have a global assessment of functioning, though the Children's Global Assessment Scale (CGAS) has been produced for use with children between the age of 4 and 16, and is now well validated for use within community and clinical populations (Bird et al., 1990; Green et al., 1994; Weissman et al., 1990). It has also been used by the author and others for inpatient adolescent populations.

Deliberate self-harm and assault

The closest that DSM-IV comes to a self-harm scale is in the overdose section of the associated medical conditions section of Axis III, where 24 subcategories of possible drug poisons are listed. ICD-10 has 25 categories of self-harm (X60–X84) including various categories of drug overdosage (though no specific drugs), other poisons (including alcohol, organic solvents, gases and vapours, and pesticides), self-harm including hanging, drowning, shooting (various), explosives, fire, hot objects, sharp or blunt objects, jumping, and self-harm involving vehicles (various) and other specified means.

COMPARISON OF CHILD AND ADOLESCENT DIAGNOSES IN DSM-IV AND ICD-10

ICD-10 differs from DSM-IV in having a conceptual description of each disorder category, as well as specific diagnostic criteria. The diagnostic criteria themselves are perhaps more rigorous in DSM-IV than in ICD-10, although neither specify how the information is to be collected. DSM-IV criteria are also less technical in some instances. For example, ICD-10 refers to the cardinal features of overactivity and impaired attention, briefly describing them in separate paragraphs. DSM-IV identifies inattention (nine criteria, e.g. 'often does not seem to listen when spoken to directly'), hyperactivity (six criteria, e.g. 'Often fidgets with hands of feet or squirms in seat') and impulsivity (three criteria, e.g. 'Often blurts out answers before questions have been completed'), as well as three more general criteria for fulfilment of the diagnosis.

USING A CLASSIFICATION IN CLINICAL PRACTICE

The two main classificatory systems each have strengths and weaknesses as indicated above. DSM-IV gives considerable assistance to the thoughtful user and uses more everyday criteria. ICD-10, however, has the advantage of being more compact, has a more comprehensive self-harm coding and is the system predominant within the UK. Whichever classification you choose, it is probably best to stick to one and become really familiar with it.

GATHERING INFORMATION AND MAKING A DIAGNOSIS

Cantwell (1988) described nine important questions in the diagnostic process and six major types of instruments to answer them:

- Does the child have a psychiatric disorder (a problem in behaviour, emotions, relationships or cognition of sufficient severity and duration to cause distress, disability or disadvantage)?
- Does it meet criteria for a clinical syndrome?
- What are the intra-psychic, family, social–cultural and biological roots of the disorder, and what are their relative strengths?
- What forces maintain the problem?
- What forces facilitate the child's normal development?
- What are the strengths and competencies of the child and the family?
- What is the likely outcome without treatment?
- Is intervention necessary in this case?
- What types of intervention are most likely to be effective?

Information is usually gathered using an interview with the parents about the child, which may include the child or significant others in a position to observe the child on a daily basis, and interviews with the child. These core techniques will often be sufficient but may be supplemented by physical and neurological examinations, and further information gathered using laboratory studies (including psychometric testing for diagnosis of mental retardation and specific developmental disorders, blood tests and X-rays, etc). Finally, behaviour rating scales completed by parents, teachers and significant others may be useful in confirming hyperactivity disorders, and other disorders that are situation specific.

When validated against overall psychiatric judgement, the parental interview is found to be the best if used alone (Rutter *et al.*, 1970), whilst the child interview adds little in terms of detecting disorders missed by the other methods. The child interview is useful in helping to distinguish between types of disorders and in picking up some disorders that the others miss (e.g. minor depressive episodes). Parent and teacher rating scales are both good at detecting children with psychiatric illness, but tend to have little overlap in the disorders detected.

EPIDEMIOLOGY OF ADOLESCENT DISORDERS

Epidemiological studies provide statistics on the extent of morbidity (i.e. specific disorders) within a population, and attempt to relate these statistics both to the environment and the population itself (e.g. age, social class, gender) with a view to detecting associations with possible causal factors (see Table 3.4).

Table 3.4 Epidemiology of adolescent disorders

Disorder		Prevalence	Age	Reference	Notes
Attention deficit hyperactivity disorder		3–6%	school age	Goldman et al. (1998)	Broadening criteria for attention deficit hyperactivity disorder (ADHD) with a growing appreciation of the persistence into adolescence and adulthood. Some children are being diagnosed and treated on insufficient grounds, but there is little evidence of widespread over-prescription of ritalin.
Affective disorders	bipolar	rates likely to be at least those of the adult population 1%	14–18	Geller and Luby (1997) Lewinsohn et al. (1995)	Pre-pubertal onset is a non-episodic, chronic, rapid cycling, mixed manic state that may be co-morbid with, or have features of, ADHD and/or conduct disorder. Significant functional impairment and high rates of co-morbidity, particularly with anxiety and behaviour disorders, suicide attempts, and usage of mental health services. Bipolar disorder in children commonly presents with ADHD which makes diagnosis difficult. Irritability, chronicity and mixed symptoms of mania and depression give an atypical picture when compared to adults (Wozniak and Biederman, 1997).
		0.5% of an established adult sample had onset aged 5–9 years, and 7.5% between 10–14 years	5–9 10–14	Loranger and Levine (1978)	

Table 3.4 Continued

Disorder		Prevalence	Age	Reference	Notes
	depression	0.4–2.5% 0.4–8.3%	children adolescent	Birmaher et al. (1996)	Depression increases in frequency with age in children and adolescents, often coexists with anxiety and behaviour disorders, and is associated with long-term morbidity and risk of suicide (Pataki and Carlson, 1995). Children identify their depression more often than their parents. Early-onset major depressive disorder and dysthymic disorder are frequent, recurrent and familial disorders that tend to continue into adulthood. These disorders have poor psychosocial and academic outcomes. Risk is increased for substance abuse, bipolar disorder, and suicide. Rates of depression are probably increasing, and both major depression and bipolar disorder are occurring at a younger age (Bland, 1997).
	dysthymic disorder	0.6–1.7% 1.6–8.0%	children adolescent	Birmaher et al. (1996)	Seventy percent of early-onset dysthymic disorder patients have a superimposed major depressive disorder, and 50% have other psychiatric disorders, including anxiety disorders (40%), conduct disorder (30%), ADHD (24%) and enuresis or encopresis (15%), with 15% having two or more co-morbid disorders.
Anxiety disorders	general	10–15% 10–20%	children and adolescent	Black (1995) Pine (1997)	Anxiety disorders are more common in girls than boys. Co-morbidity is found in up to 39% of children with an anxiety disorder and 14% of adolescents in the community have two or more anxiety disorders. Additional diagnoses may be depression, attention deficit disorder and conduct disorder (Craske, 1997).

Disorder	Prevalence	Age	Source	Notes
separation anxiety disorder	0.7–12.9% 2.0–3.6% 2.4%	pre-adolescent adolescent 12–16	Craske (1997) Bowen et al. (1990)	Has the highest recovery rate (96%) over 3–4 years.
over-anxious or generalised anxiety disorder	2.7–12.4% 2.4–7% 3.6%	pre-adolescent adolescent 12–16	Craske (1997) Bowen et al. (1990)	Has the highest rate of co-morbidity. High overlap between the presence of OAD and SAD, and externalising disorder and depression. One half with OAD and SAD have pure anxiety disorder. Youngsters with OAD and SAD are just as impaired as youngsters with conduct disorder and depression, except that they admit to less social isolation, and their schoolwork is less affected.
simple phobia	2.4–9.2% 3.6%	pre-adolescent adolescent	Craske (1997)	These tend to be associated with the least additional pathology. Common specific fears include heights, dark, loud noises, injections, insects, dogs and other small animals, and school.
obsessive-compulsive disorder (OCD)	0.3% 1.9–4.0% 1.9%	pre-adolescent adolescent adolescent	Craske (1997) Wallace et al. (1995)	Juvenile OCD has a bimodal incidence, male preponderance, and may occur with ADHD and other developmental disorders (Geller et al., 1998). Co-morbidity may also occur with tic, anxiety and affective disorders (March and Leonard, 1996).
social phobia	0.9–1.1% 1.1%	pre-adolescent adolescent	Craske (1997)	When socially phobic and specifically phobic children are compared, socially phobic children report more fears and more commonly display multiple phobias. They also experience more loneliness and depression.

Table 3.4 Continued

Disorder		Prevalence	Age	Reference	Notes
	panic disorder	0–1.1%		Pine (1997)	Atypical presentations include fainting, shortness of breath, palpitations, seizures, or other psychological or behavioural complaints, including fear of vomiting, or choking (sometimes with weight loss), separation anxiety, school avoidance, tempers or disturbed sleep (Black, 1995).
Asperger syndrome		20 per 10 000	2–15	Wing and Gould (1979)	Male to female ratio 3:1.
		10–26 per 10 000		Gillberg and Gillberg (1989)	Minimum figures for children with normal intelligence.
		36 per 10 000	7–16	Ehlers and Gillberg (1993)	Minimum figures. Male to female ratio 4:1.
Child sexual abuse		10% abused by age 16. Thus 4.5 million adults were abused as children	15+	Baker and Duncan (1985)	A total of 2019 men and women aged 15 years and over interviewed as part of a MORI survey of a nationally representative sample of Great Britain. 8% of males, 12% of females. No increased risk by social class or residence area.
		7–36% women 3–29% men 10–12% girls	<14	Finkelhor (1994) Feldman et al. (1991)	Review of studies from 19 countries. Male to female ratio 1.5–3:1. Data from the 1940s (Kinsey) compared to 1970s and 1980s. Prevalence has not changed, but increased reporting due to changes in legislation and social climate.
Chronic fatigue		rare	child and adolescent	Khawaja and Van Boxel (1998)	There are no community surveys in this age group. Overall prevalence in primary care estimated to be 0.5–1.5%.

Disorder	Subtype	Prevalence	Age	Reference	Notes
Conduct disorder		8.3% 14%	4–11 12–16	Offord et al. (1987)	Male to female ratio 3.5:1. Male to female ratio 2.5:1.
Creutzfeldt–Jacob disease (CJD)		Unknown	<17	Nigro and Nigro (1997)	The name paediatric CJD is proposed for those cases appearing in childhood and adolescence. Twenty European cases feature a mean course of 14–35 months and early onset psychiatric symptoms.
Drug, alcohol and addictive disorders	alcohol in previous week	29.0%	13	Kurtz (1996)	The majority of adolescents that use drugs do not progress to abuse, or dependence. Adolescent substance abuse clusters with delinquency, early sexual behaviour, and pregnancy. It may also be linked to accidents, violence and school dropout, as well as engagement in risky sexual behaviour and risk of contracting human immunodeficiency virus (Weinberg et al., 1998).
	solvents and illegal drugs	2.0%	11	Pearce and Holmes (1995)	
	regular drug use	8.0%	16	Light and Bailey (1992)	
	heroin and cocaine	0.9%	15–16	Wallace et al. (1995)	
Eating disorders	anorexia nervosa	0.36–0.83% 0.04–0.17%	12–19 girls 12–19 boys	Wallace et al. (1995)	Prevalence of substance abuse or depression amongst family members is higher in bulimic anorectics than restricting ones. Substance abuse occurs more frequently in bulimic anorectics, and is associated with stealing, self-mutilation, suicidality, laxative abuse, diuretic abuse and impaired social relationships (Bailly, 1993).

Table 3.4 Continued

Disorder		Prevalence	Age	Reference	Notes
	bulimia nervosa	2.5%	12–19 girls	Wallace et al. (1995)	
	binge eating disorder	1.7% (normal weight) 14.3% (obese)	16–35 girls	Fairburn and Cooper (1993)	
Epilepsy		4%	all children	Hauser (1995)	The most frequently occurring disorder is febrile convulsion, which shows a wide geographic variation and is usually benign. Epilepsy affects 1% of the population by age 20. Rates rise to 30% in patients with mental retardation and 50% of those with multiple handicaps in institutional settings (Sunder, 1997).
Gender identity disorder		(1.3%) (5.0%)	4–5 boys 4–5 girls	Achenbach and Edelbrock (1983)	There are no formal epidemiological studies of prevalence or incidence of this disorder in children. The original child behaviour checklist standardisation sample gave mothers report rates for sometimes wanting, or frequently wanting, to be the opposite sex. These figures may represent the upper limit of prevalence and are hence in brackets. Clinic samples consistently have referral rates of boys to girls of around 7:1 (Zucker et al., 1997).
Mental retardation		1% 5%	children school age children	Gillberg (1997) Lyon (1996)	Rates depend on the inclusiveness of the criteria used.

Condition			Reference	Notes
Schizophrenia	very very rare (1%)	before 6 general population	Werry (1996) Loranger (1984)	At least two clinical phenotypes, one with longstanding neuro-behavioural difficulties of early onset, the other developing in a normal personality. Around 39% males and 23% females had their first symptoms before 19 years of age.
Sleep disorders			Anders and Eiben (1997)	Sleep problems are more common in children of Indian subcontinent descent than in white children and in children whose mothers did not reach secondary education. Behavioural and supportive measures remain the best methods of treatment (Anders and Eiben, 1997).
general	4%	at 5		
	1%	at 9		
	<2%	childhood		
nightmares	20%	childhood		
sleepwalking	15%	4–12		
night terrors	3%	18/12–6		
narcolepsy	0.4–0.7%	early adolescent		
Smoking	28%	12th grade girls	French and Perry (1996) Perez-Stable and Fuentes-Afflick (1998)	Highest rates amongst whites, lowest in African-Americans and Asians. Adolescent girls that do not go to college are more likely to smoke than those that do. Effective school-based interventions have been developed but are usually not appropriately implemented.
	19.9% white 10.9% Latino 7.2% African-American	high school students		
Specific maths difficulty (SMD)			Lewis et al. (1994)	There are equal numbers of males and females in the two groups with arithmetic difficulties.
Pure SMD	1.3%	9–10		
SMD + SRD	2.3%			
pure SRD	3.9%			

Table 3.4 Continued

Disorder	Prevalence	Age	Reference	Notes
Specific reading difficulty (SRD)	9.3%	8–18	Esser and Schmidt (1994)	No correlation with pre or perinatal complications. Mothers have lower educational level. Note frequent co-morbidity with SMD (Lewis et al., 1994). School-identified samples are subject to referral bias in favour of boys, whereas research identified cases show an equal sex distribution (Shaywitz et al., 1990).
Specific spelling difficulty	6–9%	adolescent and young adult	Haffner et al. (1998)	Academic achievement is considerably affected despite sufficient non-verbal intelligence.
Speech articulation disorder	32.5% 18.4% 7.4%	at age 5 at age 7 at age 9	Luotonen (1995)	90% of all errors are in sounds /r/ and /s/. Errors in two or more sounds is rare. Early speech development is slower in boys than girls. Boys have more articulation problems.
Stuttering	2%	1st to 8th grade	Ardila et al. (1994)	The prevalence of minor brain injury, developmental dyslexia history, word-finding difficulties and depressive symptoms is higher amongst self-reported stutterers than non-stutterers.
Suicide attempted	2.0–4.0%	adolescent	Wallace et al. (1995)	The suicide rate in England and Wales in 15–24 year old males rose by 80% between 1980 and 1992, though New Zealand presently has the highest rate in the world (Hawton, 1998). Similarly rates of deliberate self-harm rose by 194% in the same age group in an Oxford sample between 1985 and 1995, although females changed very little.

	completed	0.0075%	15–19 boys	Pearce and Holmes (1995)	
	completed	0.0025%	15–19 girls	Pearce and Holmes (1995)	
Teenage pregnancy and sexual health	live births	1.1–9.9/1000	<16 girls	Nicoll et al. (1999)	Rates by health district for girls under 16. Highest rates in urban districts. Teenage birth rates in England and Wales are the highest in Western Europe.
	terminations	2.2–10.5/1000	16–19 girls		
	gonorrhoea	1.07/1000	girls		
	chlamydia	4.45/1000	girls		
	genital herpes	1.39/1000	girls		
	genital warts	5.84/1000	girls		
	gonorrhoea	0.71/1000	boys		
	chlamydia	1.15/1000	boys		
	genital herpes	0.22/1000	boys		
	genital warts	1.68/1000	boys		
Tourette's disorder		2.99%	13–14	Mason et al. (1998)	Tourette's disorder is more common, and milder, in secondary school than in secondary or tertiary health care service settings (Mason et al., 1998). Male to female risk varies from 1.6:1 to 10:1 (Tanner and Goldman, 1997).
		0.043%	16–17	Apter et al. (1993)	

Epidemiological statistics are usually expressed as incidence and prevalence rates. The term incidence relates to the number of new cases appearing in the defined population within a specified time period (usually a year) and is usually written as the rate per 100 000 population. Prevalence refers to the actual number of cases in a community at the time of measurement. Rates may be adjusted for age or sex, or are expressed in 'crude' form. Some adolescent disorders, particularly eating disorders, pose special challenges by virtue of the tendency of subjects to conceal their illness and avoid professional help.

PREVALENCE OF PSYCHOPATHOLOGY

Over 50 studies in the past 40 years have attempted to estimate overall prevalences of childhood and adolescent psychiatric disorders (Roberts *et al.*, 1998). Over 20 countries have been involved, although most frequently the US and the UK. Subjects' ages ranged from 1 to 18 years and the most frequently used criteria for case definition were those of Rutter or, more recently, the DSM criteria. The range of prevalence rates found by Roberts extended from 1 to 51% with a mean of 15.8%. Median rates across age the age range were:

- Pre-school = 8%
- Pre-adolescent = 12%
- Adolescent = 15%

Studies taking a wider age range had a median rate of 18%. The evidence is less informative than expected because of the familiar issues of sampling differences, the definition of caseness, the data analyses and presentation. Epidemiological research has a long history. The earliest school-based survey of child maladjustment was published in 1928, the first survey of child mental health took place in 1941 and the first large-scale epidemiological study in child psychiatry was performed in the early 1950s (Roberts *et al.*, 1998). The previous lack of standardized definitions of mental illness, procedures to collect standardized information about the most severe conditions and a widespread reluctance to label adolescents as suffering from chronic mental illness has also impeded research (Florenzano, 1991). Since the early 1980s, however, a new generation of studies has emerged using more systematic strategies aimed at minimising the effects of sampling and non-sampling errors. Hence, more use has been made of standardized diagnostic criteria like DSM-III to reduce criterion variance and structured diagnostic interviews like the Diagnostic Interview Schedule for Children to reduce information variance. As expected, these studies have produced more homogeneous results than earlier surveys, and have confirmed childhood and adolescent disorders as being relatively common.

Roberts' excellent survey of 52 epidemiological studies published between 1963 and 1996 highlighted the following challenges for future research.

SAMPLING

Representativeness and sample size both have difficulties. Only a few of the studies to date have actually used probability sampling designs, and the samples studied do not cover the diversity of the child and adolescent population generally. Most studies focus on narrow (e.g. middle school or high school) or specific age ranges so that we cannot tell how prevalence changes over the lifespan of childhood.

CASE ASCERTAINMENT

There are essentially two types of standardised interviews, structured (e.g. the Diagnostic Interview Schedule for Children) and semi-structured (e.g. K-SADS). It can be argued that structured interviews require less judgement or expertise to use and may produce more cases. Similarly semi-structured interviews may produce fewer cases. This appears to be borne out by those studies using the different methodologies finding prevalence rates of 21–25% and around 14%, respectively. A further issue is that there is no agreement on how best to use information from multiple informants to make diagnoses.

CASE DEFINITION

There is little consensus on the inclusion of a severity rating to further define caseness. The majority of studies use DSM criteria which, in the absence of a severity criteria, produces prevalence rates in the range of a quarter to a third (or more) children. Yet a substantial number of the individuals meeting these criteria for disorder are functioning adequately in their lives. There is understandable concern that the DSM criteria alone produce such high illness rates.

DATA ANALYSES

Prevalence rates are reported as either point or period prevalences. Where period prevalences are used, the time period may vary, though would typically be either 1 month, 6 months, 1 year or lifetime. The precision of the result also needs to be explicitly stated. Increased comparability across studies would be facilitated by greater use of more general epidemiological techniques, such as the presentation of prevalence rates for groups based on age, gender and socioeconomic status, and the indication of relative risk in different subgroups such as middle adolescents, males, or lower socioeconomic youngsters.

Strategies for future research should include:

- Extended prevalence data on ethnic minorities, different socioeconomic strata and urban versus rural rates

- Incidence, duration and recurrence data (i.e. natural history of disorder)
- Epidemiological data on co-morbid disorders
- Epidemiological data relating developmental stage to psychiatric disorders
- Prospective longitudinal studies to illuminate aetiology by looking at multiple psychosocial and biological risk factors
- Community studies looking at factors influencing duration, recurrence and help seeking
- Further work on biological factors including genetic variables
- Research on the links between having a disorder, and using mental health and other services; the relationship between diagnosis plus impairment in the need for services

GENDER DIFFERENCES

See Table 3.5.

Table 3.5 Gender differences

Disorder	Gender differences
Anxiety disorders	Females are more at risk of fears than males (Craske, 1997). The gender bias is noticeable even as early as age 9–12 years. Other studies show that girls report more distress after natural disasters than boys. Girls also meet criteria for specific phobias and separation anxiety in community samples more often than boys. The ratio of females to males for generalised anxiety disorder among adolescents is estimated at 6:1. There seems little gender difference in OCD and the results for social phobia are mixed. These gender differences may be less apparent in clinic samples, either because shyness and social withdrawal are seen as more normative for girls or because males and females diverge with increasing age (adult clinic sex differences mimic community samples).
Bipolar disorder	In adults the risk ratio of female to male cases is close to 1. In paediatric-onset cases using pooled data from 34 studies (2168 patients), the risk ratio was 1134:1033 in favour of females. In pre-pubertal cases, however, the ratio was 3.85:1 in favour of males (50 male, 13 female in 63 cases). It is uncertain whether this represents a true gender difference in age of onset, or to differences in presenting symptoms. Disruptive and aggressive behaviour in boys may lead to earlier intervention. Alternatively co-morbid ADHD may call attention to the boys (Faedda *et al.* 1995).
Depression	In several studies of depression in children the rates were either equal in boys and girls or more common in boys. In adolescents the results for depression are much more variable (Pataki and Carlson, 1995). The rates for major depressive disorder in adolescents seem to have a sex ratio of 2:1, female to male which parallels the ratio in adults (Birmaher *et al.*, 1996).

Table 3.5 Gender differences – continued

Disorder	Gender differences
Drug and alcohol	In cross-European surveys, 15-year-old boys living in Wales and Northern Ireland are most likely to drink alcohol at least weekly, though it is the girls in Wales and Scotland who have the highest positions for females (McKee, 1999). Studies in California have also shown gender differences. Amongst Californian teens, boys reported significantly higher rates of alcohol, tobacco and marijuana in seventh grade, though these gender differences disappear, except for alcohol use, by the 11th grade. Rates rise generally through the 7th to 11th grades. There are no significant differences between boys and girls use of methamphetamines (Young, 1997).
Eating disorders	An American nutrition study of 40 000 subjects found that amongst blacks and whites, females tend to be fatter than males (as measured by triceps fat fold) at all ages (Garn and Clark, 1975). They also found that females tend to gain, and males tend to lose, fat during adolescence. Amongst white females there is an income-related reversal of fatness during adolescence, with adolescent females in high-income families starting out fatter, but ending up leaner than those of lower income families. Finally, there is also a reversal of fatness during adolescence of white and black females. White females start out being fatter, but end up being leaner, than black females during adolescence. Studies of anorexia nervosa that examine both males and females have consistently found a ratio of about 1:10. In children the figure appears to be much greater, with figures of between 19 and 30% of boys being representative of a number of smaller studies of younger (pre-pubertal) adolescents. This finding merits further investigation.
Obsessive-compulsive disorder	The Geller et al. 1998 review of extant literature showed a male to female predominance of 3:2. The mean age of onset ranged from 7.5 to 12.5 years, though boys may be more likely to have a pre-pubertal onset. Neither gender nor age at onset predict the type, severity or number of obsessive compulsive symptoms.
Schizophrenia	A sex difference in early onset schizophrenia of 1.3:1 in favour of males, has been found in under 21s by the recent ABC study (Häfner et al., 1998), though it has long been recognised that, on average, women fall ill 3–4 years later than men (Häfner and Heiden, 1997). This finding was reported by Emil Kraepelin as early as 1909, and has been replicated since in a majority of more than 50 studies. These gender differences disappear in familial cases of schizophrenia.

RACIAL DIFFERENCES

See Table 3.6.

Table 3.6 Racial differences

Disorder	Racial differences
Anxiety disorders	Very little is known.
Depression	Race is not a risk factor for depression in adolescence (Kandel and Davies, 1982).
Drug and alcohol	In 1998 the European Drugs Monitoring Centre reported that British teenagers were more likely to have used all categories of illicit drugs than those in any other European Union country; 15-year-old boys living in Wales and Northern Ireland are most likely to drink alcohol at least weekly, with highest rates amongst girls going to Wales and Scotland (McKee, 1999). The situation is slightly better with smoking, although Welsh girls still come close to the top, with over a quarter smoking at least once a week. The reasons for these differences remain to be clarified, although there may well be links with poverty, education and home life. Extended education is a major factor in delaying pregnancy and education level is an important factor in smoking rates. Pre-school education may also reduce harmful behaviour in adolescence and early adulthood. Britain lags behind the rest of Europe at the lower end of the educational spectrum in terms of literacy, numeracy and basic skills, though compares well at the top. Poverty rates have increased markedly over the last 20 years, with many more families living in poverty in the UK than in the rest of the EU. British parents also work the longest hours in Europe, alongside a trend towards more shift working with the growth in 24 h service industries. The highest rates of alcohol use in the US are generally found in American Indians, followed in decreasing order by whites, Hispanics, African-Americans and Asian-Americans (Edwards et al., 1995).
Eating disorders	Increasingly reports of anorexia nervosa in people of African and Asian racial backgrounds, both in their countries of origin and elsewhere, are helping to dispel the notion that anorexia is a disease of people of white ethnic origin. In non-Western cultures, the prevalence of eating disorders has increased where dieting behaviours have become more common. Within Western cultures it may be that the children from different ethnic backgrounds that do develop eating disorders, come from those families that maintain their own beliefs and practices and socialise primarily with others of the same racial origins. In other words, it is the children where there is a struggle to accommodate their experience at school and elsewhere with their home life that are at greater risk, rather than those from more Westernised families (Bryant-Waugh, 1993).
Obsessive-compulsive disorder	International studies report prevalence rates of juveniles of 2.3% in Israel, 3.9% in New Zealand and 4.1% in Denmark. Lifetime co-morbidity rates for other psychiatric disorders were high at 75–84%. Obsessive compulsive disorder is more common in Caucasian than African-American children in clinical samples, though epidemiological data suggests no differences in prevalence as a function of ethnicity or geographic region (March and Leonard, 1996)

Table 3.6 Racial differences – continued

Disorder	Racial differences
Schizophrenia	When restrictive and precise definitions of schizophrenia and standardised assessment methods are used on large, representative populations, the incidence rates for schizophrenia appear stable across countries and cultures over time, at least for the last 50 years (Häfner and Heiden, 1997).
Teenage pregnancy	Throughout the 1990s the UK has had the highest teenage pregnancy rate in Western Europe, with birth rates seven times those in the Netherlands amongst 15–19 year olds (McKee, 1999). Rates of sexual activity are comparable in the Netherlands, but adolescents use more contraception. In ranked order the live birth rates per 1000 women amongst 15–19 year olds in Western European countries is England and Wales (29.8), Portugal (20.9), Ireland (16.1), Austria (15.6), Norway (13.5), Greece (13.1), Finland (9.8), Germany (9.4), Belgium (9.1) Denmark (8.3), Spain (8.2), Sweden (7.7), Italy (7.3), France (7), Netherlands (4.1), and Switzerland (4) (Nicoll et al., 1999).

URBAN VERSUS RURAL

Very few studies have investigated the impact of urban living, compared to that of rural life, on the prevalence of psychiatric disorder in adolescence. It is known that child psychiatric referral rates tend to be higher in areas of low social status, although not whether these differences arise from prevalence differences, detection or referral differences (Gath et al., 1972). Reading backwardness has also been associated with low social class areas. Work on delinquency in the field of criminology has repeatedly shown higher rates in urban environments, with the highest rates in industrial cities, followed by non-industrial towns. Suicide tends to be more frequent in socially disorganised and isolated areas, but not in overcrowded areas or ones with high unemployment. Studies with young schizophrenic adults have typically shown higher admission rates in poor working class areas adjacent to business districts and lower rates in middle class suburbs. It is now apparent that these findings are largely due to selective migration and downward drift, as their fathers' social class does not differ from that in the general population. It is also currently thought premature to state that there is a social class bias in early onset anorexia nervosa, though there are a number of small scale studies showing an over-representation of social classes I and II (e.g. Gowers et al., 1991).

Rutter's important Isle of Wight study (Rutter et al., 1975a) showed rates of psychiatric disorder in non-immigrant 10 year olds to be twice as high in London as on the Isle of Wight itself, with similar results for both specific reading retardation and behavioural problems. Lavik's 1977 comparison of 15 year olds living in a suburb of Oslo and a rural Norwegian valley found rates of 20 and 8%, respectively, for psychiatric disorder. Most of this difference was due to cases of conduct disorder, and Oslo had a much higher rate of family breakdown. In the Isle of Wight study the higher urban rates were largely accounted for by the much higher levels of family and school disadvantage. Family disadvantage was reflected in lack of home ownership, overcrowding, family size, discord and breakdown, parental mental illness, criminal activity, and a care history. Educational disadvantage was indicated by high teacher and pupil turnover, pupil absenteeism, and a high proportion of children receiving free school meals.

SPECIAL GROUPS

Externalising disorders such as disruptive behaviour are more prevalent among children in foster family care, even compared to children with backgrounds of similar deprivation (Pilowsky, 1995).

Table 3.7 Trends over time

Disorder	Trend
Delinquency and crime	With the exception of Japan, it is generally accepted that crime statistics have risen in most countries by a factor of 5 since the World War II. There has also been a steeper rise amongst females committing crimes than in males. Most crimes are committed by teenagers and young adults who tend to stop criminal activities in their mid-20s. Rates of conduct disorder and antisocial personality seem to be rising over time, which may well relate causally to the increasing crime rates.
Depression	Findings from large family genetic studies and community surveys in different countries suggest increasing rates with an earlier age of onset across the century. Repeat surveys of 7- to 16-year-old American children over a period of 13 years indicated increased parent and teacher reports of depressed mood, and scores of depressive syndromes. Other cross-sectional surveys of mental health on representative samples of American adults in 1957 and 1976 showed that young adult respondents reported fewer feelings of happiness in the more recent survey. In addition, levels of reported happiness in 15 surveys of US nationally representative samples, reduced between the late 1950s and early 1970s, particularly so in young respondents. The trend appears to apply to mild and moderate depressions but not for more severe depressions, and has not been found in dysthymic disorder (Birmaher et al., 1996).
Drug and alcohol	Alcohol consumption has risen in most countries between 1950 and 1980. Rates of alcohol consumption rise steadily throughout the adolescent years and tend to decline in early adulthood. 90% of teenagers have experienced alcohol by the age of 16. Even though the rates of under age drinking have not increased in the UK, they are associated with larger quantities of alcohol consumption in recent years (Newcombe et al., 1994) and a rise in official NHS statistics for hospital discharges of 11–17 year olds with a diagnosis of non-dependent abuse of alcohol over the same time period. The increasing popularity of designer drinks,

Table 3.7 Trends over time – continued

Disorder	Trend
Drug and alcohol continued	particularly amongst 14–16 year olds, has led to a pattern of drinking in less secure environments, greater drunkenness and heavier consumption (Hughes *et al.*, 1997). Similar rises in illicit drug use from the 1950s have been shown, with epidemiological data tending to show increasing rates of substance misuse, and abuse among young people, together with a trend towards a younger age of onset of addictive behaviours in most countries. The flattening of rates seen in the 1980s has been replaced by a further upward trend over the last 5 years.
Eating disorders	Studies using a rigorous methodology have consistently reported a recent increase in the incidence of anorexia nervosa (Hsu, 1996). Other studies also support an increasing rate, but have been criticised for having problems with diagnosis, improved availability of service, poor data reporting, demographic changes in the population and erroneous inclusion of re-admissions (Fombonne, 1995). Earlier reports that eating disorders may have reached epidemic proportions were based on questionnaire studies using over inclusive diagnostic criteria, however. There is no current evidence for a rising rate of bulimia nervosa, although this conclusion is based on a limited number of studies (Fombonne, 1998).
Schizophrenia	Given the even distribution of morbidity across countries and cultures, it seems unlikely that there will be a great variation over historical time, though this is a difficult assumption to verify. Such studies that have been performed on case register data in Norway, Iceland and Victoria (Australia) have found fairly stable rates (Häfner and Heiden, 1997).
Suicide and para-suicide	Almost all European countries have seen increased rates of suicide over the last century, with most of the increase due to more young men committing suicide, since rates in older men have fallen. Indeed suicide is the leading cause of death amongst 15–24 year olds in the UK, France and North America. There is also evidence of increasing rates in 10–14 year olds in the US, where there has been 120% increase between 1980 and 1992. Black adolescents are catching up with whites and rates are also increasing in minority youth in the US. Rates for girls vary much more by country. Para-suicide is also increasing. Fombonne's survey of 1300 male adolescents referred to psychiatric services for suicidal behaviours in a London hospital found an increase from 6.5% in 1970–1972 to 16% in 1988–1990, with most of the increase accounted for by greater abuse of substances, particularly alcohol. The girls rates of suicidal behaviour were higher than for the boys, but did not show an upward trend (Fombonne, 1998).
Teenage pregnancy and sexual health	In the early 1990s both pregnancy rates and termination rates were falling, but the most recent data for 1995–1996 shows a rise of 14.5% for terminations amongst the under 16s and 12.5% for 16–19 year olds. Similarly maternity rates rose by 6.7 and 4.6% in the two groups, respectively. In 1996, teenage girls accounted for 20% of all terminations, though only 9% of the births and had the second highest termination rates behind 20–24 year olds (Nicoll *et al.*, 1999). Older 16–19 year old girls had the highest rates of gonorrhoea, genital chlamydial infection and warts, and the second highest rate for genital herpes simplex behind 20- to 24-year-old women (Nicoll *et al.*, 1999).

TRENDS OVER TIME

Findings from prospective studies, family genetic studies, community surveys, repeated cross-sectional surveys, and data from mortality and police statistics suggest that suicide, delinquency, addictive behaviours and depression are all increasing (Fombonne, 1998). Similarly incidence rates for anorexia nervosa and bulimia nervosa have also probably increased in recent years (Hsu, 1996; Pyle, 1983/85). See preceding Table 3.7.

REFERENCES

Achenbach, T. M. and Edelbrock, R. C. (1978) The classification of child psychopathology: a review and analysis of empirical efforts. *Psychological Bulletin*, **85**, 1275–1301.

Achenbach, T. M. and Edelbrock, R. C. (1983) *Manual for the Child Behaviour Checklist and Revised Child Behaviour Profile*. Burlington, VT: University of Vermont.

Anders, T. F. and Eiben, L. A. (1997) Pediatric sleep disorders: a review of the past 10 years. *Journal of the American Academy of Child and Adolescent Psychiatry*, **36**, 9–20.

Apter, A., Pauls, D. L., Bleich, A., Zohar, A. H., Kron, S., Ratzoni, G., *et al.* (1993) An epidemiologic study of Gilles de la Tourette's syndrome in Israel. *Archives of General Psychiatry*, **50**, 734–738.

Ardila, A., Bateman, J. R., Nino, C. R., Pulido, E., Rivera, D. B. and Vanegas C. J. (1994) An epidemiologic study of stuttering. *Journal of Communication Disorders*, **27**, 37–48.

Bailly, D. (1993) Epidemiological research, disorders of eating behaviour and addictive behaviour. *Encephale*, **19**, 285–292.

Baker, A. W. and Duncan, S. P. (1985) Child sexual abuse: a study of prevalence in Great Britain. *Child Abuse and Neglect*, **9**, 457–467.

Bird, H. R., Yager, T. J., Staghezza, B., Gould, M. S., Canino, G. and Rubio-Stipec, M. (1990) Impairment in the epidemiological measurement of childhood psychopathology in the community. *Journal of the American Academy of Child and Adolescent Psychiatry*, **29**, 796–803.

Birmaher, B., Ryan, N. D., Williamson, D. E., Brent, D. A., Kaufman, J., Dahl, R. E., Perel, J. and Nelson, B. N. (1996) Childhood and adolescent depression: a review of the past 10 Years. Part I. *Journal of the American Academy of Child and Adolescent Psychiatry*, **35**, 1427–1439.

Black, B. (1995) Anxiety disorders in children and adolescents. *Current Opinion in Paediatrics*, **7**, 387–391.

Bland, R. C. (1997) Epidemiology of affective disorders: a review. *Canadian Journal of Psychiatry/Revue Canadienne de Psychiatrie*, **42**, 367–377.

Bowen, R. C., Offord, D. R. and Boyle, M. H. (1990) The prevalence of overanxious disorder and separation anxiety disorder: results from the Ontario Child Health Study. *Journal of the American Academy of Child and Adolescent Psychiatry*, **29**, 753–758.

Bryant-Waugh, R. (1993) Epidemiology. In B. Lask and R. Bryant-Waugh (eds), *Childhood Onset Anorexia Nervosa and Related Eating Disorders*. London: Erlbaum, pp. 55–68.

Cantwell, D. P. (1988) DSM-III studies. In M. Rutter, A. H. Tuma and I. S. Lann (eds), *Assessment and Diagnosis in Child Psychopathology*. New York: Guilford Press, pp. 3–36.

Cantwell, D. P. and Baker L. (1988) Issues in the Classification of Child and Adolescent Psychopathology. *Journal of the American Academy of Child and Adolescent Psychiatry*, **27**, 521–533.

Caron, C. and Rutter, M. (1991) Comorbidity in child psychopathology: concepts, issues and research strategies. *Journal of Child Psychology and Psychiatry*, **32**, 1063–1080.

Craske, M. G. (1997) Fear and anxiety in children and adolescents. *Bulletin of the Menninger Clinic*, **61** (2 Suppl. A), A4–A36.

Edwards, R. W., Thurman, P. J. and Beauvais, F. (1995) Patterns of alcohol use among ethnic minority adolescent women. *Recent Developments in Alcoholism*, **12**, 369–386.

Ehlers, S. and Gillberg, C. (1993) The epidemiology of Asperger syndrome. A total population study. *Journal of Child Psychology and Psychiatry and Allied Disciplines*, **34**, 1327–1350.

Endicott, J., Spitzer, R. L., Fleiss, J. L. and Cohen, J. (1976) The Global Assessment Scale: a procedure for measuring overall severity of psychiatric disturbance. *Archives of General Psychiatry*, **33**, 766–771.

Esser, G. and Schmidt, M. H. (1994) Children with specific reading retardation – early determinants and long-term outcome. *Acta Paedopsychiatrica*, **56**, 229–37.

Faedda, G. L., Baldessarini, R. J., Suppes, T., Tondo, L., Becker, I. and Lipschitz, D. S. (1995) Paediatric-onset bipolar disorder: a neglected clinical and public health problem. *Harvard Review of Psychiatry*, **3**, 171–195.

Fairburn, C. G. and Cooper, Z. (1993) The eating disorder examination, ED 12. In C. G. Fairburn and G. T. Wilson (eds), *Binge Eating*. New York: Guilford Press, pp. 317–360.

Feighner, J., Robins, E., Guze, S. B., Woodruff, R. A., Winokur, G. and Munoz, R. (1972) Diagnostic criteria for use in psychiatric research. *Archives of General Psychiatry*, **26**, 57–63.

Feldman, W., Feldman, E., Goodman, J. T., McGrath, P. J., Pless, R. P., Corsini,

L. and Bennett S. (1991) Is childhood sexual abuse really increasing in prevalence? An analysis of the evidence. *Paediatrics*, **88**, 29–33.

Finkelhor, D. (1994) The international epidemiology of child sexual abuse. *Child Abuse and Neglect*, **18**, 409–417.

Florenzano, R. U. (1991) Chronic mental illness in adolescence: a global overview. *Paediatrician*, **18**, 142–149.

Fombonne, E. (1995) Anorexia nervosa. No evidence of an increase. *British Journal of Psychiatry*, **166**, 462–471.

Fombonne, E. (1998) Increased rates of psychosocial disorders in youth. *European Archives of Psychiatry and Clinical Neuroscience*, **248**, 14–21.

French S. A. and Perry C. L. (1996) Smoking among adolescent girls: prevalence and etiology. *Journal of the American Medical Womens Association*, **51**, 25–8.

Freud, A. (1965) *Normality and Pathology in Childhood*. New York: International Universities Press.

Garn, S. M. and Clark, D. C. (1975) Nutrition, growth, development, and maturation: Findings from the ten-state nutrition survey of 1968–1970. *American Academy of Paediatrics*, **56**, 306–319.

Gath, D., Cooper, B. and Gattoni, F. E. G. (1972) Preliminary communication: child guidance and delinquency in a London borough. *Psychological Medicine*, **2**, 185–191.∫

Geller, B. and Luby, J. (1997) Child and adolescent bipolar disorder: a review of the past 10 years. *Journal of the American Academy of Child and Adolescent Psychiatry*, **36**, 1168–1176.

Geller, D., Biederman, J., Jones, J., Park, K., Schwartz, S., Shapiro, S. and Coffey, B. (1998) Is juvenile obsessive-compulsive disorder a developmental subtype of the disorder? A review of the pediatric literature. *Journal of the American Academy of Child and Adolescent Psychiatry*, **37**, 420–427.

Gillberg, C. (1997) Practitioner review: physical investigations in mental retardation. *Journal of Child Psychology and Psychiatry and Allied Disciplines*, **38**, 889–897.

Gillberg, I. C. and Gillberg, C. (1989) Asperger syndrome – some epidemiological considerations: a research note. *Journal of Child Psychology and Psychiatry and Allied Disciplines*, **30**, 631–638.

Goldman, L. S., Genel, M., Bezman, R. J. and Slanetz, P. J. (1998) Diagnosis and treatment of attention-deficit/hyperactivity disorder in children and adolescents. *Journal of the American Medical Association*, **279**, 1100–1107.

Gowers, S. G., Crisp, A. H., Joughin, N. and Bhat, A. (1991) Pre-menarcheal anorexia nervosa. *Journal of Child Psychology and Psychiatry*, **32**, 515–524.

Green, B., Shirk, S., Hanze, D. and Wanstrath, J. (1994) The Children's Global Assessment Scale in clinical practice: an empiracle evaluation. *Journal of the American Academy of Child and Adolescent Psychiatry*, **33**, 1158–1164.

Group for the Advancement of Psychiatry (1966) *Psychopathological Disorders in Childhood: Theoretical Considerations and a Proposed Classification (Research Report 62)*. New York: Group for the Advancement of Psychiatry, pp. 229–230,.

Haffner, J., Zerahn-Hartung, C., Pfuller, U., Parzer, P., Strehlow, U. and Resch, F. (1998) Impact and consequences of specific spelling problems of young adults – results of an epidemiological sample. *Zeitschrift fur Kinder- und Jugendpsychiatrie und Psychotherapie*, **26**, 124–135.

Häfner, H. and Heiden, W. (1997) Epidemiology of schizophrenia. *Canadian Journal of Psychiatry*, **42**, 139–151.

Häfner, H., Heiden, W., Behrens, S., Gattaz, W. F., Hambrecht, M., Löffler, W. *et al.*, (1998) Causes and consequences of the gender difference in age at onset of schizophrenia. *Schizophrenia Bulletin*, **24**, 99–113.

Hauser, W. A. (1995) Epidemiology of epilepsy in children. *Neurosurgery Clinics of North America*, **6**, 419–429.

Hawton, K. (1998) Why has suicide increased in young males? *Crisis*, **19**, 119–124.

Hsu, L. K. (1996) Epidemiology of the eating disorders. *Psychiatric Clinics of North America*, **19**, 681–700.

Hughes, K., MacKintosh, A. M., Hastings, G., Wheeler, C., Watson, J. and Inglis, J. (1997) Young people, alcohol, and designer drinks: quantitative and qualitative analysis. *British Medical Journal*, **314**, 414–418.

Jaspers, K. (1962) *General Psychopathology*. Translated by J. Hoening and M. W. Hamilton. Manchester: Manchester University Press.

Kandel, D. B. and Davies, M. (1982) Epidemiology of depressive mood in adolescents: an empirical study. *Archives of General Psychiatry*, **39**, 1205–1212.

Khawaja, S. S and Van Boxel, P. (1998) Chronic fatigue syndrome in childhood: seven-year follow-up study. *Psychiatric Bulletin*, **22**, 198–202.

Kramer, T. and Garralda, M. E. (1998) Psychiatric disorders in adolescents in primary care. *British Journal of Psychiatry*, **173**, 508–513.

Kurtz, Z. (1996) *Treating Children Well: A Guide to using the Evidence Base in Commissioning and Managing Services for the Mental Health of Children and Young People*. London: The Mental Health Foundation.

Lavik, N. (1977) Urban–rural differences in rates of disorder. A comparative psychiatric population study of Norwegian adolescents. In P. Graham (ed.), *Epidemiological Approaches in Child Psychiatry*. London: Academic Press.

Lewinsohn, P. M., Klein, D. N. and Seeley, J. R. (1995) Bipolar disorders in a community sample of older adolescents: prevalence, phenomenology, comorbidity, and course. *Journal of the American Academy of Child and Adolescent Psychiatry*, **34**, 454–463.

Lewis, C., Hitch, G. J. and Walker, P. (1994) The prevalence of specific arithmetic difficulties and specific reading difficulties in 9- to 10-year-old boys and girls.

Journal of Child Psychology and Psychiatry and Allied Disciplines, **35**, 283–292.

Light, D. W. and Bailey, V. (1992) A needs based purchasing plan for Child Based Mental Health Services. London: NW Thames RHA.

Loranger, A. and Levine, P. (1978) Age at onset of bipolar affective illness. *Archives of General Psychiatry*, **35**, 1345–1348.

Loranger, A. W. (1984) Sex difference in age of onset of schizophrenia. *Archives of General Psychiatry*, **41**, 157–161.

Luborsky, L. (1962) Clinicians' judgements of mental health. *Archives of General Psychiatry*, **7**, 407–417.

Luotonen, M. (1995) Early speech development, articulation and reading ability up to the age of 9. *Folia Phoniatrica et Logopedica*, **47**, 310–317.

Lyon, G. R. (1996) Learning disabilities. *Future of Children*, **6**, 54–76.

March, J. S. and Leonard, H. L. (1996) Obsessive-compulsive disorder in children and adolescents: a review of the past 10 years. *Journal of the American Academy of Child and Adolescent Psychiatry*, **35**, 1265–1273.

Mason, A., Banerjee, S., Eapen, V., Zeitlin, H. and Robertson, M. M. (1998). The prevalence of Tourette syndrome in a mainstream school population. *Developmental Medicine and Child Neurology*, **40**, 292–296.

McKee, M. (1999) Sex and drugs and rock and roll: Britain can learn lessons from Europe on the health of adolescents. *British Medical Journal*, **318**, 1300–1301.

Newcombe, R., Measham, F. and Parker, H. (1994) A survey of drinking and deviant behaviour among 14/15 year olds in North West England. *Addiction Research*, **2**, 319–341.

Nicoll, A., Catchpole, M., Cliffe, S., Hughes, G., Simms, I. and Thomas, D. (1999) Sexual health of teenagers in England and Wales: analysis of national data. *British Medical Journal*, **318**, 1321–1322.

Nigro, N. and Nigro, G. (1997) Pediatric forms of Creutzfeldt–Jacob disease (nvCJD). *Minerva Pediatrica*, **49**, 529–531.

Offord, D. R., Boyle, M. H., Szatmari, P., Rae-Grant, N. I., Links, P. S., Cadman, D. T. *et al.* (1987) Ontario Child Health Study II: Six-month prevalence of disorder and rates of service utilization. *Archives of General Psychiatry*, **44**, 832–836.

Pataki, C. S. and Carlson, G. A. (1995) Childhood and adolescent depression: a review. *Harvard Review of Psychiatry*, **3**, 140–151.

Pearce, J. and Holmes, S. P. (1995). Health Gain Investment Programme, Lead Document for People with Mental Health Problems (Part 4). Nottingham: NHS Executive (Trent).

Perez-Stable, E. J. and Fuentes-Afflick, E. (1998) Role of clinicians in cigarette smoking prevention. *Western Journal of Medicine*, **169**, 23–29.

Pilowsky D. (1995) Psychopathology among children placed in family foster care. *Psychiatric Services*, **46**, 906–910.

Pine, D. S. (1997) Childhood anxiety disorders. *Current Opinion in Paediatrics*, 9, 329–338.

Pyle, R. L. (1983/5) The epidemiology of eating disorders. *Paediatrician*, 12, 102–109.

Roberts, R. E., Attkisson, C. C. and Rosenblatt, A. (1998) Prevalence of psychopathology among children and adolescents. *American Journal of Psychiatry*, 155, 715–725.

Rutter, M., Lebovici, S., Eisenberg, L., Sneznevskij, A. V., Sadoun, R., Brooke, E. and Lin, T.-Y. (1969) A triaxial classification of mental disorders in childhood. *Journal of Child Psychology and Psychiatry and Allied Disciplines*, 10, 41–61.

Rutter, M., Tizard, J. and Whitmore, K. (eds) (1970) *Education, Health, and Behaviour*. London: Longmans. (Reprinted 1981. New York: Krieger).

Rutter, M., Cox A., Tupling, C., Berger, M. and Yule, W. (1975a) Attainment and adjustment in two geographical areas. I: The prevalence of psychiatric disorder. *British Journal of Psychiatry*, 126, 493–509.

Rutter, M., Shaffer, D. and Shepherd, M. (1975b) *A Multiaxial Classification of Child Psychiatric Disorders*. Geneva: World Health Organisation.

Shaywitz, S. E., Shaywitz, B. A., Fletcher, J. M. and Escobar M. D. (1990) Prevalence of reading disability in boys and girls. Results of the Connecticut Longitudinal Study. *Jouranl of the American Medical Association*, 264, 998–1002.

Sunder, T. R. (1997) Meeting the challenge of epilepsy in persons with multiple handicaps. *Journal of Child Neurology*, 12 (Suppl. 1), S38–43.

Tanner, C. M. and Goldman, S. M. (1997) Epidemiology of Tourette syndrome. *Neurologic Clinics of North America*, 15, 395–402.

Wallace, S. A., Crown, S., Cox, A. and Berger, M. (1997) *Health Care Needs Assessment: Child and Adolescent Mental Health*. Oxford: Radcliffe Medical Press.

Weinberg, N. Z., Rahdert, E., Colliver, J. D. and Glantz, M. D. (1998) Adolescent substance abuse: a review of the past 10 years. *Journal of the American Academy of Child and Adolescent Psychiatry*, 37, 252–261.

Weissman, M. M., Warner, V. and Fendrich, M. (1990) Applying impairment criteria to children's psychiatric diagnosis. *Journal of the American Academy of Child and Adolescent Psychiatry*, 29, 789–795.

Werry, J. (1996) Childhood schizophrenia. In F. Volkmar (ed.), *Psychoses and Pervasive Developmental Disorders in Childhood and Adolescence*. Washington, DC: American Psychiatric Press, pp. 1–56.

Wing, L. and Gould, J. (1979) Severe impairments of social interaction and associated abnormalities in children. *Journal of Autism and Developmental Disorders*, 9, 11–30.

World Health Organization (1978) *Mental Disorders: Glossary and Guide to their Classification in Accordance with the Ninth Revision of the International Classification of Diseases*. Geneva: World Health Organization.

World Health Organization (1992) *The ICD-10 Classification of Mental and Behavioural Disorders. Clinical Descriptions and Diagnostic Guidelines.* Geneva: World Health Organization.

Wozniak, J. and Biederman, J. (1997) Childhood mania: insights into diagnostic and treatment issues. *Journal of the Association for Academic Minority Physicians*, **8**, 78–84.

Young, N. K. (1997) Effects of alcohol and other drugs on children. *Journal of Psychoactive Drugs*, **29**, 23–42.

Zucker, K. J., Bradley, S. J. and Sanikhani, M. (1997) Sex differences in referral rates of children with gender identity disorder: some hypotheses. *Journal of Abnormal Child Psychology*, **25**, 217–227.

Chapter 4

AFFECTIVE AND EMOTIONAL DISORDERS

Tania Stanway
and Andrew J. Cotgrove

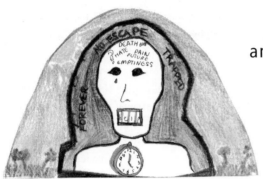

INTRODUCTION

Affective and emotional disorders are a wide ranging group of conditions, including depression, anxiety disorders, adjustment and post-traumatic disorders, and obsessive-compulsive disorder. We have also included deliberate self-harm, whether or not it is associated with depression, as it is not covered elsewhere in the book. These disorders, along with conduct disorder, make up by far the largest group of disorders diagnosed in adolescence, and when 'partial disorders' and other emotional symptoms are included, can affect the majority of adolescents at some time during this stage of their lives.

In this chapter we systematically review each of the main affective and emotional disorders, where possible looking at their epidemiology, evidence of aetiology, classification, clinical features, management and prognosis. Affective disorders with psychotic features, including bipolar affective disorder and mania, are dealt with separately in Chapter 8.

DEPRESSION

Although there are significant differences, it is now widely believed that depressive disorders akin to those seen in adults occur in both children and adolescents (Harrington and Wood, 1995).

They are an important group of disorders often being recurrent (Harrington, 1992), and causing significant levels of psychosocial impairment (Puig-Antich *et al.*, 1985) and scholastic failure (Forness, 1988). They are difficult to treat and have links with suicidal behaviour (Brent *et al.*, 1988; Kovacs *et al.*, 1993; Myers *et al.*, 1991).

EPIDEMIOLOGY

There is a suggestion that rates of depression have increased over the last generation (Fombonne, 1995; Klerman, 1988); however, it is as yet unclear whether this is a true increase or merely a reflection of increased diagnosis. Prevalence rates rise through adolescence, with estimates in pre-adolescents of the order of 0.5–2.5% increasing up to 8% in adolescence (Harrington, 1994). At the age of 11 there is no difference between the rates of depression for boys and girls, but although prevalence rates for both sexes increase steadily through adolescence, these increases are most marked in girls. By the end of adolescence the rates resemble those of the adult disorder, with it being twice as likely for females to have significant depressive symptomatology as males (Angold and Rutter, 1992).

It is important to view symptoms in a developmental context, and depression in adolescence differs from that in adulthood in that there is a greater blurring of the boundary between a disorder and subclinical symptomatology. Adolescence is often seen as a time of 'emotional turmoil' and most adolescents feel sad, frustrated and despondent at times. One community survey of 11- to 16-year-old girls showed the prevalence rate for a major depressive disorder in the past year was 6%, but the equivalent rate for depressive symptoms was 20.7% (Cooper and Goodyer, 1993). These 'partial depressive disorders' may be less severe in terms of the symptomatology, more short-lived and often reactive to external events; however, they undoubtedly cause much subjective distress and present to services on a regular basis.

AETIOLOGY

There are clear familial links in adolescent depression. Children of depressed parents have greater than expected rates of depression (Radke-Yarrow *et al.*, 1992). Harrington *et al.* (1993) demonstrated that lifetime prevalence rates of depression in the relatives of depressed children were twice that of relatives of non-depressed controls. Sadowski *et al.* (1999) have shown that multiple family disadvantages in childhood such as family or marital instability, a combination of poor mothering and poor physical care, and a combination of dependence on social welfare and overcrowding all predispose for depression later in life. For females in particular, major depression was linked to the quality of parenting in early life.

Whilst there is a wealth of evidence to suggest environmental influences on and within the family predispose to depression, there have not been any definitive twin or molecular genetic studies to demonstrate a genetic component. Many, however, believe that the inheritance of depression is likely to come from a combination of genetic and environmental predispositions (Rutter *et al.*, 1999).

A link between adverse events and depressive symptoms has been demonstrated. Specific events, including loss, divorce and exposure to suicide, have been associated with the onset of depression (Brent *et al.*, 1993; Reinherz *et al.*, 1993). Friendship difficulties may also be relevant (Goodyer *et al.*, 1989), as well as schooling difficulties and bullying. These links are non-specific with those experiencing an event being as likely to develop anxiety as depression.

Despite clear environmental influences, the majority of those experiencing an adverse event do not become depressed or develop other psychiatric disorders, and the concepts of resilience and vulnerability are important. Vulnerability to developing a depressive disorder is likely to be multi-faceted. Sufferers often come from families where there is a high rate of dysfunction and psychopathology (Harrington, 1992). Some vulnerability will be a consequence of chronic adversity whilst some may be mediated by biological mechanisms.

Despite the relative ineffectiveness of antidepressant therapy in adolescents, the monoamine hypothesis is still influential. This theory proposes that depression results from hypoactivity of monoamine reward systems (Deakin and Crow, 1986) and arose from observations that drugs which deplete monoamines can cause depression, whilst those that inhibit monoamine re-uptake can have an antidepressant effect. Studies investigating biological mechanisms in young people with depression are equivocal and it is likely that sufferers are a biologically heterogeneous group. For example, some young people with depression show abnormalities in basal cortisol levels whilst others do not (Goodyer *et al.*, 1991), and some have abnormal sleep EEGs, usually relating to abnormal REM sleep (Kutcher *et al.*, 1992), whilst in others these are normal (Giles *et al.*, 1992).

CLASSIFICATION

Various approaches can be applied to the classification of depressive disorders in adolescents and, as yet, there is little empirical evidence to suggest which have the most validity (Harrington and Wood, 1995).

The subdivision of depression into bipolar (episodes of depression and mania) and unipolar (depression only) is well accepted in adults, and there is increasing evidence of its validity in younger people. Juvenile probands with bipolar disorder are more likely to have relatives with bipolar disorder than probands with unipolar depression (Kutcher and Marton, 1991). The diagnosis of bipolar disorder has prognostic implications in that there is an increased risk of a subsequent psychotic episode, most often mania (Werry and McClellan,

1992). The distinction also has therapeutic implications in that naturalistic studies suggest that lithium prophylaxis reduces the risk of further episodes of illness in adolescents with bipolar disorder (Strober *et al.*, 1990) and there is some evidence that tricyclic antidepressants may induce an episode of mania in adolescents with bipolar disorder or a family history of this disorder (Geller *et al.*, 1993).

An alternative system of subclassification distinguishes between those depressive disorders with somatic symptoms (e.g. appetite disturbance, early morning wakening and psychomotor retardation) and those without. In adults this distinction has some validity with those suffering severe somatic symptoms having a worse prognosis (Lee and Murray, 1988) and a different response to physical treatments (Paykel, 1989). However, in younger people studies have been less conclusive (Berney *et al.*, 1991; Puig-Antich *et al.*, 1989), and the distinction between somatic and non-somatic depression appears to be one of severity rather than representing qualitatively different disorders.

DSM-IV (American Psychiatric Association, 1994) makes a distinction between acute depression (major depressive disorder) and chronic depression (dysthymia) which lasts for more than 1 year but has fewer symptoms. This has resulted in some confusion in that some investigators have included both dysthymia and chronic major depressive disorder in the same group. It is also possible for a single case to have both dysthymia and a more acute major depressive disorder. Young people with dysthymia tend to have an earlier age of onset (Kovacs *et al.*, 1994), a slower rate of improvement (Shain *et al.*, 1991), and higher rates of social impairment and co-morbidity with behavioural disorders. However, on long-term follow-up the two disorders have similar outcomes (Kovacs *et al.*, 1994), and the distinction may just be one of severity and duration.

Many researchers have classified depression as to whether it had its onset before or after puberty. However, there are difficulties in accurately dating the onset of disorders and the onset of puberty, and studies have failed to link changes in hormonal levels in adolescence to changes in mood (Buchanan *et al.*, 1992). Social or cognitive changes might be just as significant as biological change at this time. Despite this there is evidence to support the validity of a distinction between pre-adolescent and adolescent onset depression. The most obvious of these is the shift to a female preponderance of the disorder as adolescence progresses. Studies have also shown that pre-adolescent cases have a lower risk of recurrence in adulthood (Harrington *et al.*, 1992) and go into new episodes more quickly than adolescents (Kovacs *et al.*, 1989). Differences have been shown in family studies in that individuals with pre-adolescent-onset depressive disorder have a non-specific familial loading for depression, criminality and alcoholism (Harrington and Wood, 1995; Puig-Antich *et al.*, 1989), whilst those with adolescent-onset disorders show a specific familial loading for depression.

Finally, it is also possible to subclassify depressive disorders according to co-morbidity. In particular, children with co-morbid depression and conduct disorder have been found to have lower rates of depression in adulthood (Harrington *et al.*, 1994), lower rates of depression amongst relatives (Puig-Antich *et al.*, 1989) and a greater variability of mood (Costello *et al.*, 1991) when compared to depressed children with no conduct problems. In contrast, those with both anxiety disorder and depressive disorder tend to have increased severity and duration of depressive symptoms, increased suicidality, increased risk for substance abuse, poor response to psychotherapy, and increased psychosocial problems (Brent *et al.*, 1988; Clarke *et al.*, 1992; Kendall *et al.*, 1992).

DIAGNOSIS AND CLINICAL FEATURES

The presentation of a depressive disorder varies according to the developmental stage of the adolescent. However, diagnosis is made using the same criteria as in adults (see Table 4.1)

Lowered mood may vary little from day to day and is often unresponsive to circumstances. Sleep problems are common and there may be diurnal variation of mood. Irritability, anxiety or motor agitation and social withdrawal may be more prominent in depressed adolescents when compared with their adult counter-parts. In younger adolescents separation anxiety or school refusal may occur, and in later years there may be loss of libido.

ICD-10 (World Health Organisation, 1992) requires symptoms to be present for at least 2 weeks in order to make a diagnosis and describes mild (F32.0), moderate (F32.1) and severe (F32.2) forms of the disorder. ICD-10 also makes the distinction between unipolar and bipolar disorders, a distinction supported by family and genetic studies (Rutter *et al.*, 1990). In severe cases there may be psychotic symptoms (F32.3) such as delusions and hallucinations, the content of which typically reflect the depressive symptomatology.

Adolescent depression differs from the disorder in adulthood in the higher rates of co-morbid disorders that occur (Rohde *et al.*, 1991). The most common of these are anxiety disorders (38%), conduct disorders (15–30%) and substance abuse (20–50%). Adolescents with a depressive disorder are, therefore, likely to

Table 4.1 Typical symptoms of a depressive episode (ICD-10 F32)

Depressed mood
Loss of interest and enjoyment
Reduced energy leading to increased tiredness and diminished activity
Reduced concentration and attention
Reduced self-esteem and self-confidence
Ideas of guilt and unworthiness
Bleak and pessimistic views of the future
Ideas or acts of self-harm or suicide
Disturbed sleep
Diminished appetite and weight loss

have multiple problems. They are usually experiencing difficulties with school-work, social withdrawal is common and they are likely to have significant problems relating to peers.

MANAGEMENT

In view of the serious consequences of adolescent depression it is important that assessment and treatment can be delivered quickly and efficiently. As always, management should start with a full assessment. Multiple sources of information should be sought, including information from the school and family. An attempt should be made to assess psychopathology in family members and any associated problems that may be maintaining the disorder. It is vital that the young person is seen individually to assess their mental state. Studies consistently show that family members underestimate the presence of depressive symptoms, many of which are purely subjective (Barrett et al., 1991). Sufferers are often reticent to discuss how they are feeling with parents for fear of upsetting them, and this may be exacerbated by their feelings of guilt and low self-worth. It is important to ask about ideas of self-harm as these may not be readily forthcoming and are particularly common. Clinical interview may be supplemented by the use of questionnaire measures of mood-related symptoms. These can help provide a relatively objective measure of response to treatment.

Treatment depends on the nature of the problems identified at assessment. If the disorder is mild it may respond to supportive therapy and an amelioration of any maintaining factors. More severe disorder will need a more focused approach and therapy needs to be individually tailored to the needs of the patient. Specific and realistic treatment goals should be agreed with the patient and their family. An aim of reducing depression should go hand in hand with strategies designed to address related problems such as academic difficulties or peer relationship difficulties that may be serving to maintain the disorder.

Many different psychosocial interventions have been used to treat young people with depression. These include cognitive-behavioural therapy (CBT), interpersonal therapy, psychodynamic psychotherapy, family therapy, psycho-drama and art therapy, and social skills training programmes. Most evidence exists to support the efficacy of CBT, although large-scale trials are still needed to confirm this. CBT treatment programmes aim to treat the cognitive distortions identified in depressed adolescents. There are usually 8–12 weekly sessions and the therapist and sufferer work together to solve problems. The young person is encouraged to monitor their feelings and thoughts by means of a diary and cognitive distortions can then be challenged (Harrington et al., 1998a). Behavioural components of the programme include such things as offering strategies to improve sleep problems. See Chapter 19 for more details.

In cases where family pathology seems to be contributing to the disorder it is sensible to offer family therapy, though studies have yet to demonstrate its effectiveness. Most families will benefit from sessions intended to educate them about the disorder and provide general support.

In view of the well-demonstrated psychosocial problems related to depressive disorders strategies aimed at improving social skills may be helpful. These may be targeted specifically or offered as a component of CBT or supportive therapy.

In some cases, unresponsive to psychotherapeutic strategies it may be worth considering the use of antidepressant medication. Numerous studies have failed to demonstrate the effectiveness of tricyclic antidepressants (Hazell *et al.*, 1995). These drugs have a problematic side effect profile and are cardiotoxic in overdose. In view of this it is wise to use one of the newer selective serotonin reuptake inhibitors (SSRIs) as a first-line treatment. Whilst large-scale trials demonstrating the effectiveness of these drugs are as yet unavailable, there are some preliminary findings which suggest that fluoxetine may be more effective than placebo (Emslie *et al.*, 1997) and SSRIs are generally better tolerated and are safer in overdose than tricyclics (Kutcher, 1997). Newer still are the noradrenergic and specific serotonergic antidepressants such as mirtazapine which work by blocking central α_2-adrenoreceptors leading to enhanced secretion of noradrenaline and serotonin. In addition, mirtazapine blocks post-synaptic 5-HT_2 and 5-HT_3 receptors. Data on the efficacy of such drugs is as yet limited and there are no reported trials in adolescents; however, such drugs may prove to be useful in the future.

If there is a good response to medication it is wise to continue it for 6 months after the resolution of symptoms before a gradual withdrawal is considered. During the stage of withdrawal the patient will need to be seen regularly to monitor for a recurrence of symptoms as well as to continue with any psychotherapeutic strategies that have been used. If there is a failure to respond to medication a review of diagnosis may be necessary as well as a check for compliance. Medication should not be discounted until it has been tried at the maximum dose possible without undue side effects (Kutcher, 1997).

In severe cases lithium augmentation may be useful and studies suggest that lithium reduces the risk of further episodes of illness in adolescents with bipolar disorder (Strober *et al.*, 1990). If there are psychotic symptoms, in addition to an antidepressant, the use of an antipsychotic should be considered. If medication fails and severe symptoms persist, electroconvulsive therapy (ECT) can be considered (Walter *et al.*, 1999).

In some cases resistant to outpatient treatment, particularly where environmental factors appear to be perpetuating the disorder, then admission to an adolescent unit can be useful, both diagnostically and therapeutically. If a dramatic improvement follows this intervention then further consideration needs to be given as to how to bring about change in aspects of the adolescents environment, such as their home or school situation (see Chapter 14).

PROGNOSIS

The vast majority of adolescents with a depressive disorder will recover from the index episode. For example, in one study of adolescents with severe depression requiring inpatient treatment, 90% had recovered in 2 years (Strober *et al.*, 1993). However, there is a high rate of recurrence and continuity of depressive symptoms into adulthood (Garber *et al.*, 1988). The best predictor of recurrence into adult life is a severe adult-like presentation and the absence of co-morbid conduct disorder (Harrington, 1992). A small but significant number of cases will go on to develop a bipolar affective disorder. Follow-up studies indicate that a small number of cases will also go on to kill themselves.

DELIBERATE SELF-HARM AND SUICIDE

EPIDEMIOLOGY

The incidence of deliberate self-harm shows it to be extremely common place, with approximately 19 000 young people in England and Wales aged 10–19 years referred to hospital each year (Hawton and Fagg, 1992). The number of recorded deaths from suicide are much smaller, 73 male and 19 female aged 15–19 years in England and Wales in 1997 (Office of Population Census and Surveys, 1998), although this figure is probably an underestimate because coroners are reluctant to burden bereaved parents with a stigmatising label. Despite this, suicide still represents the fourth most common cause of death in this age group in the UK and the suicide rate for young males continues to increase (Fombonne, 1998; Hawton, 1992).

Although the gender ratio of deaths from suicide in the 15–19 year age group is approximately 4:1 male:female (Office of Population Census and Surveys, 1998), the sex ratio for deliberate self-harm is reversed at approximately 1:6 male:female (Cotgrove *et al.*, 1995).

METHODS OF DELIBERATE SELF-HARM

Probably the commonest form of deliberate self-harm is cutting or scratching. This is characteristically seen in young females and is not usually associated with suicidal ideation. Cutting behaviour rarely presents to hospital for treatment and so does not feature in medical statistics of deliberate self-harm such as those quoted above. The most frequently recorded form of deliberate self-harm in the UK is from self-poisoning (Hawton *et al.*, 1996) and the majority of this in the adolescent age group is from paracetamol overdose.

In the UK self-poisoning also represents the commonest means of completed suicide amongst young females, whilst for males it is hanging. In the US guns are used in over 50% of adolescent suicides, reflecting their easy availability.

CHARACTERISTICS OF DELIBERATE SELF-HARMERS

Adolescents who self-harm are a heterogeneous group, ranging from those who scratch or cut themselves to relieve a sense of inner tension, to those that have a clear intent to kill themselves. Whilst those that have an unequivocal wish to die are rare, there are many who have suicidal ideation (27% of 14–17 year olds; Centers for Disease Control, 1991), some of whom go on to put themselves at considerable risk. It would, therefore, be extremely useful if clinicians have at their disposal a means of assessing that risk. Table 4.2 summarises the main characteristic features which predispose to completed suicide in adolescence. An awareness of these features can help predict those at highest risk.

The role of mental illness, particularly major depressive disorder and to a lesser extent conduct disorder and substance misuse, as predisposing factors to deliberate self-harm is still unclear. Some studies based on routine clinical practice suggest a relatively small proportion of adolescent self-harmers have a psychiatric disorder, e.g. Hawton and Fagg (1992) found only 3.5% and Cotgrove et al. (1995) 6%. Others, however, using detailed research evaluations have reported high rates, e.g. Kerfoot et al. (1996) and Burgess et al. (1998) diagnosed 75 and 100%, respectively, as having a psychiatric disorder at, or soon after, the time the adolescent harmed themselves.

Immediate precipitants to deliberate self-harm and suicide have some overlap with the predisposing characteristics shown in Table 4.2. They include interpersonal conflicts with family and friends, losses through bereavement or relationship breakdown, and external stressors such as bullying, disciplinary problems, legal difficulties, unemployment, abuse/neglect and exposure to deliberate self-harm or suicide. In addition, the adolescent's emotional state, such as feelings of hopelessness, anxiety and anger, is relevant.

Table 4.2 Characteristics predisposing to completed suicide

Individual factors	Family and Environment
Psychiatric disorder	Loss of parent in childhood
• depression	Family dysfunction
• psychosis	Abuse and neglect
• substance misuse	Family history of psychiatric illness or suicide
• conduct disorder	
Isolation	
Low self-esteem	
Physical Illness	

THE MEANING OF DELIBERATE SELF-HARM

An act of deliberate self-harm can have a range of meanings. It can be a serious attempt to die in order to escape from unbearable feelings or an unbearable situation. However, rather than death, an overwhelming wish to escape may be the main intention, the adolescent knowing that they want things to change but feeling powerless to bring this about without taking dramatic action. In this case it can be helpful to view the act of deliberate self-harm as a communication. This communication may include a 'cry for help', but may also involve feelings of hostility or anger directed to others or themselves.

Alternatively, there might be no suicidal intent, the act helping to release feelings of inner tension. There may be an associated sense of low self-worth and guilt, the deliberate self-harm being seen as a means of self-punishment.

Exploring its meaning and considering alternatives to deliberate self-harm as a means of communication can play an important role in working with adolescents to reduce repetition.

MANAGEMENT

The immediate management of an act of deliberate self-poisoning should generally include admission to a paediatric or medical ward overnight to facilitate a considered assessment, even if there are no medical indications for this (Royal College of Psychiatrists, 1998). Further management is strongly influenced by the risk assessment, there being a need for more pro-active management, with an emphasis on safety, if the risk of repetition is considered high. Factors suggestive of a high risk of repetition include:

- The circumstances of the attempt
  - the degree of isolation
  - the potential lethality of the means used
  - precautions to avoid detection
  - leaving a suicide note
- The presence of a psychiatric disorder
- The degree of premeditation and expressed degree of suicide intent
- A past history of deliberate self-harm

Rating scales such as the Pierce Suicide Intent Score (Pierce, 1981) can help with such an assessment, although it has been shown that a clinician's crude impression of the level of risk alone is highly predictive of repeated deliberate self-harm (Cotgrove et al., 1995).

Practical methods such as reducing the availability of the means of self-harm can be helpful on both an individual and societal level. For example, in the UK the switch from coal to natural gas reduced suicide rates significantly. Repackaging of paracetamol into smaller blister packs is a recent attempt to reduce the quantities easily available for overdosing. Other social measures such as attempting to reduce the availability and consumption of drugs, particularly alcohol, have been shown to have an impact on suicide rates in adults.

Underlying psychiatric disorder should be treated, for example, with CBT for depression and feelings of hopelessness. Other predisposing or precipitating factors should be addressed wherever possible, although little can be done about some of these, e.g. relationship break-ups, except through the offer of support. Evidence of abuse or neglect should be addressed and if there is a suggestion that this is ongoing in the adolescent's home, they should not be discharged from hospital until their safety can be assured.

Adolescent suicide attempters and their families are often not compliant with follow-up treatment and so any intervention needs to address this issue to have any likelihood of success. Interventions need to be both convenient and acceptable to the adolescent and their families. On reviewing a range of treatments, both with adults and adolescents, Brent (1997) concludes that treatment goals such as improved social adjustments, reduced suicidal ideation and reduced suicidal attempts can best be achieved by more aggressive outreach, and therapy focused on dysfunctional cognitions, problem solving and interpersonal skills.

To date there have been only two randomised control trials evaluating specific interventions with adolescents to reduce repetition. Cotgrove et al. (1995) used a 'green card' to allow a youngster immediate access to a paediatric bed should they feel suicidal. Whilst the results were not statistically significant, fewer adolescents repeated self-harm with the green card. A similar study with adults (Morgan et al., 1993) allowing patients to contact a doctor 24 h a day was shown to be effective in reducing the rate of repeated self-harm (when both threats and acts of self-harm were considered). Harrington et al. (1998b) evaluated a home-based family intervention. Whilst this achieved a greater compliance with treatment with good parental satisfaction, there was no reduction in repetition.

There is not a large role for inpatient psychiatric treatment, but occasionally, when there is an underlying psychiatric disorder and the immediate risk from repetition is judged to be high, admission may be indicated.

In conclusion, there remains considerable uncertainty about which forms of psychosocial interventions are most effective for adolescents who deliberately harm themselves.

PROGNOSIS

Following an episode of deliberate self-harm, approximately 10% will go on to repeat within a year (Cotgrove et al., 1995; Goldacre and Hawton, 1985; Spirito et al., 1989) and a significant proportion in this group will go on to kill themselves. Estimates of this latter group vary, but at the extreme Otto (1972) found as many as 4% of girls and 11% of boys had killed themselves at 5 years follow up.

ANXIETY DISORDERS

The experience of anxiety is a normal phenomenon and its expression varies with development. In infancy, fear and anxiety are provoked mainly by sensory stimuli. In early childhood they can be evoked by fear of strangers and separation anxiety. Later in childhood fears of the dark, of animals and imaginary creatures are more common. In adolescence it is performance anxiety and fear of social situations which predominate. These changes may reflect cognitive development but may also be a function of the differential threat that various stimuli pose at different ages. These same age patterns are also reflected in the onset of pathological manifestations of anxiety with social phobia and agoraphobia being most common in adolescence (Ost, 1987).

AETIOLOGY

Over the years many models have been used to help explain and understand anxiety. These include psychodynamic theory, attachment theory, learning theory, cognitive theory and neurophysiology. Evidence of a genetic inheritance is equivocal with few studies of childhood-onset anxiety syndromes. Studies of anxiety in adults suggest there may be some familial linkage though this requires further research (Noyes *et al.*, 1987).

It is likely that in the majority of cases there is a multi-factoral aetiology with temperamental traits and experience playing a part. At times there is an obvious precipitant, but this is not necessarily the case.

EPIDEMIOLOGY

Epidemiological studies suggest a high prevalence of anxiety disorders in non-referred adolescents. For example, lifetime prevalence rates of 3.7% have been reported for generalized anxiety disorder and prevalence rates for separation anxiety disorder of 3.6% (Bowen *et al.*, 1990). However, they are much less common in clinical samples, cases only being referred when symptoms are very severe or worrying to others.

At least 50% of adult cases of anxiety syndromes had their onset in childhood. The median age of onset is said to be 16 with an earlier age of 12 for syndromes of social anxiety and simple phobias (Klein, 1994).

CLASSIFICATION

ICD-10 (World Health Organisation, 1992) distinguishes anxiety disorders found specifically in childhood from those found in adulthood. Although the diagnoses

Table 4.3 Summary of ICD-10 classification of anxiety disorders

Anxiety disorders specific to childhood

- Separation Anxiety Disorder of Childhood F93.0
- Phobic Anxiety Disorder of Childhood F93.1
- Social Anxiety Disorder of Childhood F93.2

Phobic Anxiety Disorders

- Agoraphobia F40.0
- Social Phobias F40.1
- Specific (isolated) phobias F40.2

Other anxiety disorders

- Panic Disorder F41.1
- Generalised Anxiety Disorder F41.1
- Mixed Anxiety and Depressive Disorder F41.2

used in childhood appear to overlap with those used for adults, as summarised in Table 4.3, they are usually only used in those disorders which seem to constitute exaggerations of normal developmental trends rather than phenomena that are quantitatively abnormal in themselves.

CLINICAL FEATURES

Generally, anxiety disorders specific to childhood do not appear for the first time in adolescence. For example, in childhood, separation anxiety may manifest as school refusal (or phobia). However, in adolescence, school refusal arising for the first time should not be diagnosed as separation anxiety unless there are clear features of this dating back to pre-school years. If an anxiety disorder is underlying the school refusal it is more likely due to a social phobia or other anxiety disorder.

In phobic anxiety disorders anxiety is evoked by well-defined situations. One such disorder particularly common in adolescents is social phobia. This is a fear centred on scrutiny by other people when in small social groups, e.g. when in a restaurant. It is often associated with low self-esteem and, in contrast to other anxiety disorders, which have a preponderance of female sufferers, the sex incidence is equal. Another phobic anxiety syndrome which becomes prevalent in adolescence is agoraphobia, classically the fear of 'the market place', but now used more widely to apply to the fear of open spaces, crowds and other experiences associated with leaving the house. Marked avoidance of anxiety provoking situations often occurs.

Panic attacks may be associated with phobic anxiety disorders such as agoraphobia or, alternatively, they may occur unpredictably and not associated with a particular set of circumstances. In this latter case a diagnosis of panic disorder alone can be made. Symptoms of panic can vary widely but typically include a sudden onset of tachycardia, palpitations and a sensation of chest tightening. There may be choking sensations, dizziness and feelings of unreality, and sometimes a secondary fear of dying or losing control.

In a generalised anxiety disorder the sufferer experiences excessive anxiety and worrying associated with apprehension, motor tension, tiredness, poor concentration, irritability and sleep disturbance. There may also be associated experiences of depersonalisation.

There is a high rate of co-morbidity, with anxiety symptoms frequently co-existing or occurring with other disorders, in particular depression.

MANAGEMENT

A full account of the symptoms should be elicited from the young person and this can be supplemented where possible by a more objective account from someone who has observed the anxiety attacks. The history might give pointers to any precipitating or maintaining factors, although these are not always evident. Physical causes such as hyperthyroidism should be excluded. Evidence of any co-morbid disorders should be sought and treated appropriately. During assessment the interviewer should note any attempts the sufferer has made to control their symptoms and the effectiveness of these attempts. Any small successes can then be built upon during therapy.

There are no large-scale studies to guide treatment. In general, pharmacological treatments, with either antidepressants or benzodiazepines have proved to be ineffective, although some advocate the use of SSRIs in the treatment of social phobias and panic disorder. The most promising therapies seem to be those based on cognitive behavioural theories, using the principles of relaxation, exposure to anxiety provoking stimuli, response prevention and reinforcement of progress (King and Ollendick, 1997).

Adolescent sufferers of anxiety are usually obviously in distress. This can be difficult for families to bear and parents often blame themselves for their offspring's symptoms. Sufferers may have involved their parents in complex rituals as a means of avoiding anxiety-provoking situations. Parents will need support in encouraging gradual reintroduction of exposure to these situations.

PROGNOSIS

Available evidence suggests that anxiety syndromes in the young frequently remit but may recur again. Some studies suggest that there may be a link between separation anxiety in childhood and panic disorder later. However, this finding awaits replication (Klein, 1994).

ADJUSTMENT DISORDERS

CLINICAL FEATURES

ICD 10 defines an adjustment reaction as a state of subjective distress and emotional disturbance, usually interfering with social functioning and performance, and arising in the period of adaptation to a significant life change or to the consequences of a stressful life event (World Health Organisation, 1992).

Individual predisposition or vulnerability plays a role in the risk of occurrence of adjustment disorder. However, it is assumed that the symptomatology would not have occurred without the presence of the stressor. Onset of symptoms should be within 1 month of the stressful event and symptoms should not last more than 6 months.

Symptoms may be those of anxiety, depression or a disturbance of conduct. They may occur individually or in combination with each other. Psychopathology is generally moderate rather than severe and it is assumed that the symptoms are not an exacerbation of a pre-existing disorder.

NATURE OF VULNERABILITY

Chronic adversities appear to predispose individuals to difficulties in coping with more acute stressful events. Work on attachment suggests that the quality of early relationships has an effect on the development of psychopathology later in life. There is also evidence to suggest that vulnerable individuals act in such ways that predispose them to experience more than the average number of adverse life events.

It is important to remember that an individuals response to a stressor will be dependent on the vulnerability of the system that surrounds them as well as vulnerabilities within themselves, and that the system and the individual will be interacting with each other at all times.

NATURE OF POTENTIAL STRESSORS

Adolescence is a time of change and the vast majority of individuals experience many potentially stressful events without developing psychopathology. Conversely individuals may develop psychiatric disorder without experiencing a stressful life event. Care should be taken in assuming a causal link between stressors and psychopathology.

Definition of an adjustment disorder is reliant on making a subjective assessment of what would be a normal reaction to the stressful life event that has occurred. A single stressful event will have different meanings for different individuals dependent on their past experience and internal world. In order to fulfil the definition of an adjustment disorder the potential stressor should be a relatively circumscribed event. Many stressors in a young person's life develop over a period of time and inter-relate with each other. For example, a parental divorce is likely to follow a prolonged period of marital discord. The young person may have had to leave the family home and perhaps change schools, a situation that may have resulted in academic problems or bullying from peers. It can be seen that making an assessment of potential stressors is fraught with difficulty.

MANAGEMENT

An individual interview will allow the young person to reveal stressful events the parents may be unaware of or trying to hide, e.g. bullying at school or sexual abuse. An attempt should be made to assess the mental state of other family members on whom the young person is dependent for support.

There is little evidence to suggest the most effective treatment and this might be different for different clinical presentations. A strategy designed to eliminate or reduce the stressors whilst offering support and coping strategies to the individual and their family seems the most appropriate.

It may be possible to prepare vulnerable individuals for predictable stressors such as examinations or a change of school. However, the efficacy of such strategies is untested.

PROGNOSIS

By definition an adjustment disorder is time limited. However, adolescents may go on to develop other psychiatric disorders, though data is lacking to say how often this occurs.

POST-TRAUMATIC STRESS DISORDER

Post-traumatic stress disorder (PTSD) arises as a delayed or protracted response to a stressful event or situation of an exceptionally threatening or catastrophic nature, which is likely to cause pervasive distress in most people. Predisposing factors such as personality or previous neurotic illness may exacerbate the condition but are not in themselves sufficient to explain its occurrence. The diagnosis is usually made if psychological symptoms occur in the 6 months following a major trauma (World Health Organisation, 1992). These features can be contrasted with those of an adjustment disorder (see Table 4.4).

PREVALENCE

PTSD was originally a disorder described in adults, but there have been numerous studies that support its validity with children and adolescents (e.g. McFarlane *et*

Table 4.4 Comparison of adjustment disorder and PTSD

	Adjustment disorder	PTSD
Onset	Usually within 1 month of stressful event	Usually within 6 months of stressful event
Precipitant	Yes, but not necessarily severe	Traumatic event of exceptional severity
Predisposition	Usually vulnerable individual	Not necessarily vulnerable
Symptoms	Depression, anxiety or conduct disturbance, feeling unable to cope; no symptoms severe enough to warrant separate diagnosis	Flashbacks, anxiety, depression, sleep disturbance, nightmares, feelings of numbness, avoidance of stimuli reminiscent of trauma and autonomic hyperarousal with hypervigilance
Prognosis	Resolves within 6 months	May be prolonged, but recovery can be expected in the majority of cases

al., 1987; Pynoos *et al.*, 1987). Estimates of prevalence rates vary widely according to the disaster involved, the life threat to individuals involved, the measures used, and the time elapsed between the event and the study. Studies have quoted rates between 10 and 100% of those experiencing a major trauma.

CLINICAL FEATURES

The cardinal symptoms of PTSD are repetitive, intrusive recollections or re-enactments of the event in memory (so called flashbacks) and nightmares. There may also be emotional detachment, numbing of feeling, avoidance of stimuli which might trigger flashbacks, autonomic disturbance, mood disorder and other symptoms of anxiety. Flashbacks are often vivid and are most likely to occur at times of quiet such as when lying in bed trying to sleep. Sleep problems are particularly common and sufferers are often awakened by nightmares, reliving the event (Yule, 1994). There may be a fear of the dark and problems related to separation from parents.

Sufferers often want to talk about their traumatic experience but conversely may find it difficult to discuss with those close to them. Family and peers may have been involved in the traumatic events and young people may wish to protect them or sometimes, particularly in adolescence, sufferers are ashamed of their symptoms and seek to hide them. There is often a feeling of isolation as a consequence of this. Sufferers may experience increased irritability that may serve to further isolate them. Young people report difficulties with concentration and memory that may result in academic problems.

Rates of depression and anxiety symptoms are increased, particularly in adolescent sufferers, who may also describe a lack of faith in the future or a change in priorities in their life. Sufferers may experience physiological as well as psychological symptoms. A life-threatening event will have precipitated a flight or fight response and the physiological elements of this may be re-experienced involving increased secretion of noradrenaline and endogenous opiates in the brain. Better understanding of these reactions may hold out hope for targeted pharmacological therapy in the future.

NATURE OF STRESSORS

PTSD in young people has been described in relation to a whole range of traumatic events, including war, natural disasters, technological accidents, road and maritime accidents, and witnessing or experiencing violent attack. There has been an ongoing debate whether the sequelae of child abuse should be understood in terms of PTSD (Wolfe *et al.*, 1989). This seems more useful in instances of one-off abuse, which are not usually associated with the chronic adversity experienced by sufferers of chronic abuse (Cotgrove and Kolvin, 1996). Studies suggest that there is a dose–response relationship between the stressor and the subsequent psychopathology. In any one event it seems that individuals exposed to more loss or more threat to life experience more severe symptoms.

Adult studies suggest that natural disasters produce less emotional reactions than man-made ones and that accidental man-made accidents have less serious effects than those where deliberate violence is involved (Yule, 1994). However, it is important to remember that there is a subjective element to any stressful event and an individual will experience a trauma differently according to their circumstances. For example, in a study of reactions following a sniper attack on a Californian school, a boy was very deeply affected after having left early and avoided directly experiencing the trauma but having left his sister behind (Pynoos *et al.*, 1987).

Reactions to a particular stress are also affected by the support systems surrounding the young person. It is often the case that important others have also been traumatised and this will affect their ability to be supportive.

MANAGEMENT

There have been few evaluative studies of the effects of preventative critical incident debriefing following disasters. Studies in adults suggest this may be helpful and self-report data following debriefing of adolescent girls following the sinking of the *Jupiter* suggested that this may have been helpful particularly in relation to intrusive thoughts (Yule and Udwin, 1991). However, debriefing should not be expected to be a panacea for everyone and some have questioned its value.

Pharmacological treatments do not have a major role to play in the treatment of PTSD. Cognitive-behavioural approaches seem most helpful, with sufferers being encouraged to re-experience the event and its associated emotions in a supportive environment where they can learn to master their feelings. Using drama or drawings may help facilitate the discussion of their feelings if this is difficult. Sleep problems will need careful evaluation. Initial insomnia may be aided by relaxation training whilst there are behavioural techniques which may alleviate nightmares.

Family and social support is a vital protective factor in alleviating the effects of stress on young people. Attention should be given to helping families and schools come to terms with trauma for themselves and to providing them with the skills necessary for their supportive role. In situations where natural groupings such as schools or communities are involved in a trauma it makes sense to use this group as a means of sharing feelings or coming to a shared understanding of what has happened.

It is important not to overlook practical means of offering support for difficulties related to the trauma. For example, sufferers can hardly be expected to come to terms with their symptoms if they are refugees with nowhere to stay or are still under threat of harm.

PROGNOSIS

The majority of sufferers improve between 6 weeks and 6 months (Mirza *et al.*, 1998). However, PTSD may run a long and disabling course (Yule, 1994). There is evidence that early levels of distress are related to outcome and that the more severe the trauma, the more likely it is that its effects will last for 6 months or more. Symptoms such as intrusive memories seem to decrease over time whilst it is more likely that depression and symptoms of anxiety will increase over the first 6 months. Mediating variables such as good family support have a greater effect following less serious trauma and it seems that the severity of the stressor is the most reliable predictor of the severity of later psychopathology.

OBSESSIVE-COMPULSIVE DISORDER

Obsessive-compulsive disorder (OCD) is characterised by recurrent, intrusive thoughts and/or repetitive, compulsive urges or behaviours that are distressing, time consuming or significantly interfere with daily functioning. Adolescents presenting with this disorder are a heterogeneous group with a wide range of clinical presentations and course.

EPIDEMIOLOGY

OCD is relatively common with a lifetime prevalence of 1–3% (Black, 1996). Studies suggest that between one- and two-thirds of cases have their onset in childhood or adolescence (Bolton *et al.*, 1996; Rasmussen and Eizen, 1990). As in adult cases there is a high rate of co-morbidity, particularly with depressive and anxiety disorders. There are also reported associations with eating disorders, conduct disorder, substance abuse, trichotillomania (hair pulling), body dysmorphophobic disorder and habit disorders such as nail biting (March and Leonard, 1996). There is a well-recognised association between OCD and Tourette's syndrome, and an increased incidence of chorieform movements in cases of OCD with their onset in childhood or adolescence.

The mean age of onset of symptoms is 10 years (Swedo *et al.*, 1989). Males are more likely to have an earlier age of onset, and cases with a very early onset are more likely to be familial and to have an association with neurological conditions such as Tourette's syndrome.

AETIOLOGY

It is generally accepted that behavioural explanations are not of major significance in the aetiology of this disorder. However, reported cases of OCD following a traumatic experience and the fact that cognitive behavioural therapy is effective suggest some psychological mechanisms are influential in the expression of symptomatology. In contrast, there is strong evidence that genetic and biological factors are of importance (Lenane *et al.*, 1990) with genetic studies showing a familial link for OCD. In a study of 46 cases of childhood onset OCD 25% had a first degree relative with the disorder. In a study of 15 monozygotic and 15 dizygotic twin pairs the concordance rate for treated OCD was 33 and 7%, respectively. When the phenotype was widened to include obsessional and compulsive symptoms regardless of treatment status the rates increased to 87 and 47% (Carey and Gottesman, 1981).

Biological research suggests that the basal ganglia and fronto-striatal tracts may have an aetiological role in development of the disorder (Rapoport *et al.*, 1994). The association with tics and chorieform movements is also suggestive of basal ganglia pathology. It is not surprising, then, that diseases with underlying basal ganglia dysfunction such as Sydenham's chorea, post-encephalitic Parkinson's disease and Tourette's syndrome show an association with OCD. It is hypothesised that group A β-haemolytic streptococcal infections may provoke an autoimmune response in this part of the brain. It is thought that this may be the cause of a subgroup of childhood onset OCD (Allen *et al.*, 1995). Surgical lesions that disconnect the basal ganglia from the frontal lobes are also known to be therapeutic in OCD. Computed tomography and functional imaging studies also implicate frontal lobes and basal ganglia.

The efficacy of clomipramine and fluoxetine has led to the hypothesis that serotonin is implicated in the disorder, and the association with movement disorders has led to the suggestion that dopamine may also be involved. However, although various studies have suggested that these neurotransmitters may be involved, as yet their role is unclear.

CLINICAL FEATURES

The essential feature of this disorder is recurrent obsessional thoughts or compulsive acts. ICD-10 (World Health Organisation, 1992) suggests that in order to make the diagnosis obsessional thoughts or compulsive acts, or both, should be present on most days for at least 2 successive weeks and be a source of distress or interference with activities.

Obsessional symptoms should have the following characteristics:

- They must be recognised as the individuals own thoughts or actions
- There must be at least one thought or act that is still resisted unsuccessfully, even though others may be present which the sufferer no longer resists
- The thought of carrying out the act must not in itself be pleasurable
- The thought, images or impulses must be unpleasantly repetitive

A significant proportion of cases may have compulsive thoughts or urges with no associated rituals.

Adolescents with OCD may go unrecognised. There are large differences between the number of cases identified in epidemiological surveys and those in treatment. Sufferers are often ashamed of their symptoms, and may go to great lengths to hide them from parents and others.

In the majority of cases symptoms change over time. Washing rituals are the most common though repeating and checking rituals also frequently occur. Sexual thoughts and rituals become more common in later adolescence, and may be a cause of particular distress. Sufferers may involve parents in their rituals and families may find this difficult to resist because of the distress caused. Stressful situations tend to make symptoms worse and sufferers often find that if they keep busy their obsessions are easier to resist.

MANAGEMENT

Except in the most severe cases it is unusual for sufferers to present to clinicians with their obsessional symptoms (Riddle, 1998). It is important to question patients about obsessional symptomatology when they present with other problems. Because of the high rates of co-morbidity for the disorder it is equally important to assess patients presenting with OCD for other disorders such as tics, depression and anxiety. Most young people with OCD require multiple treatments and this is likely to need the involvement of the multi-disciplinary team. Gaining cooperation may be a difficulty and it is vital that a strong therapeutic alliance is created from the outset. The patient and his family should be given information about the disorder and its treatment.

It is worthwhile making an attempt to assess parents and other family members for obsessional symptoms and to encourage them to seek treatment if necessary. Sometimes they become involved in the adolescent's OCD symptoms, such as rituals, in a way that can perpetuate or even exacerbate them. Parental counselling then, in some form, is a key part of any treatment package.

Behavioural techniques, in particular exposure and response prevention, have been shown to be effective in OCD in adults (Greist, 1996). Beyond case reports there have been few studies of such techniques in younger people but those there have been suggest they may also be effective in this age group (March et al., 1994). This treatment involves exposing the adolescent to the feared situation until their anxiety decreases whilst blocking the rituals or avoidance behaviour (response prevention). The efficacy is reliant on the young person being able to understand and cooperate with instructions, and with younger adolescents or in those with a learning difficulty this may be a problem, in which case a greater reliance on family involvement may be needed.

Where obsessions predominate or where psychotherapy is ineffective it may be necessary to give a trial of medication. Clomipramine and the SSRIs have been shown to be effective in the treatment of OCD in children and adolescents (Flament et al., 1985; Leonard et al., 1989). As with adults, it is difficult to predict who will respond to medication but the efficacy is not dependent on the presence of co-morbid depression (Riddle, 1998). Patients should be started on a low dose of medication and increases should be made at intervals until a therapeutic effect is observed or side effects are intolerable. In one study a mean dose of Clomipramine of 140 mg per day was effective in 75% of adolescent cases of OCD. This effect could generally be seen by 3 weeks (Flament et al., 1985). The effectiveness of clomipramine is limited by common and significant side effects such as sedation and weight gain, and there are risks of cardiotoxicity, particularly in overdose. For these reasons, an SSRI such as fluoxetine would normally be the drug of first choice.

PROGNOSIS

Retrospective data from adult studies suggests the course may be chronic or episodic. Spontaneous remission may occur in up to a third of patients. There have been few prospective studies of childhood onset cases of OCD and those there have been suggest that up to 50% of cases still have symptoms at follow-up (Leonard et al., 1993). Treatment seems to make little difference to these figures and no clear predictive factors have been identified (Bolton et al., 1996).

However, most young people with the disorder are able to lead full lives despite their symptoms.

CONCLUSIONS

Affective and emotional disorders are a varied group of conditions, but ones which commonly present to child and adolescent mental health services. They have wide ranging aetiologies, often being predisposed by childhood adversity and precipitated by environmental events, but sometimes, as with OCD, with clear biological and genetic factors.

Treatments are also varied, with psychosocial interventions predominating but there is also a role for pharmacotherapy with some disorders. Much further work is still needed to acquire evidence to support the efficacy of many of the treatments currently used in routine clinical practice.

REFERENCES

Allen, A. J., Leonard, H. L. and Swedo, S. E. (1995) Case study: a new infection-triggered auto-immune subtype of paediatric OCD and Tourette's syndrome. *Journal of the American Academy of Child and Adolescent Psychiatry*, 34, 307–311.

American Psychiatric Association (1994) *Diagnostic and Statistical Manual of Mental Disorders*, 4th edn (DSM-IV). Washington, DC: American Psychiatric Association.

Angold, A. and Rutter, M. (1992) Effects of age and pubertal status on depression in a large clinical sample. *Development and Psychopathology*, 4, 5–28.

Barrett, M. L., Berney, T. P., Bhate, S., Famuyiwa, O., Fundudis, T., Kolvin, I. *et al.* (1991) Diagnosing childhood depression: who should be interviewed-parent or child? The Newcastle Child depression Project. *British Journal of Psychiatry*, 159 (Suppl. 11), 22–27.

Berney, T. P., Bhate, S. R., Kolvin, I., Famuyiwa, O. O., Barrett, M. L., Fundudis, T. *et al.* (1991) The context of childhood depression. The Newcastle Childhood Depression Project. *British Journal of Psychiatry*, 159, 28–35.

Black, D. W. (1996) Epidemiology and genetics of OCD: a review and discussion of future directions and research. *CNS Spectrums*, 1, 10–16.

Bolton, D., Luckie, M. and Steinberg, D. (1996) Obsessive-compulsive disorder treated in adolescence: 14 long-term case histories. *Clinical Child psychology and Psychiatry*, 1, 409–430.

Bowen, R. C., Offord, D. R. and Boyle, M. H. (1990) The prevalence of over-anxious disorder and separation anxiety disorder: results from the Ontario Child Health Study. *Journal of the American Academy of Child and Adolescent Psychiatry*, 29, 753–758.

Brent, D. A. (1997) Practitioner review: the aftercare of adolescents with deliberate self-harm. *Journal of Child Psychology and Psychiatry*, 38, 277–286.

Brent, D. A., Perper, J. A., Goldstein, C. E., Kolko, D. J., Allan, M. J., Allman, C. J. *et al.* (1988) Risk factors for adolescent suicide. A comparison of adolescent suicide victims with suicidal inpatients. *Archives of General Psychiatry*, 45, 581–588.

Brent, D. A., Perper, J. A. and Moritz, G. (1993) Psychiatric risk factors for adolescent suicide: a case-control study. *Journal of the American Academy of Child and Adolescent Psychiatry*, 32, 521–529.

Buchanan, C. M., Eccles, J. S. and Becker, J. B. (1992) Are adolescents the victims of raging hormones: evidence for activational effects of hormones on moods and behaviour at adolescence. *Psychology Bulletin*, 111, 62–107.

Burgess, S., Hawton, K. and Loveday, G. (1998) Adolescents who take overdoses: outcome in terms of changes in psychopathology and the adolescent's attitudes to care and to their overdose. *Journal of Adolescence*, 21, 209–218.

Carey, G. and Gottesman, I. I. (1981) Twin and family studies of anxiety, phobic, and obsessive disorders. In D. F. Klein and J. Rabkin (eds), *Anxiety: New Research and Changing Concepts*. New York: Raven Press, pp. 117–136.

Centers for Disease Control (1991) Attempted suicides among high school students – United States 1990. *Morbidity and Mortality Weekly Report*, 40, 633–635.

Clarke, G. N., Hops, H., Lewinsohn, P. M., Seely, J. R. and Williams, R. (1992) Cognitive behavioural group treatment of adolescent depression: prediction of outcome. *Behaviour Therapy*, 23, 341–354.

Cooper, P. J. and Goodyer, I. (1993) A community study of depression in adolescent girls. I: Estimates of symptom and symptom prevalence. *British Journal of Psychiatry*, 163, 369–374.

Costello, E. J., Benjamin, R., Angold, A. and Silver D. (1991) Mood variability in adolescents: a study of depressed, nondepressed and comorbid patients. *Journal of Affective Disorders*, 23, 199–212.

Cotgrove, A. J. and Kolvin, I. (1996) Child sexual abuse. *Hospital Update*, 22, 401–406.

Cotgrove, A. J., Zirinsky, L., Black, D. and Weston, D. (1995) Secondary prevention of attempted suicide in adolescence. *Journal of Adolescence*, 18, 569–577.

Deakin, J. F. W. and Crow, T. J. (1986) Monoamine, rewards and punishments – the anatomy and physiology of the affective disorders. In J. F. W. Deakin (ed.), *The Biology of Depression*. London: Royal College of Psychiatrists, pp. 1–25.

Emslie, G., Rush, A., Weinberg, W., Kowatch, R., Hughes, C., Carmody, T., *et al.* (1997) A double-blind, randomized placebo-controlled trial of fluoxetine in depressed children and adolescents. *Archives of General Psychiatry*, 54, 1031–1037.

Flament, M. F., Rapoport, J. L., Berg, C. J., Sceery, W., Kilts, C., Mellstrom, B. et al. (1985) Clomipramine treatment of childhood compulsive disorder: a double-blind controlled study. *Archives of General Psychiatry*, **42**, 977–983.

Fombonne, E. (1995) Depressive disorders: time trends and putative explanatory mechanisms. In M. Rutter and D. Smith (eds), *Psychosocial Disorders in Young People: Time Trends and their Origins*. Chichester: Wiley, pp. 544–615.

Fombonne, E. (1998) Suicidal behaviours in vulnerable adolescents: time trends and their correlates. *British Journal of Psychiatry*, **173**, 154–159.

Forness, S. R. (1988) School characteristics of children and adolescents with depression. In R. B. Rutherford, C. M. Nelson and S. R. Forness (eds), *Bases of Severe Behavioural Disorders in Children and Youth*. Boston, MA: Little Brown, pp. 177–203

Garber, J., Kriss, M. R., Koch, M. and Lindholm, L. (1988) Recurrent depression in adolescents: a follow-up study. *Journal of the American Academy of Child Psychiatry*, **27**, 49–54.

Geller, B., Fox, L. W. and Fletcher, M. (1993) Effect of tricyclic antidepressants on switching to mania and the onset of bipolarity in depressed 6- to-12- year-olds. *Journal of the American Academy of Child and Adolescent Psychiatry*, **32**, 43–50.

Giles, D. E., Roffwarg, H. P., Dahl, R. E. and Kupfer, D. J. (1992) Electroencephalographic sleep abnormalities in depressed children: a hypothesis. *Psychiatric Research*, **41**, 53–63.

Goldacre, M. and Hawton, K. (1985) Repetition of self-poisoning and subsequent death in adolescents who take overdoses. *British Journal of Psychiatry*, **146**, 395–398.

Goodyer, I. M., Wright, C. and Altham, P. M. E. (1989) Recent friendships in anxious and depressed school-age children. *Psychological Medicine*, **19**, 165–174.

Goodyer, I., Herbert, J., Moor, S. and Altham, P. (1991) Cortisol hypersecretion in depressed school-aged children and adolescents. *Psychiatry Research*, **37**, 237–234.

Greist, J. H. (1996) New developments in behaviour therapy for obsessive-compulsive disorder. *International Clinical Psychopharmacology*, **II** (Suppl. 5), 63–73.

Harrington, R. (1992) Annotation: the natural history and treatment of child and adolescent affective disorders. *Journal of Child Psychology and Psychiatry*, **33**, 1287–1302.

Harrington, R. (1994) Affective disorders. In M. Rutter, E. Taylor, and L. Hersolv (ed.), *Child and Adolescent Psychiatry*. London: Blackwell Science, pp. 330–374.

Harrington, R. C. and Wood, A. J. (1995) Validity and classification of child and adolescent depressive disorders. Review of the field circa. 1995. In G. Forrest (ed.), *Childhood Depression. ACPP Occasional Paper 11*. London: Association for Child Psychology and Psychiatry, pp. 3–22.

Harrington, R. C., Fudge, H., Rutter, M., Bredenkamp, D., Groothues, C. and Pridham, J. (1993) Child and adult depression: a test of continuities with data from a family study. *British Journal of Psychiatry*, **162**, 627–633.

Harrington, R. C., Bredenkamp, D. and Groothues, C., Rutter, M., Fudge, H. and Pickles, A. (1994) Adult outcomes of childhood and adolescent depression III. Links with suicidal behaviour. *Journal of Child Psychology and Psychiatry*, **35**, 1380–1391.

Harrington, R., Whittaker, J. and Shoebridge, P. (1998a) Psychological treatment of depression in children and adolescents: a review of treatment research. *British Journal of Psychiatry*, **173**, 291–298.

Harrington, R. C., Kerfoot, M., Dyer, E., McNiven, F., Gill, J., Harrington, V., Woodham, A. and Byford, S. (1998b) Radomized trial of home-based family intervention for children who have deliberately poisoned themselves. *Journal of the American Academy of Child and Adolescent Psychiatry*, **37**, 512–518.

Hawton, K. (1992) By their own young hand. *British Medical Journal*, **304**, 1000.

Hawton, K. and Fagg, J. (1992) Deliberate self-poisoning and self-injury in adolescents: a study of characteristics and trends in Oxford, 1976–89. *British Journal of Psychiatry*, **161**, 816–823.

Hawton, K., Fagg, J . and Simkin, S. (1996) Deliberate self-poisoning and self-injury in children and adolescents under 16 years of age in Oxford, 1976–1993. *British Journal of Psychiatry*, **169**, 202–208.

Hazell, P., O'Connell, D., Heathcoat, D., Robertson, J. and Henry, D. (1995) Efficacy of tricyclic drugs in treating child and adolescent depression. *British Medical Journal*, **310**, 897–90

Kendall, P. C., Kortlander, E., Chansky, T. E. and Brady, E. U. (1992) Comorbidity of anxiety and depression in youth: treatment implications. *Journal of Consulting Clinical Psychology*, **60**, 869–880.

Kerfoot, M., Dyer, E., Harrington, V., Woodham, A. and Harrington, R. (1996) Correlates and short-term course of self-poisoning in adolescents. *British Journal of Psychiatry*, **168**: 38–42.

King, N. J. and Ollendick, T. O. (1997) Annotation: treatment of childhood phobias. *Journal of Child Psychiatry and Psychology*, **38**, 389–400.

Klein, R. G. (1994) Anxiety disorders. In M. Rutter, E. Taylor and L. Hezov (eds), *Child and Adolescent psychiatry: Modern Approaches*, 3rd edn. Oxford: Blackwell Science, pp. 351–374

Klerman, G. L. (1988) The current age of youthful melancholia: evidence for increase in depression among adolescents and young adults. *British Journal of Psychiatry*, **152**, 4–14.

Kovacs, M., Gatsonis, C., Paulauskas, S. and Richards, C. (1989) Depressive disorders in childhood. IV: A longitudinal study of co-morbidity with and risk for anxiety disorders. *Archives of General Psychiatry*, **46**, 776–782.

Kovacs, M., Goldston, D. and Gatsonis, C (1993) Suicidal behaviours and childhood-onset depressive disorders: a longitudinal investigation. *Journal of the American Academy of Child and Adolescent Psychiatry*, **32**, 8–20.

Kovacs, M., Akiskal, S., Gatsonis, C. and Parrone, P. L. (1994) Childhood-onset dysthymic disorder. *Archives of General Psychiatry*, **51**, 365–374.

Kutcher, S. (1997) Practitioner review: the pharmacotherapy of adolescent depression. *Journal of Child Psychology and Psychiatry*, **38**, 755–767.

Kutcher, S. and Marton, P. (1991) Affective disorders in first degree relatives of adolescent onset bipolars, unipolars, and normal controls. *Journal of the American Academy of Child and Adolescent Psychiatry*, **30**, 75–78.

Kutcher, S., Williamson, P., Marton, P. and Szalai, J. (1992) REM latency in endogenously depressed adolescents. *British Journal of Psychiatry*, **161**, 399–402.

Lee, A. S. and Murray, R. M. (1988) The long-term outcome of Maudsley depressives. *British Journal of Psychiatry*, **153**, 741–751.

Lenane, M. C., Swedo, S. E., Leonard, H. L., Pauls, D. L., Sceery, W. and Rapoport, J. L. (1990) Psychiatric disorders in first degree relatives of children and adolescents with obsessive compulsive disorder. *Journal of the American Academy of Child and Adolescent Psychiatry*, **29**, 407–412.

Leonard, H. L., Swedo, S. E. and Rapoport, J. L., et al. (1989) Treatment of childhood obsessive-compulsive disorder with Clomipramine and desipramine; a double-blind crossover comparison. *Archives of General Psychiatry*, **46**, 1088–1092.

Leonard, H. L., Swedo, S. E., Lenane, M. C., et al. (1993) A 2–7-year follow-up study of 54 obsessive-compulsive children and adolescents. *Archives of General Psychiatry*, **50**, 429–439.

March, J. S., Mulle, K. and Herbel, B. (1994) Behavioural psychotherapy for children and adolescents with obsessive-compulsive disorder: an open trial of a new protocol-driven package. *Journal of the American Academy of Child and Adolescent Psychiatry*, **33**, 333–341.

March, J. S. and Leonard, H. L. (1996) Obsessive-compulsive disorders in children and adolescents: a review of the past 10 years. *Journal of the American Academy of Child and Adolescent Psychiatrists*, **34**, 1265–1273.

McFarlane, A. C., Policansky, S. and Irwin, C. P. (1987) A longitudinal study of the psychological morbidity in children due to natural disaster. *Psychological Medicine*, **17**, 727–738.

Mirza, K. A. H., Bhadrinath, B. R., Goodyer, I. M. and Gilmour, C. (1998) Post-traumatic stress disorder in children and adolescents following road traffic accidents. *British Journal of Psychiatry*, **172**, 443–447.

Morgan, H. G., Jones, E. M. and Owen, J. H. (1993) Secondary prevention of non-fatal self-harm: the green card study. *British Journal of Psychiatry*, 163, 111–112.

Myers, K., McCauley, E., Calderon, R. and Treder, R. (1991) The 3-year longitudinal course of suicidality and predictive factors for subsequent suicidality in youths with major depressive disorder. *Journal of the American Academy of Child and Adolescent Psychiatry*, 30, 804–810.

Noyes, R., Jr, Clarkson, C., Crowe, R. R., Yates, W. R. and McChesney, C. M. (1987) A family study of generalized anxiety disorder. *American Journal of Psychiatry*, 144, 1019–1024.

Office of Population Census and Surveys (1998) *1997 Mortality Statistics. Cause: England and Wales*. London: HMSO.

Ost, L. G. (1987) Age of onset in different phobias. *Journal of Abnormal Psychology*, 96, 223–229.

Otto, U. (1972) Suicidal acts by children and adolescents: a follow-up study. *Acta Psychiatrica Scandinavia Supplement*, 233, 5–23.

Paykel, E. S. (1989) Treatment of depression: the relevance of research for clinical practise. *British Journal of Psychiatry*, 155, 754–763.

Pierce, D. W. (1981) The predictive validation of the suicide intent scale: a five year follow-up. *British Journal of Psychiatry*, 139: 391–396.

Puig-Antich, J., Lukens, E., Davies, M., Goetz, D., Brennan-Quattrock, J. and Todak, G. (1985) Psychosocial functioning in prepubertal major depressive disorders. Interpersonal relationships during the depressive episode. *Archives of General Psychiatry*, 42, 500–507.

Puig-Antich, J., Goetz, D., Davies, M., Kaplan, T., Davies, S., Ostrow, L. *et al.* (1989) A controlled family history study of prepubertal major depressive disorder. *Archives of General Psychiatry*, 46, 406–418.

Pynoos, R. S., Frederick, C., Nader, K., Arroyo, W., Steinberg, A., Eth, S., Nunez, F. and Fairbanks, L. (1987) Life threat and post-traumatic stress in school-age children. *Archives of General Psychiatry*, 44, 1057–1063.

Radke-Yarrow, M., Nottelmann, E., Martinez, P., Fox, M. B. and Belmont, B. (1992) Young children of affectively ill parents: a longitudinal study of psychosocial development. *Journal of the American Academy of Child Psychiatry*, 31, 68–77.

Rapoport, J. L., Swedo, S. E. and Leonard, H. L. (1994) Obsessive-compulsive disorder. In M. Rutter, E. Taylor and L. Herzov (eds), *Child and Adolescent Psychiatry: Modern Approaches*, 3rd edn. Oxford: Blackwell Science.

Rasmussen, S. A. and Eisen, J. L. (1990) Epidemiology of obsessive compulsive disorder. *Journal of Clinical Psychiatry*, 53 (Suppl.), 10–14.

Reinherz, H. Z., Giaconia, R. M., Pakis, B., Silverman, A. B., Frost, A. K. and Lefkowitz, E. S. (1993) Psychosocial risks for major depression in late adolescents: a longitudinal community study. *Journal of the American Academy of Child and Adolescent Psychiatry*, 32, 1155–1163.

Riddle, M. (1998) Obsessive-compulsive disorder in children and adolescents. *British Journal of Psychiatry*, **173** (Suppl. 35), 91–96.

Rohde, P., Lewinsohn, P. M. and Seeley, J. R. (1991) Co-morbidity of unipolar depression: II. Co-morbidity with other mental disorders in adolescents and adults. *Journal of Abnormal Psychology*, **100**, 214–222.

Royal College of Psychiatrists (1998) *Managing Deliberate Self-Harm in Young People*. London: Royal College of Psychiatrists.

Rutter, M., MacDonald, H., Le Couteur, A., Harrington, R. C., Bolton, P. and Bailey, A. (1990) Genetic findings in child psychiatric disorders. II. Empirical findings. *Journal of Child Psychology and Psychiatry*, **31**, 39–83.

Rutter, M., Silberg, J., O'Connor, T. and Simonoff, E. (1999) Genetics and child psychiatry: II. Empirical research findings. *Journal of Child Psychology and Psychiatry*, **40**, 19–55.

Sadowski, H., Urgarte, B., Kolvin, I., Kaplan, C. and Barnes, J. (1999) Early life family disadvantages and major depression in adulthood. *British Journal of Psychiatry*, **174**, 112–20.

Shain, B. N., King, C. A., Naylor, M. and Alessi, N. (1991) Chronic depression and hospital course in adolescents. *Journal of the American Academy of Child and Adolescent Psychiatry*, **30**, 428–433.

Spirito, A., Brown, L., Overholser, J. and Fritz, G. (1989) Attempted suicide in adolescence: a review and critique of the literature. *Clinical Psychology Review*, **9**, 335–363.

Strober, M., Morrell, W., Lampert, C. and Burroughs, J. (1990) Relapse following discontinuation of lithium maintenance therapy in adolescents with bipolar I illness: a naturalistic study. *American Journal of Psychiatry*, **147**, 457–461.

Strober, M., Lampert, C., Schmidt, S. and Morrell, W. (1993) The course of major depressive disorder in adolescents: recovery and risk of manic switching in a follow-up of psychotic and non-psychotic subtypes. *Journal of the American Academy of Child and Adolescent Psychiatry* 32, 34–42.

Swedo, S., Rapoport, J. L., Leonard, H. L., Lenane, M. and Cheslow, D. (1989) Obsessive compulsive disorder in children and adolescents: clinical phenomenology of 70 consecutive cases. *Archives of General Psychiatry*, **46**, 335–341.

Walter, G., Rey, J. M. and Mitchell, P. B. (1999) Practitioner review: electroconvulsive therapy in adolescents. *Journal of Child Psychology and Psychiatry*, **40**, 325–334.

Werry, J. S. and McClellan, J. M. (1992) Predicting outcome in child and adolescent (early onset) schizophrenia and bipolar disorder. *Journal of the American Academy of Child and Adolescent Psychiatry*, **31**, 147–150.

Wolfe, V. V., Gentile, C. and Wolfe, D. A. (1989) The impact of sexual abuse on children: a PTSD formulation. *Behaviour Therapy*, **20**, 215–228.

World Health Organisation (1992) *The ICD-10 Classification of Mental and behavioural Disorders. Clinical Descriptions and Diagnostic Guidelines*. Geneva: World Health Organisation.

Yule, W. and Udwin, O. (1991) Screening child survivors for post-traumatic stress disorders: experiences from the 'Jupiter' sinking. *British Journal of Clinical Psychology*, 30, 131–138.

Yule, W. (1994) Post-traumatic stress disorders. In M. Rutter, E. Taylor and L. Herzov (eds), *Child and Adolescent Psychiatry. Modern Approaches*, 3rd edn. Oxford: Blackwell Science, pp. 392–406.

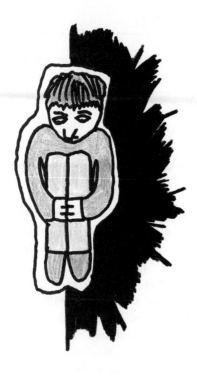

Chapter 5

CONDUCT DISORDER AND DELINQUENCY

Michael Venables

INTRODUCTION

Antisocial behaviours constitute the most frequent reason for referring young people to mental health services. However, these adolescents also make large and expensive demands on other agencies such as education, social services and the juvenile justice system. Despite the size of the problem, society in general and child mental health services in particular have achieved little in stemming the year-on-year increase in such behaviours. There is an urgent need to develop more effective interventions for helping these young people and their families, and thus reduce their multiple levels of handicap and the transmission of their difficulties to future generations. The part that mental health perspectives and services can play in understanding and supporting the roles played by other community agencies in helping adolescents with antisocial behaviours is the focus of this chapter.

DEFINITIONS

Mental health professionals intervening with antisocial adolescents are increasingly likely to conceptualise their behaviours as a mental disorder – conduct disorder – and apply the diagnostic criteria of DSM-IV (American Psychiatric Association, 1994) or ICD-10 (World Health Organisation, 1992). The former lists 15 antisocial behaviours under category headings of aggression, destructiveness, deceitfulness, theft and serious violations of rules. To qualify for the diagnosis the young person must show at least three of the 15 potential symptoms within the last 12 months, with at least one symptom within the last 6 months.

Delinquency simply refers to antisocial behaviour which breaks the law.

Young people demonstrate a range of antisocial behaviours, any one of which is likely to be continuously distributed with 'normal' behaviour. Any cut-off point for diagnostic purposes is made on the basis of clinical pragmatism and as a research heuristic device. However, a categorical or diagnostic approach should not lead to oversimple assumptions and stereotypes. Social dysfunction, proximal and distal causal processes, the variety of interventions and influences which affect these processes, and long-term prognosis need to be assessed individually in relation to each adolescent. Behaviours falling short of diagnosis can clearly be a source of significant distress and handicap for the young person and their family, and may eventually worsen to reach the threshold for diagnosis. Finally, it is important to be aware of the therapeutic nihilism and stigma associated with the diagnosis of conduct disorder in the minds of many professionals.

The diagnosis of oppositional defiant disorder (ODD) was first introduced in DSM-III and is probably best viewed as a developmental precursor of conduct disorder. If a young person fulfils criteria for both diagnoses, ODD is subsumed under the diagnosis of conduct disorder. A second related diagnosis is antisocial personality disorder, which cannot be made until a young person reaches 18 years.

DSM-IV treats conduct disorder as a polythetic diagnostic category, i.e. no one criterion is specific. For this reason adolescents with a diagnosis of conduct disorder constitute a very heterogeneous group. Various subclassifications have fallen in and out of favour over the years. A recent meta-analysis of factor analyses of symptoms of conduct and oppositional defiant disorders suggested two dimensions – overt versus covert and more versus less destructive (Hinshaw et al., 1993). The covert end of the dimension covers the less visible behaviours of stealing, truancy and vandalism. In addition Dodge (1991) and Berkowitz (1993) have argued persuasively for differentiating between affective/reactive versus instrumental/proactive aggression, even though the majority of aggressive youth may demonstrate both types. This distinction is useful partly because anger management training can be used to treat affective aggression and behaviour modification to treat instrumental aggression.

EPIDEMIOLOGY

Cohen et al. (1993) reported prevalence rates for conduct disorder across late childhood and adolescence. Those for boys dropped steadily over the teen years – from 16% at 10–13 years, 15.8% at 14–16 years to 9.5% at 17–20 years. For girls rates increased from 3.8% at 10–13 years to 9.2% at 14–16 years, dropping again to 7.1% at 17–20 years. As can be seen, there is an equalling up of the sex ratio with increased age.

There is a marked intercountry variation in violence and crime for young people. The US homicide rate in the age range 15–24 years is 18 times higher than for the UK and 73 times higher than for Austria. Within the US the homicide rate for black males is more than seven times higher than for white males (Fingerhut and Kleinman, 1990). By contrast estimated prevalence rates for diagnosed conduct disorder do not show large variations between the countries in which epidemiological surveys have been carried out, such as the US, Canada, New Zealand, UK, etc. This discrepency may be explicable in terms of political and social factors. For example, in the US the ready availability of firearms is clearly important, given that 75% of US homicides committed by 15–24 year-olds involve firearms, compared with 23% for other 'developed' countries (Fingerhut and Kleinman, 1990).

RISK FACTORS

No single risk factor is either necessary or sufficient alone to bring about the development of conduct disorder in a young person. Rather the influences of various risk factors seem to act in an approximately additive way to bring about the disorder (Loeber *et al.*, 1993).

INDIVIDUAL RISK FACTORS

GENETICS

DiLalla and Gottesman (1989) reviewed studies of criminal arrest or conviction in adult twin pairs. The weighted concordance across studies proved to be 51% for monozygotic twins and 22% for dizygotic twins. By contrast, the weighted concordance rates for juvenile delinquency were 87% for monozygotic twins and 72% for dizygotic twins. This suggests a lower genetic effect and a stronger 'shared environment' effect for juvenile delinquency. This and other research seems to demonstrate that genetic influences are stronger for conduct disorder which persists into adult life as antisocial personality disorder (Lyons *et al.*, 1995).

Plausible mediating factors include temperament, hyperactivity, and attentional deficits. There is now strong evidence for the heritability of attention deficit hyperactivity disorder (ADHD), which in turn predisposes towards the development of conduct disorder. Eaves *et al.* (1997) suggest a heritability estimate of 70% for ADHD. Silberg *et al.* (1996) demonstrated a strong genetic influence for mixed conduct disorder/ADHD, with little heritability for pure conduct disorder.

GENDER

The male:female ratio increases from ODD, through conduct disorder, delinquency to a highest value for crimes of violence. The gender ratio peaks in early adulthood and is less strong for adolescence-limited disorder. In the UK and other countries there has been a reduction in this ratio over the last four decades (Rutter et al., 1998).

BRAIN DYSFUNCTION

Brain disorders are associated with increased rates of emotional and behavioural disorders, although this increase is not specific for conduct disorder (Rutter et al. 1970).

PUBERTAL HORMONAL CHANGES

Adolescence brings temporary increases in antisocial behaviour and violence in particular (Moffitt, 1993a). Inoff-Germain et al. (1988) report that onset of puberty in particular is associated with an increase in aggression.

Inoff-Germain et al. (1988) found an association between raised oestradiol and androstenedione sex hormone levels in adolescent girls and aggressive behaviour in their interactions with family members. However, they found no hormonal effect on behaviour for boys. Olweus et al. (1980, 1988) found only a small, indirect effect of circulating testosterone on general antisocial behaviour and self-reported aggression in males, but did find a larger direct association with provoked aggression. Moreover, testosterone levels and aggression clearly influence each other in a reciprocal fashion.

NEUROTRANSMITTER FUNCTION

There is consistent evidence for lowered serotoninergic functioning in adults with a history of impulsive behaviour. Pliszka et al. (1988) found higher levels of whole blood serotonin (inversely related to cerebospinal fluid 5-hydroxyindoleacetic acid (HIAA) – the main serotonin metabolite) among adolescents with conduct disorder compared to adolescents with anxiety and depressive disorders.

AUTONOMIC NERVOUS SYSTEM FUNCTIONING

Raine (1993) has reviewed studies on autonomic nervous system activity and violence. Low resting heart rate seemed to relate to violent behaviour in all 13 studies reviewed. Magnussen et al. (1993) reported low levels of adrenaline secretion as predictive of persisting criminal behaviour up to 18 years, and persistant and sporadic offending after 18 years. Venables (1988) has argued that violent individuals are dominated by parasympathetic rather than sympathetic activity, suggesting that antisocial youth lack fear responses in situations normally calculated to evoke fear.

INTELLIGENCE

There is a lowering of IQ by approximately 8 points for adolescents with conduct disorder and juvenile delinquency, with verbal subscores particularily reduced (Moffitt, 1993b).

ACADEMIC UNDERACHIEVEMENT

Academic underachievement and general school failure are strongly associated with delinquency and early-onset conduct disorder, but not for adolescence-limited conduct disorder (Moffitt, 1993b).

TEMPERAMENT

The Dunedin Multidisciplinary Health and Development Study showed low but significant correlations between experimenter ratings of 'Lack of Control' at 3–5 years and parent, teacher ratings of antisocial behaviour at 9–11 years and ratings of conduct disorder at 13–15 years (Caspi et al., 1995). By 18 years, children who had been temperamentally 'undercontrolled' at 3 years differed to a small extent from a well adjusted group on self-reports of 'Aggression', and to a larger extent for self-reported 'Constraint' and 'Negative emotionality' (Caspi and Silva, 1995).

Although 'difficult' temperament predicts behavioural problems in childhood, particularly if there is associated poor parenting (Coon et al., 1992), such predictions weaken for the adolescent years. Temperamental factors, mainly, clearly seem to influence quality of parenting and other socialising influences in the early years.

SOCIAL INFLUENCES

FAMILY DEMOGRAPHIC AND SOCIAL FACTORS

Large family size, overcrowding, parental unemployment, poverty and poor housing are all objective measures which statistical associations with conduct disorder and juvenile lawbreaking. However, the strengths of these associations are outweighed by the stronger associations of the more specific and proximal family influences described below (Rutter et al., 1998).

INDIVIDUAL PARENTAL FACTORS

Parents of conduct disordered adolescents are more likely to have a history of mental disorder, personality disorder, aggressive and criminal behaviour, and alcoholism. There is an increased chance that their marital relationship is disturbed, conflicted and violent. The pregnancy is more likely to have taken place in teenage years and the associated teenage relationships are more likely to involve partner violence (Rutter et al., 1998). Such violence may well be witnessed by children in the household.

These parental factors may promote the development of antisocial behaviour via a number of mechanisms, including genetics, role modelling, neglectful and abusive parental care, and disordered parent-child attachments.

PARENT-CHILD RELATIONSHIPS AND QUALITY OF PARENTAL CARE

Disciplinary styles of parents of conduct disordered adolescents are more likely to be coercive, hostile, critical, harsh, lax, erratic and inconsistent (Patterson, 1982; Patterson et al., 1992). In the extreme this becomes frank physical abuse, rejection and neglect.

Parents of aggressive children may also demonstrate less warmth and affection towards their children (Eron et al., 1991). By contrast, provision of cognitively structured and emotional support predicts decreased antisocial behaviour (Dubow and Ippolito, 1994).

Quality of parenting continues to exert a direct influence on aggressive and antisocial behaviour once a young person enters adolescence. Two of the above factors seem to be particularily crucial – disciplinary style and supervision. Both these factors appear to influence the involvement of the adolescent in antisocial peer groups.

Hostility between parents and antisocial sons can work in both directions (Florsheim et al., 1996). Aggressive behaviour in sons makes it more likely that mothers will emotionally withdraw, supervise less well and become more harsh in parenting (Kandel and Wu, 1995).

PEER RELATIONSHIPS

Aggressive and antisocial behaviours are individual characteristics which, depending on other factors and circumstances, lead to rejection by the adolescent's peer group. Such rejection predisposes the adolescent to greater antisocial behaviour and associated school failure, thus propelling him into the company of antisocial peers. These 'friendships' are less stable and more aggressive than conventional friendships.

Of recorded juvenile offences, 63% are committed by groups of two to three adolescents. Offending rates are higher during membership of a gang compared to the period after leaving the gang (Thornberry *et al.*, 1993). Finally, deviant peer group influences appear to be stronger for older adolescents.

SCHOOL

Rutter and colleagues (1979) showed that the influence of school appears to be strongest for behaviours within the classroom, with much less influence for delinquency outside of the school environment. School factors which exerted a positive influence included classroom management skills, teacher modelling of behaviour, use of rewards and encouragement, giving of responsibility to pupils, and academic expectations for pupils. However, the strength of the school's influence on deliquency is small compared to the influence of the academic ability mix of the peer group, an effect which is mediated via peer group factors. The differing school distribution of intellectual ability of pupils does not appear to affect teacher behaviour, which compounds the detrimental effects of delinquent adolescents clustering in certain schools.

URBAN ENVIRONMENT

Most studies show higher prevalence rates for conduct disorder for children and adolescents living in urban as opposed to rural environments. The mechanisms of influence may include family adversity factors (Rutter *et al.*, 1975), antisocial peer influences and exposure to 'soft drugs' (Wichstrøm *et al.*, 1996).

ETHNIC BACKGROUND

Racial differences for aggression do not become significant until early adolescence. Black American teenagers are much more likely to be arrested for murder, rape, assault, robbery, burglary and car theft than their white peers. However, the black:white ratio reduces significantly when self-report rates are considered.

MEDIA

There is fairly clear evidence that the more a young person watches violence on television, the more aggressive he is likely to be, both in the short and longer term, even after controlling for aggressiveness at the same age. Meta-analytic reviews have demonstrated that the effects of TV violence account for 10% of the variance in childhood aggression (Wood *et al.*, 1991). Various factors affect the degree of influence, including early age, belief in reality of violence, lack of parental supervision and harsh parental discipline. The learning mechanisms may involve the acquisition of new aggressive strategies, experience of the vicarious thrill of the aggressor, belief that aggression is justified, distortion of social realities, increased violent fantasising and desensitisation to the negative effects of violence.

AVAILABILTY OF WEAPONS

There is a clear link between the prevalence of serious violence amoung young people and the availability of firearms. Sadowski *et al.* (1989) reported that 48% of US non-urban adolescent males and 4% of females owned guns.

LIFE EVENTS AND TRANSITION POINTS

There are a number of life events which may function as triggers or exacerbating/ameliorating factors in the development of conduct disorder. These include parental loss by parental separation, expulsion from school, change of home, separation from neighbourhood, physical assault, loss or gain of employment, entry or exit from sexual relationships and detention by the legal system. However, careful research has usually identified factors preceding or following such life events which are more relevant to the development, persistance or desistance of behavioural problems.

Burton *et al.* (1994) reported high levels of post-traumatic symptoms in males with conduct disorder. This is probably not surprising given the number of traumatic experiences to which they are likely to be exposed.

MENTAL PROCESSES

SOCIAL ATTRIBUTIONAL BIAISES AND COGNITIVE DISTORTIONS

Aggressive children attend to few cues when interpreting the meaning of the behaviour of others (Dodge and Newman, 1981) report higher rates of hostile cues (Milich and Dodge, 1984), and attribute other's behaviour in ambiguous situations to their hostile intentions (Dodge *et al.*, 1986, 1990). Finally, they underperceive their own level of aggressiveness and their responsibility for early stages of dyadic conflict (Lochman, 1987).

POOR AFFECT LABELLING AND AROUSAL MANAGEMENT

Garrison and Stolberg, (1983) describe aggressive children as anticipating that they will have fewer feelings of fear or sadness in difficult social situations. When they suddenly experience these emotions, they are more likely to label the generalised arousal as anger.

DEFICITS IN PROBLEM SOLVING SKILLS

Aggressive adolescents tend to have difficulties in the following areas:

- They generate fewer and less socially competent behavioural responses
- They evaluate aggressive behaviour more positively
- They fail to inhibit accessed aggressive responses
- They have relative deficits in using non-aggressive behavioural skills (such as verbal ability and negotiation skills) as alternatives to aggressive responses
- They are less concerned about the negative consequences of their aggression.

Crick and Dodge (1996) showed that distortions in encoding and attributions relate more strongly to reactive aggression, whereas distortions in later stage processes, such as response evaluations, are more typical of proactive aggression.

PSYCHIATRIC CO-MORBIDITY

The majority of adolescents with a diagnosis of conduct disorder also have a co-morbid diagnosis.

ATTENTION DEFICIT HYPERACTIVITY DISORDER (ADHD)

The Ontario Child Health Study showed that 6.7% of boys aged 12–16 years had pure conduct disorder, 3.8% had pure ADDH and 2.9% had both disorders (Szatmari et al., 1989). The corresponding figures for girls were 2.7, 1.6, and 1.6%. Given this degree of overlap, it is not surprising that ICD-10 has created the new diagnosis of hyperkinetic conduct disorder.

ADHD is probably best viewed as a developmental risk factor for later conduct disorder (Taylor et al., 1996). Co-occuring conduct disorder and ADHD predict poorer social adjustment than ADHD or conduct disorder alone. The risk for conduct disorder is greater for adolescents whose ADHD symptoms have persisted rather than abated. Barkley (1997) argued that children with ADHD develop aggressive behaviour problems because of their inability to inhibit aggressive behavioural responses.

DEPRESSIVE DISORDER

Kovacs et al. (1988) estimated that the co-morbidity between depression and conduct disorder in children and adolescents varies from 23 to 36%.

Early psychoanalysts claimed that conduct disorder and delinquency functioned as a form of 'acting out' or psychic defense against depression threatened by early parental 'object loss'. Kovacs *et al.* (1988) showed that depression did indeed develop first, but also that conduct disorder symptoms did not usually reduce after the disappearance of the depressive symptoms with treatment.

Harrington *et al.* (1991) showed that, in contrast to depression, the mixed combination of depression and conduct disorder has no raised risk for adult depression. There is also a lower familial loading for the mixed disorder (Hinshaw *et al.*, 1993; Puig-Antich *et al.*, 1982). To date it would appear that depression in the presence of conduct disorder may be fundamentally different to depression without conduct disorder.

SUBSTANCE MISUSE

Antisocial behaviour precedes substance misuse for both male and female adolescents (Windle, 1990). Substance misuse is also more associated with adolescence-limited conduct disorder. Whatever the mechanisms of onset, adolescent alcohol and drug misuse clearly help to precipitate or perpetuate adolescent behaviour problems for a number of obvious reasons. Intoxication impares social judgements and makes for greater impulsivity. Aggressive tendencies are also likely to be exaggerated. The lifestyle and peer group affiliations of adolescents who misuse substances is also likely to be more generally delinquent, not helped by the illegal status of most recreational drugs. Finally the lifestyle is also likely to impair functioning in school, college or work environments.

DEVELOPMENTAL PATHWAYS

The symptoms of conduct disorder become more diverse with increasing age. Frequency of physically aggressive acts decreases but the potential for inflicting serious harm through violence increases before and through adolescence. The tendency towards antisocial and aggressive behaviours remains very stable over time (Olweus, 1979). Although law-breaking gradually reduces after early adulthood, social and personality dysfunction continues (Farrington, 1995).

Moffitt (1993a) describes two distinct developmental patterns: early onset or life-course-persistant and adolescence–limited. Conduct disorder which develops for the first time in adolescence is less associated with neuropsychological disorder, lower intelligence, AHD, family clustering of externalising disorders and male bias. This subtype is more related to peer influences and substance misuse. By contrast, the early onset group is more likely to be involved in violence and delinquency in adolescence, and to break the law in adulthood.

West and Farrington (1977) showed that a minority of adult criminals were free of conduct disorder during childhood, and that late onset was associated with low social status and criminality of parents.

PROGNOSIS

PREDICTORS

Only a few conduct disorder symptoms are required to yield prediction of adult social dysfunction (Zoccolillo *et al.*, 1992).

Overall severity
Severity can be measured in several ways – symptom count, frequency, pervasiveness, dangerousness, persistance and associated social handicaps. It is the best predictor of persistance into adulthood.

Age of onset
The earlier the age of behavioural disturbance the more likely that antisocial behaviours will persist into adulthood.

Aggression
The best single symptom predictor of poor prognosis is early aggression.

Hyperactivity and attentional difficulties
Loeber *et al.* (1997) showed that hyperactivity was not associated with severity of subsequent antisocial behaviours but rather with their persistence.

Employment
Rutter *et al.* (1998) suggested that young adults who can establish a stable work record can usually escape their previous criminal career.

OUTCOMES

Adult offending
Most adults gradually move away from criminal offending and violence as they move through their 20s. Those who continue have shown violent behaviours from early in childhood and are more likely to be of African-American origin if in the US. This continuation appears to be linked to unemployment and poverty, providing little escape from a delinquent subculture.

Educational/occupational functioning

West and Farrington (1977) showed that young people who developed delinquency in childhood are much more likely to have frequent periods of unemployment as adults. They are more likely to end up in unskilled jobs and to be given the sack.

Teenage pregnancy

Girls with a history of delinquency and conduct disorder are more likely to engage in early sexual activity and become pregnant during their teens (Rutter et al., 1998).

Adult psychiatric morbidity

Of children with conduct disorder, approximately one third develop adult antisocial personality disorder (Robins, 1966). Associated hyperactivity and inattention may predict the conduct disorder most likely to develop into adult antisocial personality disorder (Farrington, 1995).

Alcohol and substance misuse

Alcohol and substance misuse often develops out of earlier antisocial behaviours but in turn exacerbates these behaviours. Windle (1990) reported on data from the National Longitudinal Youth Survey which showed that antisocial behaviour in early adolescence (14–15 years) predicted alcohol and drug use 4 years later – more strongly for males than for females.

Parenting failure

With time antisocial and violent behaviour become less evident on the streets, but also more evident within the family environment. Huesmann et al. (1984) showed continuity between peer-directed aggression at 8 years and partner and child abuse at 30 years. Children of these relationships are also at a heightened risk of developing antisocial behaviours, thus fuelling further cycles of deprivation and behavioural disturbance.

Injury and death

Rydelius (1988) showed a five- to ten-fold increase in death rates of young persons admitted to Swedish probationary schools over a 19 year period. Of the deaths, 88% of boys and 77% of girls died sudden violent deaths – accidents, suicides, death from uncertain causes, murder/manslaughter, or alcohol/drug abuse. However, death as a direct result of drug/alcohol abuse occurred only in boys.

ASSESSMENT AND TREATMENT PLANNING

Parents and adolescent should be interviewed together and separately. Additional information should always be sought from school or college. These sources will be more accurate for specific behavioural areas. Home-based aggression and oppositional behaviour will usually be more accurately rated by parents. Subjective and affective symptoms, peer-related behaviours, and alcohol and substance use will usually be reported more accurately by the adolescent. An interview with the adolescent alone is also important to begin to defuse feelings of mistrust and antagonism, particularily if the young person has been brought to the interview very much against his/her will. Academic performance, social skills, school attendance, and school-based aggression and non-compliance may be reported most accurately by teaching staff.

A systematic review for the possible presence of the frequent co-morbid diagnoses of ADHD, depressive and substance misuse disorders should always be made. In addition, assesment should also be made of the positive strengths and motivation for change in both the young person and family.

Treatment planning should consider all domains of dysfunction. It is important to liaise with school, social worker and probation officer in order to coordinate a treatment package. A professional network planning meeting may be a helpful way of achieving this.

INTERVENTIONS

There is now a large literature describing and evaluating educational, social, legal and community interventions which purport to prevent or ameliorate antisocial behaviours (Rutter *et al.*, 1998). Space here permits only a description of the treatments which mental health professionals are likely to use with adolescents. Inpatient and forensic psychiatric interventions are described in separate chapters.

SPECIFIC PSYCHOLOGICAL TREATMENTS

PARENT MANAGEMENT TRAINING (PMT)

Parent management training (PMT) is based for the most part on social learning theory. In particular it views antisocial behaviour as learned and sustained by positive and negative attention the child receives from social agents, especially parents (Patterson, 1982). That is, PMT uses a predominantly operant model. Although applicable to adolescents as to younger children, evidence suggests that PMT is less effective for adolescents (Dishion and Patterson, 1992). For younger children there is less direct involvement with the child, although for adolescents they may become more involved in negotiating and developing the programme.

Bank *et al.* (1991) compared PMT to court provided family treatment (family therapy, group therapy and drug counselling) for adolescent delinquents (less than 16 years). Parents were trained to use age appropriate rewards and punishments. Offence rates for both groups declined after the onset of interventions. The decline was greater for the parent training group. However, this difference disappeared by 2–3 year follow-up. Non-status offences at 3 years were less for the parent training group.

Social isolation and deprivation are predictors of treatment failure. There are also doubts as to whether treatment gains are maintained at follow-up. There are particular dangers of failing to address the treatment context, e.g. by ignoring parental psychopathology.

FAMILY THERAPIES

The various schools of family therapy conceptualise the problem behaviour of the 'identified patient' as reflective of generalised dysfunction in family relationships. For this reason empirical evaluation of family therapy approaches requires that measures of process and outcome should demonstrate reciprocal relationships between individual and family relationship measures.

Alexander and Parsons (1973) compared 'functional family therapy' (Alexander and Parsons, 1982) with client-centred and psychodynamically orientated family treatment and no-treatment controls. This study included male and female adolescents referred to juvenile court for behaviours such as running away, truancy, theft and unmanageability. Over a 18 month follow-up period the functional family therapy group showed greater improvement on family interaction measures and lower recidivism rates. Interestingly siblings also showed lower rates of referral to juvenile courts over a 2.5 year follow-up. Alexander *et al.* (1976) showed that the effectiveness of treatment is influenced by therapist warmth and directiveness. Process measures of family functioning were related to subsequent recidivism, lending support for the specific mechanisms of functional family therapy.

COGNITIVE PROBLEM-SOLVING SKILLS TRAINING

This approach targets the antisocial beliefs and abnormal cognitive processes described above. The techniques used include self-monitoring, self-instruction, perspective taking, social problem solving, affect labelling and relaxation. These techniques can be used either individually or with groups of adolescents.

A number of outcome evaluations have shown that this approach can produce significant therapeutic change in impulsive, aggressive and antisocial behaviours at home and at school (Baer and Nietzel, 1991).

CONFLICT NEGOTIATION/ANGER MANAGEMENT SKILLS

Feindler and Ecton (1986) have written a short monograph on anger management for adolescents. The approach used builds on Novaco's innovative approach to anger management with adults, and uses a mixture of cognitive and behavioural strategies, both individually and with groups in a style suitable for adolescents. Specifically addressed is the difficult problem of encouraging adolescents to carry out monitoring and homework tasks outside of sessions, crucial to achieve if strategies are to be applied in many different settings and when anger arousal is likely to impede rational thought processes.

'MULTI-SYSTEMIC THERAPY'

This term was coined by Henggeler *et al.* (1998) to describe the coordinated application of different therapeutic approaches to adolescents across different social systems. In particular, they argue that it is crucial to target the adolescent in the family, school and peer environments, and also to address the ways in which events and issues in one system impact on functioning in other systems. For example, family conflict may impact on school functioning, requiring interventions in both systems.

Henggeler's group has also undertaken several evaluation studies (Borduin *et al.*, 1995; Henggeler *et al.*, 1992). Broadly they have been able to report significant positive change both for the individual adolescent (in terms of offending behaviour and other emotional and behavioural measures) and for family relationships, in comparison to more traditional criminal justice interventions. They also showed links between these outcome measures and theoretically important family process measures such as verbal communication and conflict negotiation. The multisystemic approach seems to show good promise although replication by different research groups will be important. However, the approach requires high levels of professional time and resources.

SOCIAL SKILLS TRAINING (SST)

Given the widespread difficulties which conduct disordered adolescents experience in maintaining relationships with non-conduct disordered peers, social skills training (SST) would seem to be a logical intervention. However, there has not been much in the way of empirical validation of SST to date. Beelman et al's (1994) meta-analysis was able to show significant short-term gains for 'social competence training', although these benefits did not tend to persist for the longer term.

SST uses a mixture of techniques, including modelling, behavioural rehearsal, coaching, video feedback, homework tasks and other strategies aiming to promote generalisation of learnt skills across different situations. More recently cognitive strategies have been added, such as developing awareness of affects, promoting thinking aloud to assist self-monitoring, encouraging positive rather than negative cognitions, promoting problem solving and self-control skills. Generally a balance is struck between encouraging prosocial behaviours and discouraging antisocial behaviours.

OTHER GROUP THERAPY APPROACHES

Other non-behaviourally orientated group therapy approaches have been used over the years with delinquent adolescents. There is virtually no scientific evidence for their effectiveness. Unfortunately there is also evidence that group work can worsen antisocial behaviour and substance use (Dishion and Andrews, 1995).

SUBSTANCE MISUSE THERAPIES

Co-morbid substance misuse needs to be treated in its own right and because it exacerbates antisocial behaviours. Various treatment models have been advocated, partly deriving from the adult literature, e.g. response prevention models.

TREATMENT OF OTHER CO-MORBID CONDITIONS

Clearly it is important to provide help in other problem areas identified. However, it is uncertain whether benefits gained in these other problem areas will necessarily spill over into improvements in antisocial behaviours. The specific example of co-morbid depression is discussed briefly in the section on co-morbid disorders. Some have argued that co-morbid anxiety disorder may protect against conduct disorder. By contrast ADHD and substance misuse are disorders whose treatment does seem to bring positive benefits for co-morbid conduct disorder.

DRUG TREATMENTS

The following medications have been advocated as treatment for antisocial behaviours in general and aggression in particular – psychostimulant, antipsychotic. antiepileptc, and antidepressant drugs, lithium and benzodiazepines. However, with the exception of psychostimulants, there is very little in the way of relevant double-blind, placebo-controlled research evidence for their effectiveness.

Short-term investigations have clearly shown that stimulant medication can improve social behaviour in young people with ADHD. There are fewer studies examining the effects of stimulants on oppositional and aggressive behaviours

(Cunningham *et al.*, 1985; Whalen *et al.*, 1987). Hinshaw *et al.* (1989) showed a dose-related effect of methylphenidate on both non-compliance and verbal and physical aggressiveness in 25 boys with ADHD, reducing both to levels comparable with normal controls. Interestingly, there was no effect on non-social or prosocial behaviours. Hinshaw's (1991) review concludes that stimulants seem effective in reducing aggression, although it is unclear whether reactive aggression is more amenable to medication than instrumental aggression.

CONCLUSIONS

Antisocial behaviours in adolescence constitute a very large problem for individual adolescents, their families and society. The efforts of mental health workers will only constitute a drop in the ocean if our efforts are restricted to direct therapeutic work with adolescents and families. I would suggest that we should take a much more proactive role in helping develop innovative interventions and services to be delivered by professional and voluntary groups outside of adolescent mental health teams. Such advice and consultation should be based on the slowly emerging body of research on treatment interventions that work and being clear about those that do not. It may be necessary to advocate protocol-driven treatment packages which nevertheless target the assessed needs of individual adolescents. Finally, the mental health profession should take a strong line with policy makers over public health policy in relation to factors such as preventative programmes, alcohol pricing and availability, and the availability of firearms, particularily within the US.

REFERENCES

Alexander, J. F., Barton, C., Schiavo, R. S. and Parsons, B. V. (1976) Systems behavioural interventions with families of delinquents: therapist character-istics, family behaviour, and outcome. *Journal of Consulting and Clinical Psychology*, **44**, 656–664.

Alexander, J. F. and Parsons, B. V. (1973) Short-term behavioural interventions with delinquent families: impact on family process and recidivism. *Journal of Abnormal Psychology*, **81**, 219–225.

Alexander, J. F. and Parsons, B. V. (1982) *Functional Family Therapy*. Monterey, CA: Brooks/Cole

American Psychiatric Association (1994) *Diagnostic and Statistical Manual of Mental Disorders*, 4th edn (DSM-IV). Washington, DC: American Psychiatric Association.

Baer, R. A. and Nietzel, M. T. (1991) Cognitive and behavioral treatment of impulsivity in children: a meta-analytic review of the outcome literature. *Journal of Clinical Child Psychology*, 20, 400–412.

Bank, L., Marlowe, J. H., Reid, J. B., Patterson, G. R. and Weinrott, M. R. (1991) A comparative evaluation of parent training interventions for families of chronic delinquents. *Journal of Abnormal Child Psychology*, 19, 15–33.

Barkley, R. A. (1997) Behavioural inhibition, sustained attention and executive function: constructing a unified theory of ADHD. *Psychological Bulletin*, 121, 60–94.

Beelman, A., Pfingsten, U. and Lösel F. (1994) Effects of training social competence in children: a meta-analysis of recent evaluation studies. *Journal of Clinical Child Psychology*, 23, 260–271.

Berkowitz, L. (1993) *Aggression: Its Causes, Consequences, and Control.* New York: McGraw-Hill.

Borduin, C. M., Mann, B. J., Cone, L. T., Henggeler, S. W., Fucci, B. R., Blaske, D. M. *et al.* (1995) Multisystemic treatment of serious juvenile offenders: long term prevention of criminality and violence. *Journal of Consulting and Clinical Psychology*, 63, 569–578.

Burton, D., Foy, D., Bwanuasi, C. and Johnson, J. (1994) The relationship between traumatic exposure and post-traumatic symptoms in male juvenile offenders. *Journal of Trauma and Stress*, 7, 83–93.

Caspi, A., Henry, B., McGee, R. O., Moffitt, T. E. and Silva, P. A. (1995) Temperamental origins of child and adolescent behaviour problems: from age three to age fifteen. *Child Development*, 66, 55–68.

Caspi, A. and Silva, P A. (1995) Temperamental qualities at age 3 predict personality traits in young adulthood: longitudinal evidence from a birth cohort. *Child Development*, 66, 486–498.

Cohen, P., Cohen, J., Kasen, S., Velez, C. N., Hartmark, C., Johnson, J. *et al.* (1993) An epidemiological study of disorders in late childhood and adolescence. I. Age and gender specific prevalence. *Journal of Child Psychology and Psychiatry*, 34, 851–867.

Coon, H., Carey, G., Corley, R. and Fulker, D. W. (1992) Identifying children in the Colorado Adoption Project at risk for conduct disorder. *Journal of the American Academy of Child and Adolescent Psychiatry*, 31, 503–511.

Crick, N. R. and Dodge, K. A. (1996) Social information processing mechanisms in reactive and proactive aggression. *Child Development*, 67, 993–1002.

Cunningham, C. E., Siegel, L. S. and Offord, D. R. (1985) A developmental dose-response analysis of the effects of methylphenidate on the peer interactions of attention deficit disordered boys. *Journal of Child Psychology and Psychiatry*, 26, 955–971.

DiLalla, L. F. and Gottesman, I. I. (1989) Heterogeneity of causes of delinquency and criminality: life-span perspectives. *Development and Psychopathology*, 1, 339–349.

Dishion, T. J. and Andrews, D. W. (1995) Preventing escalation in problem behaviours with high-risk and young adolescents: immediate and one-year outcomes. *Journal of Consulting and Clinical Psychology*, **63**, 538–548.

Dishion, T. J. and Patterson, G. R. (1992) Age effects in parent training outcomes. *Behaviour Therapy*, **23**, 719–729.

Dodge, K. A. (1991) The structure and function of reactive vs proactive aggression. In D. J. Pepler, and K. H. Rubin (eds), *The Development and Treatment of Childhood Aggression*. Hillsdale, NJ: Lawrence Erlbaum, pp. 201–218.

Dodge, K. A. and Newman, J. P. (1981) Biased decision-making processes in aggressive boys. *Journal of Abnormal Psychology*, **90**, 375–379.

Dodge, K. A., Pettit, G. S., McClaskey, C. L. and Brown, M. M. (1986) Social competence in children. *Monographs of the Society for Research in Child Development*, **51** (2, Serial no. 213) pp. 1–85.

Dodge, K. A., Price, J. M., Bachorowski, J. A. and Newman, J. P. (1990) Hostile attributional biases in severely aggressive adolescents. *Journal of Abnormal Psychology*, **99**, 385–392.

Dubow, E. F. and Ippolito, M. F. (1994) Effects of poverty and quality of home environment on changes in the academic and behavioural adjustment of elementary school age children. *Journal of Clinical Child Psychology*, **23**, 401–412.

Eaves, L., Silberg, J., Meyer, J., Maes, H., Simonoff, E., Pickles, A., Rutter, M. *et al.* (1997) Genetics and developmental psychopathology: The main effects of gene and environment on behavioural problems in the Virginia Twin Study of Adolescent Development. *Journal of Child Psychology and Psychiatry*, **38**, 965–980.

Eron, L. D., Huesmann, L. R. and Zelli, A. (1991) The role of parental variables in the learning of aggression. In D. J. Pepler and K. H. Rubin (eds), *The Development and Treatment of Childhood Aggression*. Hillsdale, NJ: Lawrence Erlbaum, pp. 169–188.

Farrington, D. P. (1995) The development of offending and antisocial behaviour from childhood: key findings from the Cambridge Study in Delinquent Development. *Journal of Child Psychology and Psychiatry*, **36**, 929–964.

Feindler, E. L. and Ecton, R. B. (1986) *adolescent Anger Control: Cognitive Behavioural Techniques*. New York: Pergamon.

Fingerhut, L. A. and Kleinman, J. C. (1990) International and interstate comparison of homicides among young males. *Journal of the American Medical Association*, **263**, 3292–3295.

Florsheim, P., Tolan, P. H. and Gorman-Smith, D. (1996) Family processes and risk for externalising behaviour problems among African-American and Hispanic boys. *Journal of Consulting and Clinical Psychology*, **64**, 1222–1230.

Garrison, S. T. and Stolberg, A. L. (1983) Modification of anger in children by affective imagery training. *Journal of Abnormal Child Psychology*, **11**, 115–130.

Harrington, R. C., Fudge, H., Rutter, M., Pickles, A. and Hill, J. (1991) Adult outcomes of child and adolescent depression. II: Links with antisocial disorders. *Journal of the American Academy of Child and Adolescent Psychiatry*, **30**, 434–439.

Henggeler, S. W., Melton, G. B. and Smith, L. A. (1992) Family preservation using multisystemic therapy: an effective alternative to incarcerating serious juvenile offenders. *Journal of Consulting and Clinical Psychology*, **60**, 953–962.

Henggeler, S. W., Schoenwald, S. K., Borduin, C. M., Rowland, M. D. and Cunningham, P. B. (1998) *Multisystemic Treatment of Antisocial Behavior in Children and Adolescents*. New York: Guilford Press.

Hinshaw, S. P. (1991) Stimulant medication and the treatment of aggression in children with attentional deficits. *Journal of Clinical Child Psychology*, **20**, 301–312.

Hinshaw, S. P., Henker, B., Whalen, C. K., Erhardt, D. and Dunnington, R. E., Jr. (1989) Aggressive, prosocial, and non-social behavior in hyperactive boys: dose effects of methylphenidate in naturalistic settings. *Journal of Consulting and Clinical Psychology*, **57**, 636–643.

Hinshaw, S. P., Lahey, B. B. and Hart, E. L. (1993) Issues of taxonomy and comorbidity in the development of conduct disorder. *Development and Psychopathology*, **5**, 31–49.

Huesmann, L. R., Eron, L. D., Lefkowitz, M. M. and Walder, L. O. (1984) Stability of aggression over time and generations. *Developmental Psychology*, **20**, 1120–1134.

Inoff-Germain, G., Arnold, G. S., Nottelman, E. D., Susman, E. J., Cutler, G. B., Jr and Chrousos G. P. (1988) Relations between hormone levels and observational measures of aggressive behaviour of young adolescents in family interactions. *Developmental Psychology*, **24**, 129–139.

Kandel, D. B. and Wu, P. (1995) Disentangling mother-child effects in the development of antisocial behavior. In J. McCord (ed.), *Coercion and Punishment in Long-term Perspectives*. Cambridge: Cambridge University Press, pp. 106–23.

Kovacs, M., Paulaskas, S., Gastoris, C. and Richards, G. (1988) Depressive disorders in childhood III A longitudinal study of comorbidity with and risk for conduct disorder. *Journal of Affective Diseases*, **15**, 205–217.

Lochman, J. E. (1987) Self and peer perceptions and attributional biases of aggressive and non aggressive boys in dyadic interactions. *Journal of Consulting and Clinical Psychology*, **55**, 404–410.

Loeber, R., Wung, P., Keenan, K., Giroux, B., Strouthamer-Loeber, M., van Kammen, W. B. *et al.* (1993) Developmental pathways in disruptive child behaviour. *Development and Psychopathology*, **5**, 103–133.

Loeber, R., Keenan, K. and Zhang, Q. (1997) Boys' experimentation and persistence in developmental pathways toward serious delinquency. *Journal of Child and Family Studies*, 6, 321–357.

Lyons, M. J., True, W. R., Eisen, S. A., Goldberg, J., Meyer, J. M., Faraone, S. V. et al. (1995) Differential heritability of adult and juvenile antisocial traits. *Archives of General Psychiatry*, 52, 906–915.

Magnusson, D., Klinteberg, B. and Stattin, H. (1993) Autonomic activity/reactivity, behaviour, and crime in a longitudinal perspective. In J. McCord (ed.), *Facts, Framework, and Forecasts: Advances in Criminological Theory*. New Brunswick, NJ: Transaction, pp. 287–318.

Milich, R. and Dodge, K. A. (1984) Social information-processing patterns in child psychiatric populations. *Journal of Abnormal Child Psychology*, 12, 171–189.

Moffitt, T.E. (1993a) Adolescence-limited and life-course-persistent antisocial behaviour: a developmental taxonomy, *Psychological Review*, 100, 674–701.

Moffitt, T.E. (1993b) The neuropsychology of conduct disorder. *Development and Psychopathology*, 5, 135–52.

Olweus, D. (1979) Stability of aggressive reaction patterns in males: a review. *Psychological Bulletin*, 86, 852–875.

Olweus, D., Mattson, Å., Schalling, D. and Löw, H. (1980) Testosterone, aggression, physical, and personality dimensions in normal adolescent males. *Psychosomatic Medicine*, 42, 253–269.

Olweus, D., Mattson, A., Schalling, D. and Löw H. (1988) Circulating testosterone levels and aggression in adolescent males: a causal analysis. *Psychosomatic Medicine*, 50, 261–272

Patterson, G. R. (1982) *Coercive Family Process*. Eugene, OR: Castalia.

Patterson, G. R., Reid, J. B. and Dishion, T. J. (1992) *Antisocial Boys*. Eugene OR: Castalia.

Pliszka, S. R., Rogeness, G. A., Renner, P., Sherman, J. and Broussard, T. (1988) Plasma neurochemistry in juvenile offenders. *Journal of the American Academy of Child and Adolescent Psychiatry*, 27, 588–594.

Puig-Antich, J. (1982) Major depression and conduct disorder in pre-puberty. *Journal of the American Academy of Child Psychiatry*, 21, 118–128.

Raine, A. (1993) *The Psychopathology of Crime: Criminal Behaviour as a Clinical Disorder*. San Diego, CA: Academic Press.

Robins, L. N. (1966) *Deviant Children Grown Up*. Baltimore, MD: Williams & Wilkins.

Rutter, M., Graham, P. and Yule, W. (1970) *A Neuropsychiatric Study in Childhood*. London: SIMP/William Heinemann.

Rutter, M., Yule, B., Quinton, D., Rowlands, O., Yule, W. and Berger, M. (1975) Attainment and adjustment in two geographical areas: III. Some factors accounting for area differences. *British Journal of Psychiatry*, 126, 520–533.

Rutter, M., Maughan, B., Mortimore, P. and Ouston, J. (1979) *Fifteen Thousand Hours: Secondary Schools and their Effects on Children*. London: Open Books.

Rutter, M., Giller, H. and Hagell, A. (1998) *Antisocial Behaviour in Young People*. New York: Cambridge University Press.

Rydelius, P. A. (1988) The development of antisocial behaviour and sudden violent death. *Acta Psychiatrica Scandanavica*, **77**, 398–403.

Sadowski, L. S., Cairns, R. B. and Earp, J. A. (1989) Firearm ownership among non-urban adolescents. *American Journal of Diseases of Children*, **143**, 1410–1413.

Silberg, J. L., Rutter, M. L., Meyer, J., Maes, H., Hewitt, J., Simonoff. E. *et al.* (1996) Genetic and environmental influences on the covariation among symptoms of hyperactivity and conduct disturbance in juvenile twins. *Journal of Child Psychology and Psychiatry*, **37**, 803–816.

Szatmari, P., Boyle, M. and Offord, D. R. (1989) ADDH and conduct disorders: degree of diagnostic overlap and differences among correlates. *Journal of the American Academy of Child and Adolescent Psychiatry*, **28**, 865–872.

Taylor, E., Chadwick, O., Heptinstall, E. and Danckaerts, M. (1996) Hyperactivity and conduct problems as risk factors for adolescent development. *Journal of the American Academy of Child and Adolescent Psychiatry*, **35**, 1213–1226.

Thornberry, T. P., Krohn, M. D., Lizotte, A. J. and Chard-Wierschem, D. (1993) The role of juvenile gangs in facilitating delinquent behavior. *Journal of Research in Crime and Delinquency*, **30**, 55–87.

Venables, P. H. (1988) Psychophysiology and crime: theory and data. In T. Moffitt and S. A. Mednick (eds), *Biological Contributions to Crime Causation*. Dordrecht: Martinus Nijhoff, pp. 3–13.

West, D. J. and Farrington, D. P. (1977) *The Delinquent Way of Life*. London: Heineman Educational.

Whalen, C. K., Henker, B., Swanson, J. M., Granger, D., Kliewer, W. and Spencer, J. (1987) Natural social behaviors in hyperactive children: dose effects of methylphenidate. *Journal of Consulting and Clinical Psychology*, **55**, 187–193.

Wichstrøm, L., Skogen, K. and Øia, T. (1996) Increased rate of conduct problems in urban areas: what is the mechanism? *Journal of the American Academy of Child and Adolescent Psychiatry*, **35**, 471–471.

Windle, M. (1990) A longitudinal study of antisocial behaviours in early adolescence as predictors of late adolescence substance use: gender and ethnic group differences. *Journal of Abnormal Psychology*, **99**, 86–91.

Wood, W., Wong, F. Y. and Chachere, G. (1991) Effects of media violence on viewers aggression in unconstrained social interaction. *Psychological Bulletin*, **109**, 371–383.

World Health Organisation (1992) *The ICD-10 Classification of Mental and Behavioural Disorders: Clinical Descriptions and Diagnostic Guidelines.* Geneva: World Health Organisation.

Zoccolillo, M., Pickles, A., Quinton, D. and Rutter, M. (1992) The outcome of childhood conduct disorder: implications for defining adult personality disorder and conduct disorder. *Psychological Medicine*, **22**, 971–986.

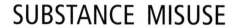

Chapter 6

SUBSTANCE MISUSE

John Merrill and Lesley Peters

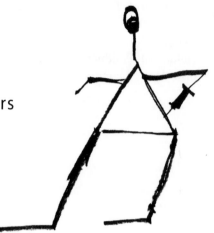

INTRODUCTION

The increasing and widespread use of chemical substances by young people in order to alter mood states has been a feature of the 1990s. Western society's most accepted mood-altering substance, alcohol, is specifically marketed to the young in the form of 'alcopops'. In many areas those that have not taken an illegal drug before leaving school are in the minority. Stimulants and hallucinogens ('dance drugs') were fundamental to the emergence of the predominant youth culture – the 'rave' scene. Heroin addiction among adolescents has become endemic in towns not previously known for their drug problems. Sniffing glue and inhaling aerosol gas remains a major cause of mortality amongst the young.

Official costs of illicit drug misuse in the UK are conservatively estimated at between £3–4 billion a year. For alcohol the costs are £2–3 billion. Neither figure takes into consideration incalculable costs, such as educational underachievement, family break-up and social disharmony.

Although there is now abundant data on the prevalence of adolescent substance use, little is known about its consequences, how it can be prevented and how it should be treated. Compared to treating adults, substance misuse by adolescents is less likely to require medical treatment of dependence and is more likely to be a symptom of a behavioural or conduct disorder. As such, treatment involves a range of therapeutic interventions pursued by multiple disciplines and is less substance orientated.

TERMINOLOGY

There is no universally accepted terminology for describing the various facets of substance misuse.

In this chapter, 'substance use' means the non-medical use of chemical substances in order to achieve alterations in psychological functioning. Substances include alcohol, nicotine, illegal drugs, prescription drugs when not used for medical purposes and volatile substances.

Substance use may be:

Experimental Initial use usually prompted by curiosity

or

Recreational Continued use after initial experimental use that may be infrequent or regular but does not amount to dependent use

or

Dependent Characterised by a compulsion to take the drug in order to experience its psychic effects or avoid the discomfort of abstinence.

Problem or *harmful substance use* refers to the presence of social, psychological or physical problems resulting from the use of substances.

Substance misuse has been interpreted variously as meaning socially unsanctioned use, non-medical use and potentially harmful or harmful use. In this chapter, 'substance misuse' refers to the latter, i.e. substance use that has or may well result in social, psychological or physical problems.

The term 'substance abuse' has been avoided because of its various interpretations and pejorative connotations.

Traditionally, dependence has been divided into physical and psychological dependence – physical dependence being characterised by the presence of observable physical symptoms when the drug is withdrawn, psychological dependence comprising urges to continue using ('craving') or changes in mood states when a drug is stopped. Increased scientific knowledge of the neurobiological basis of substance use has rendered the division into physical and psychological dependence obsolete.

The international diagnostic criteria DSM-IV and ICD-10 have not been validated for adolescent substance misuse and are of little relevance amongst this age group.

PREVALENCE OF ADOLESCENT SUBSTANCE USE

There is now consistent data available from an impressive array of large population studies on the use of both legal and illegal substances (Balding, 1998;

Health Education Authority, 1996; Parker *et al.*, 1995; Ramsay and Spillar, 1997). Whether relying upon household or school surveys, their results will underestimate prevalence rates because substance users will be over-represented amongst the 10–20% that surveys miss, i.e. the homeless and those absent from school as a result of illness or truanting.

DRINKING

By the age of 15–16, 94% of British schoolchildren have drunk alcohol, 78% have been intoxicated and more than half have had more than 5 drinks in a row within the previous month (Miller and Plant, 1996). Four percent of 11–15 year olds drink more than the upper limits recommended for adults. There is good evidence that over the last decade young people drink more frequently and get drunk more often (Royal College of Physicians and British Paediatric Association, 1995) and that excessive drinking is now as common for girls as it is for boys (Miller and Plant, 1996).

SMOKING

Over two-thirds of 15–16 year olds have smoked cigarettes, with 36% smoking within the last month of being questioned and 6% smoking more than 10 cigarettes every day in the last month (Miller and Plant, 1996). Smoking is more common in girls than boys and the prevalence of smoking amongst girls is increasing.

VOLATILE SUBSTANCE ABUSE

Inhalation of volatile substances appears to be increasing with one recent survey reporting 21% of young people ever having done so (Miller and Plant, 1996). The increase is mainly amongst girls who now are just as likely as boys to have inhaled volatile substances.

ILLEGAL DRUGS

About one in twelve 12 year olds, one in three 14 year olds and, by the age of 16, two in five schoolchildren will have taken an illegal drug. Once they have left school, young people's exposure to drug misuse increases further. Of those in their late teens and early 20s, 50% will have used an illegal drug and 25% will use illegal drugs on a regular basis. The proportion of 15–16 year olds who have ever used illegal drugs rose six-fold between 1987 and 1997 (Balding, 1998), and girls are as likely as boys to have used drugs.

The vast majority of illicit drug use is experimental use of cannabis, although more than 10% of 15–16 year olds have smoked cannabis on 40 occasions or more. So-called 'dance drugs' have been used by a minority of 15–16 year olds, with 15% having taken LSD, 13% amphetamine and 8% Ecstasy. Although less than 1% of school children have injected a drug, 1.6% have tried heroin and 2.5% crack cocaine (Miller and Plant, 1996).

INTERNATIONAL COMPARISONS

Adolescent drug use is higher in the UK than the rest of Europe. A survey of nearly 75 000 European 15–16 year olds found 42% of British school children had taken an illegal drug – similar to 41% found using similar methodology in the US. After the UK, the highest lifetime prevalence of drug use was found in Ireland (37%) and the Czech Republic (23%). More ominous for the UK was the greater lead in the proportion of those who had taken a drug 10 times or more – 22% of UK school children, compared to 9% of the second-placed Italians (European Drug Monitoring Centre, 1998).

AETIOLOGY

There is a healthy literature on predisposing and preventative factors for substance misuse (Brook and Brook, 1990; Newcomb *et al.*, 1986; Tsuang *et al.*, 1998) but little is known about their relative importance or how they interact. Harmful substance misuse in young adolescents usually occurs in the context of behavioural disorder and most of the risk factors for substance misuse are also predictive of problem behaviour.

Reducing risk factors and enhancing protective factors is important both for preventing and managing substance misuse.

RISK FACTORS

Risk factors may be classified under environmental factors, interaction with family, peers and school, and individual factors

Environmental risk factors
- Widespread drug availability
- High crime rate
- Poverty and industrial decline
- Acceptance of drug use within community
- Neighbourhood disorganisation

Interaction with family, peers and school
- Low parental affection
- Childhood abuse
- Parental substance misuse
- Family conflict

- Drug using peers
- Peer rejection
- Failure at school
- Low commitment to school
- Dropping out of school

Individual risk factors
- Low self-esteem
- High sensation seeking or risk taking behaviour
- Attitudes favourable to drug use
- Self-destructive behaviour
- Early and persistent behavioural problems
- Genetic vulnerability
- Mental health problems
- Precocious sexual behaviour
- Homeless or in foster care

PROTECTIVE FACTORS

- Positive temperament
- Intellectual ability
- Supportive family environment
- Caring relationship with at least one adult
- External support system that encourages positive values
- Social support system that encourages personal efforts

ASSOCIATED PROBLEMS

Problems associated with substance use arise through a variety of often inter-related ways. They may be due to intrinsic properties of the substance or as a result of dependence, intoxication or withdrawal states. Alternatively they may result from the illegality of a drug, from actions taken in order to fund substance use, from the route of administration of the substance, or from the consequences of leading a 'drug lifestyle'. There is considerable overlap between risk factors and substance-related harm. Establishing cause and effect may not be possible.

Initiation of substance use at a young age is strongly associated with continued use and the development of substance-related harm.

SOCIAL, EDUCATIONAL AND LEGAL PROBLEMS

Substance misuse in adolescence is strongly associated with family dysfunction, childhood abuse, educational underachievement, behavioural problems, dropping out of school, having antisocial attitudes and precocious sexual behaviour.

Substance misusers are over-represented in local authority or foster care and in youth custody facilities.

The prevalence of sexually transmitted diseases is highest amongst adolescents and alcohol use in the young is associated with unsafe sex. Amongst 16–21 year olds the probability of having unsafe sex was directly related to the intensity of drinking (McEwan *et al.*, 1992).

Few dependent substance misusers are able to fund their use through legitimate means. Acquisitive crime, drug dealing and prostitution are common means of raising funds to buy substances. Criminal activity frequently precedes substance use but the onset of regular use is associated with increased offending and substance use is a predictor of re-offending. Violent offences may be carried out in the context of theft but are more often associated with alcohol intoxication or, to a lesser extent, intoxication with benzodiazepines, amphetamine or cocaine. Violence may also be a consequence of paranoia induced by stimulants.

PSYCHOLOGICAL PROBLEMS

The relationship between substance misuse and psychiatric disorder is complex. Both may share common aetiological factors and the presence of one predisposes to the development of the other. It has been suggested that substance misuse may develop as a form of self-medication for those with pre-existing mental illness (Khantzian, 1985). Psychiatric co-morbidity is especially common amongst young adolescents. In a study of adolescents referred to psychiatric services after detoxification, 42% had conduct disorder, 35% major depression, and 21% a combination of attention deficit, hyperactivity and impulsive disorder (DeMilio, 1989).

Substance misuse has been shown to be a significant factor in suicide attempts, repeated attempts and completed suicide. Most countries have witnessed a significant rise in male suicide rates over the last 20 years. The increase has been greatest for young men aged 15–24. Non-fatal suicide attempts are most common amongst young women of similar age. Excessive drinking is an important factor in attempted suicide and subsequent completed suicide in young people (Hawton *et al.*, 1993). One-third of adolescents who kill themselves are intoxicated at the time of death and it has been suggested that 'focussing on drug and alcohol abuse would have a greater impact on adolescent suicide rates than any other primary prevention programme' (Williams and Morgan, 1994).

PHYSICAL PROBLEMS

Substance misuse is associated with both acute and chronic physical problems. Acute problems may result from intoxication, e.g. accidents or overdose. Maintaining a drug lifestyle is associated with poor nutritional status, increased vulnerability to infections and general physical ill health.

Both accidental and non-accidental injury commonly result from substance misuse. A significant proportion of road traffic accident fatalities (both to pedestrians and vehicle occupants) are alcohol-related and adolescents' driving skills are impaired at a lower blood alcohol concentration than that of an adult (Royal College of Physicians and British Paediatric Association, 1995).

Abscesses, cellulitis, septicaemia and deep venous thrombosis are common amongst those who inject drugs. Young injectors may be particularly vulnerable to hepatitis B, C and HIV as they may have limited access to clean injecting equipment and be less aware of routes of viral transmission. Hepatitis C has been detected in about 70% of adult injecting drug users and, like hepatitis B, has a worse prognosis in those who continue to drink alcohol.

Substance misusers die at an earlier age than non-users. Substance-related deaths include the well-recognised morbidity from tobacco, alcohol and blood-borne viruses, accidents, overdoses, suicide, septicaemia, and deaths from natural causes brought about by poor physical health.

ASSESSMENT

All adolescents presenting to psychiatric services must be assessed for substance misuse.

The assessment must be comprehensive and cover the following areas (The Children's Legal Centre and Standing Conference on Drug Abuse, 1999):

- The range of problems the individual has including their use of substances, physical and mental health, and their social, family and educational context
- The needs and requirements for intervention, treatment and care
- The competence of services and its staff to meet the identified needs of the young person
- The young person's capacities, capabilities, development and competence to consent to treatment

SCREENING

Several screening instruments in the form of questionnaires or structured interviews are available for assessing adolescent substance use (Weinberg et al., 1998). A more detailed instrument that assesses substance use in the context of overall psychological functioning and indicates treatment needs and monitoring of progress is also available (Tarter, 1990).

TAKING A HISTORY OF SUBSTANCE USE

The manner in which a history of substance use is elicited is of crucial importance. Minimisation or denial of substance use is common and is facilitated by a brusque or judgmental attitude. The exact pattern and emphasis of the history will vary depending on, amongst other things, the age of the individual, the substances used and the nature of the presenting problem. It may take several appointments before a full history is obtained. In all cases supplementary information should be obtained from others, e.g. parents, partners, social workers and teachers.

The history of substance use should begin with legal substances that are likely to have been used (cigarettes and alcohol), progressing through solvents and cannabis to stimulants, hallucinogens and opiates. Use of prescription drugs (whether prescribed for the individual or not) must be included.

For each substance, the age of first use, frequency of use, amount taken, route of use and periods of abstinence should be established. Enquiries should follow about the problems – physical, psychological, at school/work, familial, social or legal – that the substance has caused. The situations where current use occurs and the reasons for such use should be discussed. Questions should be asked about the positive as well as the negative effects of substance use. Does the individual want to continue, reduce or stop using? What makes stopping difficult? Is there evidence of tolerance, craving or dependence?

Sensitive enquiries should be made about how current use is being funded, e.g. theft, selling drugs, prostitution. For those who inject, the health complications of intravenous use (e.g. abscesses, septicaemia, thrombosis, hepatitis) need to be explored. Where do they get their needles from? Have they ever shared injecting equipment? Where appropriate, evidence of risky sexual behaviours and STDs should be sought. A history of general physical health must be taken.

A psychiatric history should also be taken including details of the adolescent's development, education, mental health, family and social circumstances.

PHYSICAL EXAMINATION

The extent of physical examination will depend on the findings from the history but key areas should always be covered. The arms (and if indicated legs and groin) should be examined for injection sites and sequelae of injecting such as bruising and abscesses. An estimation should be made of whether weight is in accordance with height and age. A low body mass index may be a non-specific sign of poor health secondary to drug use or a specific sign of stimulant-induced weight loss. Dilation or constriction of the pupils may give an indication of recent drug use. An overall assessment should be made as to whether the patient appears intoxicated or to be experiencing withdrawal symptoms.

MENTAL STATE EXAMINATION

Where there is reason to suspect mental health problems a full mental state examination is required.

LABORATORY AND OTHER INVESTIGATIONS

Laboratory investigations are an essential supplement to the assessment and treatment of substance misuse.

Drug urinalysis

Drug urinalysis is an essential adjunct to the history. Enzyme immunoassays using dipstick tests give instantaneous results, but test only for drug classes, and their high sensitivity not uncommonly produces false positives. They may, however, be useful preliminary screens with positive tests being sent to the laboratory for more detailed chromatographic analysis. Urinalysis is limited by the half-life and metabolism of the drug. Use of heroin, cocaine or amphetamine may not be detected more than 48 h after last taken. Metabolites of methadone and benzodiazepines may be detected for 1 week after last use and chronic heavy cannabis use may produce detectable metabolites for up to 1 month.

Hair analysis for drugs

Hair analysis is expensive but has the advantage of providing quantitative analyses over a long period. Hair grows at approximately one cm per month so a 6 cm length of hair can be used to determine drug use over a 6-month period.

Testing for blood-borne viruses

Tests for hepatitis B or C and HIV should never be undertaken without the consent of the adolescent. Testing must be preceded by pre-test counselling by an expert in this area and results must only be given face to face with post-test counselling.

Investigations for alcohol misuse

The most simple and under-used investigation where alcohol misuse is suspected is that of breath alcohol measurement. Breath alcohol meters provide an accurate and inexpensive measurement of breath alcohol concentration which is then converted into the equivalent blood alcohol concentration. A high alcohol concentration produced when an individual is not obviously intoxicated indicates tolerance. Where alcohol intake is chronic, tests of liver function are indicated.

NOTIFICATION OF DRUG MISUSE

Most Western countries have systems of monitoring trends in drug misuse. In the UK this used to involve compulsory notification by doctors to the Home Office of all individuals known or suspected to be addicted to heroin, cocaine and some other drugs. This system has now been superseded by completing forms for the Regional Drug Misuse Databases. Regional Database forms are anonymous, collate information on all substances used, and are completed by the range of professionals concerned with drug misuse and not just doctors.

CASE STUDY 1

An 18-year-old man presented to drug services requesting methadone. He claimed to be injecting 1 g of heroin daily. His General Practitioner had taken a urine sample which was positive for morphine. He aroused suspicion as physical examination did not show injection sites consistent with injecting three or four times per day. A subsequent urine test was negative for morphine. He was not prescribed methadone.

TREATMENT

Whilst older adolescents not uncommonly present for treatment at their own initiative, younger adolescents are more likely to be referred by a parent or a concerned professional. This could include teachers, youth workers, social workers, probation officers, educational psychologists, school health workers, hospital accident and emergency departments, family doctors, and child psychiatrists. At least some of these disciplines are likely to have important roles in treatment which usually entails addressing multiple targets through a coordinated multiagency approach with statutory and non-statutory, specialist and generic services.

Services for treating the younger adolescent are poorly developed and in many areas do not exist. Further, there is a definite lack of training in the recognition and management of substance misuse by those professionals most likely to be in contact with and in a position to help young substance misusers.

REQUIREMENTS OF YOUNG PEOPLE'S SUBSTANCE MISUSE SERVICES

There are considerable risks in providing adolescent substance misuse services at adult-orientated services. Unlike adults, younger adolescents who present for treatment have only rarely developed dependence and there is a considerable risk that youngsters may find the lifestyles of adults attending the service glamorous and appealing.

Young people's substance misuse services should (Health Advisory Service, 1996):

- Provide advice and treatment that is sensitive to the specific needs of children and young people and is separate from adult services
- Be appealing to young people to encourage self-referral
- Be available out of school hours and at convenient and non-stigmatising sites

- Have staff who are experienced with working both with young people and substance misuse
- Provide a holistic approach to treatment within the context of addressing other needs the young person is likely to have
- Have established routes of referral, coordination and collaboration between education, social services, voluntary services, youth services, youth justice service, police, family doctors, paediatricians and child psychiatrists
- Routinely involve the family in treatment

CONFIDENTIALITY AND CONSENT

An important factor in determining whether a young person will divulge their substance use to others or present for treatment is whether confidentiality will be maintained. To be able to offer treatment (be it in the form of medication, provision of clean injecting equipment, counselling or advice), consent to treatment must be obtained. In UK law there is an assumption that those aged under 16 years old are not competent to give informed consent which must be obtained from a parent or those with parental responsibility for the young person (e.g. social services). Those aged under 16 may be 'competent' to consent depending on factors which include their age, maturity and the treatment concerned (The Children's Legal Centre and Standing Conference on Drug Abuse, 1999).

Confidentiality is not an absolute, especially in matters affecting children. The 1989 United Nations' 'Convention on the Rights of the Child' considers the welfare of the child as paramount and young people may not be the best judges of what is in their best interest. Confidential information may have to be disclosed if there are concerns that a child or adolescent is suffering, or at risk of suffering, significant harm. This applies whether the child is the substance misuser or the child of a substance misuser.

Adolescents should always be encouraged to allow the involvement of parents and significant others in their treatment. Whether confidentiality is maintained or breached will depend upon the seriousness of the substance misuse, the multiplicity of problems and agencies involved, and whether the problem is static, worsening or getting better.

GENERAL INTERVENTIONS

Harm reduction

The aim of treatment is to prevent harm resulting from substance misuse. For most misused substances eliminating harm would entail stopping substance use completely. Whilst abstinence may be a goal of treatment, especially in younger adolescents and for the more dangerous substances, to restrict treatment to those who are willing or able to stop using would exclude the vast majority of users, and so ignore most of the harm to individuals and society that results from substance use.

Harm reduction (or harm minimisation) is a pragmatic response to substance misuse which often uses a series of intermediate goals. For a heroin injector, the immediate goal might be to stop using injecting equipment used by others. Subsequent intermediate goals might be to reduce and stop injecting by undergoing a period of methadone maintenance, followed ultimately by gradual detoxification from methadone. Intermediate goals will also usually be required to address other areas.

Principles of harm reduction may be applied outwith a treatment context. Examples include public media broadcasts on the dangers of drinking and driving, providing information to club-goers on how to avoid dehydration if taking Ecstasy, and instructing drug users what action to take if a friend overdoses.

Needle and syringe exchange

The threat of an HIV epidemic catalysed rapid expansion in drug treatment services. An influential UK government advisory group summarised the then prevailing situation as 'The spread of HIV is a greater threat to individual and public health than drug misuse. Accordingly, we believe that services which aim to minimise HIV risk behaviour by all available means should take precedence in development plans' (Advisory Council on the Misuse of Drugs, 1988).

The most important development in HIV (and hepatitis) prevention amongst drug users has been the widespread development of needle and syringe exchange schemes. They operate from a variety of settings including drug treatment services, non-statutory street agencies, community pharmacies and may be provided by outreach workers. The provision of injecting equipment to those aged under 16 is fraught with issues of competency and confidentiality. Nevertheless, young injectors who are unable to stop need to be provided with clean equipment and exchange schemes offer valuable opportunities to engage young people in treatment. This process can be enhanced and the danger of mixing with adult drug users minimised by arranging for young people to have injecting equipment supplied at appointments with professionals involved in their care.

Motivational enhancement

Adolescents may show no motivation to address their substance misuse. Indeed, their use of drugs and alcohol may be their main or only source of pleasure. Further, substance misuse runs a chronic relapsing course and motivation waxes and wanes. A 'stages of change' model has been proposed which recognises pre-contemplation, contemplation and action phases (Prochaska and DiClemente, 1992). Motivational interviewing techniques (Miller and Rollnick, 1991) accept that ambivalence to change is the norm with there being advantages and

---

CASE STUDY 2

A 15-year-old who funded heroin use through prostitution attended a needle exchange service requesting needles, syringes and condoms. She told the voluntary worker that she was having unprotected sex and sharing injecting equipment. She understood the risks of her behaviours. She was judged competent to consent to treatment and given a limited supply of injecting equipment and condoms on condition that she returned the next day for a full assessment. At her subsequent appointment it was agreed that confidentiality would not be breached by telling her parents. She would continue to receive injecting equipment and condoms until detoxification and rehabilitation could be arranged. Efforts would continue to be made to persuade her to involve her parents who would be able to administer naltrexone after detoxification.

---

disadvantages to continued substance use. By examining and challenging adolescent's perceptions of the advantages and disadvantages, the balance may be shifted in the direction of change.

Family therapy

A fundamental tenet of treating young substance misusers is to involve the family. There may be obstacles including reluctance by the adolescent or by parents, because of parental substance misuse, childhood abuse, or the family may have fragmented. Nevertheless, such issues are likely to be relevant to the young person's substance misuse and the family's acceptance of being involved in treatment is likely to be therapeutic in itself.

Several theory-based family therapies have been shown to be effective in improving parent–adolescent relationships and reducing substance use including systems-based, strategic and behavioural models (Weinberg *et al.*, 1998). Families are also likely to benefit from practical advice on issues such as setting limits and conflict resolution. Attendance at family support groups is likely to be helpful.

Relapse prevention

Relapse prevention is an important component of treatment which involves examining factors implicated in previous relapses, anticipating 'high-risk' situations, devising strategies to deal with these situations and putting them into practice (Marlatt and George, 1979). Behavioural techniques involving contingency contracting may be useful. In the US high value is placed on attendance at '12-step' groups, although elsewhere such groups are uncommon.

Management of co-morbidity

The management of co-existing substance misuse and mental illness begins with diagnosis. This is seldom straightforward. Symptoms of mental illness are common features of both intoxication and withdrawal states. The most difficult diagnostic dilemma is distinguishing between a psychotic illness arising solely from drug use and schizophrenia in a young person misusing drugs, most notably stimulants. Substance-induced psychotic symptoms will usually subside within a few days of abstinence. Persisting psychotic symptoms in the absence of continued drug use indicates alternative causation. Whatever the aetiological factors, there is a need to alleviate distress and behavioural disturbance with antipsychotic medication.

Both the substance misuse and psychiatric disorder will need treatment plans. The presence of substance misuse should not mean that accepted treatments are withheld but, conversely, psychiatric disorders may require more intense treatment. Special vigilance is required with pharmacological treatments (Myles and Wilner, 1999). Methylphenidate has a high potential for abuse, some antidepressants may have adverse interactions with stimulants and precautions should be taken to prevent overdose of prescribed medication. There is an identified role for psychological treatments. Depressive disorders in substance misusers may respond well to cognitive behaviour therapy (Kaminer et al., 1998). Co-morbidity requires intensive treatment to all aspects of the adolescent's problems.

Meeting the treatment needs of patients with co-morbidity presents problems with service delivery. Psychiatric and substance misuse services rarely have the requisite knowledge or facilities to manage all aspects of treatment independently. Specialist 'dual diagnosis' services are emerging for the treatment of co-morbidity in adults. Similar service development for adolescents needs evaluation.

SPECIFIC INTERVENTIONS

Alcohol detoxification

In the relatively infrequent instances where adolescents have become dependent on alcohol and experience withdrawal symptoms, detoxification is required. This is best achieved using reducing doses of benzodiazepines (typically chlordiazepoxide or diazepam). Vitamin B supplements should also be prescribed. With daily support from a health worker, detoxification can often be achieved without admission to hospital.

Disulfiram (Antabuse) may be a useful adjunct to relapse prevention. Disulfiram acts as a deterrent by producing unpleasant physical symptoms if alcohol is consumed. Compliance with disulfiram treatment is best achieved by ensuring the drug is administered daily by a parent or carer. Acamprosate is a relatively new medication which reduces relapse following detoxification and is thought to have an anti-craving effect. The role of these drugs in treating adolescents is, as yet, uncertain.

Heroin detoxification

Heroin dependence in young adolescents is not uncommon. Over one-third of teenage heroin users are aged under 16 (Parker *et al.*, 1998b). Whilst detoxification using reducing doses of methadone remains the most common method amongst adults, the potential for fatal overdose, prolonged withdrawal symptoms from methadone and a tendency for reducing doses to become maintenance makes methadone far from ideal in this age group.

Lofexidine is a clonidine analogue that has proved effective in reducing most of the symptoms of opiate withdrawal and is the treatment of choice in adolescents. Detoxification can usually be achieved in community settings with daily support and monitoring of blood pressure. Adjuncts to lofexidine in the form of anti-diarrhoeals and night sedation may be required.

Failure at completing detoxification in the community may require inpatient admission. Rapid methods of opiate detoxification using opiate antagonists (naltrexone or naloxone) may offer the best chance of completing detoxification but should only be used in hospitals.

A daily dose of 50 mg of naltrexone will prevent relapse into opiate dependence. Compliance is enhanced if naltrexone administration is supervised by an adult. Unless following rapid detoxification using antagonists, naltrexone will precipitate severe withdrawal symptoms if initiated less than a week following last opiate use.

Methadone maintenance

Methadone maintenance substantially reduces illicit drug use, injecting and crime, whilst improving physical health, mental health and social functioning of heroin users (Ward *et al.*, 1998). It should not be a first-line treatment for adolescents but may have an invaluable role if detoxification is not feasible as it 'buys time' to allow progress to be made on other issues. Extreme caution must be taken when initiating treatment in young heroin misusers. Dependence must be established beyond doubt by sequential drug urinalysis and observation of withdrawal symptoms. The starting dose of methadone should be low and titrated upwards slowly according to response. Methadone should be dispensed on a daily basis and its administration should be supervised by a parent, carer, pharmacist or health professional.

Buprenorphine has recently been introduced as an alternative to methadone. It has the advantage of being safer in overdose and is easier to withdraw from. Buprenorphine is likely to be increasingly used for the treatment of adolescent heroin dependence.

Inpatient and residential facilities

Inpatient treatment is indicated for adolescents who are suicidal, acutely psychotic, severely impaired because of their substance misuse or psychiatric illness, a danger to themselves or others, or unable to receive appropriate assessment or treatment in the community (American Academy of Child and Adolescent Psychiatry, 1997). Specialist inpatient adolescent substance misuse services are scarce. Adolescent psychiatric units may be more appropriate for some. Alternatively next-best options including adult substance misuse units, general hospital or psychiatric beds may have to be considered.

Residential adolescent substance misuse services are helpful for those who lack psychosocial support or have relapsed after inpatient treatment. Usually a stay of several months is recommended. Sadly residential facilities are also scarce.

CASE STUDY 3

A school teacher referred a 15-year-old boy who was sniffing glue and drinking 2 litres of strong cider each day. He was truanting, had recently had *grand mal* fits and described hearing voices. Immediate inpatient treatment was required for alcohol detoxification and physical investigations. There was no local adolescent substance misuse unit. Admission to an adult medical ward was thought more appropriate than a paediatric ward or psychiatric unit. Auditory hallucinations resolved rapidly and physical investigations showed no abnormality. He described intense social anxiety at school. A case conference was arranged involving his teacher, parents and adolescent psychiatrist to establish a treatment plan.

PREVENTION

Preventing substance misuse involves reducing both supply and demand. Reducing supply is essentially about legislation and law enforcement. For legal substances, e.g. alcohol and tobacco, there is good evidence that increasing their price, restricting advertising and limiting availability (e.g. by having limited licensing hours) reduces overall consumption. Reducing demand is about education and treatment: stopping initial use (primary prevention) and preventing escalation of substance use (secondary prevention). A further aim of prevention is to reduce the harms to individual substance users and the general population that are a consequence of substance misuse (tertiary prevention).

EDUCATION

More is known about what has been shown to be ineffective in preventing substance misuse than what is effective. Using fear as a deterrent to using drugs merely reinforce anti-drug attitudes in those least likely ever to use, leaving those most at risk unaffected. Some programmes aim to prevent cannabis use on the over-simplistic assumption that cannabis is a gateway drug into illicit drug use. There is merit in preventing early use of substances but drinking and smoking are also strongly predictive of subsequent illicit drug use and are more harmful than cannabis. 'Just say No' campaigns based on the unsupported premise that adolescents use drugs because of peer pressure ignore the reality which is that most young people see at least some attraction in drug taking and 'peer preference' seems a more apt concept (Coggans and McKellar, 1994).

There is now widespread acceptance that prevention initiatives should start in primary school. This would seem essential in order to influence children before they have started using substances. Further, whist older children take more notice of what their peers think, younger children are more influenced by teachers. Programmes should be delivered by teachers and include factual information on legal and illegal substances and their associated harms. They should be a component of ongoing education in life skills aimed at personal and social development including problem solving, decision making, increasing self-esteem and constructive use of leisure time.

Prevention initiatives should be flexible and adapted to suit local circumstances and cultures. There is scope for targeting highly intensive programmes to those at particular risk, e.g. adolescents in custody or in the care of social services, and involving out-of-school interventions through youth clubs and parents.

As yet, the most effective school-based prevention programmes have been shown only to bring about a short-term delay in initial substance use and a short-term reduction in use by current users (Dorn and Murji, 1992; White and Pitts, 1998). Given the strong association between early substance use and the development of substance-related and other problems, delaying the onset of substance use is a worthy goal. It is, however, only a proxy for the true test of success which is reducing future harmful drug use.

SUBSTANCES USED

Features of the most commonly used substances are listed according to their predominant actions – depressants, stimulants, hallucinogens – with those that are not easily categorised described under 'others'.

DEPRESSANTS

Alcohol

Alcohol depresses the central nervous system, releasing inhibitions and reducing social anxiety. In higher doses reflexes, co-ordination and judgement are impaired, and aggression may be released leading to violence. Alcohol also potentiates effects of other drugs, e.g. opiates and benzodiazepines. The young are more susceptible to toxic effects of alcohol than adults, and drinking less than one bottle of spirits may result in toxic overdose with loss of consciousness, seizures and death.

Alcohol problems in the young are more likely to be caused by intoxication than dependence. Between a quarter and a half of 15 year olds drink to experience the perceived social benefits of alcohol including fun, reducing shyness, helping 'chat up' prospective partners. About 20% drink to relieve boredom and up to one-third drink with the intention of getting drunk (Parker et al., 1998b).

The relationship between adolescent and adult drinking is uncertain; however, early onset of drinking is predictive of later illicit drug use (Bagnall, 1988).

Volatile substances

Volatile substance abuse (VSA) is also referred to as 'inhalant abuse', 'solvent abuse' or 'glue sniffing'. Easily obtainable products containing volatile substances include adhesives, typewriter correction fluids, aerosols, bottled gas, petrol, paint strippers and thinners, and lighter fuel. Substances are inhaled from plastic bags, typically an empty crisp packet, or poured onto a sleeve or cloth and inhaled, 'huffing'. Aerosols can be sprayed directly into the throat. This is especially dangerous as the resulting sudden cooling of the pharynx can cause cardiac arrhythmias and death. VSA may be detected by a characteristic sweet smelling breath or a facial rash covering areas exposed through inhalation from a plastic bag.

Whilst all volatile substances have an onset of action occurring seconds after inhalation and similar behavioural effects, metabolism and elimination vary depending on their specific chemical properties (Dinwiddie, 1994). The duration of intoxication produced by butane gas lasts only a few minutes whereas the effects of toluene (from glue) take 30 to 60 min to subside (Evans and Raistrick, 1987a). Typically doses are 'topped up' when the effects subside. One reason for the popularity of VSA amongst school children is the ability to become intoxicated between lessons or after school and return to class or home completely sober.

The effects of volatile substances are similar to alcohol intoxication. They include: euphoria, disinhibition, impulsiveness, giddiness, nausea, vomiting, tinnitius, ataxia, slurred speech, disordered perception of the passing of time, illusions, and (occasionally) transient visual hallucinations and persecutory delusions. There may be partial or total amnesia for events that occurred whilst intoxicated. Extreme intoxication may lead to disorientation, fits, unconscious-ness, coma and death. Following acute intoxication feelings of drowsiness, lethargy, nausea and headaches may last for a further 30 min or so. Chronic use has been associated with neurological effects including memory impairment, poor concentration, cerebellar disease, peripheral neuropathy and myopathy.

Chronic use may result in tolerance and a withdrawal syndrome comprising sleep disturbance, nausea, tremor, sweating, irritability, chest and abdominal discomfort lasting from 2 to 5 days (Evans and Raistrick, 1987b).

In the UK there are 50–100 deaths annually from VSA, the majority aged under 18. Causes of death include cardiac arrhythmias, inhalation of vomit, asphyxia (through inhaling from a plastic bag placed over the head) and trauma or accidents occurring whilst intoxicated. There have been isolated reports of death due to hepatic or renal toxicity.

VSA typically occurs amongst adolescents and rarely persists into adulthood. The prognosis is worse for those whose VSA is a solitary activity than for those who use with friends.

Cannabis

Cannabis is usually smoked in the form of resin (the concentrated sap of the *Cannabis sativa* plant) which is mixed with tobacco in a reefer or 'joint'. Alternatively, cannabis leaves ('grass') may be rolled into a reefer and smoked. After smoking, acute subjective effects peak between 20 and 30 min and last 2–3 hours. When cannabis is taken by mouth, the onset of action is slower. The principal psychoactive ingredient is Δ^9-tetrahydrocannabinol (Δ^9-THC). Varia-tions in breeding and cultivation techniques of the cannabis plant have resulted in cannabis preparations that vary widely in Δ^9-THC content.

Acute effects of the drug include euphoria and a feeling of well-being, relaxation, heightened sensitivity to external stimuli, a distorted sense of time, increased appetite, increased heart rate, and bloodshot eyes. Adverse effects include anxiety (particularly in novice users), slowed psychomotor perform-ance, and impaired attention, concentration and coordination. Depersonalisa-tion and derealisation, hallucinations and paranoid ideas may occur. Psycho-logical set and social setting are extremely important to the subjective experience.

Although by the end of their teens most people in the UK, US and Australia will have tried cannabis, most will stop using the drug in their 20s. About one in 10 who have ever used cannabis become daily users at some time. Amongst regular users, tolerance to the effects of the drug is recognised and a dependence syndrome with a mild withdrawal reaction may occur (Hall and Solowij, 1998).

Toxic confusional states with psychotic features and short-lived psychotic episodes in clear consciousness may occur with high doses or in those who are especially sensitive to the drug's effects. Cannabis may precipitate a relapse of acute schizophrenia, but there is no convincing evidence that cannabis use causes schizophrenia. Chronic intoxication may cause amotivation and apathy.

Cannabis may cause diseases of the respiratory tract, including bronchial carcinoma. There are no known cases of death from cannabis poisoning.

Opiates

The term 'opiates' refers to natural drugs derived from the opium poppy, *Papaver somniferum*, and includes morphine and codeine. Synthetic derivatives of morphine such as heroin (diacetylmorphine) and entirely synthetic drugs with morphine-like actions, e.g. methadone, are correctly termed 'opioids'. In practice the two terms are used interchangeably.

Acute effects of opiates include euphoria, analgesia, drowsiness, miosis, respiratory depression, nausea, vomiting and decreased gastric motility. Respiratory depression is the most common cause of death in opiate overdose. Tolerance and dependence develop rapidly. The withdrawal syndrome begins with craving for the drug, dilated pupils, lacrimation, rhinorrhoea, yawning, sweating, and is followed by anorexia, gooseflesh, restlessness, irritability, tremor, nausea and vomiting, diarrhoea, stomach cramps, increased blood pressure and heart rate, muscle and bone pain, insomnia, and hot and cold flushes. Although acute withdrawal symptoms subside in 1–2 weeks, dysphoria and sleep disturbance may linger for much longer.

In the UK, heroin ('brown' or 'gear') is commonly bought in 'bags' which contain about 0.1 g of 40% purity. Bags cost about £10 but greater quantities attract discount so 1 g costs £50–80. Initial heroin use is usually by smoking – inhaling the fumes when heroin powder is heated on tin foil, 'chasing the dragon'. Injecting ('fixing') the drug enhances the initial feelings of intoxication ('the rush') and is more cost-effective. Heroin can also be snorted intranasally, but this is uncommon in the UK. The effects of heroin last 4–6 h so three or four doses each day are needed to prevent withdrawal symptoms.

Other commonly misused opiates include codeine, dihydrocodeine, dextromoramide, pethidine, buprenorphine, morphine sulphate, dipipanone and methadone. Methadone prescribed for the treatment of heroin addiction all too frequently is sold on the street. For many young people methadone is the first opiate drug they have used and fatalities from overdose are not uncommon.

Sedatives

Just as benzodiazepines have replaced barbiturates as the most commonly prescribed sedative in clinical practice, they have also replaced barbiturates as the most commonly misused sedative.

Benzodiazepines are usually taken by mouth although tablets are frequently crushed and injected. They may be taken alone, used in conjunction with other depressants (e.g. alcohol or opiates) to enhance the effect, used with stimulants to reduce anxiety that may be produced by stimulants, or taken to relieve withdrawal symptoms from other drugs.

The effects sought from intoxication are similar to those from alcohol. Accidents may result from sedation and psychomotor impairment. Aggression may be released and acts of extreme violence have been committed whilst under the influence of benzodiazepines. Amnesia for the period of intoxication may occur.

Suddenly stopping benzodiazepines after regular use can result in a withdrawal syndrome. A variety of psychological, physiological and perceptual symptoms occur with different constellations of symptoms occurring in different people. The original symptoms for which the drugs were prescribed can return and can be difficult to disentangle from true withdrawal symptoms. Withdrawal symptoms are uncommon amongst adolescents who are more likely to binge on benzodiazepines rather than take them on a daily basis.

Gamma hydroxybutyric acid

Gamma hydroxybutyric acid (GHB) occurs naturally in the central nervous system, although its function is unknown. It is taken by mouth, usually dissolved in water to produce a euphoric effect which may last for more than 24 h. GHB has also been used by body builders to increase muscle bulk. The dose needed to achieve euphoria is close to that which induces coma, and deaths from using GHB have been reported.

STIMULANTS

Nicotine

Nicotine is one of the most addictive substances known. Smoking tobacco is the greatest cause of preventable illness and premature death in the Western world. Smoking is closely associated with illicit drug use. Few who have never smoked have tried illegal drugs. Whilst overall smoking is becoming less popular, smoking in adolescent girls is becoming more common. Tobacco companies have been criticised for directing marketing towards the young. There is also strong evidence that points towards adolescent girls using the anorexic properties of nicotine to control their weight.

Amphetamine

After cannabis amphetamine is the most commonly used illicit drug in the UK. Its popularity amongst adolescents is due to its prominence within the 'rave' dance culture, ready availability, low cost and, amongst girls, its anorectic properties.

Amphetamine is a synthetic analogue of adrenaline. Illicit amphetamine ('speed', 'whizz' or 'sulphate') is usually amphetamine sulphate in the UK and methylamphetamine (methamphetamine) in the US. Amphetamine sulphate is cheap, costing about £5–8 for 1 g of low purity (typically 5%) powder in the UK. It is also available as more potent 'paste'. Amphetamine can be taken by mouth, snorted through the nose or injected. A smokeable form of methylamphetamine is popular in some areas of the US. Methylphenidate and pemoline are amphetamine-related drugs with abuse potential.

Effects include enhanced wakefulness, decreased fatigue, decreased appetite, elevation of mood and increased self-confidence that last about 4 h. Adverse physical effects are generally due to the sympathomimetic actions of amphetamine, and include headaches, sweating, tension in the jaw muscles, grinding of the teeth, chest pain, hypertension, palpitations, cardiac arrhythmias and hyperthermia. Delirium, convulsions and coma may occur. Of particular importance to children is a risk of growth retardation with regular use. Adverse psychological effects include agitation, panic attacks, automatic stereotyped behaviour and paranoia. Psychotic episodes with hallucinations and paranoid delusions can occur. Such an amphetamine psychosis resembles an acute schizophrenic episode. Amphetamine psychosis usually settles within a few days of stopping the drug but cases have been reported which last several weeks.

Most amphetamine use is recreational. After such use, withdrawal symptoms are minimal. Heavy amphetamine users typically take the drug in 'runs', delaying withdrawal symptoms by repeatedly using several grams of illicit amphetamine without sleeping over a few days. This is followed by the 'crash', a period of exhaustion, lethargy, low mood, sleepiness and excessive appetite. When amphetamine is used on most days, tolerance and dependence develop. Withdrawal symptoms can be severe with pronounced craving for the drug, agitation, depression and suicidal ideation.

Cocaine

Cocaine is a stimulant drug with properties very similar to amphetamine. Although available in powder form which is snorted or injected, most cocaine use in the UK is the smokeable form of 'crack' cocaine ('base', 'rock' or 'wash'). In the UK cocaine use is less prevalent than that of amphetamine, but in the US the reverse is true.

When snorted, the effects of cocaine are relatively long-lasting and the drug's vasoconstrictive action limits the amount absorbed. Injecting or smoking cocaine produces immediate, short-lived effects with marked withdrawal symptoms ensuing 10–15 min later. Subsequent cravings to repeat the high are intense.

Cocaine is more cardiotoxic than amphetamine and sudden death may occur through respiratory failure, cardiac arrhythmias or intracerebral haemorrhage. Smoking crack may burn the respiratory tract causing black or bloody sputum. Snorting cocaine may cause necrosis of the nasal septum. A cocaine psychosis similar to that seen with amphetamine can occur. Tactile hallucinations and the belief that the skin is infested leads to itching: this is formication, 'cocaine bug'.

MDMA (Ecstasy)

MDMA (3,4-methylene dioxymethamphetamine) is an amphetamine analogue. The most sought after effect of MDMA is to increase openness and empathy towards others. The stimulant and 'empathogenic' effects have made MDMA central to the 1990s dance music culture.

MDMA sells for about £10–15 for a 125 mg tablet. It is taken orally and the effects last for about 4 h. Withdrawal symptoms after one or two tablets are mild and similar to withdrawal from amphetamine. MDMA is rarely, if ever, taken on a daily basis.

Anxiety, panic attacks, depression and paranoid psychoses have been attributed to MDMA use but with little substantiating evidence. Deaths from taking MDMA are rare but attract widespread publicity. They are usually the result of malignant hyperthermia ('heatstroke') resulting from a combination of dancing in a hot environment and MDMA's actions of increasing body temperature and impeding hypothalamic temperature control. These are largely avoidable by 'chilling out' from the dance floor and taking regular non-alcoholic drinks. Some deaths appear to have resulted from MDMA-induced liver failure.

MDMA causes serotonergic neurone loss in animals. There is concern that this may occur in humans. As yet, there is little clinical evidence of long-term damage. However, surveys of MDMA users show empathogenic qualities of the drug diminish the more the drug is taken, and subtle cognitive deficits and impaired neurotransmitter functioning proportional to lifetime MDMA use have been reported. That an estimated half a million young people take MDMA in the UK every week gives cause for concern.

Methylene dioxyamphetamine (MDA) and methylene dioxyethamphetamine (MDEA) have similar effects to MDMA but are less emphathogenic.

HALLUCINOGENS

Lysergic acid diethylamide (LSD)

LSD ('acid') is the archetypal hallucinogen. It is extremely potent and taken by mouth on paper squares ('blotters' or 'trips') impregnated with 50–150 µg of the drug that sell for as little as £2. Effects may last up to 12 h and include elation/euphoria, depersonalisation, derealisation, a slowing of sense of time, dream-like imagery, visual distortions and synaesthesias, e.g. 'seeing' smells or 'hearing' colours and feelings of having great insight. Adverse effects include experiencing a 'bad trip' with feelings of panic and frightening imagery/sensory distortions. The set and setting have a profound bearing on the drug's effect. 'Flashbacks' where part of a previous 'trip' is relived sometimes occur, usually when the subject is under the influence of other drugs, most notably cannabis. The relationship between acute and chronic psychoses and LSD is open to conjecture. There are no reports of deaths due to LSD toxicity, but suicides and accidental deaths have occurred during periods of intoxication.

LSD was a cornerstone of the 'hippy' counterculture and has re-emerged with the 1990s dance scene. Doses taken tend to be lower than in the 1960s as profound 'hallucinatory' experiences are not generally sought.

Psilocybe mushrooms

Psilocybin and psilocin, the psychoactive ingredients in 'magic' mushrooms, have similar effects to LSD but are less potent. The mushrooms grow abundantly in temperate climates during the autumn. They are either eaten shortly after picking, cooked or preserved for later use by drying or freezing. More poisonous mushrooms may be consumed in error. Mescaline derived from the Mexican peyote cactus has similar effects.

Phencyclidine and ketamine

Phencyclidine (PCP or 'Angel Dust') was used as a dissociative anaesthetic but the high incidence of hallucinations produced resulted in its replacement by ketamine. Phencyclidine use is rare in the UK but relatively common in the USA. In the UK, ketamine ('K', 'Special K') has emerged as a popular drug on the rave dance scene. The actions and effects of phencyclidine are similar to but stronger than those of ketamine. Both drugs cause pronounced sympathetic stimulation, increased muscle tone, repetitive movements, disorientation, distorted body image, euphoria, hallucinations and anxiety. The dissociative effects can be controlled by experienced users to cause insightful 'trips'. Adverse effects include hyperthermia, violence, catalepsy and coma, bad trips, flashbacks, psychosis, depression, memory impairment and visual disturbance.

OTHERS

Nitrites

Nitrites are popular within club culture. They are bought from sex shops and known as 'poppers' because of the sound made when breaking the glass ampoules. They are inhaled and produce intense feelings of excitement that last only a few minutes. If used during sexual intercourse the vasodilation produced may intensify orgasm. Poppers may be used by homosexual men to relax the anal sphincter. Unwanted effects include dizziness, facial flushing, headache and palpitations.

Anabolic steroids

Anabolic steroids are taken by mouth or injection to increase muscle bulk. Their use is common amongst those who work out in gyms. Up to 2% of those in their mid teens in the UK and up to 10% of similar aged adolescents in the US have taken anabolic steroids with use being twice as common in males than females. They may cause increased aggression with outbursts of violence 'roid rage'.

Depression and paranoia following their use have been reported. Chronic anabolic steroid use may lead to a range of cardiovascular and hormonal disorders.

REFERENCES

Advisory Council on the Misuse of Drugs (1988) *AIDS and Drug Misuse. Part 1.* London: HMSO

American Academy of Child and Adolescent Psychiatry (1997) Practice parameters for the assessment and treatment of children and adolescents with substance use disorders. *Journal of the American Academy of Child and Adolescent Psychiatry*, **36**, 140S–156S.

Balding, J. (1998) *Young People and Illegal Drugs in 1998.* Exeter: Schools Health Education Unit.

Bagnall, G. (1988) Use of alcohol, tobacco and illicit drugs amongst 13 year olds in three areas of Britain. *Drug and Alcohol Dependence*, **22**, 242–251.

Brook, D. and Brook, J. (1990) The etiology and consequences of adolescent drug use. In R. Watson (ed.), *Drug and Alcohol Abuse Prevention*. Clifton, NJ: Umana Press, pp 339–362

The Children's Legal Centre and Standing Conference on Drug Abuse (1999) *Young People and Drugs: Policy Guidance for Drug Interventions.* London: SCODA.

Coggans, N. and McKellar, S. (1994) Drug use amongst peers: peer pressure or peer preference? *Drugs: Education, Prevention and Policy*, **1**, 15–26.

DeMilio, L. (1989) Psychiatric syndromes in adolescent substance abusers. *American Journal of Psychiatry*, **146**, 1212–1214.

Dinwiddie, S. H. (1994) Abuse of inhalants: a review. *Addiction*, **89**, 925–939.

Dorn, N. and Murji, K. (1992) *Drug Prevention: A Review of the English Language Literature. Institute for the Study of Drug Dependence Research Monograph 5*. London: Institute for the Study of Drug Dependence.

European Drug Monitoring Centre. (1998) *Annual Report on the State of the Drugs Problem in the European Union.* Lisbon: EMCDDA.

Evans, A. C. and Raistrick, D. (1987a) Patterns of use and related harm with toluene-based adhesives and butane gas. *British Journal of Psychiatry*, **150**, 773–776.

Evans, A. C. and Raistrick, D. (1987b) Phenomenology of intoxication with toluene-based adhesives and butane gas. *British Journal of Psychiatry*, **150**, 769–773.

Hall, W. and Solowij, N. (1998) Adverse effects of cannabis. *Lancet*, **352**, 1611–1616.

Hawton, K., Fagg, J., Platt, S. and Hawkins, M. (1993) Factors associated with suicide after parasuicide in young people, *British Medical Journal*, **306**, 1641–1644

Health Advisory Service (1996) *Children and Young People Substance Misuse Services: The Substance of Young Needs.* London: HMSO.

Health Education Authority (1996) *Drug Realities.* London: HMSO.

Kaminer, Y., Burtesen, J. A., Blitz, C., Sussman, J. and Rounsaville, B. J. (1998) Psychotherapies for adolescent substance abusers: a pilot study. *Journal of Nervous and Mental Disorder*, **186**, 684–690.

Khantzian, E. (1985) The self-medication hypothesis of addictive disorders: focus on heroin and cocaine dependence. *American Journal of Psychiatry*, **142**, 1259–1264.

McEwan, R., McCallum, A., Bhopal, R. and Madhok, R. (1992) Sex and the risk of HIV infection: the role of alcohol. *British Journal of Addiction*, **87**, 577–584

Marlatt, G. A. and George, G. W. (1979) Relapse prevention: introduction and overview of the model. *British Journal of Addiction*, **79**, 261–273.

Miller, P. M. and Plant, M. (1996) Drinking, smoking, and illicit drug use among 15 and 16 year olds in the United Kingdom. *British Medical Journal*, **313**, 394–397.

Miller, W. R. and Rollnick, S. (1991) *Motivational Interviewing: Preparing People to Change Addictive Behaviour.* New York: Guilford Press.

Myles, J. A. and Wilner, P. (1999) Substance misuse and psychiatric comorbidity in children and adolescents. *Current Opinion in Psychiatry*, **12**, 287–290.

Newcomb, M., Maddahian, E. and Bentler, P. (1986) Risk factors for drug use among adolescents: concurrent and longitudinal analyses. *American Journal of Public Health*, **76**, 525–530.

Parker, H., Measham, F. and Aldridge, J. (1995) *Drug Futures: Changing Patterns of Drug Use Amongst English Youth.* London: Institute for the Study of Drug Dependence.

Parker, H., Bury, C. and Egginton, R. (1998) *New Heroin Outbreaks amongst Young People in England and Wales.* London: Home Office.

Prochaska, J. O. and DiClemente, C. C. (1992) Stages of change in the modification of problem behaviors. *Programs of Behaviour Modification*, **28**, 183–218.

Ramsay, M. and Spillar, J. (1997) *Drug Misuse Declared in 1996: Latest Results from the British Crime Survey, Research Study 172.* London: HMSO.

Royal College of Physicians and British Paediatric Association (1995) *Alcohol and the Young.* London: Royal College of Physicians.

Tarter, R. E. (1990) Evaluation and treatment of adolescent substance abuse: a decision tree method. *American Journal of Drug and Alcohol Abuse*, **16**, 1–46.

Tsuang, M. T., Lyons, M. J., Meyer, J. M., Doyle, T., Eisen, S. A., Goldberg, J. *et al.* (1998) Co-occurrence of abuse of different drugs in men. The role of drug-specific and shared vulnerabilities. *Archives of General Psychiatry*, 55, 967–972

Ward, J., Mattick, R. and Hall, W. (1998) *Methadone Maintenance Treatment and other Opioid Replacement Therapies*. Amsterdam: Harwood Academic Publishers.

Weinberg, N. Z., Rahdert, E., Colliver, J. D. and Glantz, M. D. (1998) Adolescent substance abuse: a review of the past 10 years. *Journal of the American Academy of Child and Adolescent Psychiatry*, 37, 252–261.

White, D. and Pitts, M. (1998) Educating young people about drugs: a systematic review. *Addiction*, 93, 1475–1487.

Williams, R. and Morgan, H. G. (1994) *Suicide Prevention – The Challenge Confronted*. NHS Health Advisory Service. London: HMSO.

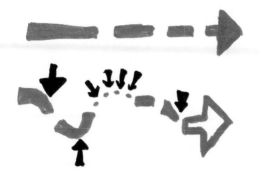

Chapter 7

ADOLESCENT PERSONALITY DEVELOPMENT – DIFFERENCES, DEPARTURES AND DEVIATIONS

Jonathan Hill

INTRODUCTION

The concept of personality is often referred to, but seldom adds clarity. A major reason is that there are quite contrasting meanings of the term, and because it refers to an amalgam of phenomena and processes that need to be separated. Adolescence provides a particular challenge to the concept because personality is generally taken to imply consistency across time and place, and yet adolescence is a period of substantial biological, psychological and social change. In this chapter, I will review briefly some key concepts of personality and personality disorder, then indicate some ways in which these are in need of revision. Then, I will consider a range of phenomena and processes in adolescence each of which are candidates for inclusion under the general heading of personality and its disorders, and then go on to clinical implications.

PERSONALITY AND PERSONALITY DISORDER

Stability over time and circumstance is fundamental to the concept of personality. However, it is not clear how stable and consistent we should expect individuals to be. It probably depends on what we mean by personality. Behavioural traits such as shyness or honesty have been investigated extensively and in general stability has been found to be modest. More recent formulations of personality have placed an emphasis on factors that underpin the organisation of behaviours such as neural systems, beliefs or representations of the external world. At the same time these formulations have tended to focus on particular aspects of functioning rather than the sum total of a person's psychological and behavioural make-up. A major advantage of investigating more specific aspects of personality functioning is that it allows for the possibility that there may be different answers to questions concerning different processes. This can be illustrated with reference to two approaches to the organisation of behaviours, those referring to temperament and attachment. Infants show early differences in the ways in which they interact with the external world. Some infants react generally to unfamiliar events with interest and pleasure, whilst others withdraw and appear anxious. These temperamental differences tend to persist through childhood and into adolescence (Kagan *et al.*, 1999), and they may be underpinned by inherited variations in brain neurochemistry (Gray, 1987). Similarly security of attachment to key care givers (usually, but not necessarily, parents) can be assessed reliably at 1 year and shows moderate stability to middle childhood. Attachment security is predictive of a wide range of cognitive and social competencies later in childhood (Sroufe *et al.*, 1999), many of which are relevant to personality functioning. Equally whether or not security of attachment in early childhood remains stable is related to changes in life stressors (Egeland and Farber, 1984). There is far more to personality, as we normally think of it, than temperament and attachment; however, by narrowing the focus more, specific questions concerning stability, and influences on it over development, can be asked.

If the identity and the functioning of 'personality' were clearer then we would be in a good position to define 'personality disorder'. However, as we shall see, there are numerous problems with the concept and the measures, arising in part because there is not a satisfactory empirical background concerning personality on which to build. The problem is widely recognised and there are continuing attempts to improve upon current systems (Westen and Shedler, 1999). An alternative approach, taken in this chapter, is to define more specifically some of the relevant clinical phenomena, and then consider associated processes and causal mechanisms.

WHAT IS TO BE EXPLAINED? THE ROLE OF INTERPERSONAL FUNCTIONING

There is general agreement that personality disorder refers to relatively enduring and pervasive maladaptive behaviour. Furthermore the DSM and ICD systems propose subtypes that are distinguished by differences in assumed personality traits. It is not clear how many of these will turn out to be valid and distinctive. Current research, predominantly into the DSM personality disorders, is hampered by problems of measurement which include low agreement across raters and instruments. Co-occurrence of personality disorder types is very common which generally frustrates attempts to investigate the causes and consequences of any particular type (Oldham et al., 1992). Inspection of the DSM subtypes shows that markedly contrasting items are included. For instance, antisocial personality disorder is characterised by antisocial behaviours and interpersonal difficulties, whilst borderline personality disorder by a pattern of instability of interpersonal relationships, uncertain self-image and labile affects, and marked impulsivity. These differences may reflect the rather contrasting origins of the proposed personality disorders. Antisocial personality disorder has its origins in the well-replicated findings that aggressive and disruptive behaviours in childhood are often followed in adult life by a constellation of antisocial behaviours and instability of employment and relationships. Borderline personality disorder is an attempt to define behaviourally a psychoanalytic formulation of a pattern of disorganised personality We have argued that deficits in interpersonal functioning may be common to a number of the proposed personality disorders including the antisocial and borderline types (Hill and Rutter, 1994; Hill et al., 1989). This is supported mainly by evidence from longitudinal studies. Whilst conduct disordered boys and girls differ in many respects in their adult outcomes, they resemble each other in having poor interpersonal functioning (Robins, 1986). Continuities between conduct disorder in childhood and performance in work and interpersonal functioning in adult life appear to be stronger than those with antisocial behaviour in adult life (Zoccolillo et al., 1992). Monozygotic–dizygotic differences in adulthood of twins with conduct disorder in childhood are stronger for interpersonal functioning than for antisocial behaviours. Where personality disorder has been assessed in terms of deficits in interpersonal functioning it has shown substantial stability (Quinton et al., 1995; Rutter and Quinton, 1984). A survey in the US of the methods clinicians use to assess personality disorder found that they generally regard persistent interpersonal difficulties as central to the concept (Westen, 1997).

The identification of interpersonal functioning as central to the idea of personality disorder may appear to depart from the original concept. However, from a developmental perspective this is not so evident. From birth infants give priority to social stimuli and individual development is embedded in interactions with others (Stern, 1985). The quality of the child's attachment representations is associated with the quality of his/her interactions with parents and in turn this is predictive of peer relationships (Sroufe et al., 1999). Disruptive behaviour problems in childhood, with their substantially increased risks of antisocial personality problems in adolescence and adult life, are also embedded in poor relationships with parents and with other children.

EPISODIC DISORDERS

It is commonly assumed that, although we may not know what should be included in our ideas of personality disorder, episodic disorders such as depression or eating disorder should be seen as different and distinct. In the DSM system episodic disorders are referred to as Axis I disorders and personality disorders as Axis II disorders. However, a re-evaluation of personality disorder should also include examination of the distinction between (DSM Axis I) episodic disorders and (DSM Axis II) personality disorders. To a certain extent a blurring has already occurred in that borderline personality disorder includes altered mood states and whether these are seen as forming part of the personality disorder or episodes of major depression often hinges on how long each episode lasts. In clinical practice with adolescents and adults, individuals with personality problems manifest as persistent interpersonal difficulties, and often also have depression, anxiety disorders, eating disorders and substance misuse. From a developmental perspective, childhood conduct problems are often followed by antisocial behaviours, interpersonal difficulties *and* Axis I disorder. Similarly, maltreatment in childhood, such as sexual abuse, physical abuse or neglect, increases the risk for persistent interpersonal dysfunction, and for depression and anxiety disorders (Fergusson *et al.*, 1996; Mullen *et al.*, 1993). The general point is that some childhood disorders or experiences may predispose individuals to personality difficulties and episodic disorders, and that we should perhaps see some episodic disorders as part of the personality problems. We cannot assume that because symptoms come and go, in a manner that resembles the onset and offset of illness, they do not reflect aspects of personality functioning.

WHAT ARE THE PROCESSES?

The phenomenon of personality disorder, however defined, is static, whilst the relevant processes are more dynamic and bring us closer to causal explanation. Processes refer to the factors that are associated with variations in development and the ways they are associated with each other, often providing pointers to explanations of outcomes. However, they stop short of specifying how one factor impacts upon another. In general terms there are individual, environmental and interactional processes. We are referring here both to processes that at any one time may work together to create a constellation of beliefs, emotions and behaviours, and to processes that link influences, behaviours and experiences at one point in development to subsequent functioning.

Individual processes in development are all those where the links between genetic or environmental influences and functioning are mediated by character-istics of the individuals. A good example is provided by Cloninger's theory of personality disorder (Cloninger, 1987). He argues that there are three basic temperamental qualities, which in normal individuals perform complementary functions in regulating emotions and behaviours. Personality disorder arises where there is an imbalance of these temperamental systems. The disorder therefore arises directly from the characteristics of the individual. Behaviour patterns identifiable early in childhood are later seen as personality disorder and this therefore represents a continuity of individual functioning, without the addition of other processes. The environment may affect the likelihood that the abnormalities may be seen, but does not have a role in generating or maintaining them.

By contrast, environmental processes are those where what is seen at any particular time is a direct reflection of current environmental factors and continuities of the individual's behaviours, from one time to another, are accounted for by continuities in the environment. Interactional processes entail the contribution of two or more participants. For example, tension between a parent and a child can arise from the interaction between parental irritability and the child's impulsivity. Accumulation of such tension may contribute to depression in the parent or outbursts of aggressive behaviour in the child. What appears as an individual problem has occurred because of the accumulated effect of interactions between two people. Evocative person–environment interactions are those where the behaviour of one individual evokes particular behaviours in another (Caspi and Moffitt, 1995). The parent of a child who has difficulty with impulse control, or whose mood is predominantly negative, may find that her supportive behaviours are not reinforced and may start to respond to her child with anger or criticism. Then the child has evoked these new behaviours in his parent and these in turn may increase the likelihood that he will respond negatively. For example, boys who are frequently oppositional seem to provoke family members to counter with punitive or angry responses which are likely to escalate into aggressive interactions (Patterson and Bank, 1989). Interactions in which the behaviours of an individual lead to selection of particular environments are referred to as proactive person–environment interactions. Disruptive children often fail academically and are placed in classes with similar children where academic opportunities are few and teachers may anticipate failure. This in turn increases the likelihood of leaving school without academic skills. Girls with behaviour problems in adolescence are more likely to become pregnant without a supportive partner (Quinton et al., 1993). Unsupported teenage motherhood reduces educational and social opportunities.

CAUSAL LINKS

In general terms, causal explanations in psychological development refer to the way the individual processes information about events, ascribes meaning to them and acts on them (Bolton and Hill, 1996). Much of this goes on within an interpersonal context, and so interpreting the actions and the meanings of others, and responding appropriately is a crucial human skill. Difficulties in representing the external world and responding accurately may arise because of deficits in neural systems. For instance, deficits in understanding the meaning of the behaviours and emotions of others are found in autism. Deficits in understanding the context of events or in monitoring actions, or a combination of the two, may give rise to symptoms of schizophrenia (Frith, 1996). Alternatively, maladaptive ways of interpreting events or acting may be generated in circumstances in which such perceptions and actions have been essential to coping. For example, children who have been physically abused are more likely to perceive threat in the actions of others (Pettit et al., in press) and in turn this is associated with higher levels of aggression. This readiness to perceive threat may be useful if the child is at risk of physical harm; however, it may lead him to misinterpret the benign actions of others under different circumstances. If this misinterpretation leads to action, then the child may act aggressively in situations where aggression is inappropriate. We turn now to specific findings on processes and causal mechanisms in relation to personality difficulties in adolescence.

INDIVIDUAL PROCESSES AND ADOLESCENT PERSONALITY DEVELOPMENT

Links between temperamental differences seen at age three and violence in adolescence were demonstrated in the Dunedin Multidisciplinary Health and Development Study (Henry et al., 1996). Those boys who at the age of 3 were impulsive, liable to react to stress and challenge with negative emotions, and who were not persistent in problem solving, were more likely than other boys to be convicted for a violent offence by age 18. Cloninger's theory when applied to antisocial behaviours predicts that problems will arise in individuals who have high novelty seeking, which is not modified by the effects of anxious inhibition (low harm avoidance), and who are not oriented to social rewards (low reward dependence). This was tested in the Montreal longitudinal experimental study (Kerr et al., 1997). Children who at ages 10–12 were disruptive and also inhibited, did not have increased rates of delinquency at age 13–15, whilst children who were disruptive and withdrawn, but not inhibited, were more likely to be delinquent by mid-adolescence.

The causal links are at this stage speculative. One possibility is that these temperamental differences arise from differences in activity of neurotransmitters. Identifying such differences is difficult because brain transmitters have many varied functions depending on their location and the nature of receptors. Neurotransmitter levels measured in the cerebrospinal fluid, or more commonly in blood or urine, are very indirect reflections of what is happening within the brain. Nevertheless, there are some pointers. Gray (1985) has proposed that behavioural inhibition (in Cloninger's model 'harm avoidance') is mediated by neuronal circuitry involving the hippocampus, and the lateral nucleus of the amygdala, both of which are involved in labelling fearful stimuli. The neurotransmitter serotonin [5-hydroxytryptamine (5-HT)] is thought to be particularly important to these circuits. Moffit *et al.* (1997) found that at age 21 violent males had higher levels of blood 5-HT – indicating lower levels in the brain – than the non-violent. In other words violent males had lower levels of the neurotransmitter that is thought to play a part in inhibiting aggressive behaviours. It is likely that differences in neurotransmitter activity are influenced by genetic factors. Equally there is substantial evidence, primarily from work on monkeys, that early social and maternal deprivation leads to persistent alterations in brain biogenic amines (Schneider *et al.*, 1998).

The study of the biological basis of personality development has not been confined to antisocial behaviours. Individual differences in fearful, inhibited behaviour are evident towards the end of the first year of life, and stability of fearful inhibition from the second to the eighth year of life and from pre-school to the age of 18 have been demonstrated (Caspi and Silva, 1995). In a follow up study of 13-year-old adolescents, Schwartz *et al.* (1999) found that, compared to uninhibited controls, children who had been assessed as inhibited at age 21 months were more likely to suffer from social anxiety.

Causal mechanisms in individual continuities from childhood to adolescence are likely also to entail representations of early attachment relationships and cognitive styles acquired in early life. Attachment is a complex phenomenon that includes the way emotions and information are regulated by the individual in the context of close relationships, and the extent to which the individual is able to deal with and enjoy intimacy. Insecure individuals have been characterised as either down-regulating the significance and emotional implications of events in close relationships (avoidant or dismissing attachment) or experiencing height-ened and overwhelming, especially negative, emotions (ambivalent or pre-occupied attachment). Infants who show contradictory or confused (dis-organised) behaviours in relation to caregivers appear to have not developed a clear attachment strategy, possibly as a consequence of their parents' frightening or frightened behaviours (Main and Hesse, 1990; Van Ijzendoorn *et al.*, 1999). Attachment theory predicts that security of attachment in infancy provides the basis of later psychosocial adaptation and that this adaptation influences and in turn is influenced by experiences later in development. Although the theory hypothesises that interactional processes will be important, it also that predicts that security of attachment in infancy remains a causal factor in adaptation in adolescence. Findings from Sroufe *et al.* (1999) support this. They followed children from low socioeconomic status families in Minnesota from infancy into adolescence. After controlling for more recent adaptation and experiences, avoidant attachment and disorganised attachment in infancy were associated with psychopathology at age 17.5 years. Disorganisation in infancy was also associated with higher scores on the Dissociative Experiences Scale at age 19 (Carlson, 1998). This scale documents difficulties such as recurrent memory disturbances and alterations of conscious awareness, which are likely to reflect failures to integrate memories, thoughts and emotions into a coherent and unified sense of consciousness.

Studies of children with multiple caretakers in early childhood also support a long-term effect of disrupted attachments on individual functioning. Hodges and Tizard (1989) followed up adolescents who had been in institutions with multiple caretakers for the first 4 years of their lives, some of whom were adopted and some returned to their biological families. Those who were adopted, were doing well educationally and had fewer behaviour problems than those who returned home. However, compared to a normally reared control group at age 16 they tended to be over-friendly with strangers, were less popular and had fewer friends.

The limited available evidence suggests that associations with relationship difficulties and psychiatric problems in adults are most likely to occur where the insecure pattern is accompanied by unresolved loss or trauma (Fonagy et al., 1996; Patrick et al., 1994) and this may be true also in adolescence. Although the mechanism is not clear, it is possible that where an individual has developed an avoidant coping strategy in response to a loss or trauma, she may be vulnerable in relationships where there is a need to be emotionally responsive or where faced with life events that threaten his or her emotional equilibrium. By contrast the person who has become preoccupied and angry following a trauma may be overwhelmed or confused in relationships, especially where it is difficult for her to separate the emotions that are still evoked from relationships with parents and those aroused within the current relationships.

The combination of interpersonal difficulties and psychiatric conditions such as depression may be associated with particular patterns of memory and information processing. Studies of adults have showed that a history of depression is associated with difficulties in retrieving specific memories. Williams (1996) has suggested that, in the face of trauma or neglect, having general memories may be a way of coping with the negative emotions associated with specific memories, and that this could become maladaptive in adolescence and adult life. The use of general characterisations of events, which are not updated with specific examples, may lead to generalized assumptions about the self and others. Support for a link between abuse in childhood and the development of generalized attributions in relationships comes from a recent study by McCarthy and Taylor (1999). They found that young adults who had been abused in childhood had more problems in intimate relationships and were more likely to attribute difficulties to general aspects of the partner rather than the particulars of interactions. The use of such general characterisations within relationships, which are not updated with specific examples, may then contribute to ineffective problem solving in relationships, and hence to depression. Where general characterisations about the self are negative these also are likely to increase the likelihood of depression. Lack of specific memories has also been associated with borderline personality disorder and with dissociation in young adults (Jones *et al.*, 1999), which further suggests that early patterns of remembering, often associated with abuse, may affect the integration of memory and affect many years later.

INTERACTIONAL PROCESSES AND ADOLESCENT PERSONALITY DEVELOPMENT

Even where there is a clear effect of individual factors such as early temperament, attachment or information processing, generally there are also interactional processes. This will be particularly likely to occur where the parents and the child share a genetic risk, e.g. for irritable or impulsive behaviour. However, a child with poor impulse control and predominantly negative moods may also induce irritability or anger from otherwise more placid parents. Similarly young aggressive children are often rejected by sociable children and gain peer groups of children with similar difficulties, with whom aggressive exchanges increase. Dishion *et al.* (1996) demonstrated how interactional processes in adolescents can contribute to the maintenance of antisocial behaviours. A group of 13- and 14-year-old boys, some of whom were already antisocial, and their closest friends participated in a videotaped problem-solving discussion. These videotapes were analyzed using a coding system that focused on verbal content and affective reactions. Two topics were defined: rule-breaking talk and normative talk. The possible reactions were *laugh* and *pause*. Rule-breaking talk occurred four times more frequently in antisocial dyads. Whereas non-antisocial and mixed (antisocial and non-antisocial) dyads responded to normative talk with a laugh, antisocial dyads were found to respond to rule-breaking talk with a laugh. Friendship dyads that provided positive reinforcement for rule-breaking talk were more likely to report increased delinquent behavior during the following 2 years, even controlling for prior levels (Dishion *et al.*, 1996).

The interplay between the individual's characteristics and the quality of the family environment is exemplified in studies of genetic and environmental influences. For instance Cadoret *et al.* (1995) showed that aggression in adolescence among adoptive children was associated both with having had an antisocial biological parent and with the presence of problems in the adoptive home environment, such as marital difficulties or psychiatric problems in the adoptive parent. There was an interaction between the inherited characteristics and the adoptive environment whereby the likelihood of adolescent aggression was increased by the combination of these factors. In the study of longitudinal predictors of adolescent violence described earlier (Moffitt *et al.*, 1997), abnormal 5-HT levels were most strongly associated with violence in the presence of high family conflict, underlying the need to attend simultaneously to individual and interactional processes even where individual biological factors contribute.

Generally, antisocial behaviour is manifest in early childhood as impulsiveness and negative affect, and aggressive and disruptive behaviours, and these are seen repeatedly through childhood and into adolescence. However, other aspects of personality may be manifest at particular life stages and in relation to particular developmental demands stressors. For instance, it has been hypothesised that eating disorders in adolescence are often preceded by perfectionist traits, which are predominantly adaptive before puberty (Srinivasagan et al., 1995). For the young person, for whom maintenance of control has been important, puberty and emerging sexuality, increased academic challenges, and the impending increased responsibilities associated with adulthood may threaten control. Severe dieting and regulation of body weight may restore sense of control. Thus a condition which is seen mainly in adolescence may be understood as the outcome of personality development in relation to the demands of adolescence. Furthermore, following recovery from the condition personality traits may still be evident and different episodic conditions may take the place of the one seen in adolescence. Srinivasagan et al. (1995) followed up women after they had been treated for anorexia nervosa. They found that only a small minority still met diagnostic criteria for the condition; however, among those who were not anorexic, perfectionism was common, and there were high rates of depression, anxiety disorders and alcoholism.

Studies of children who have been in care illustrate further the complexity of interactional processes in adolescence. Girls who were in children's homes in the mid-1960s have been shown to have increased rates of psychosocial difficulties in their 20s and 30s. These difficulties appear to arise from genetic factors, from early disruptive experiences and the in-care experience. These girls were also more likely to experience family discord if they returned home in adolescence, to have a deviant adolescent peer group and to get pregnant in adolescence outside a supportive relationship. All of these factors in turn were associated with poor adult outcomes. A central factor associated with the likelihood of going down the disadvantaging pathway was whether or not they planned for work or marriage/cohabitation. Those girls who knew what they wanted to do before leaving school and those who knew their partners for 6 months or more before starting a cohabitation were less likely to have a deviant partner or early unsupportive pregnancy. Put another way, impulsive behaviour with respect to work or cohabitation was a personality attribute in adolescence that formed part of the process that led to clear psychosocial difficulties in adult life (Quinton et al., 1993). Disentangling cause and effect here is difficult. Where a young person has difficulty appraising the quality of developing relationships or where powerful and confusing emotions are aroused by relationships, he/she maybe vulnerable to lack of 'planning'. Thus it could be that a factor such as insecure attachment made it more likely that a girl would start a cohabitation before getting to know her partner, and also make it more likely that she would choose a deviant partner and hence more likely to have later difficulties. Alternatively, circumstances such as having nowhere to live may have contributed to the speed of cohabitation, giving less time to appraise a partner's qualities and hence increased risk of deviance. Once she had a deviant partner other adversities followed and hence adult difficulties. Often these processes are seen in adolescence where the individual has clear behaviour problems. For instance, in their study of aggressive children and adolescents, Moffitt *et al.* (1997) found that persistent violence in late adolescence was associated with an increased likelihood of leaving school early, which was likely in turn to contribute to reduced employment opportunities later in life.

A substantial body of research links mental health problems in adolescents and young adults to previous trauma and neglect. No doubt some of this reflects common genetic influences on parenting and on the risk of psychiatric disorder in the children. Equally where it has been possible to study childhood adversities within twin studies there has been evidence that trauma such as child sexual abuse has long-term consequences (Statham *et al.*, 1998). The consequences of childhood abuse and neglect in adult life cross the personality disorder–episodic disorder boundary, in that there is an increased likelihood of persistent interpersonal problems, depression, anxiety disorders and substance misuse. Similar findings in late adolescence come from the Christchurch Health and Development Study in New Zealand (Fergusson *et al.*, 1996). Over 1000 children were studied at birth, 4 months and at annual intervals to the age of 16, and then at age 18. The findings underline the extent to which family adversities cluster together, so that, for instance, children exposed to harsh physical treatment were also more likely to come from families where there was inter-parental violence, parental criminality and substance misuse, and were more likely to be exposed to sexual abuse from within or outside the family. Sexual abuse was associated with an increased risk of a wide range of mental health problems including depression, anxiety and substance misuse, *and* in girls with an increased likelihood of early consensual sexual intercourse, multiple sexual partners and sexually transmitted disease in adolescence, and teenage pregnancy. This constellation of difficulties clearly was itself already a problem in adolescence and also entailed processes that increased the likelihood of later psychosocial difficulties, e.g. for girls through having children with unsupportive or violent partners. Processes within family relationships are also likely to have contributed to difficulties. For instance, we have shown (Hill *et al.*, 1999) that there are strong associations between recalled childhood relationships with parents and the quality of current relationships with parents in late adolescence and early adult life. It is therefore likely that these young people whose relationship and mental health problems were associated with adverse parenting in childhood, also in adolescence, experienced unsupportive or rejecting relationships with their own parents.

INDIVIDUAL, ENVIRONMENTAL AND INTERACTIONAL PROCESSES IN CLINICAL PRACTICE

An adolescent girl has multiple problems. She is frequently verbally aggressive and regularly provokes fights. She is an expert shoplifter, mainly to raise money to buy drugs. She has brief relationships with older boys and men, many of whom have a criminal record. Her mood is labile, at times she is depressed and suicidal, and at others appears confident and invulnerable. She has taken five overdoses over the past year.

What is the phenomenon? It is a mixture of antisocial behaviours, poor peer relationships, mood changes and substance misuse. When she is 13, our clinical description may refer to these features separately, probably adding further relevant information such as truanting and few educational achievements. By age 18 she might be seen clinically in terms of personality disorder. Her difficulties cross the traditional boundaries of what is often thought of as personality and yet it is not difficult to see how they may be linked. Many of the processes that we have reviewed earlier are seen. She has already closed down most educational options, both because she has acquired few skills and most schools will not take her. Her peer group centres on drug taking and the boys in it are antisocial. She takes risks sexually with boys who would not support her if she became pregnant. She lacks support from parents and from peers. This has multiple effects. She has no source of comfort when upset and therefore has to appear invulnerable through being aggressive. She does not have others with whom she can rehearse alternative ways of solving problems, and this is another reason that she is aggressive and challenging in interpersonal situations. Not only does she lack support from parents, her mother is, in fact, hostile, and there are frequent arguments. She is more likely to provoke a fight after she has had an argument with her mother. Lack of problem solving when feeling low also increases the likelihood that she will take an overdose.

Part of the causal explanation involves her early temperament which has had much in common with that of her biological father who had a long history of violence and spent much of her childhood in prison. As a young child she was active, impulsive and easily upset, and this irritated her mother who had two other children and no partner. This was in contrast to her sister and brother who were placid and friendly and favoured by her mother. Her mother did hit her, but not her sister and brother. Early coping strategies included avoidance of painful memories of being hurt and of the associated emotions, avoidance of intimacy, and a precocious independence, with increased vigilance for signs of threat. She has brought all of these coping mechanisms into relationships in adolescence. This has a paradoxical effect. In some respects she fails to notice danger, e.g. with boys. She becomes involved with people who it is clear will harm her. In other respects she sees threat where there is none and responds aggressively. Most of this can be understood as learnt. Equally it may be that her early experiences have affected neurochemical systems, so that she is more vulnerable to become depressed. Even when she is not depressed her relatively low mood reduces further her problem solving capabilities.

Once we identify the phenomena and the processes, we begin to see how they conspire to stack the odds against a young person. It becomes clearer also that our research and clinical strategies need to examine which are the key components of the picture: the ones that have the major effects, and the ones that, if changed might lead to wider change. Or perhaps there are processes that in combination are most damaging and so need attention together. It is likely that we will need to consider individual, environmental and interactional processes, and biological, psychological and social mechanisms.

NOTE ON THE GENDER OF PRONOUNS

In discussions of antisocial problems, male pronouns have been used, and in relation to non-antisocial problems, female pronouns. This reflects the gender distribution for these difficulties, without implying that they are exclusive to either males or females.

REFERENCES

Bolton, D. and Hill, J. (1996) *Mind, Meaning and Mental Disorder: The Nature of Causal Explanation in Psychology and Psychiatry.* Oxford: Oxford University Press.

Cadoret, R. J., Yates, W. R., Troughton, E., Woodworth, G. and Stewart, M. A. (1995) Genetic–environmental interaction in the genesis of aggressivity and conduct disorders. *Archives of General Psychiatry,* **52**, 916–924.

Carlson, E. (1998) A prospective longitudinal study of attachment disorganiza-tion/disorientation. *Child Development,* **69**, 1107–1128.

Caspi, A. and Moffitt, T. E. (1995) The continuity of maladaptive behaviour: from description to understanding in the study of antisocial behaviour. In D. Cicchetti and D. J. Cohen (eds), *Developmental Psychopathology.* New York: Wiley, vol. 2, pp. 472–511.

Caspi, A. and Silva, P. A. (1995) Temperamental qualities at age 3 predict personality traits in young adulthood: longitudinal evidence from a birth cohort. *Child Development*, **66**, 486–498.

Cloninger, C. R. (1987) A systematic method for clinical description and classification of personality variants: a proposal. *Archives of General Psychiatry*, **44**, 573–588.

Dishion, T. J., Spracklen, K. M., Andrews, D. W. and Patterson, G. R. (1996) Deviancy training in male adolescent friendships. *Behavior Therapy*, **27**, 373–390.

Egeland, B. and Farber, E. (1984) Infant–mother attachment, factors related to its development and changes over time. *Child Development*, **55**, 753–771.

Fergusson, D., Horwood, L. J. and Lynskey, M. T. (1996) Childhood sexual abuse and psychiatric disorders in young adulthood: part II. Psychiatric outcomes of sexual abuse. *Journal of the American Academy of Child and Adolescent Psychiatry*, **35**, 1365–1374.

Fonagy, P., Leigh, T., Steele, M., Steele, H., Kennedy, R., Mattoon, G. *et al.* (1996) The relation of attachment status, psychiatric classification, and response to psychotherapy. *Journal of Consulting and Clinical Psychology*, **64**, 22–31

Frith, C. (1996) The neuropsychology of schizophrenia, what are the implications of intellectual and experiential abnormalities for the neurobiology of schizophrenia? *British Medical Bulletin*, **52**, 618–626.

Gray, J. A. (1987) *The Psychology of Fear and Stress*, 2nd edn. New York: McGraw-Hill.

Henry, B., Caspi, A., Moffitt, T. and Silva, P. A. (1996) Temperamental and familial predictors of violent and nonviolent criminal convictions: age 3 to age 18. *Developmental Psychology*, **32**, 614–623.

Hill, J. and Rutter, M. (1994) Personality disorders. In M. Rutter, E. Taylor and L. Hersov (eds), *Child and Adolescent Psychiatry, Modern Approaches*. Oxford: Blackwell Science, pp. 688–696.

Hill, J., Harrington, R., Fudge, H., Rutter, M. and Pickles, A. (1989) The adult personality functioning assessment: development and reliability. *British Journal of Psychiatry*, **155**, 24–35.

Hill, J., Mackie, E., Banner, L., Kondryn, H. and Blair, V. (1999) Relationship with Family of Origin Scale (REFAMOS). Interrater reliability and associations with childhood experiences. *British Journal of Psychiatry*, **175**, 565–570.

Hodges, J. and Tizard, B. (1989) Social and family relationships of ex-institutional adolescents. *Journal of Child Psychology and Psychiatry*, **30**, 77–97.

Jones, B., Heard, M., Startup, M., Swales, M., Williams, J. M. G. and Jones, R. S. P. (1999) Autobiographical memory and dissociation in borderline personality disorder. *Psychological Medicine*, **29**, 1397–1404.

Kagan, J., Snidman, N., Zentner, M. and Peterson, E. (1999) Infant temperament and anxious symptoms in school age children. *Development and Psychopathology*, **11**, 209–224.

Kerr, M., Tremblay, R. Pagani, L. and Vitaro, F. (1997) Boys' behavioural inhibition and the risk of later delinquency. *Archives of General Psychiatry*, **54**, 809–816.

McCarthy, G. and Taylor, A. (1999) Avoidant/ambivalent attachment style as a mediator between abusive childhood experiences and adult relationships difficulties. *Journal of Child Psychology and Psychiatry*, **40**, 465–478.

Main, M. and Hesse, E. (1990) Parents' unresolved traumatic experiences are related to infant disorganized attachment status: is frightened and/or frightening parental behaviour the linking mechanism? In M. T. Greenberg, D. Cicchetti and M. Cummings (eds), *Attachment in the Preschool Years: Theory, Research and Intervention*. Chicago, IL: Chicago University Press.

Moffitt, T., Caspi, A., Fawcett, P., Brammer, G. L., Raleigh, M., Yuwiler, A. *et al.* (1997) Whole blood serotonin and family background relate to male violence. In A. Raine, P. A. Brennan, D. P. Farrington and S. A. Mednick (eds), *Biosocial Bases of Violence*. New York: Plenum, pp. 321– 240.

Mullen, P. E., Martin, J. L., Anderson, J. C., Romans, S. E. and Herbison, P. (1993) Childhood sexual abuse and mental health in adult life. *British Journal of Psychiatry*, **163**, 721–732.

Oldham, J. M., Skodol, A. E., Kellman, H. D., Hyler, S. E., Rosnick, L. and Davies, M. (1992) Diagnosis of DSM-III-R personality disorders by two structured interviews: patterns of comorbidity. *American Journal of Psychiatry*, **149**, 213–220.

Patrick, M., Hobson, P., Castle, D., Howard, R. and Maughan, M. (1994) Personality disorder and the mental representation of early social experience. *Development and Psychopathology*, **6**, 375–388.

Patterson, G. R. and Bank, L. (1989) Some amplifying mechanisms for pathologic process in families. In M. R. Gunar and E. Thalen (eds), *Minnesota Symposium in Child Psychology. Vol. 22. Systems and Development*. Hillsdale, NJ: Erlbaum, pp. 167–200.

Pettit, G., Polaha, J. and Mize, J. (In press) Perceptual and attributional processes in aggression and conduct problems. In J. Hill and B. Maughan (eds) *Cambridge Monographs in Child and Adolescent Psychiatry – Conduct Disorders*. Cambridge: Cambridge University Press.

Quinton, D., Pickles, A., Maughan, B. and Rutter, M. (1993) Partners, peers, and pathways: assortative pairing and continuities in conduct disorder. *Development and Psychopathology*, **5**, 763–783.

Quinton, D., Gulliver, L. and Rutter, M. (1995) A 15–20 follow-up of adult psychiatric patients. Psychiatric disorder and social functioning. *British Journal of Psychiatry*, **167**, 315–323.

Robins, L. N. (1986) The consequences of conduct disorder in girls. In D. Olweus, J. Block and M. Radke-Yarrow (eds), *Development of Antisocial and Prosocial Behaviour: Research, Theory and Issues*. New York: Academic Press, pp. 385–414.

Rutter, M. and Quinton, D. (1984) Parental psychiatric disorder: effects on children. *Psychological Medicine*, **14**, 853–880.

Schneider, M. L., Clarke, A. S., Kraemer, G. W., Roughton, E. C., Lubach, G. R., Rimm-Kaufman, S. *et al.* (1998) Prenatal stress alters brain biogenic amine levels in primates. *Development and Psychopathology*, **10**, 427–440.

Schwartz, C. E., Snidman, N. and Kagan, J. (1999) Adolescent social anxiety as an outcome of inhibited temperament in childhood. *Journal of the American Academy of Child and Adolescent Psychiatry*, **38**, 1008–1015.

Srinivasagan, N., Kaye, W., Plotnikov, K., Greeno, C., Weltzin, T. and Rao, R. (1995) Persistent perfectionism, symmetry and exactness after long term recovery from anorexia nervosa. *American Journal of Psychiatry*, **152**, 1630–1634.

Sroufe, L. A., Carlson, E. A., Levy, A. K. and Egland, B. (1999) Implications of attachment theory for developmental psychopathology. *Development and Psychopathology*, **11**, 1–14.

Statham, D. J., Heath, A. C., Madden, P. A. F., Bucholz, K. K., Bierut, L., Dinwiddie, S. H. *et al.* (1998) Suicidal behaviour: an epidemiological and genetic study. *Psychological Medicine*, **28**, 839–856.

Stern, D. N. (1985) *The Interpersonal World of the Infant*. New York: Basic Books

Van Ijzendoorn, M. H., Schuengel, C. and Bakermans-Kranenberg, M. J. (1999) Disorganised attachment in early childhood: meta-analysis of precursors, concomitants, and sequelae. *Development and Psychopathology*, **11**, 225–249.

Westen, D. (1997) Divergences between clinical and research methods for assessing personality disorders: implications for research and the evolution of axis II. *American Journal of Psychiatry*, **154**, 895–903.

Westen, D. and Shedler, J. (1999) Revising and assessing axis II, part II: toward an empirically based and clinically useful classification of personality disorders. *American Journal of Psychiatry*, **156**, 273–285.

Williams, J. M. G. (1996) Depression and the specificity of autobiographical memory. In D. C. Rubin (ed.), *Remembering Our Past: Studies in Autobiographical Memory*. Cambridge: Cambridge University Press.

Zoccolillo, M., Pickles, A., Quinton, D. and Rutter, M. (1992) The outcome of childhood conduct disorder: implications for defining adult personality disorder and conduct disorder. *Psychological Medicine*, **22**, 971–986.

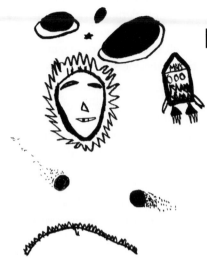

Chapter 8

PSYCHOTIC DISORDERS

Andrew Clark

INTRODUCTION

The term psychotic disorder has been variably used within child and adolescent psychiatry to include a wide variety of disorders including those now classified as the pervasive developmental disorders. It is now used in a more restrictive sense for only those disorders in which the individual suffers from such severe distortions and deviancies of cognitions and perceptions that they lose sight of the morbid nature of their experience and their reality testing become significantly impaired. In this chapter, the nature, causes, assessment, management and outcomes of the following disorders will be considered: drug-induced and other organic psychoses; schizophrenia and other schizophrenia-like psychoses (taken to include the schizo-affective disorders); and bipolar psychoses (predominantly focusing upon manic disorder; depressive disorders with psychotic features will be discussed in Chapter 4). Drug treatments will be covered in outline, but readers should also refer to Chapter 18 for greater detail on these.

DIAGNOSTIC CRITERIA

ORGANIC AND DRUG-INDUCED PSYCHOSES

A wide variety of organic conditions can present with the signs and symptoms of a psychotic disorder. It is obviously important that these are separately diagnosed from the schizophrenias and from bipolar disorder, and that prompt treatment of the underlying cause is given where possible. Pointers to an underlying organic cause are those of associated physical symptoms and of fluctuations in mental state, particularly if associated with variable disturbance in cognitive functioning. For an unequivocal diagnosis there needs to be clear evidence of an underlying physical disorder potentially associated with the psychotic state and a temporal relationship with its development rather than a chance co-morbidity of a psychotic disorder developing in the context of a longer-standing unassociated physical disorder. Drug-induced psychosis should always be considered, irrespective of whether a history of substance misuse is initially given. Symptoms of mania ['organic mania disorder' (World Health Organisation, 1992)] can be produced by neurological disorders (e.g. tumours, encephalitis, temporal lobe epilepsy, subdural haematoma), metabolic and systemic disorders (e.g. hyperthyroidism, Wilson's disease, uraemia, porphyria), prescribed medications (e.g. antidepressants, steroids, stimulants) and by non-prescribed psychoactive substances (e.g. amphetamines, cocaine, ecstasy) (American Academy of Child and Adolescent Psychiatry, 1997). A similarly wide range of disorders can produce symptoms indistinguishable from a schizophrenia like psychosis ['organic delusional disorder' (World Health Organisation, 1992)]. Disorders provoked by substance misuse rather than by underlying illness are classified separately. Although a primary organic cause for psychotic disorder in adolescence is found only rarely, this does make full physical assessment including a complete neurological examination mandatory.

SCHIZOPHRENIA, SCHIZOPHRENIA-LIKE AND SCHIZO-AFFECTIVE PSYCHOSES

Criteria for a diagnosis of schizophrenia have steadily been refined over time (Kafantaris, 1996; Kolvin, 1972). ICD-10 (World Health Organisation, 1992) requires specific symptoms to have been present for at least 1 month and for there to be no evidence of major affective symptoms or organic brain disease. These are either at least one of the following major symptoms or two of the minor symptoms. Major symptoms are typically Schneiderian: thought echo, insertion, withdrawal and broadcasting; control or passivity delusions or delusional perception; running commentary, auditory hallucinations in the third person or emanating from some part of the body; and other persistent delusions of an inappropriate or impossible nature. Minor symptoms are less specific: persistent hallucinations associated with fleeting or half-formed delusions; disruption of train of thought causing incoherence, irrelevance or neologism; catatonic features (excitement, posturing, waxy flexibility, negativism, etc.); and 'negative' symptoms (apathy, paucity of speech, emotional blunting, etc.). There is also an alternative criteria of significant and consistent behavioural change (self-absorption, social withdrawal, aimlessness, loss of interest, idleness, etc.) over a duration of at least 1 year although this applies solely to a diagnosis of simple schizophrenia and its reliability is uncertain (World Health Organisation, 1992). DSM-IV has similar requirements although requiring the illness to have been present for at least 6 months (American Psychiatric Association, 1994). This should mean only more persistent and severe cases are so diagnosed (Volkmar, 1996; Werry, 1992), although there is in fact little difference in predictive validity (Mason *et al.*, 1997).

There is also a group of young people presenting with psychotic symptoms whose illness is relatively brief but otherwise indistinguishable from schizophrenia. These acute schizophrenia-like psychoses may or may not be associated with significant environmental stresses and may or may not subsequently go on to develop into the full schizophrenia syndrome. Treatment of the acute episode is identical to that for schizophrenia but the longer-term outcome slightly better. Schizo-affective disorders, or disorders presenting with the simultaneous symptoms of both schizophrenia and bipolar disorder presenting together, are of uncertain nosological status

MANIC DISORDER

Manic disorder is characterised by symptoms of elevation of mood, overactivity, overtalkativeness, grandiosity, flight of ideas and a generalised sense of well-being (Carlson, 1994; World Health Organisation, 1992). Symptoms should be present for at least 1 week. Psychotic symptoms of grandiose or persecutory delusions may occur as may auditory or visual hallucinations. Exaggerated belief in sporting, intellectual or physical prowess is often seen with a young person believing against all the evidence that they will become an international footballer, a famous rock musician, a television star or some other unreachable aspiration. Irritability often follows any challenge to these statements and can result in physical aggression. Sexual disinhibition and overfamiliarity are not uncommon, as is involvement in other risk-taking behaviours. On occasion this can even mean that law-breaking and police involvement may lead to the first recognition of the disorder although unless the offence has been particularly serious criminal prosecution is not necessarily likely to follow.

EPIDEMIOLOGY

Schizophrenia is a rare disorder in adolescent psychiatric practice but the incidence increases markedly through the teenage years. Adult studies suggest that the prevalence within the adult general population is about 0.5% and that the annual incidence per year of new cases amounts to 2/10 000 population. The commonest age of onset of first episode is in the mid-20s with women falling ill slightly later than men. However, the initial descriptions of Kraepelin and Bleuler describe up to 5% of adult sufferers experiencing their first episode of illness before the age of 15 years (Asarnow and Asarnow, 1994), whilst Hafner and Nowotny (1995) using a retrospective diagnostic instrument suggested that as many as 20% of adult sufferers had their onset aged 20 years or less. Gillberg *et al.* (1986) estimated a population prevalence in the 13–19 year old age group for psychotic disorders of 0.54% and that schizophrenia accounted for 40% of these cases. Prevalence of psychosis increased from 0.9/10 000 at age 13 years to 17.6/10 000 at 18 years. In their study, Remschmidt *et al.* (1994) also demonstrate a similar marked increase in prevalence with increasing age across the teenage years. There is a consistent finding that the disorder is commoner in males than females (Werry, 1992), although this difference becomes less marked with later age of onset or when less restrictive definitions such as ICD-10 are used.

Precise epidemiological data regarding bipolar disorders amongst adolescents are not available. Its prevalence in adult life is approximately 1%. Community studies of adolescents suggest figures of up to 0.5–1.0%, although this varies with age and definitions of severity and duration used. There is additionally considerable concern that many milder cases may go undetected until later in life (Carlson, 1990; Geller and Luby, 1997; Volkmar, 1996). Retrospective information from adult sufferers regarding age of first episode gives similar figures to those for schizophrenia, with up to 20% of individuals having an onset before the age of 20 years (American Academy of Child and Adolescent Psychiatry, 1997). The incidence appears equal between males and females.

ASSESSMENT OF YOUNG PEOPLE WITH SUSPECTED PSYCHOSIS

The diagnosis of a psychotic disorder in a young person carries considerable implications and should therefore be reached only after careful assessment. This should include information from the young person themselves, from their immediate carers (usually but not always parents) and, subject to consent having been obtained, from other significant areas of their lives (e.g. school or work) where possible. Both current history, with an emphasis upon any recent changes, and a longer-term developmental background are necessary. There should be specific enquiry for salient symptoms such as mood disturbance, persecutory ideation, abnormal perceptual experiences, cognitive or social impairment and precise examples of these recorded. The individual, their family, their friends and their colleagues may each attempt either to minimise symptoms and explain them away in social or psychological ways or to emphasise the abnormality of the sufferer without reference to their previous development or experiences. The interviewer should be alert to both of these possibilities and attempt to obtain as dispassionate account as possible. A detailed history of any substance misuse and its chronology should also be sought. The developmental history should include questions regarding any family history of psychiatric disorder and particularly psychotic disorders, with if possible details of diagnoses and treatment interventions and efficacies. The young person's own early development should be reviewed with particular emphases upon their cognitive, social and emotional developmental pathways.

The interview with the young person should include a detailed assessment of mental state with clear recording of any abnormalities found. Use of a semi-structured interview (either in its entirety or merely in specific parts) such as the K-SADS-PL (Kaufman *et al.*, 1996) may be helpful in ensuring that symptoms are most accurately and fully ascertained and recorded (Rapoport and Ismond, 1996). The young person's understanding of their experiences should be explored in the light of their background cultural and social beliefs and previous experience, and with reference to their developmental stage. The pathoplastic effects of age should be remembered and possibly normal adolescent concerns regarding topics such as sensitivity regarding physical appearance, existential questions and the meaning of life or strong concern for environmental issues should neither be disregarded as non-significant nor automatically elevated to pathological import without fuller exploration.

Physical examination, including a full neurological examination, is mandatory in any young person presenting with the first episode of a psychosis. Evidence of thyroid, adrenal or pituitary dysfunction, of any ophthalmic (e.g. Kayser–Fleisher rings in Wilson's disease) or focal neurological abnormality, or other systemic disease (e.g. systemic lupus erythematosus) should all be actively sought. Psychosis secondary to an organic state is rare but well recognised as possibly occurring secondary to a wide variety of conditions. More questionable is how far to pursue laboratory and neuroimaging investigations routinely or purely upon other clinical findings. Urinary or hair drug screening should probably be performed routinely, even in the absence of any history of relevant misuse, in view of the potential unreliability of information. Many would additionally routinely undertake blood investigations (e.g. full blood count, urea and electrolytes, thyroid function and liver function), EEG and computed tomography or magnetic resonance imaging scan (Clark and Lewis, 1998), although the benefits of this approach have been disputed (Adams *et al.*, 1996). Additional investigations (e.g. autoantibody screen, serum calcium, chromosome studies, serum copper, arylsulphatase A and cerebrospinal fluid examination) should only be pursued in response to specific clinical indications.

Treatment of an organic psychosis is that of the underlying condition where possible. Close liaison with a paediatrician or adult physician may be necessary dependent upon the nature of the disorder and it may be important to consider whether the young person is treated primarily within a physical or mental health setting. This will depend upon the particular health care needs and requirements of the young person, and on the skills, expertise and resources of the various options. Full explanation of the primary condition and of the mechanisms underlying the psychotic experiences is essential but symptomatic management of the psychotic symptoms by appropriate prescription of antipsychotic medications is also necessary. Psychosis secondary to substance misuse poses particular challenges as the treatment goal of abstinence is not always readily achieved, even within an inpatient environment.

DIAGNOSTIC DIFFICULTIES

There will often be a history of substance misuse in an adolescent presenting with an episode of psychotic disorder. This poses particular diagnostic and management problems. The psychotic disorder may be entirely secondary to direct biochemical effects of the ingested substance or it may be indicative of an underlying illness process either unrelated to the substance misuse or exacerbated by it. This is true of both schizophrenia-like and manic-like psychoses. Detailed information about the timing and nature of substances used may help to clarify the relationship but confusion frequently remains. A false diagnosis of schizophrenia or manic disorder when the true diagnosis is that of psychotic disorder secondary to psychoactive drug usage carries major social and treatment implications for both the young person and for health services. Where psychotic symptoms persist longer than 7–10 days in a controlled setting of no continued misuse then an underlying illness becomes more likely. Continued substance misuse in the context of an established diagnosis of schizophrenia or bipolar affective disorder is associated with a poorer prognosis (American Academy of Child and Adolescent Psychiatry, 1997; American Psychiatric Association, 1997; McClellan and Werry, 1994).

Conduct disorder or severe emotional disorder will not usually be confused for a psychotic disorder, although it must be remembered that in childhood and adolescence non-specific hallucinatory experiences can occur in a wide variety of non-psychotic conditions, most typically as a part of a dissociative process (Altman *et al.*, 1997). Accurate history taking and strict adherence to diagnostic criteria should avoid most confusions. However, the increased oppositional and challenging behaviours and attitudes and the inflated self-importance of the hypomanic teenager can in its early stages be mistaken as behavioural disturbance rather than illness in nature, especially if there is any prior history of conduct disturbance (American Academy of Child and Adolescent Psychiatry, 1997; Carlson, 1990, 1994).

On occasions the clinician will be asked 'Is this the prodrome or pre-psychotic phase of a psychotic illness?'. Most young people suffering from a bipolar illness and many of those suffering from a schizophrenic disorder will have had unremarkable developmental pathways prior to the onset of the first psychotic symptoms of their illness. Some, however, particularly those with a schizophrenia or schizophrenia-like illness, will have shown previous developmental and interpersonal difficulties. Excessive social anxiety and sensitivity, an oddness or gaucheness in social relationships and a mistrust of others of an overvalued nature may all reflect either a combination of developing personality traits and environmental experiences, or pre-existing ways of relating, or the prodromal stages of a psychotic episode. Attempts at identification of this schizophrenia prodrome in the months before frank psychotic symptoms appear is highly unreliable (Yung et al., 1996). Other than attempting to facilitate the early recognition of that minority who may eventually develop schizophrenia, any intervention in this group is limited to practical and psychotherapeutic supports (Birchwood, McGorry et al., 1997).

AETIOLOGICAL AND PREDISPOSING FACTORS

The precise aetiologies of both schizophrenia and bipolar disorder are not clearly established. Multi-factorial processes play a part in both with an interaction of both intrinsic and environmental factors. Genetic predisposition is clearly important with suggestions that a positive family history is more commonly found in those cases of schizophrenia or bipolar disorder with early onset than those with onset delayed into adult life (Werry, 1992). For schizophrenia there is additionally accumulating evidence of a deviant and abnormal developmental pathway throughout infancy and childhood (Done et al., 1994; Hollis, 1995; Jones et al., 1994), although the significance of this is not fully understood; it may reflect underlying vulnerability or it may reflect part of the disease process itself. These findings have lead to the increasingly held view of schizophrenia as a neurodevelopmental disorder which finds its major expression in adult life once central neural myelination of cortical pathways is completed (Volkmar, 1996; Weinberger, 1995). This maturational aspect of cortical functioning may also explain the apparent differences between manic disorders in adolescents and those rarer cases in younger children. The neurodevelopmental hypothesis is further supported by the demonstration of decreased cortical volumes and increased ventricular sizes from neuroimaging studies amongst children and adolescents with similar findings to those amongst adult sufferers (Frazier et al., 1996; Jacobsen et al., 1996; Peterson, 1995).

MANAGEMENT

The management and treatment of a young person suffering from a psychotic disorder is complex and needs to involve a multi-disciplinary and multi-modal approach. Different issues are faced at the different stages of the disorders irrespective of the precise diagnosis. In the acute phase the issues are those of immediate assessment and treatment in the least intrusive manner whilst ensuring the safety of the young person and others. After resolution of the acute episode comes a more prolonged recuperative phase in which slow continued improvement often continues. Finally, is the recovery phase in which maintenance of health, prevention of relapse and rehabilitation are the main goals of treatments.

ACUTE PHASE

Early recognition is important both in reducing immediate handicap and distress for the sufferer and their family, and potentially in reducing long-term morbidity. Many episodes of first onset psychosis go unrecognised by professionals for some months after the development of acute symptoms despite the concerns of carers (Johnstone et al., 1986) and an appropriate index of suspicion for what is admittedly a rare disorder is vital. Additionally there seems to be an association between the duration of untreated psychosis and a poorer long-term outcome, leading to the hypothesis that enduring untreated psychosis may of itself exert a toxic effect upon cerebral functioning (Wyatt, 1995).

Once the diagnosis is suspected the first task is to gain the cooperation of the sufferer and their family in further assessment and treatment. In some cases this may not be possible despite attempts at engagement, explanation and appropriate reassurances. Where the health or safety of a young person or others is at significant risk it may be necessary to consider mandatory treatment through mental health legislation (in England and Wales via the Mental Health Act 1983; other jurisdictions will have their own legislation) (Department of Health and Welsh Office, 1993; Nicholls et al., 1996). In most cases, however, this will not be necessary, and it will be possible to obtain adequate consent for informal treatment from both the young person and their carer. The developmental stage and level of understanding of the young person when well is an important factor in considering the level of consent or assent needed from the young person themselves (McClellan and Werry, 1994; Pearce, 1994). The information given in obtaining consent must include not merely likely benefits of treatment but also its potential risks (Brabbins et al., 1996).

The next decision is whether treatment can be undertaken as an outpatient or whether day or inpatient admission to hospital may be required. This needs careful discussion with the individual and with their carers. If there is no evidence of significant risk of aggression, unpredictability or suicide and if full compliance with investigation and treatment can be anticipated then it may be possible to continue as an outpatient, albeit at very regular review, possibly even daily in the first instance (Clark and Lewis 1998; Tolbert, 1996). Where the level of risk is too great or when full compliance is unlikely then day or inpatient care should be considered. Ideally this should be within the age-appropriate setting of an adolescent mental health service (Department of Health and Welsh Office, 1993;

Jaffa, 1995; Parry-Jones, 1991). The reality, however, is that too few adolescent units offer an emergency admission or even assessment response and often the only possible venue for admission will be to an adult mental health ward, or for younger teenagers perhaps a paediatric ward (Health Advisory Service, 1995). In such circumstances parents and young people may elect to continue in outpatient treatment despite advice towards admission. On very rare occasions the level of disturbance of a young person and their nursing care needs may mean that a high dependency setting is needed or even, *in extremis*, a period of seclusion in order to ensure safety (Angold and Pickles, 1993).

Psychopharmacological interventions are discussed more fully in Chapter 18, but some outline consideration is necessary here. Additional detail can also be found in texts of child and adolescent psychopharmacology (e.g. Green, 1995; Kutcher, 1997; Weiner, 1996). In any young person presenting with signs and symptoms of a psychotic disorder a period of observation and assessment prior to instituting any drug treatment is desirable, although this may not always be possible in the face of high levels of disturbance or distress (Clark and Lewis 1998).

In schizophrenia and the schizophrenia-like psychoses the mainstay of drug treatment is antipsychotic medication (Findling *et al.*, 1996; McClellan and Werry, 1994). Historically antipsychotic medication has meant the prescription of one of the older neuroleptic agents such as chlorpromazine, haloperidol or thioridazine despite their extensive side effect profile and particularly their risk of producing an irreversible tardive dyskinesia (Casey, 1993; Remschmidt, 1993a,b; Sachdev, 1995). Although in the past there has been a tendency to use high dosages of these, there is little evidence that this practice has greater therapeutic effect than lower dosages and certainly it carries increased side effects (Kane, 1994; Lowe *et al.*, 1996; Thompson, 1994; Will *et al.*, 1994). Daily dosages of above 10 mg haloperidol equivalent should therefore now be the exception (Clark and Lewis, 1998; McClellan and Werry, 1994). With the development of the newer 'atypical' antipsychotic drugs (risperidone, olanzepine and quetiapine) which carry a much lesser risk both of side effects in general and of tardive dyskinesia in particular, whilst still appearing to have at least equal efficacy, there is now an alternative (Thomas and Lewis, 1998). Reduced side effects are likely to be associated with better compliance and therefore better overall long-term outcome, although the studies to show this are not yet available. These 'atypicals' appear to now be becoming the drugs of first choice despite their greater cost. If they do mean better outcome then even this greater initial cost may be offset by subsequent lower health care needs and overall costs may in fact be reduced. This has already been shown to be the case in treatment of treatment-resistant schizophrenia with clozapine (Aitchison and Kerwin, 1997; Davies and Drummond, 1993, 1994; Knapp, 1997; Robert and Kennedy, 1997). Regardless of whether an atypical agent or a neuroleptic is chosen, it should be continued for 6–8 weeks before being considered ineffective and a change of medication considered. Where sedative effects are required over and above those provided by the antipsychotic agent chosen then a benzodiazepine could be added for a limited period (Clark and Lewis, 1998). When two antipsychotic drugs each for adequate time periods have failed to produce therapeutic benefit then prescription of clozapine, which is of proven benefit in treatment resistant schizophrenia, should be considered (American Psychiatric Association, 1997; Kumra et al., 1996).

In those patients who do not comply with oral medication despite all attempts at encouragement and enlistment of other supports (information and explanation, community psychiatric nursing involvement, parents, school, once daily dosages, adjustment of daytime routine, etc.), it may be necessary to prescribe a depot preparation (Lowe et al., 1996; Remschmidt, 1993b; see Fenton et al., 1997, for a detailed discussion of compliance and non-compliance). These are oily preparations of neuroleptic agents given by deep intramuscular injection at intervals of between 1 week and 1 month. None of the 'atypical' agents are currently available in this form and therefore the benefits of greater compliance must be weighed against the increased risk of side effects.

The considerations regarding decisions about inpatient or outpatient care, the preference for drug-free observation and on occasions the need for compulsory treatment apply equally to episodes of manic disorder. However, whilst the acute phase of a manic disorder can be treated with antipsychotic medication, the prescription of a mood stabiliser is generally to be preferred as first-line treatment (Kafantaris, 1995). There is some evidence for the efficacy of each of lithium, carbamazepine and sodium valproate (American Academy of Child and Adolescent Psychiatry, 1997; Carlson, 1994; Cookson, 1997; Freeman and Stoll, 1998; Moncrieff, 1997; Post et al., 1997), both as single agents or in various combinations with each and with other agents. If an additional sedative effect is still required the adjunctive prescription of a benzodiazepine alongside the mood stabiliser is often a useful strategy, although should not be used over the longer term in view of the risks of producing dependency. Very rarely electroconvulsive treatments (ECT) may be considered in the treatment of severe and life-threatening manic disorder not responding to pharmacological intervention alone (Freeman, 1995; Rey and Walter, 1997).

Individual and family supports are an essential component of management through this phase as both the young person and their family (including any siblings, who may additionally have fears and anxieties for their own mental health) seek to make sense of the nature and effects of the illness. Information giving about the diagnosis, the treatments and the likely course will need to be repeated on a number of occasions as the process of bereavement for the loss of the healthy individual takes place. It may be useful for this to be given in writing as well as verbally so as to be available for future reference. This work provides a basis for greater likelihood of subsequent treatment compliance and for any more formal individual or family based interventional packages to be delivered during later phases of the disorder (see below).

RECUPERATIVE/RECOVERY PHASE

The acute psychotic symptoms can be expected to be resolving with antipsychotic drug treatment by 6–8 weeks, although a proportion of cases may prove resistant to one or more agents necessitating the choice of second- or even third-line treatments. Whilst a very few may remain severely ill despite all interventions there then usually follows a more prolonged phase in which concentration, social functioning, and vocational and educational abilities gradually all continue to improve. Liaison and planning around post-recovery educational or vocational arrangements are important here, possibly with a graded or phased transition from adolescent unit-based schooling to that out of hospital. Additional supports (often both to the young person and to educational staff), reduced timetabling and/or decreased academic demands may be necessary parts of any aftercare plan.

Family interventional packages with an emphasis upon giving of information, improving communications and clarifying expectations have been well developed in adult mental health practice (Frances et al., 1996), and shown to be associated with improvements in the subsequent course of the disorder by reducing relapse rates and improving social functioning (de Jesus Mari and Streiner, 1994; Dixon and Lehman, 1995; Penn and Mueser, 1996). These have not been formally evaluated for use within adolescent populations (Dixon and Lehman, 1995), and there may be specific adaptations necessary to take account of the young person's developmental stage and what would be appropriate autonomy and independence for them. Strategies aimed at the reduction of high levels of 'expressed emotion' in the form of hostility and criticism directed to the young person, however, are likely to be beneficial irrespective of age. Arranging appropriate vocational or educational provision can also be a useful means of reducing time spent in such an environment, alongside its other aims of offering achievement, success and social integration. Family interventions also play an important role in managing the questions and anxieties of siblings, and in enabling the family together to develop a common language and understanding around the psychotic disorder.

Specific individual psychological therapies have been shown to be of some benefit for some adult sufferers of psychotic disorders. Again these have not been formally evaluated in adolescents. Problems-solving skills, social skills training, coping strategy enhancements (Tarrier et al., 1993) and cognitive-behavioural approaches (Drury et al., 1996a,b) have all been advocated although benefits seem to be confined to limited effects upon improved social functioning rather than to any effect upon relapse rates (Penn and Mueser, 1996). Continued supportive work around the impact of the disorder upon the young person's life and upon their development of adult identity is also important in maintaining treatment engagement and compliance.

The voluntary sector can often be an additional source of valuable individual and family supports. A variety of organisations including MIND (Granta House, 15–19 Broadway, Stratford, London E15 4BQ; Tel: 020 8519 2122), the

National Schizophrenia Fellowship (28 Castle Street, Kingston upon Thames, Surrey KT1 1SS; Tel: 020 8547 3937; www.nsf.org.uk) and the Manic Depression Fellowship (6–10 High Street, Kingston upon Thames, Surrey KT1 1EY; Tel: 020 8974 6550) may have active local groups which could prove useful to either young people or their carers. They also produce a range of useful and informative factsheets and booklets (e.g. National Schizophrenia Fellowship, 1998).

RESIDUAL/MAINTENANCE PHASE

The focus here is upon maintaining treatment compliance over time, and upon maximising the functioning and well-being of the individual. There is no clear consensus on how long any young person should remain either on medication or subject to psychiatric monitoring after apparent recovery from a psychotic episode. Where symptoms persist or functioning remains impaired the need for continued collaborative health and social care planning is more clear-cut, together with an eventual planned transition into adult mental health services. This transition should be carefully managed so that the young person and their family do not find themselves abandoned by all familiar workers simultaneously on, for example, the young person's 18th birthday, but rather that some continuity is always maintained through each change. The principles of the Care Programme Approach, with its emphasis upon appointment of a key worker, full assessment of needs and regular review of progress, should be implemented early in the treatment planning with a young person and their family. In practice, rigid age criteria and artificial service demarcations can act as barriers to smooth transitions of care and a pro-active approach which highlights the young person's particular needs from both adult and child oriented services is often necessary. A period of dual involvement is often helpful if it can be negotiated, provided of course that channels of clinical responsibilities are clearly agreed and communicated to all professionals and the young person and their carers.

The asymptomatic individual on medication who has appeared well for some time poses considerable dilemmas in treatment planning. Most authorities would concur that a first episode of psychosis (whether manic or schizophrenic in nature) should be treated for at least 12 months before considering discontinuation of medication. Reduction should be gradual and closely monitored for any deterioration in the young person's mental state. The timing should be discussed fully with both them and their carers, and the unquantifiable risk of relapse clearly stated. Some young people and families may not wish to take such a risk, and these wishes should be respected and treatment continued. Where there is a wish to stop medication a period of minimal other change in a young person's life should be chosen in so far as possible (i.e. not to coincide with a change of school or college or other major disruption to a young person's routine and support system). Early warning signs of potential relapse should be discussed and avenues of psychiatric help clarified. Remaining in outpatient follow-up for period post-withdrawal may be an important part of providing effective aftercare arrangements.

OUTCOMES

Distinguishing manic disorders and schizophrenias from each other at first presentation is often unreliable, and the pattern of the illness may only become apparent with time. Short-term follow-up studies indicate that a substantial number of young people will 'switch' diagnosis subsequently, particularly from a diagnosis of schizophrenia to one of affective disorder (Carlson, 1990; McClellan et al., 1993; Werry et al., 1994). This makes giving accurate prognostic information to young people and their families difficult although the range of possible outcomes should be discussed.

Longer-term follow-up studies of the outcome of young people diagnosed as suffering from psychotic disorders are not encouraging. Cawthron et al. (1994) followed up 58 young people who had been admitted to an inpatient adolescent psychiatric unit suffering from a psychotic disorder and compared them to a group of non-psychotic inpatients. Nineteen of the psychotic group were diagnosed as suffering from schizophrenia and a further nine from a schizo-affective disorder. After a mean follow-up period of 11 years, the schizophrenic group had a significantly poorer outcome either than the bipolar group or than the schizo-affective group (only 36% of the originally matched pairs completed the study). Seven of the nine followed up who were diagnosed as suffering from schizophrenia had remained continuously ill. Gillberg et al. (1993) reported an extremely poor outcome in 18 out of 23 cases of schizophrenia with no better outcome for bipolar or schizo-affective disorders in a follow-up study of teenage psychosis to age 30 years. These studies obviously relate to treatment interventions before some of the newer drugs (particularly the atypical antipsychotics but also the more extensive usage of carbamazepine and sodium valproate as mood stabilisers) now available were developed. Whilst follow-up studies of young people currently under treatment might therefore be slightly more encouraging, it is doubtful that the picture would be radically different.

REFERENCES

Adams, M., Kutcher, S., Antoniw, E., Bird, D. and Ryan, N. D. (1996) Diagnostic utility of endocrine and neuroimaging screening tests in first-onset adolescent psychosis. Journal of the American Academy of Child and Adolescent Psychiatry, 35, 67–73.

Aitchison, K. J. and Kerwin, R. W. (1997) Cost-effectiveness of clozapine. *British Journal of Psychiatry*, **171**, 125–130.

Altman, H., Collins, M. and Mundy, P. (1997) Subclinical hallucinations and delusions in nonpsychotic adolescents. *Journal of Child Psychology and Psychiatry*, **38**, 413–420.

American Academy of Child and Adolescent Psychiatry (1997) Practice parameters for the assessment and treatment of children and adolescents with bipolar disorder. *Journal of the American Academy of Child and Adolescent Psychiatry*, **36** (10 Suppl.), 157S–176S.

American Psychiatric Association (1994) *Diagnostic and Statistical Manual of Mental Disorders*, 4th edn (DSM-IV). Washington, DC: American Psychiatric Association.

American Psychiatric Association (1997) Practice guideline for the treatment of patients with schizophrenia. *American Journal of Psychiatry*, **154** (Suppl. April), 1–63.

Angold, A. and Pickles, A. (1993) Seclusion on an adolescent unit. *Journal of Child Psychology and Psychiatry*, **34**, 975–989.

Asarnow, R. F. and Asarnow, J. R. (1994) Childhood-onset schizophrenia: Editors' introduction. *Schizophrenia Bulletin*, **20**, 591–597.

Birchwood, M., McGorry, P. and Jackson, H. (1997) Early intervention in schizophrenia. *British Journal of Psychiatry*, **170**, 2–5.

Brabbins, C., Butler, J. and Bentall, R. (1996) Consent to neuroleptic medication for schizophrenia: clinical, ethical and legal issues. *British Journal of Psychiatry*, **168**, 540–544.

Carlson, G. A. (1990) Annotation: child and adolescent mania – diagnostic considerations. *Journal of Child Psychology and Psychiatry*, **31**, 331–341.

Carlson, G. A. (1994) Adolescent bipolar disorder. In W. M. Reynolds and H. E. Johnston (eds), *Handbook of Depression in Children and Adolescents*. New York: Plenum, pp. 41–60.

Casey, D. E. (1993) Neuroleptic induced acute extrapyramidal syndromes and tardive dyskinesia. *Psychiatric Clinics of North America*, **16**, 589–610.

Cawthron, P., James, A., Dell, J. and Seagrott, V. (1994) Adolescent onset psychosis. A clinical and outcome study. *Journal of Child Psychology and Psychiatry*, **35**, 1321–1332.

Clark, A. F. and Lewis, S. W. (1998) Practitioner review: the treatment of schizophrenia in childhood and adolescence. *Journal of Child Psychology and Psychiatry*, **39**, 1071–81.

Cookson, J. (1997) Lithium: balancing risks and benefits. *British Journal of Psychiatry*, **171**, 120–125.

Davies, L. M. and Drummond, M. F. (1993) Assessment of costs and benefits of drug therapy for treatment-resistant schizophrenia in the United Kingdom. *British Journal of Psychiatry*, **162**, 38–42.

Davies, L. M. and Drummond, M. F. (1994) Economics and schizophrenia: the real cost. *British Journal of Psychiatry*, **165** (Suppl. 25), 18–21.

de Jesus Mari, J. and Streiner, D. L. (1994) An overview of family interventions and relapse on schizophrenia: meta-analysis of research findings. *Psychological Medicine*, **24**, 565–578.

Department of Health and Welsh Office (1993) *Code of Practice Mental Health Act 1983*. London: HMSO.

Dixon, L. B. and Lehman, A. F. (1995) Family interventions for schizophrenia. *Schizophrenia Bulletin*, **21**, 631–643.

Done, D. J., Crow, T. L., Johnstone, E. C. and Sacker, A. (1994) Childhood antecedents of schizophrenia and affective illness: social adjustment at ages 7 and 11. *British Medical Journal*, **309**, 699–703.

Drury, V., Birchwood, M., Cochrane, R. and Macmillan, F. (1996a) Cognitive therapy and recovery from acute psychosis: a controlled trial. I: Impact upon psychotic symptoms. *British Journal of Psychiatry*, **169**, 593–601.

Drury, V., Birchwood, M., Cochrane, R. and Macmillan, F. (1996b) Cognitive therapy and recovery from acute psychosis: a controlled trial. II: Impact upon recovery time. *British Journal of Psychiatry*, **169**, 602–607.

Fenton, W. S., Blyler, C. R. and Heinssen R. K. (1997) Determinants of medication compliance in schizophrenia: empirical and clinical findings. *Schizophrenia Bulletin*, **23**, 637–651.

Findling, R. L., Grcevich, S. J., Lopez, I. and Schulz, S. C. (1996) Antipsychotic medications in children and adolescents. *Journal of Clinical Psychiatry*, **57** (Suppl. 9), 19–23.

Frances, A., Docherty, J. P. and Kahn, D. A. (1996) Expert concensus guideline series: treatment of schizophrenia. *Journal of Clinical Psychiatry*, **57** (Suppl 12B), 5–58.

Frazier, J. A., Giedd, J. N., Hamburger, S. D., Albus, K. E., Kaysen, D., Vaituzis, A. C. *et al.* (1996) Brain anatomic magnetic resonance imaging in childhood onset schizophrenia. *Archives of General Psychiatry*, **53**, 617–624.

Freeman, C. P. (1995) ECT in those under 18 years old. In C. P. Freeman (ed.), *The ECT Handbook*. London: Royal College of Psychiatrists, pp. 18–21.

Freeman, M. P. and Stoll, A. L. (1998) Mood stabilizer combinations: a review of safety and efficacy. *American Journal of Psychiatry*, **155**, 12–21.

Geller, B. and Luby, J. (1997) Child and adolescent bipolar disorder: a review of the past 10 years. *Journal of the American Academy of Child and Adolescent Psychiatry*, **36**, 1168–1176.

Gillberg, C., Wahlstrom, J., Forsman, A., Hellgren, L. and Gillberg, I. C. (1986) Teenage psychoses – epidemiology, classification and reduced optimality in the pre-, peri- and neonatal periods. *Journal of Child Psychology and Psychiatry*, **27**, 87–98.

Gillberg, I. C., Hellgren, L. and Gillberg, C. (1993) Psychotic disorders diagnosed in adolescence. Outcome at 30 years. *Journal of Child Psychology and*

Psychiatry, **34,** 1173–1186.

Green, W. H. (1995) *Child and Adolescent Clinical Psychopharmacology.* Baltimore, MD: Williams & Wilkins.

Hafner, H. and Nowotny, B. (1995) Epidemiology of early onset schizophrenia. *European Archives of Psychiatry and Clinical Neurosciences,* **245,** 80–92.

Health Advisory Service (1995) *Child and Adolescent Mental Health Services: Together We Stand.* London: HMSO.

Hollis, C. (1995) Child and adolescent (juvenile onset) schizophrenia: a case control study of premorbid developmental impairments. *British Journal of Psychiatry,* **166,** 489–495.

Jacobsen, L. K., Giedd, J. N., Vaituzis, A. C., Hamburger, S. D., Rajapakse, J. C., Frazier, J. A. *et al.* (1996) Temporal lobe morphology in childhood onset schizophrenia. *American Journal of Psychiatry,* **153,** 355–361.

Jaffa, T. (1995) Adolescent psychiatry services. *British Journal of Psychiatry,* **166,** 306–310.

Johnstone, E. C., Crow, T. J., Johnson, A. L. and MacMillan, J. F. (1986) The Northwick Park study of first episodes of schizophrenia: I. Presentation of the illness and problems relating to admission. *British Journal of Psychiatry,* **164,** 431–432.

Jones, P., Rodgers, B., Murray, R. and Marmot, M. (1994) Child developmental risk factors for adult schizophrenia in the British 1946 birth cohort. *Lancet,* **344,** 1398–1402.

Kafantaris, V. (1995) Treatment of bipolar disorder in children and adolescents. *Journal of the American Academy of Child and Adolescent Psychiatry,* **34,** 732–741.

Kafantaris, V. (1996) Diagnostic issues in childhood psychosis. *Current Opinion in Psychiatry,* **9,** 247–250.

Kane, J. M. (1994) The use of higher-dose antipsychotic medication. *British Journal of Psychiatry,* **164,** 431–432.

Kaufman, J., Birmaher, B., Brent, D., Rao, U. and Ryan, N. (1996) *Kiddie–Sads– Present and Lifetime Version (K-SADS-PL).* Pittsburg, PA: Western Psychiatric Institute and Clinic.

Knapp, M. (1997) Costs of schizophrenia. *British Journal of Psychiatry,* **171,** 509–518.

Kolvin, I. (1972) Late onset psychosis. *British Medical Journal,* **3,** 816–817.

Kumra, S., Frazier, J. A., Jacobsen, L. K., McKenna, K., Gordon, C. T., Lenane, M. C. *et al.* (1996) Childhood onset schizophrenia: a double blind clozapine haloperidol comparison. *Archives of General Psychiatry,* **53,** 1090–1097.

Kutcher, S. (1997) *Child and Adolescent Psychopharmacology.* Philadelphia, PA: Saunders.

Lowe, K., Smith, H. and Clark, A. (1996) Neuroleptic prescribing in an adolescent psychiatric in-patient unit. *Psychiatric Bulletin,* **20,** 538–540.

Mason, P., Harrison, G., Croudace, T., Glazebrook, C. and Medley, I. (1997) The predictive validity of a diagnosis of schizophrenia. *British Journal of Psychiatry*, **170**, 321–327.

McClellan, J. and Werry, J. (1994) Practice parameters for the assessment and treatment of children and adolescents with schizophrenia. *Journal of the American Academy of Child and Adolescent Psychiatry*, **33**, 616–635.

McClellan, J. M., Werry, J. S. and Ham, M. (1993) A follow-up study of early onset psychosis: Comparison between outcome diagnoses of schizophrenia, mood disorders and personality disorders. *Journal of Autism and Developmental Disorders*, **23**, 243–262.

Moncrieff, J. (1997) Lithium: evidence reconsidered. *British Journal of Psychiatry*, **171**, 113–119.

National Schizophrenia Fellowship (1998) *NSF Caring and Coping Resource Pack*. Kingston upon Thames: National Schizophrenia Fellowship.

Nicholls, J. E., Fernandez, C. A. and Clark, A. F. (1996) Use of mental health legislation in a regional adolescent unit. *Psychiatric Bulletin*, **20**, 711–713.

Parry-Jones, W. Ll. (1991) Adolescent psychoses: treatment and service provision. *Archives of Diseases in Childhood*, **66**, 1459–1462.

Pearce, J. (1994) Consent to treatment during childhood. *British Journal of Psychiatry*, **165**, 713–716.

Penn, D. L. and Mueser, K. T. (1996) Research update on the psychosocial treatment of schizophrenia. *American Journal of Psychiatry*, **153**, 607–617.

Peterson, B. S. (1995) Neuroimaging in child and adolescent neuropsychiatric disorders. *Journal of the American Academy of Child and Adolescent Psychiatry*, **34**, 1560–1576.

Post, R. M., Denicoff, K. D., Frye M. A. and Leverich G. S. (1997) Re-evaluating carbamazepine prophylaxis in bipolar disorder. *British Journal of Psychiatry*, **170**, 202–204.

Rapoport, J. L. and Ismond, D. R. (1996) *DSM-IV Training Guide for Diagnosis of Childhood Disorders*. New York: Brunner/Mazel.

Remschmidt, H. (1993a) Childhood and adolescent schizophrenia. *Current Opinion in Psychiatry*, **6**, 470–479.

Remschmidt, H. (1993b) Schizophrenic psychoses in children and adolescents. *Triangle*, **32**, 15–24.

Remschmidt, H. E., Schulz, E., Martin, M., Warnke, A. and Trott, G. E. (1994) Childhood-onset schizophrenia: history of the concept and recent studies. *Schizophrenia Bulletin*, **20**, 727–745.

Rey, J. M. and Walter, G. (1997) Half a century of ECT use in young people. *American Journal of Psychiatry*, **154**, 595–602.

Robert, G. and Kennedy, P. (1997) Establishing cost-effectiveness of atypical neuroleptics. *British Journal of Psychiatry*, **171**, 103–104.

Sachdev, P. (1995) The epidemiology of drug induced akathisia: part II. Chronic tardive and withdrawal akathisias. *Schizophrenia Bulletin*, **21**, 451–461.

Tarrier, N., Beckett, R., Harwood, S., Baker, A., Yusupoff, L. and Ugarteburu, I. (1993) A trial of two cognitive behavioural methods of treating drug resistant residual psychotic symptoms in schizophrenic patients: I. Outcome. *British Journal of Psychiatry*, **162**, 524–532.

Thomas, C. S. and Lewis, S. (1998) Which atypical antipsychotic? *British Journal of Psychiatry*, **172**, 106–109.

Thompson, C. (1994) The use of high-dose antipsychotic medication. *British Journal of Psychiatry*, **164**, 448–458.

Tolbert, H. A. (1996) Psychoses in children and adolescents: a review. *Journal of Clinical Psychiatry*, **57** (Suppl. 3), 4–8.

Volkmar, F. R. (1996) Childhood and adolescent psychosis: a review of the past 10 years. *Journal of the American Academy of Child and Adolescent Psychiatry*, **35**, 843–851.

Weinberger, D. R. (1995) From neuropathology to neurodevelopment. *Lancet*, **346**, 552–557.

Weiner, J. M. (1996) *Diagnosis and Psychopharmacology of Ahildhood and Adolescent Disorders*. New York: Wiley.

Werry, J. S. (1992) Child and adolescent (early onset) schizophrenia: a review in light of DSM-IIIR. *Journal of Autism and Developmental Disorders*, **22**, 601–624.

Werry, J. S., McClellan, J. M., Andrews, L. K. and Ham, M. (1994) Clinical features and outcome of child and adolescent schizophrenia. *Schizophrenia Bulletin*, **20**, 619–630.

Will, D., Wrate, R. M., Bhate, S., Taylor, P., James, T., Rothery, D. *et al.* (1994) High-dose antipsychotic medication. *British Journal of Psychiatry*, **165**, 269–270.

World Health Organisation (1992) *The ICD-10 Classification of Mental and Behavioural Disorders. Clinical Descriptions and Diagnostic Guidelines*. Geneva: World Health Organisation.

Wyatt, R. J. (1995) Early intervention in schizophrenia: can the course of the illness be altered? *Biological Psychiatry*, **38**, 1–3.

Yung, A. R., McGorry, P. D., McFarlane, C. A., Jackson, H. J., Patton, G. C. and Rakkar, A. (1996) Monitoring and care of young people at incipient risk of psychosis. *Schizophrenia Bulletin*, **22**, 283–303.

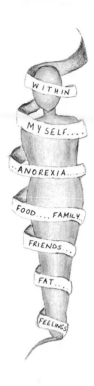

Chapter 9

EATING DISORDERS

Simon G. Gowers

INTRODUCTION

In many ways eating disorders typify adolescent mental health problems. Their origins are multifactorial, sociocultural factors and life events tending to impact on a vulnerable personality, possibly shaped by family environment against a background of genetic and biological predisposition. Within anorexia nervosa particularly, it is usually possible to identify difficulties in the areas of identity formation, independence, behavioural control and physical growth which are the essence of the teenage years.

Eating disorders can be difficult to treat and they cause considerable professional anxiety. This in part relates to the potential for a lethal outcome – anorexia nervosa has the highest mortality of any adolescent disorder – and also because patients commonly resist treatment and can be defensive about their behaviour.

Treatment can be controversial, particularly with regard to the indications for admission and where that is best provided. Obtaining informed consent is beset by difficulties.

This chapter will review issues in the aetiology, treatment and outcome of eating disorders, and provide illustrative clinical examples.

HISTORICAL BACKGROUND

Although eating disorders are of great topical interest, they are not new phenomena, medical reports date back to the 17th century (Morton 1694). The 19th century accounts (Gull, 1874; Lasegue, 1873) demonstrate that enough cases of anorexia nervosa could be drawn together to constitute a case series, whilst these clinical accounts are notable in terms of the similarity between the symptoms and concerns expressed 125 years ago and the condition we see today. Gull, in particular, was impressed by the inter-relation between family relationships and the condition, to the extent that he believed separation from family members was necessary in order to bring about a recovery. Bulimia nervosa, meanwhile, is a relatively recently described condition, originally described as an ominous variant of anorexia nervosa (Russell, 1979). It is now clear, however, that the condition occurs generally without a previous history of anorexia.

EPIDEMIOLOGY/PREVALENCE

The reported prevalence of anorexia nervosa varies somewhat with the method of ascertainment. A two-stage method involving a screening questionnaire followed by a semistructured interview of identified cases is the most widely employed. Using strict criteria, this method reveals lower rates than questionnaire surveys alone. The average point prevalence of anorexia nervosa thus determined is 280/100 000 (0.28%) (Hoek, 1995). The figure for boys is said to be about 1/2000 (Crisp et al., 1976). There are suggestions of an increase in prevalence over the past 50 years, the best evidence for which comes from Rochester, USA (Lucas et al., 1991), though this finding has been challenged by Fombonne (1995). This study suggested an increase in incidence of 36% in adolescent females every 5 years from 1950 to 1984. Case series focussing on the younger end of the age spectrum (e.g. Bryant-Waugh and Lask, 1995) suggest a more equal sex ratio in pre-pubertal cases.

There are suggestions that eating disorders may have changed over time, particularly in the increasing ratio of the purging form of anorexia nervosa to the restricting. Anorexia nervosa used to be seen as a middle class disorder of the white, Western world. This is no longer the case, although uncertainties exist as far as whether there has been a change in identification of cases in different cultures or whether the condition has spread to black immigrant populations, and to developing nations as they have taken on Western culture and aspirations. Hong Kong, in particular, seems to have seen a recent growth in eating disorders over the past 15 years (Lee and Chiu, 1989; Lee and Lee, 1996). There have been suggestions that girls who are second- or third-generation migrants from the Indian subcontinent may be at least of equal risk to the indigenous population.

Since 1980, reports of the 'new' eating disorder bulimia nervosa have suggested a growing epidemic. Surveys using questionnaires have suggested that up to 19% of female students report bulimic symptoms (Hoek, 1995). This author suggests a point prevalence of 1500 cases per 100 000 young females in the community, a rate approximately five times that for anorexia nervosa. As bulimia nervosa is easier to conceal than anorexia, the rates of the two disorders in primary care are virtually equal, whilst rates in mental health care are higher for anorexia nervosa.

CLASSIFICATION

This chapter will focus mainly on the related conditions of anorexia and bulimia nervosa. These syndromes, represented in both ICD-10 and DSM-IV systems, comprise physical, psychological, behavioural and social features which pervade all aspects of sufferers' lives. Increasingly, however, attention is being directed to the problems of obese adolescents, due to the current rapid increase in prevalence and the relationship with other eating disorders. Obesity will therefore be discussed briefly.

For completeness, mention should be made of the other eating and feeding disorders, which occur earlier in adolescence, having usually commenced in childhood. Bryant-Waugh and Kaminsky (1993) list these as selective eating, pervasive refusal, food refusal and food avoidance emotional disorder (Higgs *et al.*, 1989). Although having some features in common, these disorders are probably discontinuous with anorexia and bulimia nervosa.

ANOREXIA NERVOSA

ICD-10 criteria F50.0 (World Health Organisation, 1992) specify:

- Body weight is maintained at least 15% below that expected (lost or never achieved) or Body Mass Index [BMI = weight (kg)/height (m)^2] is below 17.5
- Weight loss is self-induced by avoidance of fattening foods. Weight loss may be induced by restriction, exercise, vomiting or purgation.
- There is a body image distortion, manifested as a dread of fatness.
- A widespread endocrine disorder involving the hypothalamic–pituitary–gonadal axis is present. In the female this is manifest as amenorrhoea and in the male as impotence and loss of sexual interest.

The ICD system addresses the difficulties of making the diagnosis in younger adolescents, allowing for failure to gain weight (and height) at puberty and for delay in the process of puberty, rather than requiring secondary amenorrhoea.

In practise the diagnosis is usually straightforward if the patient's defensiveness can be overcome by good engagement and by a parental history. It is usually possible to ascertain dietary restriction in the face of normal or increased appetite rather than through loss of appetite as in depression. Dietary restriction in depression is not usually selective, whilst the anorexic can rarely conceal her beliefs about the virtue of thinness.

Although not essential to the diagnosis, social withdrawal, regressive behaviour, rigid self-control, obsessionality and perfectionism are common. The striving for control often extends to others and the family will often report feeling controlled by their son or daughter. The ICD 10 condition 'Atypical anorexia nervosa' (F50.1) may be used if one of the key symptoms (fear of fatness or amenorrhoea) is absent in spite of marked psychogenic weight loss.

BULIMIA NERVOSA

ICD 10 criteria F50.2 (World Health Organisation, 1992) require:

- Persistent preoccupation with eating, with irresistible craving resulting in episodes of binge eating. (DSM-IV requires subjective feeling of loss of control whilst bingeing).
- Vomiting, purging or drug use (amphetamines, diet pills or diuretics) in an attempt to counteract the effect of a binge.
- Dread of fatness.

The alternating cycle of control and catastrophic loss of control is often mirrored in other areas of the subject's life, thus they may have difficulty with control of drug and alcohol use, sexual behaviour or delinquency. In extreme form, the condition has been termed the multi-impulsive form of bulimia nervosa (Lacey and Evans, 1986).

BINGE EATING DISORDER

This is not an officially recognised eating disorder. It appears as one example of an 'Eating disorder not otherwise specified' in DSM-IV, but not in ICD-10. The DSM-IV research criteria comprise:

- Recurrent episodes of binge eating, with subjective feeling of loss of control
- The binges are characterised by three or more of the following: eating very rapidly, eating until feeling uncomfortably full, eating large amounts when not physically hungry, eating alone because of embarrassment at how much one is eating and feeling disgusted, depressed or very guilty.
- Marked distress about bingeing.
- Bingeing occurs at least 2 days per week for 6 months.
- There are no (regular) compensatory purging behaviours and there is no co-existing anorexia or bulimia nervosa.

OBESITY

Although obesity is not classified as a psychiatric syndrome (it is classed in Section E of ICD-10 – E66), a number of teenagers will identify emotional factors which contribute to their over eating, whilst most will point to adverse psychosocial consequences of their condition. Difficulties with self-esteem and in peer relationships predominate. Some will be helped by psychotherapeutic measures, with or without behavioural intervention aimed at weight loss.

Desirable body weight is usually considered to be between 90 and 120% of ideal weight. Obesity can be graded according to BMI (Weinsier, 1995), as follows:

Grade of obesity	BMI
0	<25
1	25–29.9
2	30–40
3	>40

Grades 2 and 3 are clearly associated with increased health risk.

Approximately 20–30% of obese individuals report serious problems with binge eating (Marcus *et al.*, 1995).

CO-MORBIDITY

Many of those with eating disorders will be co-morbid for other disorders. Depression occurs in around 50%, obsessive-compulsive disorder in 16% and psychoses in a small number of cases. Bulimia is associated with externalising disorders such as conduct disorder, drug and substance misuse.

AETIOLOGY

The aetiology of eating disorders is widely accepted to be multidetermined (Garfinkel and Garner, 1982). In a particular case, individual personality, sociocultural and family variables are likely to be present as predisposing factors, whilst peer relationship problems, an unsatisfactory sexual experience or other life event may act as a precipitant (Gowers *et al.*, 1996).

GENETIC FACTORS

Twin and family studies have provided some support for the notion of a genetic contribution to anorexia nervosa. Holland *et al.* (1988) found 56% of monozygotic twins to be concordant for the condition, compared with only 5% of dizygotic twins. Heritability has been reported as highest in restricting anorexia and almost non-existent in bulimia nervosa (Treasure and Holland, 1990).

BIOLOGICAL FACTORS

A number of risk factors have been postulated, from pre-morbid obesity (Crisp, 1995) to excessive tallness (Joughin *et al.*, 1992). Biological vulnerability may be present as genetic predisposition to early pubertal development. It is likely that once starvation has become established, the condition may be maintained by a distortion of the hunger drive. This has been likened to models of addiction (Marrazzi and Luby, 1986).

PERSONALITY

Many children who go on to develop eating disorders in adolescence are remarkably free from neurotic traits or behavioural disturbance. They are often described as having been compliant, ideal children (Crisp, 1995). A strong sense of morality, concern about the welfare of others, conscientiousness and perfectionism have been commonly reported. It is probable that these features apply in the main to restricting anorexia. The purging form, like bulimia nervosa, is more associated with periodic loss of control, impulsivity and occasionally delinquency.

FAMILY FACTORS

Structure
Anorexia nervosa more commonly arises in intact families than other mental health problems in adolescence, although parental marital breakdown can act as a life event precipitant (Gowers *et al.*, 1996). It has been shown to occur equally in any position in the sibship (Gowers *et al.*, 1985).

Functioning
There are difficulties in extrapolating from a situation of crisis (i.e. when a family has a teenager with a life-threatening illness) and relating this to a presumed situation before the onset of disorder. Families themselves report no greater difficulties in functioning than community controls and somewhat fewer than matched families with other adolescent psychiatric disorders (North *et al.*, 1995). Adolescents with anorexia nervosa themselves do tend to be fairly critical of their families functioning, and their views and those of their treating clinicians have been shown to predict the outcome of anorexia nervosa at 1 year (North *et al.*, 1997). A recent study (Gowers and North, 1999) suggested a slight inverse relationship between family difficulties and severity of anorexia, suggesting that difficulties in family functioning were not just a result of extreme concern. Dare and Key (1999) suggest that this finding may support the notion of anorexia nervosa as an adaptive strategy to reduce family distress.

SOCIO-CULTURAL FACTORS

Most cases of anorexia nervosa occur in adolescents and young women, and they have been linked to the extreme pressure on young women to conform to today's very thin role models of feminine beauty (Garner and Garfinkel, 1980). Of course this begs the question of where societies 'choice' of model physique arises from. It is probable that the combination of availability of fast food and spending power, on the one hand, and growing aspirations (in relationships, education and employment), on the other, combine to cause a dilemma. This may result in a predicament around control symbolised by concern with restraint and fear of loss of control around eating.

PRECIPITANTS AND LIFE EVENTS

Crisp provides a compelling case for an adolescent maturational crisis underlying anorexia nervosa. In his book (Crisp, 1995), he provides a number of case illustrations in which a combination of individual and family variables lead almost inevitably to a crystallisation of the disorder. A controlled study into the role of life event precipitants (Gowers *et al.*, 1996) suggested that severe negative life events occurred in the year before onset in about one-quarter of cases only, somewhat fewer than in those with other psychiatric conditions. However where a severe negative life event had occurred, this had good prognostic power, i.e. a good outcome usually followed (North *et al.*, 1997).

MAINTAINING FACTORS

Chronicity is sadly a feature of eating disorders, although a remitting and relapsing course is rare. Full recovery is only very rarely followed by relapse. So much changes with the weight loss of anorexia nervosa that if these consequences are valued by the subject they will maintain the condition. Within the subject, weight loss usually increases concern with fatness, whilst increasing hunger usually increases the fear that loss of control may be catastrophic. The sense of effectiveness and achievement is usually hard to surrender, whilst increasing (and often united) parental concern is hard to relinquish in those who may not have felt emotionally supported. The secondary consequences of the sick role (school non-attendance, relief of obligations, social isolation) can be difficult to reverse without active steps at rehabilitation.

SOPHIE

Sophie was 15 and studying hard for her GCSE exams. At the New Year she was invited to a party at which she was shocked by a friend's sexual precocity. She noticed the disappointment in her parents' eyes when she returned home slightly intoxicated. Over the next few days they reminded her that she would now have to knuckle down and study hard if she were to achieve her required exam grades. When up in her bedroom attempting to study, however, she found difficulty concentrating and would regularly interrupt her work to slip downstairs for a couple of biscuits. When term restarted, she was shocked to find her school uniform was uncomfortably tight. She really had let herself go over the Christmas holidays! As anorexia nervosa developed, she found her will power increase and she became more single-minded. Her partying days were over – at least till her exams had passed. In any case she would not want anyone to watch her eat, so invitations had to be declined. As April came, Sophie became quite unwell with a persistent virus, which resulted in further weight loss and time off from school. She feared that she would not do as well in her exams as she should. Maybe, her parents suggested, it would be better if they got a letter from the doctor explaining her illness and took the pressure off her by postponing her exams. She could take them next year when she was fully recovered and really do justice to her abilities!

In bulimia nervosa, meanwhile, the cycle of restraint and loss of control, usually occurring on a daily basis is usually maintained by a powerful combination of physiological and psychological factors:

STEPHANIE

Stephanie was 17 when she developed bulimia nervosa. The traumatic break up of her relationship with her boyfriend had left her feeling used and physically unattractive. Her friends had never liked Steve and now their predictions had been confirmed; she was beginning to doubt her own judgement. She was left somewhat bruised by the experience and with a police caution for possession of drugs. Each day she woke with a resolution to start afresh, with a new commitment to getting her life back on track. When she restricted her eating, at least that gave her a sense of achievement; she did have some will power after all. No breakfast then and no lunch. By evening she was starving, her blood sugar was so low, it demanded she eat and calorific food too. Once she started, she found it difficult to stop. She was home much of the time now, so it was easy to pig out. At the back of her mind she knew she would easily be able to vomit back the excess, so what the heck. As she flushed the lavatory later, she reflected on the fact that her parents still did not seem to have noticed her distress. How many signals did she have to give before they gave her any time these days? As she retired to bed she chastised herself again. What a loathsome fool! She dare not think about the weight she must have put on. Tomorrow she must turn over a new leaf – no breakfast for sure. At least that would be a start and in any case all she deserved.

MANAGEMENT

ANOREXIA NERVOSA

Assessment

The general principles of assessment in adolescent psychiatry apply, with one or two differences in emphasis (see Chapter 11). Time at the assessment interview should be made for an interview with parents, the young person themselves and both together. Whilst a corroborative account of eating behaviour is important, the emphasis should not be a judgmental one, rather the parental interview can provide background personal history, the parents views of stresses impinging on their son or daughter or on their own relationship. Evidence is growing to suggest that recovery is dependent on the patient owning any changes to his or her diet and weight, i.e. recovery can rarely be imposed. This suggests that the initial engagement is very important in ensuring an effective start to treatment, a view endorsed by the pattern of progress with an outpatient approach, which suggested weight gain commenced very early or not at all (Gowers et al., 1994). Physical assessment may depend on the degree of emaciation and the extent of involvement of other physicians, but the patient should be weighed and measured, and some assessment should be made of pubertal status. Further physical and haematological investigation will be indicated by the history and degree of emaciation, but concern is aroused by those who are less than 75% of expected weight for height, those who vomit or purge, those who restrict fluids and where weight is falling rapidly, rather than remaining steady at a low level. The co-existence of a metabolic disorder such as diabetes mellitus obviously requires special attention. Sometimes the extent of malnourishment can be underestimated if height has been significantly stunted. This is nearly always the case in a subject under the age of 14 years who has been underweight for a year. It is not appropriate to consider a weight on the third centile to be healthy for a girl who is on the third centile for height, any more than a weight on the 97th centile (an obese weight) for someone who is unusually tall.

Treatment

In anorexia nervosa, a comprehensive approach, which takes account of the physical needs of the patient alongside psychiatric issues, is required. The aim should be for restoration to normal weight and eating, with appropriate psychological adjustment. The treatment of choice is unclear, though intervention has been demonstrated to be more effective than no treatment (Crisp et al., 1991) and seems to require weight restoration to normal levels if full recovery is to be achieved (Ratnasuriya et al., 1991).

Whereas in adults treatment usually aims to return the sufferer to a state of pre-morbid health, in adolescents the task frequently involves achieving a healthy post-pubertal weight for the first time. This is usually accompanied by a new experience of engagement with adolescence in all its aspects, which can be as challenging as the adjustment to increased weight. This adjustment may be perceived as a challenge by parents too.

There are no completely satisfactory guidelines at present to the choice of treatment setting. Whilst pragmatic issues suggest that admission may be the logical step for those in whom physical concerns are greatest and those who fail to make progress on an outpatient basis, the indications for hospital admission are not well established.

Case series treated as hospital inpatients (Crisp et al., 1991; Eisler et al., 1997) often lose weight after discharge, before subsequently recovering, raising the question of the part played by inpatient treatment in recovery. Where inpatient treatment is coercive and perceived by the adolescent as punitive, it may contribute to a poor outcome (Gowers et al., 2000). The only randomised controlled trial of inpatient against outpatient treatment showed a modest advantage of outpatient treatment, with continuing benefits of the outpatient approach being evident at 2 years (Crisp et al., 1991; Gowers et al., 1994). Although both the Maudsley and St George's Hospital series referred to above combined adolescents and young adults, it is not possible to say whether the benefits or unwanted effects of hospital treatment are greater or less in younger subjects. On the one hand, ensuring completion of puberty and avoiding stunting of growth may be extremely important. On the other, disruption of education and normal social development might especially harm a younger person. An individual decision about admission may rest on such issues as the wishes of the patient and family, the expertise available in any setting, and the degree of physical concern. Some would argue that where a young person is failing in all areas of life, admission to a specialist adolescent service might involve a step forward rather than a step back from normal adolescent experience and thus could be construed as rehabilitative (see Chapter 14). Although compulsory treatment is permissible in certain circumstances under the Mental Health Act, the evidence for the effectiveness of coercive treatment using behavioural methods in the long term is poor (Bruch, 1974; Tiller et al., 1993).

Day programmes for the treatment of adolescents with eating disorders are rare in the UK. They have the advantage of combining the benefits of intensive treatment, peer support and behavioural therapies (particularly around meal times) without the disadvantages (and costs) of admission.

Clinicians are increasingly drawing attention to the importance of engagement and positive motivation if short-term gains are to be maintained in the longer term whatever the treatment setting (Ward et al., 1996).

Therapeutic style

There are advocates of family systemic, cognitive behavioural and cognitive analytic approaches. Assessment should have revealed the role, if any, of family difficulties in the presentation. All cases are likely to require some parental counselling to address practical issues such as dietary planning, education and sporting activities. In some cases, where family communication seems poor, there is a difficulty in a particular relationship or the disorder appears to have been precipitated by a family issue, more formal family therapy may be helpful. The Maudsley Hospital research group have suggested that approaches which involve the family are particularly beneficial when the patient is under 19 and that these advantages are still demonstrable at 5-year follow-up (Eisler et al., 1997).

Sometimes the young person's anorexia seems to have developed against a background of attempting to satisfy parental expectation or out of an attempt to resolve marital disharmony by bringing parents together. Sometimes parents have their own very strict beliefs about the value of self-control or about weight and shape. In these cases, the therapeutic task seems to be about helping the adolescent to achieve a degree of independence from parental expectation. A therapeutic style which puts 'parents in charge' might be at odds with this approach. Sometimes young people will suggest that they should attempt to recover for their parent's sake. If the condition involves a greater than optimal concern about the opinions and expectations of others, this might be considered unhelpful; a more self-centred attitude in which the sufferer resolves to permit herself to be herself in spite of others expectations would seem to be more liberating. The notion of liberation is, I think, especially apposite. Like liberation from prison, freedom from anorexia can be paradoxically threatening. Often the patient will confuse the encouragement to make progress with restriction and a pressure to conform. This may conceal their fear of independence and abandonment. In the longer term, it will be apparent that others will intrude far less on one's life if the disorder can be relinquished; an issue that can usefully be explored in a motivational interview weighing up the 'pros and cons' of recovery.

In a similar vein, making progress can be confused with being good. Few are as morally self-conscious or indeed saintly as the restricting anorexic. Progress usually involves being 'less good' and trying less hard in aiming for perfection. The dynamics of purging anorexia are somewhat different, but the sufferer is nevertheless generally very self-critical and often ashamed of her vomiting behaviour. Therapists should aim to avoid using the language of morality when evaluating progress as it is unlikely to free up the patient who is only too aware of their strengths and failings.

Pharmacological interventions have been disappointing in anorexia nervosa, both in the treatment of the condition itself and accompanying mood disorder. The scepticism the anorexic has for medication (both in terms of its calorific value and its potential for taking away control) will likely have an impact on compliance. Recent research suggests though that fluoxetine may help prevent relapse in weight restored patients (Kaye et al., 1991).

BULIMIA NERVOSA

Assessment

A number of similarities to anorexia nervosa apply, but there are a few key differences. The young person is likely to have strong beliefs about the morality of eating and purging behaviours, which they will assume the interviewer shares. It is helpful to establish a matter of fact approach that records rates of bingeing, vomiting, etc., without judgement. This is particularly important to establish an accurate baseline against which to measure recovery, particularly as cognitive distortions can make it hard for patients to acknowledge progress and cause them to lose heart during treatment.

KATIE

Katie was 16 when she presented for treatment of her bulimia nervosa. She felt disgusted by her frequent bingeing and was secretive about her vomiting, which she knew exasperated and worried her parents. With sensitive interviewing, she was able to report an average of four binges followed by vomiting daily, i.e. a rate of 28 occurrences per week. After 6 weeks, she attended with her diary despondent that she was still regularly vomiting. Review of her diary revealed that her bulimic behaviour had in fact reduced to 16 occasions in the previous week. Her view of herself was essentially negative and she found difficulty in acknowledging her successes. The therapist's feedback helped her see her progress, which would not have been so easy without accurate recording. Later in her treatment, she had a bad weekend, during which a row with a friend precipitated a major binge, though she was able to resist compensatory purging. 'My weight has ballooned', she claimed, after her scales showed a 2 pound weight rise that week. 'At this rate I'll have gained a stone by the summer'. A review of her weight over the past 3 months reminded Katie that there had been occasions when her weight had fallen too and that the overall trend showed that her weight was steady.

Treatment

In bulimia nervosa and binge eating disorder, numerous randomised controlled trials have confirmed the efficacy both of psychotherapy and pharmacotherapy, for adults, generally delivered on an outpatient basis. Both cognitive-behavioural therapy (CBT) (Wilson and Fairburn, 1993) and interpersonal therapy (Mitchell et al., 1993) have been shown to decrease binge eating, purging and related attitudes and behaviours in women with bulimia nervosa. There is very little evidence to confirm the effectiveness of these approaches in adolescents, but with appropriate modification to allow for the young person's age, it seems appropriate to use a similar approach. The role of parents alongside such a programme is unclear, but parents will need to be kept informed of the treatment plan and progress where the patient is at the younger end of the spectrum, ideally in all cases in the presence of the young person. Family therapy may usefully be employed where the patient identifies family relationship difficulties alongside her eating disorder. Antidepressants, particularly fluoxetine and desipramine appear to be an effective adjunct to treatment in combination with CBT though much less effective alone (Walsh et al., 1997). These authors reported that CBT in combination with an antidepressant was more likely to result in complete symptom remission, including of vomiting, than CBT on its own. Hartman et al. (1997) have meanwhile reported the successful treatment of a small number of women with bulimia using ondansetron, a selective serotonin receptor antagonist.

COMPULSIVE EATING AND OBESITY

Obesity in adolescence usually results from a combination of excessive calorie intake and insufficient exercise. There have been rapid changes in both diet and exercise patterns since the 1980s in Britain, leading to an imminent epidemic following the pattern which has occurred in North America. Excessive calorie intake probably results from an increase in mean disposable income, and availability of fast foods and soft drinks marketed specifically at the young. Exercise has reduced, following a number of changes impacting on children's activity, such as the loss of school playing fields and a reduction in children's independent travelling. The number of children walking to school has reduced dramatically in the past 30 years in the UK.

Assessment

The history should attempt to identify potential factors contributing to obesity, medical or psychosocial complications and past attempts at treatment. The first will include familial, behavioural, psychological and biological factors. Family variables may include a familial pattern of overeating or poor levels of exercise, family history of eating disorders, or the use of food as an expression of love and affection. Biological aetiological factors include abnormal endocrine functioning and deficiency in leptin production or receptor sensitivity. Occasionally obesity results from congenital or acquired syndromes which are associated with delayed puberty and hypogonadism, e.g. Prader–Willi and Klinefelter syndromes.

Psychosocial variables frequently set up a vicious cycle of bullying, social withdrawal and comfort eating. The poor self-esteem of obese adolescents is often exacerbated by failures in past attempts at dieting.

Assessment should include enquiry about food intake and exercise. Often adolescents will be very wary that they will come in for criticism here, and it can be refreshing for them if their reports of a hearty appetite and lack of interest in sport can be positively connoted. One can express optimism of the possibility of change much more readily if the young person reports a high fat, junk food diet, than if they claim to be on a 1000 calorie per day diet. Similarly the TV addict might more readily increase his energy expenditure than a regular jogger.

Treatment

A balance should be struck between setting modest goals of behavioural and weight change and improvement in self-esteem. If the teenager can be helped to judge him or herself less in terms of weight, improved self-esteem and mood may result, having a later positive effect on dietary behaviour.

Brownell and Fairbairn (1995) confidently state 'If there is one universal truth in current conceptualisations about the treatment of obesity, it is that exercise is a key component of any treatment programme'. How the problem of exercise adherence is best addressed, however, is a thorny problem.

A key to a successful approach probably requires working to realistic goals identified by the young person, through changes in behaviour acceptable to them. It may also be helpful to treat attempts at weight loss as an experiment without any great expectation of change, in order that failures do not add to negative self-esteem.

Other family members must support and not undermine the young person's efforts. It is important to be clear that maintaining weight loss requires a permanent change in life-style, not just a temporary one and this may need to involve all the family.

INSTRUMENTS USED IN THE ASSESSMENT AND MONITORING OF EATING DISORDERS

SEMISTRUCTURED INTERVIEWS

The Eating Disorders Examination (Fairburn and Cooper, 1993)

A semistructured interview widely used in the assessment of all eating disorders. It has four subscales: restraint, eating concern, shape concern and weight concern.

The Morgan–Russell Outcome Assessment Schedule (Morgan and Hayward, 1988)

This is a widely used instrument, which assesses outcome of anorexia nervosa on five subscales covering physical, psychological and social areas of functioning. An average outcome score can be used to compute an outcome category.

QUESTIONNAIRES

EDI-2 (Garner, 1991)
A multiscale instrument which enables a psychological profile to be drawn up and used in clinical situations. Contains 11 subscales derived from 90 questions covering attitudes, behaviours and symptoms of eating disorders and related difficulty, such as maturity fears and perfectionism.

EAT-26 (Garner et al., 1982)
A widely used 26-item questionnaire of eating disorder symptoms, sometimes used as a screening instrument.

BITE (Henderson and Freeman, 1987)
The Bulimic Inventory Test – Edinburgh consists of 33 items divided into two subscales (symptoms and severity) for the assessment of bulimia nervosa.

BULIT-R (Thelen et al., 1991)
The bulimia test is a 28-item multiple choice questionnaire to assess the severity of bulimia nervosa.

OUTCOME

On average, longer-term follow up studies of anorexia nervosa suggest that approximately 50% of patients have a good outcome, 30% intermediate and 20% poor outcome (Herzog, 1992). The outcome is generally slightly better in younger-onset series (North, Gowers et al., 1997). One recent study using survival analysis (Strober et al., 1997) followed up anorexia nervosa patients treated in a university specialist centre over 10–15 years and found 76% met criteria for full recovery, though these figures are exceptional. The natural history may be poor, with a number of sufferers following a chronic course over many years. Although most cases present between 15 and 25, a number are still stricken by the disorder into their 30s and beyond, but if they achieve a degree of stability albeit at low weight, they may escape medical attention. The physical consequences of anorexia nervosa include infertility (usually reversible but sometimes compounded by the development of polycystic ovaries) and osteoporosis (Herzog, 1992). Psychologically, co-morbid depression is a feature in 50% of cases, whilst a restricted life with limited social life is common. Bulimia nervosa is a well-recognised outcome. The mortality in long-term follow-up studies reaches 15% (Ratnasuriya et al., 1991).

Predictors of good outcome include healthy family functioning by patient rating or clinician assessment and a severe negative life event precipitant (North et al., 1997). Achievement of a weight below 65% of expected weight seems to be a negative prognostic feature. Admission to hospital, particularly for extensive psychiatric treatment, is often associated with a poor outcome. Clearly cases with a number of adverse physical and psychological features are likely to be selected for admission, but it is probable that the negative effects of loss of schooling, on peer relationships and on self-esteem are underestimated. A recent study which included a multiple regression analysis of outcome factors (Gowers *et al.*, 2000) suggested that having been admitted to hospital was the strongest predictor of poor outcome.

Bulimia nervosa generally has a better outcome than anorexia nervosa and complete remission is more likely. Poor prognostic indicators include borderline personality functioning and multi-impulsivity. A recent long-term follow-up study by Fichter and Quadflieg (1997) showed that 71% of patients receiving intensive treatment maintained gains over a 6-year period. As the mean age of onset for bulimia is 19 there are few reports specifically focussing on adolescents.

CONCLUSIONS

Of the eating disorders, anorexia nervosa poses the greatest challenge to clinicians in adolescence. The outcome is variable and the evidence for effectiveness of interventions in the face of opposition from the patient, poor. A number of factors contribute to the aetiology in a given case. In planning treatment therefore, one should be careful not to blame parents, whether or not family difficulties seem to be present and attempt at all times, to work with sufferers to common goals.

Research into the aetiology and risk factors for eating disorders seems destined to focus on genetic factors for the foreseeable future. As far as treatment research is concerned, research in bulimia nervosa far exceeds that in anorexia and this is likely to continue. Research underway will explore both the effectiveness and cost-effectiveness of the treatment of adolescents with anorexia nervosa in different settings.

REFERENCES

Brownell, K. D. and Fairbairn, C. G. (1995) Exercise in the treatment of obesity. In K. D. Brownell and C. G. Fairbairn (eds), *Eating Disorders and Obesity.* New York: Guilford Press, pp. 473–478.

Bruch, H. (1974) Perils of behaviour modification in treatment of anorexia nervosa. *Journal of the American Medical Association*, **230**, 1419–1422.

Bryant-Waugh, R, and Kaminsky, Z. (1993) Eating disorders in children: an overview. In B. Lask and R. Bryant-Waugh (eds), *Childhood Onset Anorexia Nervosa and Related Eating Disorders.* Hove: Lawrence Erlbaum Associates, pp. 17–29.

Bryant Waugh, R. and Lask, B. (1995) Eating disorders in childhood and adolescence. Annotation. *Journal of Child Psychology and Psychiatry*, 36, 191–202.

Crisp, A. H. (1995) *Anorexia Nervosa: Let Me Be*. London: Lawrence Erlbaum Associates.

Crisp, A. H., Norton, K. W. R., Gowers, S. G., Halek, C., Levett, G., Yeldham, D. et al. (1991) A controlled study of the effect of therapies aimed at adolescent and family pathology in anorexia nervosa. *British Journal of Psychiatry*, *159*, 325–333.

Crisp, A. H., Palmer, R. and Kalucy, R. S. (1976) How common is anorexia nervosa? A prevalence study. *British Journal of Psychiatry*, 128, 549–554.

Dare, C. and, Key A. (1999) Family functioning and adolescent anorexia nervosa. *British Journal of Psychiatry*, *175*, 89.

Eisler, I., Dare, C., Russell, G. F. M., Szmukler, G. I. and Le Grange, D. (1997) Family and individual therapy in anorexia nervosa. A 5 year follow up. *Archives of General Psychiatry*, 54, 1025–1030.

Fairburn, C. G., and Cooper, Z. (1993) Binge eating: nature, assessment and treatment. In C. G. Fairburn and G. T. Wilson (eds), *The Eating Disorder Examination*, 12th edn. New York: Guilford Press, pp. 317–360.

Fichter, M. M. and Quadflieg, N. (1997) Six-year course of bulimia nervosa. *International Journal of Eating Disorders*, 22, 361–384.

Fombonne, E. (1995) Anorexia nervosa: No evidence of an increase. *British Journal of Psychiatry*, 166, 462–471.

Garfinkel, P. E. and Garner, D. M. (1982) *Anorexia Nervosa: A Multidimensional Perspective*. New York: Brunner/Mazel.

Garner, D. M. (1991) *Eating Disorders Inventory-2*. Odessa, FL: Psychological Assessment Resources.

Garner, D. and Garfinkel, P. E. (1980) Sociocultural factors in the development of anorexia nervosa. *Psychological Medicine*, 10, 647–656.

Garner, D. M., Olmsted, M. P., Bohr, Y. and Garfinkel, P. E. (1982) The Eating Attitudes Test: psychometric features and clinical correlates. *Psychological Medicine*, 12, 871–878.

Gowers, S. G., Kadambari, S. R. and Crisp, A. H. (1985) Family structure and birth order of patients with anorexia nervosa. *Journal of Psychiatric Research*, 19, 247–251.

Gowers, S. G. Norton, K R. W., Halek, C. and Crisp, A. H. (1994) Outcome of outpatient psychotherapy in a random allocation treatment study of anorexia nervosa. *International Journal of Eating Disorders*, 15, 165–177.

Gowers, S., North, C., Byram V. and Weaver, A. (1996) Life event precipitants of adolescent anorexia nervosa. *Journal of Child Psychology and Psychiatry*, 37, 469–478.

Gowers, S. G. and North, C. D. (1999) Difficulties in family functioning in adolescent anorexia nervosa. *British Journal of Psychiatry*, 174, 63–66.

Gowers, S. G., Weetman, J., Shore, A., Hossain, F. and Elvins, R. (2000) The impact of hospitalisation on the outcome of adolescent anorexia nervosa. *British Journal of Psychiatry*, **176**, 138–141.

Gull, W. W. (1874) Anorexia nervosa (Apepsia Hysterica, Anorexia Hysterica). *Transactions of the Clinical Society of London*, 7, 22–28.

Hartman, B. K., Faris, P. L., Kim, S. W., Raymond, N. C., Goodale, R. L., Meller, W. H. *et al.* (1997) Treatment of bulimia nervosa with ondansetron. *Archives of General Psychiatry*, **54**, 969–970.

Henderson, M. and Freeman, C. P. L. (1987) A self rating scale for bulimia. The BITE. *British Journal of Psychiatry*, **150**, 18–24.

Herzog, W. (1992) Long term course of anorexia nervosa: a review of the literature. In W. Herzog, H.-C. Deter and W. Vandereycken (eds), *The Course of Eating Disorders*. Berlin: Springer-Verlag, pp. 15–29.

Higgs, J. F. Goodyer, I. M. and Birch, J. (1989) Anorexia nervosa and food avoidance emotional disorder. *Archives of Disease in Childhood*, 64, 346–351.

Hoek, H. W. (1995) The distribution of eating disorders. In K. D. Brownell and C. G. Fairburn (eds), *Eating Disorders and Obesity*, New York: Guilford Press, pp. 207–211.

Holland, A. J., Sicotte, N. and Treasure, J. (1988) Anorexia nervosa – evidence for a genetic basis. *Journal of Psychosomatic Research*, **32**, 561–572.

Joughin, N., Varsou, E., Gowers, S. and Crisp, A. H. (1992) Relative tallness in anorexia nervosa. *International Journal of Eating Disorders*, **12**, 193–207.

Kaye, W. H., Weltzin, T. E., Hsu, L. K. G. and Bulik, C. M. (1991) An open trial of fluoxetine in patients with anorexia nervosa. *Journal of Clinical Psychiatry*, **52**, 464–471.

Lacey, J. H. and Evans, C. D. (1986) The impulsivist: a multi-impulsive personality disorder. *British Journal of Addiction*, **812**, 715–723.

Lasegue, C. (1873) On hysterical anorexia. *Medical Times and Gazette*, **2**, 265–266.

Lee, S. and Chiu, H. F. K. (1989) Anorexia nervosa in Hong Kong. Why not more in Chinese? *British Journal of Psychiatry*, **154**, 683–688.

Lee, A. M. and Lee, S. (1996) Disturbed eating and its psychosocial correlates among Chinese adolescent females in Hong Kong. *International Journal of Eating Disorders*, **20**, 177–183.

Lucas, A. R., Beard, C. M., O' Fallen, W. M. and Kurland, L. T. (1991) Fifty year trends in the incidents of anorexia nervosa in Rochester, Minnosota: a population based study. *American Journal of Psychiatry*, **148**, 917–922.

Marcus, M. D., Wing, R. R. and Fairburn, C. G. (1995) Cognitive treatment of binge eating versus behavioural weight control in the treatment of binge eating disorder. *Annals of Behavioural Medicine*, **17**, S090.

Marrazzi, M. A. and Luby, E. D. (1986) An auto-addiction opioid model of chronic anorexia nervosa. *International Journal of Eating Disorders*, **5**, 191–208.

Mitchell, J. E., Raymond, N. and Specker, S. (1993) A review of the controlled trials of pharmacotherapy and psychotherapy in the treatment of bulimia nervosa. *International Journal of Eating Disorders*, **14**, 229–247.

Morgan, H. G and Hayward, A. E. (1988) Clinical assessment of anorexia nervosa. The Morgan–Russell outcome assessment schedule. *British Journal of Psychiatry*, **152**, 367–372.

Morton, R. (1694) *Phthisiologia – or a Treatise of Consumptions*. London: Smith and Walford.

North, C. D., Gowers, S. G. and Byram, V. (1995) Family functioning in adolescent anorexia nervosa. *British Journal of Psychiatry*, **167**, 673–678.

North, C. D., Gowers, S. G. and Byram, V. (1997) Family functioning and life events in the outcome of adolescent anorexia nervosa. *British Journal of Psychiatry*, **171**, 545–549.

Ratnasuriya, R. H., Eisler, I., Szmukler, G. I. and Russell, G. F. (1991) Anorexia nervosa: outcome and prognostic factors after 20 years. *British Journal of Psychiatry*, **158**, 495–502.

Russell, G. F. M. (1979) Bulimia nervosa: an ominous variant of anorexia nervosa. *Psychological Medicine*, **9**, 429–448.

Strober, M., Freeman, R. and Morrell, W. (1997) The long-term course of severe anorexia nervosa in adolescents: survival analysis of recovery, relapse and outcome predictors over 10–15 years in a prospective study. *International Journal of Eating Disorders*, **22**, 339–360.

Thelen, M. H., Farmer, J., Wonderlich, S. and Smith, M. (1991) A revision of the bulimia test: the BULIT-R. *Psychological Assessment: A Journal of Consulting and Clinical Psychology*, **3**, 119–124.

Tiller, J., Schmidt, U. and Treasure, J. (1993) Compulsory treatment for anorexia nervosa: compassion or coercion. *British Journal of Psychiatry*, **162**, 679–680.

Treasure, J. and Holland, A. (1990) Genetic vulnerability to eating disorders: evidence from twin and family studies. In H. Remschmidt and M. H. Schmidt (eds), *Anorexia Nervosa*. Toronto: Hogrefe & Huber, pp 59–68.

Walsh, B. T., Wilson, G. T., Loeb, K. L., Devlin, M. J., Pike, K. M. and Roose, S. P. (1997) Medication and psychotherapy in the treatment of bulimia nervosa. *American Journal of Psychiatry*, **154**, 523–531.

Ward, A., Troop, N., Todd, G. and Treasure, J. (1996) To change or not to change; how is the question. *British Journal of Medical Psychology*, **69**, 139–146.

Weinsier, R. L. (1995) Clinical assessment of obese patients. In K. D. Brownell and C. G. Fairburn (eds), *Eating Disorders and Obesity*. New York: Guilford Press, pp. 463–468.

Wilson, D. E. and Fairburn, C. G. (1993) Cognitive treatments for Eating Disorders. *Journal of Consultant Clinical Psychology*, **61**, 261–269.

World Health Organisation (1992) *The ICD-10 Classification of Diseases. Clinical Descriptions and Diagnostic Guidelines*. Geneva: World Health Organisation.

Chapter 10

PSYCHOSOMATIC DISORDERS

Mary Eminson

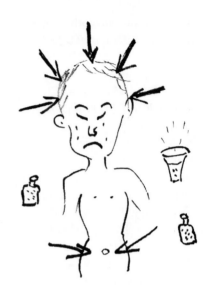

INTRODUCTION

Somatisation (a process) is the expression of psychological difficulties or distress through somatic symptoms. The process itself, of experiencing psychological distress in somatic terms, is normal, ubiquitous and familiar: the sweaty palms and palpitations experienced just prior to an examination, for example. Most people readily recognise the connection between the upsetting experience and the physical symptoms. To justify the term psychosomatic 'disorder' there must both be a failure or inability to make connections between psychological events and the physical symptoms resulting in distress and impairment, as well as a level of severity and chronicity sufficient to justify a label of disorder. It is more than a simple exaggeration of normal somatic experience of psychological upset. A psychosomatic disorder is one 'where somatic symptoms are complained of, but are unaccounted for by pathological findings, are attributed to physical illness, for which medical help is sought and on account of which lifestyle is altered' (Lipowski, 1988). This definition includes four elements: unexplained somatic complaints which the adolescent and family fail to connect with psychological stressors (*somatisation*), a conviction that a disease or illness of some kind is responsible for producing the symptom (*illness belief*), pursuit of medical treatment (*consultation behaviour*) and limitation of normal activities with adoption of a sick role (*illness behaviour*).

Presentations of psychosomatic disorders, which are both mild and severe, meeting criteria for very different ICD-10 diagnostic categories (see below, Table 10.1) and which include varied amounts of the different elements above, are included in the umbrella term 'psychosomatic disorder'. It is therefore not surprising that there are very different aetiological and maintaining factors for the various forms of disorder, wide differences in prognosis, and varying levels of severity and handicap. At one extreme are those adolescents who have a basically normal lifestyle, but are handicapped from time to time by somatic symptoms such as recurrent tension headaches or abdominal pains; at the other end of the spectrum is the teenager with severe chronic fatigue who has not attended school for several years, never leaves home except in a wheelchair and suffers an illness which constitutes a major disruption to adolescent development. The vignettes interspersed through the text illustrate the disorders, their assessment and approaches to management.

In this chapter, the term 'psychosomatic disorder' also includes those who do not fulfil all of the criteria completely and are missing some elements. For instance, there are those in whom a physical illness does explain part of their complaints (i.e. pathological findings account for some of their symptoms), but whose adoption of a limited lifestyle is grossly out of proportion to an objective assessment of the extent of their disease, e.g. an adolescent with moderately well-controlled diabetes who rarely attends school on account of worries about her health and the risk of having 'hypos', and who avoids all peer group activities because of her injections, who shows much illness belief and more illness behaviour than the physical illness warrants. There is also a group of adolescents who demonstrate substantial 'illness behaviour' with the support of their parents, but without having sought extensive medical help, i.e. consultation behaviour is minimal.

There are other uses of the term 'psychosomatic' which are not included here. One former usage was to describe situations when psychological factors were thought to influence the onset of a physical condition, e.g. asthma or ulcerative colitis. As a result of developments in understanding the physiological basis for these illnesses, the hypothesis that psychological difficulties are implicated in the primary aetiology of such conditions has been superseded. Nevertheless, psycho-social factors may have an important role in triggering particular attacks in those who already possess biological vulnerability to the disease and may delay recovery or increase the likelihood of 'illness behaviour' in response to an attack. Of course, psychological issues make some contribution to the way *all* illness is experienced and expressed, however small the part they play in aetiology (see Lask and Fosson, 1989, for an expanded discussion).

The term 'psychosomatic' has also been used to describe physical symptoms (bedwetting, eating problems) which are the symptomatic presentation of what is essentially a psychological disorder, without any significant component of unusual health beliefs or sick role adoption. Aetiologically and in management there are important differences between such psychological problems and presentations which include elements of illness behaviour: this chapter is confined to the latter.

TERMINOLOGY OF DISORDERS

Psychosomatic disorders have long been recognised and are found in all age groups (Shorter, 1992). Whilst there is a great deal of overlap between different presentations, five broad symptom clusters are recognised as predominating in adolescents: single (or few) pains or symptoms (A), losses of function (B), multiple symptoms (C), fatigue and withdrawal to an invalid lifestyle (D), and factitious symptoms (E). The letters A–E broadly denote the ICD-10 (World Health Organisation, 1996) categories (see Table 10.1).

More than most psychological conditions, these disorders continue to attract labels which imply something about their aetiology (e.g. conversion disorder, hysteria), or describe the complaints or behaviour (chronic fatigue, pervasive refusal), or use a euphemistic term ('masquerade syndrome', 'ME') which serves to obscure the psychological connections. The most obvious reason for this is because of the continued stigma of mental health problems, especially to these patients and their families, and perhaps to their doctors (Mayou, 1997). Strongly held beliefs about the exclusively physical basis for the illness, whilst often understandable, may also be another way such stigma is expressed – having a psychological condition being seen as effectively morally inferior or weak. Another reason may be because disorders of this kind are often first seen by paediatricians, resulting in a less precise use of psychiatric terminology. Perhaps a further reason is that psychiatric terms, such as 'neurasthenia', are unfamiliar and increasingly unacceptable, hence the preference for aetiologically neutral labels such as 'chronic fatigue syndrome'. A final reason may be that it is widely accepted among clinicians that the categorisations used by ICD-10 (World Health Organisation, 1996) and DSM-IV (American Psychiatric Association, 1994) are not always well fitted to the presentations of adolescents. However, despite these problems the descriptive and atheoretical principles of ICD-10, allowing use by clinicians of different theoretical persuasions, are valid, and consistent terminology is important for good communication and for research. Therefore, despite the limitations of some of the labels, the ICD-10 'somatoform' disorder categories are employed in this chapter, with the addition of two further groups: adjustment reactions, because this category may be used to include many relatively short-lived but clinically significant psychosomatic presentations, and factitious disorders.

Factitious somatic disorders, characterised by intentional production or feigning of symptoms or disabilities, are excluded from the list of ICD-10 'somatoform' disorders, only being included as an adult personality disorder. Why, then, include them in a chapter about adolescent psychosomatic illnesses? Do they satisfy Lipowski's criteria? The adolescent is certainly using a somatic route to show distress, and displays consultation and illness behaviours, and so fulfils three of Lipowski's four elements. Clearly, 'illness belief' must be absent if the symptoms have been manufactured. In practice, for many of the somatoform disorders it is often impossible to discern the extent to which a young person's complaints of symptoms are 'intentionally produced'. Clinically, a mixture of deliberate 'intentional' fabrication, with other less deliberate psychosomatic processes often seems the best explanation for many presentations. The assumed difference in motivation between the unconscious and the intentionally produced symptom is rarely relevant to the management of the difficulties, both presenting similar challenges. For these reasons factitious disorders are included in this chapter; both those instigated by the adolescent, and those which have their root in extreme beliefs and behaviours of a parent (factitious disorders by proxy).

The main diagnostic categories of somatoform disorders are listed below in Table 10.1. Generally, the presentations listed begin with the most common and decrease in number as they increase in severity.

PREVALENCE OF DISORDERS

As the cardinal feature of a psychosomatic disorder is the presentation of psychological distress through physical symptoms and as unwillingness to acknowledge psychological precipitants is common, it is to be expected that clinicians at the primary care, secondary paediatric and specialist mental health level will see patients with different types and severity of presentations. Recognition in paediatric settings of the psychological origin of the disorders varies widely. Thus prevalence figures of clinically significant presentations are hard to establish. In adults, lifetime prevalence of somatisation disorder is said to be 0.1–0.2%, with 'subthreshold' disorders about 100 times more common (Bass, 1996). In adolescents, these rates are likely to be much less, both because so little of the lifetime has passed and because some disorders, such as hypochondriasis, appear less than fully developed in the age group. It is even harder to estimate prevalences of the different specific disorders. About 10% of adolescents report multiple physical symptoms and see themselves as sickly (Aro *et al.*, 1987; Offord *et al.*, 1987), but few of these present to mental health services or reach 'disorder' criteria. If, on the other hand, one includes adjustment disorders with psychosomatic symptoms, together with the transient dissociative disorders (common and short lived presentations to a variety of specialists), psychosomatic disorders as a whole are significant in the workload of general practitioners, paediatricians and other medical specialities. In mental health services, their representation will be subject to ascertainment and referral bias, particularly the type of links with secondary or tertiary paediatricians.

BACKGROUND FACTORS AND MODELS OF ILLNESS

It has already been emphasised that the term 'psychosomatic disorders' includes very different conditions, and it is therefore not surprising that the predisposing

Table 10.1 ICD-10 diagnostic categories of psychosomatic disorders for adolescents (ICD-10 codes)

(A)	ADJUSTMENT DISORDERS (F43.2)	State of subjective distress and emotional disturbance, usually interfering with social functioning and performance, and arising in the period of adaptation to a significant life change or to the consequences of a stressful life event (including the presence or possibility of serious physical illness). The onset is usually within 1 month of the stressful event and the symptoms, by definition, time-limited. Typical examples are headaches, stomach aches, joint pains or dizzy spells, which may be recurrent. Probably the commonest form of psychosomatic disorder; there may be different symptoms on different occasions; psychological symptoms are often also present.
(B)	DISSOCIATIVE DISORDERS (F44)	Presentation usually involves losses of function. There must be no evidence of a physical disorder that can explain the characteristic symptoms; there should be convincing associations in time between the onset of symptoms of the disorder and stressful events, problems, or needs. Examples include losing the use of a limb, going deaf or having visual loss: categories include dissociative amnesia (F44.0), fugue (F44.1), stupor, trance or dissociative convulsions. No specified time length is definitive.
	Transient dissociative (conversion) disorder (F44.82)	There is a special category for 'transient' disorders in childhood and adolescence. These are usually similar to the presentations above, are by definition, time limited, and both 'isolated' and 'epidemic' forms are common. 'Epidemic' presentations are group phenomena with symptoms such as fainting or gastrointestinal complaints usually attributed to food poisoning, escaped gases or other environmental causes. These are common in girls, and for the majority of the epidemic sufferers, the episode lasts a few hours and is not associated with significant psychopathology: there is a strong element of suggestion involved. Members of the 'epidemic' group whose symptoms persist will often have the risk factors associated with more serious psychiatric disorders or with 'isolated' cases.
(C)	SOMATOFORM DISORDERS (F45)	These include a range of presentations of varying severity but all characterised by repeated presentation of physical symptoms which skilled medical assessment confirms have no basis in disease and where psychological explanations are usually rejected.
	Somatisation disorder (F45.0)	The criteria are: (a) 2 years' complaints of multiple and variable physical symptoms unexplained (or inadequately explained) by physical disorder; (b) preoccupation with symptoms leading to repeated consultations; (c) persistent refusal to accept reassurance; (d) a total of six or more symptoms, including symptoms from two or more areas of functioning including gastrointestinal, cardiovascular, genitourinary, skin and pain; and (e) exclusion criteria if symptoms only occur during a psychotic illness, panic attacks or mood disorders, or if they are intentionally produced or feigned.

Table 10.1 ICD-10 diagnostic categories of psychosomatic disorders for adolescents (ICD-10 codes) – continued

	Somatisation disorder (F45.0) continued	The time period limits the application of this category to adolescents and their symptoms are rarely genito-urinary, but in many paediatric clinics adolescents will meet the less stringent criteria below.
	Undifferentiated somatoform disorder (F45.1)	Somatisation disorder criteria (a), (b), (c) and (e) to be met, but symptoms have only lasted 6 months and either/or both (b) and (d) are incompletely fulfilled.
	Hypochondriacal disorder (F45.2)	(a) Either a 6 months (minimum) belief in the presence of physical disease or a persistent preoccupation with a presumed deformity or disfigurement (body dysmorphic disorder) and (b) preoccupation with the belief, which causes distress and leads to medical help seeking.
	Persistent somatoform pain disorder (F45.4)	Persistent severe and distressing pain (for at least 6 months and continuously on most days) in any part of the body not adequately explained by a physiological process or disorder. Unusual even in adults, both persistent somatoform pain disorder and hypochondriacal disorder are less common in adolescents than the 'undifferentiated' category. These adolescents may present in orthopaedic or pain clinics and are at risk of unnecessary surgery.
(D)	NEURASTHENIA (F48.0)	(a) Exhaustion, fatigue or weakness after minor mental or physical effort; (b) at least two of a variety of symptoms: aches and pains, dizziness, headaches, sleep disturbance, inability to relax, irritability and dyspepsia; (c) an inability to recover by rest; (d) minimum duration of 3 months; and (e) an absence of another mental disorder such as depression or anxiety. Chronic fatigue syndrome (CFS) criteria are very similar (see Sharpe, 1999).
	'Pervasive refusal syndrome' (Lask, 1996)	A variant of CFS or neurasthenia, a severe, prolonged presentation with somatic complaints, fatigue, profound withdrawal and regression (including even incontinence) and a strong passive resistance to rehabilitative efforts, sometimes to a life-threatening degree. Overlap with eating disorders may be evident, but without core features; many young people present through paediatric services requiring close liaison both to exclude primary organic difficulties and to manage secondary physical problems, such as contractures and malnutrition.
(E)	FACTITIOUS DISORDERS (F68.1)	These are defined as being intentional production or feigning of symptoms or disabilities. The motivation is said to be obscure and presumably internal, to distinguish factitious presentations from 'malingering', which is when symptoms are feigned or induced, said to be motivated by external stresses or incentives. Common factitious presentations in adolescence are of lesions in skin, eye (damaging cornea or lashes), limb extremities (damaged by application of ligatures) and joints (into which needles or other objects are inserted). The boundary with other forms of self-harm is sometimes imprecise.

Table 10.1 ICD-10 diagnostic categories of psychosomatic disorders for adolescents (ICD-10 codes) – continued

FACTITIOUS ILLNESS BY PROXY (MUNCHAUSEN SYNDROME BY PROXY ABUSE)	There is no Axis I psychiatric diagnosis for the adolescent here unless the adolescent fits another category. An Axis IV category of T68 (abuse) is made. There are often Axis V codings to be made. This disorder is characterised by parental persuasion of adolescents to join in a substantial illness behaviour presentation with corresponding illness belief. The parent may verbally fabricate complaints and insist on treatment and surgery; frank direct illness induction is rare in adolescents without learning difficulties. There may be elements of 'folie à deux' if the parent is mentally ill, but more often the parent has personality and relationship difficulties. Imagined allergies, seizures, asthma and gastroenterological problems have all been reported, in which the adolescent appears unable to distinguish their own experiences from the parental account, and drastically limits their activities and lifestyle as a result (Taylor, 1992).

and precipitating factors also vary widely, even within the same diagnostic category. The extent to which presentations emphasise the different elements (symptom experience, illness attribution, consultation seeking and sick role adoption) varies. It is also important to remember that the role of parents is a significant one: an adolescent rarely presents in a specialist medical arena without their family's encouragement and an adolescent's adoption of an invalid lifestyle is heavily determined by their parents' support or otherwise.

EPIDEMIOLOGICAL STUDIES

In epidemiological and community samples, headaches, low energy, stomach pains and joint pains are amongst the commonest symptoms experienced by Western adolescents (Egger *et al.*, 1999; Eminson *et al.*, 1996; Garber *et al.*, 1991). King and Coles (1992), in a school-based study of 11–15 year olds from 11 different countries, found wide differences between numbers of symptoms (and rates of use of medication for symptoms) reported in different countries, clearly showing sociocultural influences on symptom reporting, illness attitudes and patterns of response to symptoms, but very similar patterns of physical symptom complaints between the age group and the sexes in the different countries. At both a population level and a clinical one, some common factors are well established as increasing the likelihood of an adolescent experiencing physical symptoms, of complaining of these and of limiting activities with a sickness justification. Girls and older adolescents report more symptoms consistently; culture, gender and stage of development clearly have an influence upon how many symptoms are reported (and also on characteristic responses).

Different psychophysiological responses (which may be genetic) may also be relevant, but there is as yet little evidence.

What is associated with multiple, significant, handicapping physical symptoms? Although methodological issues confuse the picture to a certain extent, epidemiological studies in adolescence are again consistent in demonstrating an association of multiple symptoms with female gender, with all psychiatric disorders but most commonly emotional disorders (especially anxiety and depression), low self-esteem, poorer educational attainments, and acute life events and stresses (Aro et al., 1987; Eminson et al., 1996; Polkolainen et al., 1995; Rauste-von Wright and von Wright, 1992; Taylor et al., 1996). These factors are not uncommon, and they provide at least a partial explanation for what predisposes to and precipitates many of the simpler psychosomatic disorders, e.g. adjustment reactions expressed as recurrent headaches or attacks of dizziness or abdominal pain. However, is there evidence that these factors are sufficient to explain the more severe and handicapping psychosomatic illnesses? The answer to this is not clear cut. It is necessary to turn to clinical reviews of psychosomatic disorders in adolescents, and retrospective studies of adult somatisers in order to identify other factors which are important in the aetiology, precipitation and maintenance of the highly distorted attitudes, excess consulting and illness behaviour of the more serious conditions: this includes study of the family characteristics which may facilitate or limit the disorder's development or treatment. A more complex picture emerges and it is evident that there are many different pathways which may lead to a somatoform disorder.

CLINICAL SERIES

The early literature consists of case series, weakened by including a mixture of diagnoses and levels of severity (Grattan-Smith et al., 1988; Leslie, 1988), but more tightly defined series are now published, particularly for chronic fatigue syndrome (Deale et al., 1997; Sharpe, 1995), although these are studies of adults including older adolescents.

Anxiety and depression continue to be associated with all types of clinical somatic presentation, but overall, psychiatric disorders are only found in about a third of those with psychosomatic presentations (Garralda, 1996). Previous experience of illness in themselves or in other family members influences the adolescent's responses to their experience and increases the likelihood of psychosomatic disorder (Walker et al., 1993). Trouble with peer group relationships, school attendance and academic attainments act both as vulnerability factors and as sources of recent stress. Specific and mild generalised learning difficulties are, in the author's experience, associated with many presentations but especially with the transient dissociative disorders in early adolescence: often at predictable times of stressful transition, such as secondary school admission or exams. Again, this is an inconsistent finding, for previous high academic achievement is also reported by some (Lask, 1989): the vulnerability may be that whatever the level of attainment, it is being maintained with difficulty.

Temperamental and personality factors are important in some cases, and in adults personality disorders have been reported in 72% of those with somatisation disorder (Stern *et al.*, 1993). An increase in obsessional traits has been reported in adolescents with conversion reactions (Wynick *et al.*, 1997). In some studies of adolescents with chronic fatigue syndrome, sufferers have been found to be achieving, intense, perfectionistic, apparently compliant but also oppositional young people (Rangel and Garralda, 1999), who place themselves under enormous psychological pressure to achieve. In these circumstances the suggested model is that a young person with these temperamental traits finds themselves in a difficult and demanding situation with peers or at school. A coincidental minor illness provides respite from the pressures. On recovery from the physical illness the effort to resume their previous performance level proves exhausting, resulting in further withdrawal, hence setting up the vicious circle of relapse and unsuccessful attempts at return which result in further collapse.

Taylor (1986), writing of 'hysteria', described the elements of such presentations as (a) a predicament for the sufferer from which all avenues of escape are blocked, (b) a model of sickness in a relative, or the media, (c) sufficient skills to produce the 'sickness', i.e. sufficient cognitive and emotional development, (d) an ally (usually a parent) whose concern about physical illnes endorses the sick role adoption, and (e) a supporter, usually a professional who has some concern about organic illness. This constitutes a systemic formulation which can be used to analyse many of the different disorders, taking into account the factors within each of the individuals concerned (child, parent, professional) and their inter-relationships. The case example 'Drew' illustrates such a formulation: a case where the professionals' responses allowed swift resolution to be achieved.

TRANSIENT 'DISSOCIATIVE' DISORDER: DREW

Drew was a 13-year-old boy who presented as an emergency to paediatric services with a sudden onset of 'seeing and hearing things' which had started that day. He could see groups of people in the distance, talking and fighting, and could hear voices whispering in his ear.

The paediatric staff found the story became more elaborate as the evening went on. Drew denied substance abuse, and when physical examination was normal and basic investigations negative, Drew was referred to psychiatry on the day of admission with concern about the possibility of psychosis.

Drew lived with his mother, stepfather and 4-year-old stepbrother in a family without current social stresses, in a stable marriage which had occurred 9 years before. Drew's mother was extremely anxious about his illness. Drew's symptoms had begun on a day when he had been in trouble at school: that evening, unusually, he was reprimanded by his mother for fighting with his little brother.

The history was explored, looking out for predisposing and precipitating factors. Drew's early history provided some explanation. His mother was married early to a man who was physically abusive to Drew as a baby: child protection procedures were invoked and Drew was briefly in care. Mother felt intensely guilty about this history and became extremely close to and protective of Drew, with difficulty in setting firm boundaries.

Whilst in primary school Drew was noticed to be an unusual boy with an odd remote social manner which produced teasing: his abilities were low average. In middle childhood he had recurrent abdominal pain, headaches and some urinary symptoms: no serious pathology was found during several admissions. There was no significant family history of ill health otherwise. The transfer to secondary school was difficult and Drew was teased a lot, and was in trouble both for foolish rule breaking and immature strategies with his peer group. On occasion he made up dramatic stories about his life and family, to excuse failures.

Mental state assessment

Drew was aroused and rather agitated, fully oriented and increasingly vague about the content of his auditory and visual hallucinations. It was clear he did not have a psychotic illness, but that these were dissociative phenomena, preventing Drew from hearing and seeing normally.

Working formulation

This 'conversion' disorder seemed to be the most recent psychosomatic presentation in a boy who had previously experienced significant physical symptoms when distressed. He was vulnerable because of his social impairments (which failed to reach criteria for a pervasive development disorder), learning difficulty and peer group problems. The argument and reprimand from mother in the context of increasing peer group trouble and academic difficulty at school was seen as the 'final straw' causing Drew's decompensation with dissociative 'conversion' symptoms. In the past, when Drew complained of physical symptoms his mother had allowed him to avoid stressful situations (this included missing school), thus there was reinforcement for somatic presentations. His mother's chastisement on the day of admission had provoked distress and a more extreme response.

Management, progress and prognosis

Physical investigations were ceased on the day of admission and firm clear reassurance was given by the paediatric consultant and psychiatrist together about the lack of organic pathology. An explanation for his symptoms was given to Drew: the distressing events at school and at home had affected him deeply. His brain had responded with the hallucinations: a way of signalling to him that he was under stress. This was clearly serious but he was reassured that the symptoms would in time disappear as he became more confident at handling school problems. Drew's mother and stepfather (who was less protective but 'took a back seat' with Drew) were engaged in discussions of ways of managing him and they were helped to involve Drew in activities which would increase his independence and give him opportunities to practise peer group interactions. His school was given an understanding of his social impairment and psychosomatic symptoms, and encouraged to make little of his dramatic symptoms but give him more learning support. Drew responded to this approach. His auditory and visual experiences became less troublesome as he was encouraged to ignore them and his parents failed to respond to them. After about 3 weeks the hallucinations disappeared completely. In follow-up appointments, examples of earlier dissociative experiences came to light. Drew has been able to return to school, but he is likely to express his difficulties in further somatic presentations in the future, as his social interaction and learning difficulties persist.

FACTORS UNDERLYING SEVERE AND LONG-LASTING DISORDER

Studies of adults with chronic somatoform disorders (Craig et al., 1993) confirm the relevance of early adverse experience with an impact on the development of attachment: severe distortion of early relationships (e.g. by physically and emotionally abusive or neglectful parenting) are found in the backgrounds of those with severe disorders, such as pervasive regression, and in a proportion of these with somatisation and factitious disorders. It has been suggested that the combination of early neglectful and abusive parenting, combined with physical ill health which succeeds in eliciting parental care, may be a pathway to development of somatoform disorders (Craig et al., 1993). The proposed mechanisms include dissociation from emotional distress, or failure to learn to recognise the connection between emotional distress and physical symptoms. Another proposed mechanism is through 'conditional caretaking', i.e. the child learns that when he or she complains of somatic symptoms that care will be elicited from the parent who fails to respond to verbal or non-verbal emotional upset: this reinforces the tendency to express distress or need through such physical complaints. If physical illness in childhood results in hospital admission and care, this too provides a model for eliciting care in that arena in future: similar patterns may be seen at school. Clinically there is substantial support for the importance of these mechanisms to explain at least in part, some severe adolescent somatoform disorders (see case vignette: Cherry). Of course there may be lesser degrees of such early difficulties in others with less severe handicaps.

FAMILY FACTORS

Parents have a crucial role in all aspects of psychosomatic presentations, as the model outlined above has suggested. Not only are parents powerful in encouraging or discouraging any and all of the elements of the presentation: they can focus on, amplify or ignore somatic complaints, supply reassurance or increase anxiety about a physical illness cause for the symptoms, encourage or discourage medical help seeking, exaggerate, tolerate or ignore all forms of illness behaviour and promote or restrict normal activities.

Depression, anxiety, unexplained physical symptoms and psychosomatic disorders are over-represented in parents of children and adolescents with unexplained physical complaints (Hotopf *et al.*, 1998a,b; Walker *et al.*, 1994) causing increased awareness of and preoccupation with physical health. Family experience of illness is relevant: not only is a sick parent likely to worry more about a symptomatic child and to worry that a sick child may have an undiscovered serious illness suffered by another family member, but having a parent with physical ill health may provide a readily available model of sickness and demonstration of the positive benefits of illness behaviour.

Parental beliefs are also important. These relate not only to their culture with its contribution to beliefs about illnesses, their meaning, how they should be managed and the role of the medical profession, but also to the child. A child whose early life history has caused worry to their parents and made them seem particularly vulnerable will quickly trigger anxieties if physical symptoms appear in adolescence, causing difficulty for the parent in knowing how to manage illness behaviour.

The extent to which the parents can develop a trusting relationship with professionals and can accept appropriate reassurance is a further important variable. The ability to develop such trust is affected by a range of factors: the parents' own early life and experiences, both emotional and physical as well as their cultural context and previous experiences with the medical profession, and the parent's own mental and physical state at the time.

A final family characteristic which may be relevant is the extent to which a language to express emotions is available. Some families, whilst not possessing any of the psychological, social or physical risk factors already mentioned, may have difficulty in communicating openly, especially about painful or angry feelings. At its most extreme this characteristic is described as 'alexithymia' (literally, no word for feelings) (Sifneos, 1973). In a family with these traits, it is easy to understand how alternative somatic ways of communicating may develop. These traits are not, in clinical experience, necessarily the same as being antagonistic to psychological explanations which is rarely easily explained.

Table 10.2 Family and individual factors in precipitating and maintaining psychosomatic disorders

Adolescent

- Anxiety and depression
- Learning difficulties (specific / general)
- Temperamental and personality factors
- Social relating and peer group attainments
- Individual psychophysiological responses (genetic)
- Recent life events
- Experience of abuse and neglect
- Medical history: organic and psychosomatic illnesses

Family and systemic contributions

- Trust in professionals (not only those who share beliefs about the illness)
- Cultural context (all aspects of beliefs, consultation and illness behaviour)
- History of physical illness (and beliefs about it)
- History of mental health problems
- History of somatisation
- Current stresses and their relation to the adolescent's symptoms
- Emotional expression: communication about difficult emotional issues
- Psychological mindedness

'Psychological mindedness' is another poorly operationalised but useful concept which describes families who are able to consider and reflect on the connections between events, mind and bodily reactions: families who find this more difficult are harder to work with and may be more prone to indirect communication of feelings. See Table 10.2.

FACTITIOUS ILLNESS BY PROXY

Parents with extremely distorted beliefs and attributions, whether due to frank mental illness, or as an aspect of parental somatoform, factitious or other personality disorders, may focus on the health of their child or adolescent totally unnecessarily and pursue health care or a bizarre illness-focused lifestyle for the child. Sometimes there is a failure on the parent's part to differentiate between the adolescent's experience and their own, so strong may be the convictions about illness: hence the parent's needs are gratified 'by proxy'. Subjected to these powerful parental influences over many years, and persuaded to believe that they suffer from a serious and handicapping illness requiring extensive treatment, young people may be unable to separate their perceptions from their parents', and display extreme illness behaviours including pursuit of alternative treatments (Taylor, 1992). Separation of parent and adolescent may be the only way to establish the extent of the adolescent's own psychopathology and physical handicaps.

PRINCIPLES OF ASSESSMENT

The assessment of adolescents and families in these circumstances involves additions to a normal psychiatric history for this age group. Attending to the adolescent's mental health, their temperament, their peer group relationships, academic attainments and abilities in the normal way will identify relevant risk factors for *adolescent's experience of somatic symptoms*, but will not necessarily reveal adolescent and parental contributions to *illness belief*, to *consultation behaviour*, and to the adoption of a lifestyle which avoids normal activities and developmental tasks for their age group (*illness behaviour*).

The importance of parental and family beliefs, attitudes and behaviours has already been emphasised. Careful assessment of these issues is vital to achieve some understanding of aetiology: the ways in which, and the reasons for, parental responses. These are also likely to have a significant effect on future progress. Clinically many different patterns are seen: parental and family variables may be a central factor in maintaining and promoting the illness in the adolescent, or the family may demonstrate very ordinary concerns and caring responses to the somatoform presentation, with no unusual, overprotective or amplifying responses. What is found at assessment will determine the emphases of the treatment programme.

As in any psychiatric assessment, consideration of the family's subjective impressions is complimented by the observations of the clinician. Whilst it is helpful to identify and separate predisposing, precipitating and maintaining factors in the illness, the initial history rarely fully explains the puzzle of a severe and entrenched psychosomatic disorder: understanding of the interplay of aetiological and maintaining factors may only be achieved after some time. Three areas merit special consideration in history taking in order to achieve time to work with the family and to acquire some grasp of what maintains the illness, which will be the first area to be addressed clinically.

ENGAGEMENT

It is sometimes particularly difficult to overcome suspicion of mental health services in sufferers from these conditions, a suspicion which may be shared or mirrored by other medical professionals (Mayou, 1997). Some young people and their families with severe and chronic presentations, involving extensive withdrawal from normal activities, may strongly resent and resist 'psychological' interventions, with the support of some self-help groups. Antagonism towards psychological explanations, treatment and services may be extreme, despite manifest psychopathology (Garralda, 1996), and is associated with a poorer outcome in studies of adults with chronic fatigue.

As a result, it is useful to pay particular attention to engagement at the early stages. At the first appointment, careful attention should be paid to the views about, and enthusiasm for, the referral to the mental health service. If working with a familiar paediatrician, this liaison may be straightforward, but it is always important to understand the beliefs and feelings about physical investigations and any physical diagnosis which has been made. The role of possible organic disease in aetiology is often the focus of the family's attentions: the task in the first appointment is to agree a broad formulation of what precipitated the illness, but then to move on to a joint interest in what is maintaining it and what will aid recovery. The clinical example below (Ellen) illustrates many of these engagement issues. Of course, more common types of engagement processes also continue: establishing that the professional believes in the symptoms of which the patient complains: he or she is not 'putting it on'; developing trust by giving evidence that other young people have recovered through this approach; respecting the patient's and parents' fears that too much physical activity and progress will be demanded too quickly.

SOMATISATION DISORDER – OUTPATIENT TREATMENT: ELLEN

Ellen (age 14) was referred by an orthopaedic consultant whom she saw because of slipped epiphysis of her hip. This was agreed by professionals NOT to account for the extent of Ellen's disability. She reported pain, had difficulty walking, had barely attended school for a year and did not mix with other young people. Many consultations with a variety of paediatric and psychiatric services in both the NHS and private sector, with prolonged hospital stays, preceded the latest referral. Ellen also had long-standing problems of urinary urgency and frequency, for which she saw another set of specialists. A programme of rehabilitation had been commenced by a thoughtful physiotherapist but was not successful.

Ellen was obese, had many chronic symptoms of anxiety, and was truculent and obstructive with the psychiatrist. She was intellectually very able, a perfectionist, sensitive to criticisms or slights and quite indulged at home; she was not depressed.

Ellen was the only child of two wealthy parents, her mother having two children by a previous marriage, one of whom had a severe eating disorder. The family, although superficially compliant, seemed to find it difficult at a deeper level to be trusting of professionals or each other. The family history contained many examples of doctors being mistaken and of missed, subsequently serious, diagnoses: there was an entrenched pattern of needing to seek many opinions as a result. Whenever Ellen became distressed her parents gave in to her and believed pain caused her upsets.

Management

This case was initially difficult because Ellen's continued physical symptoms provided constant excuses for new opinions to be sought and for failing to adhere to any treatment programme. It was also difficult to achieve a working alliance with the orthopaedic team based on a shared management programme. Much time was spent in early appointments to establish the principles of a basic rehabilitative programme with a reassurance that Ellen's upsets and physical symptoms might be explained by fear and anxiety about both her hip and her schoolwork, and were not necessarily signs of physical disease. Little work could be done with Ellen directly. After some weeks it became possible to confront the parents about their lack of trust. This proved a turning point. A better alliance was established and an agreement was reached about limiting the search for alternative opinions. From this point the management became much easier.

A visit to Ellen's school was necessary to establish the teachers' beliefs and a possible management plan, with support for Ellen remaining in school even if she could not be in lessons. The teachers became helpful with a clear, firm and encouraging approach to Ellen.

In response to gradually increasing and firmly sustained parental expectations, Ellen's physical symptoms diminished, her ability to mix with her peers increased, setbacks in progress were quickly corrected. Ellen's anxious perfectionism and urinary symptoms proved unamenable to treatment. However, by the time of discharge, eighteen months after initial referral, Ellen was socially active, taking 10 GCSEs and challenging her parents' wishes. Ellen's increase in independence and individuation was very evident.

ATTRIBUTIONS, EMOTIONAL EXPRESSION AND COMMUNICATION AND BELIEFS

Family beliefs and attributions about health are often important in understanding parents' responses, including protective and symptom amplifying responses to a symptomatic adolescent. The physical health of other family members, over quite a substantial area of the family tree, may need to be canvassed to identify sources of worry about illness as well as models for the adolescent's presentation. Earlier perceived vulnerabilities in the child (a previous illness or other losses) may add to parental concern and hence pressure to pursue investigations. Of particular interest is the extent to which family members express emotional concerns through somatic symptoms and any evidence of 'alexithymia' in parents.

CHARACTERISTICS OF THE PROFESSIONAL NETWORK

Just as work with severe psychosomatic disorders rests on a good alliance with the family, it also relies on a rapport with other medical professionals. The helpful paediatrician will have established truly likely physical explanations, completed investigations for these, given a reasonable explanation of the findings, including the role of any co-existing physical illness which explains a part of the symptoms, and stopped all investigations. If investigations are ongoing, an agreement about the point where physical investigations will cease is essential, with a thorough airing of doubts and fears about undiscovered pathology. Persisting anxieties usually contain a kernel of distrust of doctors' judgements, often apparently arising from earlier bad experiences of parents or other family members. If these issues are not clear, it is better to seek a further medical opinion at this stage (perhaps a joint appointment with a paediatrician and psychiatrist) than to coerce a reluctant adolescent and family in to a treatment programme when they have serious underlying doubts.

The GP also has an important role and is, one hopes, fully sympathetic with the psychosomatic explanation for the difficulties, supportive of the mental health team, and will alert them if the family is dissatisfied and starts to seek new opinions.

Increasingly, self-help groups and the Internet provide sources of advice and information for parents; whilst this may provide helpful support, it may also reinforce fears and anxieties amongst those whose confidence in professionals is fragile. Particular professionals may be sought out who have formed a firm alliance with self-help groups, not on the basis of expertise in treatment to recovery, but in a shared belief system with minimal scientific basis and a prognosis of long-term invalidity. Taylor (1992) has written of some of these extreme situations which may approach the abusive in their commitment to illness behaviour and outlandish treatments.

TREATMENT AND MANAGEMENT

The principle is to establish and address systematically the maintaining factors for the psychosomatic disorder, whether in the individual, in their academic difficulties or in family relationships and communication. A wealth of clinical accounts is available (Garralda, 1999a; Nunn et al., 1998; Larsson and Mellin, 1988; Lask and Fosson, 1989; Leslie, 1988; Vereker, 1992; Wright and Beverley, 1998). Whilst poorly supported by scientific evidence, many clinical series report recovery in response to gradual rehabilitative approaches including physiotherapy and other 'face saving' methods of increasing activity and relinquishing symptoms, usually employed on an outpatient basis. Gradual encouragement to communicate distress by direct verbal or non-verbal means rather than by the indirect route of psychosomatic symptoms, reduced attention to and normalising explanations for physical symptoms and support for greater activity are common to most programmes. A clinical consensus guideline is available for chronic fatigue syndrome management (Garralda, 1999b) which has applicability to several of the severe disorders.

Liaison with school may need to be close, and a variety of supportive, explanatory, cognitive behavioural and family systemic techniques will be useful. For the common and milder disorders (adjustment reactions with headaches or abdominal pains, or transient dissociative presentations) it may be relatively easy to identify triggers for bouts of physical symptoms and use these to prevent relapse. In general, however, insight into the 'psychosomatic' nature of the symptoms is not essential, the emphasis being on working towards recovery. Treatment of any concurrent emotional disorders is important; antidepressants are used for those with frank depression or the mixed picture seen in many with fatigue or multiple pains.

It is necessary to fall back on the literature on adults in the search for randomised controlled trials of treatment approaches. Cognitive-behaviour therapy is much advocated for functional somatic symptoms, although the evidence outside fatigue and chest pain has not yet been demonstrated (Sharpe, 1995). Wessely and his colleagues, working with adolescents as well as adults, use a combined approach which involves understanding physical/psychological connections, cognitive techniques to modify attributional and cognitive factors which trigger avoidant behaviour and sustain the fatigue, a behavioural approach to enable the treatment of avoidance behaviour, a gradual return to normal physical activity, and the use of anti-depressants (Wessely et al., 1989, 1991). Substantial improvements were reported in the majority of patients, better outcome being seen in those with a less strong initial attribution of symptoms to exclusively physical causes.

Chronic headaches in adolescents have been successfully treated with relaxation and or a self-help manual (Larsson and Mellin, 1988), and similar but family-oriented cognitive behavioural techniques have been found helpful in recurrent abdominal pain (Sanders et al., 1994). In adults, psychotherapy has been found to be effective in Irritable Bowel Syndrome (Guthrie et al., 1993) and may translate to older adolescents.

WORK WITH PARENTS AND FAMILIES

With parents, worries and concerns are explored to manage and contain these: to help parents to encourage progress to recovery and to address any systemic issues which have been maintaining the symptoms or preventing parents in providing firm encouragement, e.g. a lonely parent or one in severe marital conflict may have unwittingly found the presence of a 'sick' adolescent at home provides companionship and diversion.

MORE INTENSIVE TREATMENT: DAY PATIENT AND INPATIENT MANAGEMENT

Severely affected individuals may benefit from inpatient admission, with more intensive rehabilitation than may be possible at home (Nunn *et al.*, 1998). This enables the use of a peer group milieu, which is helpful for those where individuation from parents has been difficult, and consistent encouragement of exploration of difficult predicaments with a variety of psychotherapeutic and creative techniques. Many adolescents, once engaged in treatment, may be able to acknowledge that emotional stress has a link with their experience of physical symptoms, and many of these will be able to use cognitive-behavioural techniques to find alternative solutions and responses. The case vignette, Jonathan, illustrates the use of multiple therapeutic approaches in a Day Unit setting.

PERSISTENT SOMATOFORM PAIN DISORDER/NEURASTHENIA/CHRONIC FATIGUE: JONATHAN

Referred by a paediatric rheumatologist, Jonathan (14) had a 4-month history of severe and debilitating pain in his limbs, following an acute onset of symptoms immediately after BCG vaccination. The pains, together with great fatigue, had prevented him attending school. Although a local reaction to the BCG was identified and treated, all other physical investigations were normal and the paediatrician had reassured the family about this. A rehabilitative programme with physiotherapy had had initial success but collapsed completely at the start of the new school year.

Jonathan had not had previous psychosomatic complaints, and he was intelligent and highly conscientious with enormous respect towards authority figures. The most significant event in his history was an assault by older boys, which had taken place at school a year before. Jonathan's elder brother attended special school for delicate pupils because of a minor physical handicap. Jonathan's mother had problems with her sight; his father strongly disliked his job in accountancy. The whole family was characterised by its cheerful demeanour, quick wit and much laughter. The mental health team felt that as a family they found it difficult to talk about upsetting subjects, and the atmosphere was of closeness, warmth and quite limited individuation. Jonathan had only one friend, contact with whom had diminished substantially. Jonathan's lifestyle was an extremely comfortable one for him, with time spent at home with his mother, enjoying his favourite TV programmes and new computer games.

Management and Day Unit treatment

At assessment Jonathan seemed depressed and withdrawn, and a course of antidepressants was commenced. Jonathan's rehabilitation was planned with the physiotherapy service using clear explanations for the symptoms, similar to those for chronic fatigue (Chalder, 1999). Although apparently following this programme assiduously, after 2 months there was no progress; it became evident that an important maintaining factor had been missed. Could it be that the symptoms represented a way to avoid school and the hurly burly of his peer group? Were Jonathan's symptoms necessary to justify his lifestyle and the risks of recovery greater than the benefits of more independence? Perhaps, too, his mother enjoyed his company at home, providing her with some investment in the current situation?

A decision was made to admit Jonathan to the Day Unit, but only after we gained full agreement of both parents. Once admitted, Jonathan took every possible opportunity to complain about pain and fatigue; his superior manner made him unpopular with other young people in the unit: his lack of assertiveness and extreme shyness were very obvious handicaps. These had not been so obvious before nor had his school reported them. Jonathan's difficulties were reformulated to him as being a form of mental fatigue. Jonathan was allowed to complain about his physical symptoms for only two brief periods of 15 min a day and his task at other times was to identify activities which he enjoyed, in order to give him a reason to live and a way to distract himself from pain. Individual exploratory (rather than cognitive) sessions commenced, to help Jonathan to recognise and acknowledge more directly all forms of feelings and frustrations. Didactic social skills training was given. Jonathan's parents were recruited to more active encouragement of social activities.

Jonathan, whilst not admitting this, was clearly infuriated by this change in programme. However, it was beneficial and gradually Jonathan undertook more activities, occasionally playing a game of football; peer relationships improved. Jonathan identified a goal in life, to become a teacher. His physical complaints reduced rather than disappeared. After 4 months a gradual school return commenced with reassurance that some pain and tiredness were inevitable. Jonathon was discharged after 6 months Day Unit attendance with close follow-up. Jonathan asked that family therapy also continue as the place where 'I can say what I think', perhaps an acknowledgement of the family's difficulties with emotional expression. These sessions have been used to encourage the family to speak openly, and to focus on Jonathan's future in the outside world.

Despite Jonathan's high intelligence, new skills and current good adjustment, his temperament, multiple somatic complaints and comfortable adoption of the sick role suggest a high chance of future relapse if there are new stresses.

TREATMENT ISSUES FOR FACTITIOUS DISORDERS AND FACTITIOUS DISORDER BY PROXY

These are some of the most difficult disorders to treat and those where the involvement of a psychiatrist is sometimes least welcome by patient or family. By definition, there is a lack of a trusting relationship between the patient and the professionals, and between the parent, patient and professional in the 'proxy' form. Adolescents presenting factitious disorder may demonstrate how unimportant it is to confront directly and acknowledge the fabrication – much more crucial is to understand what has maintained the behaviour and assist the young person in meeting their own needs by more direct means. Helping other health professionals who feel tricked and angered by what they may see as manipulation of their sympathy and care may be an important part of the mental health professional's role. Cherry's presentation illustrates these issues.

FACTITIOUS DISORDER AND SOMATISATION DISORDER – LIAISON /CONSULTATION: CHERRY

Cherry was 15 when referred by general surgeons to the psychiatry department. Several admissions with abdominal pain over the previous weeks had brought the possibility of an appendectomy. Back pains, bowel and urinary symptoms had resulted in a spate of investigations. Referral to psychiatry came about when Cherry was discovered to be producing lesions on her back by banging herself on surgical taps in the hospital bathroom, resulting in extensive bruising and eventually a substantial wound.

Background

Cherry had been removed from her mother and stepfather in middle childhood following emotional, physical and sexual abuse. Within-family placements had broken down, after which she had been placed in foster homes. She undoubtedly had an attachment disorder in addition to psychiatric diagnoses. Her current placement was in a foster family with several other teenage girls, where she was disliked, scapegoated and displayed unsophisticated attention-gaining manoeuvres in addition to taking and breaking items belonging to the other girls. All Cherry's relationships were superficial, ambivalent and untrusting. She had harmed herself previously by cutting and tablet ingestion. This factitious disorder had its roots in severe abuse and disruption of early relationships, Cherry probably having dissociated from many painful experiences. The most recent relationship difficulties had provoked distress and many physical complaints, which in turn resulted in Cherry's removal from the uncomfortable atmosphere she produced in her foster home to the 'nurturing' but inappropriate setting of the surgical ward.

Management

Cherry was deeply antagonistic and denigratory to direct approaches from the mental health team, who were unable to establish any form of rapport with her. Surgical ward staff were made both distressed and angry by Cherry's presentation, and they were confused because she also liked to look after younger children in the ward. Much time initially was spent helping the nurses to recognise her tremendous difficulties in communicating distress directly, to enable them to feel more sympathy rather than resentment while they nursed her.

Despite systemic work, Cherry's foster family and biological family were rejecting. Cherry moved to a different foster home. In this setting, her more extreme self-harming behaviour and physical complaints settled; she rejected further follow-up and continues to have severe relationship, psychosomatic and conduct problems. More might have been done to help Cherry directly in earlier childhood and may be possible if she has children of her own.

Indirect work in liaison with surgical ward staff, social workers and foster parents was the only way, at this time, to provide input. This liaison and consultation is not a trivial task. In the health service, the goal is to prevent unnecessary surgery, and to promote increasing understanding in ward nursing staff and in the foster home to prevent placement breakdown.

In factitious disorders *by proxy*, difficulty in identifying the extent to which an adolescent shares the parent's distorted perceptions and beliefs is usual. Whereas at their most extreme these presentations clearly constitute emotional (and sometimes physical) abuse, it is often difficult to manage less extreme forms where parental behaviour is not judged so dangerous as to necessitate removal.

'Treatment' involves allowing the adolescent to separate their own sensations, experiences and attributions from what their parent tells them and an inpatient setting may be necessary to bolster the adolescent in establishing their own identity. Eventually, if successful, treatment therefore rests on asking the child to choose between loyalty to parent and professional belief systems. The most disturbed parents will heavily resist their child making this choice. These are difficult cases which merit careful discussion with medical and social work colleagues. A formal approach to child protection agencies may be necessary, if significant physical or psychological harm is taking place.

PAEDIATRIC MANAGEMENT

Paediatricians, without need for recourse to specialist advice, manage many mild and even moderately severe psychosomatic disorders, particularly adjustment reactions or transient dissociative disorders. A good paediatric history which takes account of precipitating factors, makes connections for the family with recent stressful life events and family history, which limits investigations to those which are truly necessary to identify organic disease and gives reassurance about the lack of organic pathology, will be sufficient to achieve recovery in many mild cases without other significant psychopathology.

A second group of cases will also be managed by paediatricians, those whose antagonism to psychological explanations is such that face to face meeting with a mental health team is unacceptable (any of the severe disorders but especially factitious ones). It may be better to continue existing paediatric management than to insist on psychiatric referral and risk a move to another physical specialist likely to initiate yet more unnecessary investigations. Here the psychiatrist's role is to support the paediatrician and ensure damage limitation and regular review of potential harm.

PROGNOSIS

Difficulties in agreeing terminology in this area mean that many of the published case series are heterogeneous in terms of different disorders, severity and degree of handicap, and inevitably the resulting outcomes are also mixed (Grattan-Smith et al., 1988; Goodyer, 1981; Leslie, 1988; Nunn et al., 1998; Vereker, 1992; Wessely and Powell, 1989). More recently, small case series have started to appear with greater uniformity of characteristics, e.g. pervasive refusal and neurasthenic conditions presenting with chronic fatigue (Garralda, 1999a; Nunn et al., 1998). In general, psychosomatic disorders have a good outcome for any single bout of symptoms and illness behaviours. Adjustment disorders and dissociative disorders are particularly likely to have a time limited course, determined by the stresses which precipitated them, and to respond quickly if help is available to encourage resolution. The more chronic disorders, such as multiple physical complaints and neurasthenic presentations, if well established in late adolescence, are less likely to respond quickly or completely. They may presage lifelong difficulties, although long-term follow-up studies of these presentations in the adolescent age group have not yet been performed.

Thus the *severity* of the disability in the initial presentation is not necessarily a poor prognostic factor: worse outcomes are seen in those where the problems are long-standing and chronic. Rangel and Garralda (2000) report particular personality traits as being poor prognostic markers in chronic fatigue. Whereas, in adults, there is evidence that patients who have a conviction that the cause of the illness is purely 'physical' have a worse prognosis (Sharpe, 1999), for adolescents this is usually a family belief system. Severe attachment disorders and/ or extremely abusive early experiences (especially emotionally abusive ones); those where previous well-placed sensible interventions (including reassurance and encouragement to health) have been unsuccessful; situations where the family have persistent difficulty in establishing trusting relationships or can only do so with professionals who are perceived as reinforcing their beliefs represent a more difficult group to treat, clinically. Substantive follow up studies of the outcomes of psychosomatic disorders in adulthood are only now beginning to appear (Hotopf *et al.*, 1998b) and much more work remains to be done before confident predictions can be made.

CONCLUSION

Psychosomatic disorders are a neglected area of adolescent mental health problems, and merit much more research using robust diagnostic groupings and measurable outcomes. Whilst many have a positive prognosis and there is increasing evidence of clear treatment programmes, many areas remain to be elucidated.

REFERENCES

American Psychiatric Association (1994) *Diagnostic and Statistical Manual of Mental Disorders*, 4th edn (DSM-IV). Washington, DC: American Psychiatric Association.

Aro, H., Paronen, O. and Aro, S. (1987) Psychosomatic symptoms among 14–16 year old Finnish adolescents. *Social Psychiatry*, 22, 171–176.

Bass, C. (1996) Management of somatisation disorder. *Prescribers' Journal*, 36, 198–205.

Chalder, T. (1999) Family oriented cognitive behavioural treatment for adolescents with chronic fatigue syndrome. In E. Garralda (ed.), *Chronic Fatigue Syndrome: Helping Children and Adolescents. Occasional Papers 16.* London: Association for Child Psychology and Psychiatry, pp. 19–23.

Craig, T. K. J., Boardman, A. P., Mills, K., Daley-Jones, O. and Drake, H. (1993) The South London somatisation study I: Longitudinal course and the influence of early life experience. *British Journal of Psychiatry*, 163, 579–588.

Deale, A., Chalder, T., Marks, I. and Wessely, S. (1997) A randomised controlled trial of cognitive behaviour versus relaxation therapy for chronic fatigue syndrome. *American Journal of Psychiatry*, **154**, 408–414.

Egger, H. L., Costello, E. J., Erkanli, A. and Angold, A. C. (1999) Somatic complaints and psychopathology in children and adolescent: stomach aches, musculo-skeletal pains and headaches. *Journal of American Academy of Child and Adolescent Psychiatry* **38**, 852–860.

Eminson, D. M. (1996) The prevalence of psychosomatic disorder: moving from epidemiological to clinical samples. In M. E. Garralda (ed.), *Psychosomatic Problems in Children: Clinical Research Perspectives. Occasional Papers 12*. London: Association for Child Psychology and Psychiatry, pp. 3–12.

Eminson, D. M., Benjamin, S., Shortall, A., Woods, T. and Faragher, B. (1996) Physical symptoms and illness attitudes in adolescents: an epidemiological study. *Archives of Disease in Childhood*, **37**, 519–528.

Fritz, G. K., Fritsch, S. and Owen, H. (1997) Somatoform disorders in children and adolescents: a review of the past ten years. *Journal of American Academy of Child and Adolescent Psychiatry*, **36**, 1329–1338.

Garber, J., Walker, L. S. and Zeman, J. (1991) Somatisation symptoms in a community sample of children and adolescents: further validation of the children's somatisation inventory. *Journal of Consulting and Clinical Psychology*, **3**, 588–595.

Garralda, M. E. (1996) Somatisation in children. *Journal of Child Psychology and Psychiatry*. **37**, 13–33.

Garralda, M. E., et al (1999a) Practitioner review assessment of somatisation in childhood and adolescence: A practical perspective. *Journal of Child Psychology and Psychiatry*, **40**, 1159–1167.

Garralda, M. E. (ed.) (1999b) *Chronic Fatigue Syndrome: Helping Children and Adolescents. Occasional Papers 16*. London: Association for Child Psychology and Psychiatry.

Goodyer, I. M. (1981) Hysterical conversion reactions in childhood. *Journal of Child Psychology and Psychiatry*, **22**, 179–188

Grattan-Smith, P., Fairley, M. and Procopis, P. (1988) Clinical features of conversion disorder. *Archives of Disease in Childhood*, **63**, 408–414.

Greene, J. W., Walker, L. S., Hickson, G. and Thompson, J. (1985) Stressful life events and somatic complaints in adolescents. *Pediatrics*, **75**, 19–22.

Guthrie, E., Creed, F., Dawson, D. and Tomenson, B. (1993) A randomised controlled trial of psychotherapy in patients with refractory irritable bowel syndrome. *British Journal of Psychiatry*, **163**, 315–321.

Hotopf, M., Carr, S., Mayou, R., Wadsworth, M. and Wessely, S. (1998a) Why do children have chronic abdominal pain, and what happens to them when they grow up? Population bases cohort study. *British Medical Journal*, **316**, 1196–1200.

Hotopf, M., Mayou, R., Wadsworth, M. and Wessely, S. (1998b) Temporal relationships between physical symptoms and psychiatric disorder. *British Journal of Psychiatry*, 173, 255–261.

King, A. J. and Coles, B. (1992) *The Health of Canada's Youth: Views and Behaviours of 11-, 13- and 15 Year Olds from 11 Countries*. Canada: Minister of National Health and Welfare.

Larsson, B. and Mellin, L. (1988) The psychological treatment of recurrent headache in adolescents – short term outcome and its prediction. *Headache*, 28, 187–195.

Lask, B. (1996) Pervasive refusal syndrome. In G. Forrest (ed.), *Psychosomatic Problems in Children: Clinical Research Perspectives. Occasional Papers 12*. London: Association for Child Psychology and Psychiatry, pp. 33–36.

Lask, B. and Fosson, A. (1989) *Childhood Illness: The Psychosomatic Approach*. New York: Wiley.

Leslie, S. A. (1988) Diagnosis and treatment of hysterical conversion reactions. *Archives of Disease in Childhood*, 63, 506–511.

Lipowski, Z. J. (1988) Somatisation: the concept and its clinical application. *American Journal of Psychiatry*, 145, 1358–1368.

Mayou, R. (1997) Treating medically unexplained physical symptoms. *British Medical Journal*, 315, 561–562.

Nunn, K. P., Thompson, S. L., Moore, S. G., English, M., Burke, E. A. and Bryne, N. (1998) Managing pervasive refusal syndrome: strategies of hope. *Clinical Child Psychology and Psychiatry*, 3, 229–250.

Offord, D. R., Boyle, M. H., Szatmari, P., Rae-Grant, N. I., Links, P. S., Cadman, D. J. *et al.* (1987) Ontario child health study. II. Six month prevalence of disorder and rates of service utilisation. *Archives of General Psychiatry*, 44, 832–836.

Polkolainen, K., Kanerva, R. and Lonnquist, J. (1995) Life events and other risk factors for somatic symptoms in adolescence. *Pediatrics*, 96, 59–63.

Rauste-von Wright, M. and von Wright, J. (1992) Habitual somatic discomfort in a representative sample of adolescents. *Journal Psychosomatic Research*, 36, 383–390.

Rangel, L. and Garralda, E. (2000) Personality in adolescents with chronic fatigue syndrome. *European Journal of Child and Adolescent Psychiatry*, 9(1), 39–45.

Sanders, M. R., Shepherd, R. W., Cleghorn, G. and Woodford, H. (1994) Treatment of recurrent abdominal pain in children: a controlled comparison of cognitive behavioural family intervention and standard paediatric care. *Journal of Consulting and Clinical Psychology*, 62, 306–314.

Sharpe, M. (1995) Cognitive behavioural therapies in the treatment of functional somatic symptoms. In R. Mayou, C. Bass and M. Sharpe (eds), *Treatment of Functional Somatic Symptoms*. Oxford: Oxford University Press, pp. 122–143.

Sharpe, M. (1999) Chronic fatigue syndrome. In E. Garralda (ed.), *Chronic Fatigue Syndrome: Helping Children and Adolescents. ACPP Occasional Paper 16.* London: Association for Child Psychology and Psychiatry, pp. 5–8.

Shorter, E. (1992) *From Paralysis to Fatigue. A History of Psychosomatic Illness in the Modern Era.* New York: Free Press

Sifneos, P. (1973) The prevalence of 'alexithymic' characteristics in psychosomatic patients. *Psychotherapy and Psychosomatics,* **22,** 255–262.

Stern, J. Murphy, M. and Bass, C. (1993) Personality disorder in patients with somatisation disorder: a controlled study. *British Journal of Psychiatry,* **163,** 785–789.

Taylor, D. C. (1982) The components of sickness: disease, illnesses and predicaments. In J. Apley and C. Ounsted (eds), *One Child.* London: Spastics International Medical Publications, pp. 1–13.

Taylor, D. C. (1986) Hysteria, play-acting and courage. *British Journal of Psychiatry.* 149: 37–41.

Taylor, D. C. (1992) Outlandish factitious illness. In T. David (ed.), *Recent Advances in Paediatrics.* London: Churchill Livingstone, pp. 63–76.

Taylor, D. C., Szatmari, P., Boyle, M. and Offord, D. (1996) Somatization and the vocabulary of everyday bodily experiences and health concerns: a community study of adolescents. *Journal of the American Academy Child and Adolescent Psychiatry,* **35**(4), 491–499.

Vereker, M. (1992) Chronic fatigue syndrome: a joint paediatric–psychiatric approach. *Archives of Disease in Childhood,* **67,** 505–555.

Walker, L. S., Garber, J. and Greene, J. W. (1993) Psychosocial correlates of recurrent childhood pain: a comparison of pediatric patients with recurrent abdominal pain, organic illnes, and psychiatric disorders. *Journal of Abnormal Psychology,* **102,** 248–258.

Wessely, S. and Powell, R. (1989) Fatigue symptoms: a comparison of chronic 'postviral' fatigue with neuromuscular and affective disorders. *Journal of Neurology and Neurosurgery Psychiatry,* 52 940–948.

Wessely, S., David, A., Butler, S. and Chalder, T. (1989) Management of chronic (post-viral) fatigue syndrome. *Journal of the Royal College of General Practitioners,* **39,** 26–29.

Wessely, S., Butler, T., Chalder, T. and David, A. (1991) The cognitive behavioural management of the post-viral fatigue syndrome in 'post-viral fatigue syndrome'. In R. Jenkins and J. Mowbray (eds), *Post Viral Fatigue Syndrome.* Chichester: Wiley, pp. 305–334.

World Health Organisation (1996) *Multi-axial Classification of Child and Adolescent Psychiatric Disorders: The ICD-10 Classification of Mental and Behavioural Disorders in Children and Adolescents.* Cambridge: Cambridge University Press.

Wright, J. B., Beverley, D W. (1998) Chronic fatigue syndrome. *Archives of Disease in Childhood*, **79**, 368–374

Wynick, S., Hobson, R. P. and Jones, R. B. (1997) Psychogenic disorders of vision in childhood ('visual conversion reactions'): perspectives from adolescence: a research note. *Journal of Child Psychology and Psychiatry*, **38**, 375–379.

Chapter 11

ASSESSING ADOLESCENT MENTAL HEALTH

Simon G. Gowers

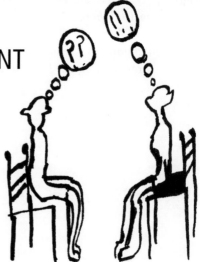

INTRODUCTION

The history of societies' concern with the mental health of adolescents, be it illness or adjustment, has been patchy. Whilst teenagers with mental disorder were frequently admitted to asylums and private madhouses 250 years ago, interest in the mental diseases of this age group increased in the mid-19th century. This followed recognition of the physiological processes of puberty as potential contributors to the development of mental illness (Parry-Jones, 1994). By the end of the 19th century, this interest had flourished with the growing attention to the phenomenology of dementia praecox and manic depressive illness. With the development of the child guidance movement in the 1930s, the new multi-disciplinary speciality of child psychiatry moved quickly into association with paediatrics. Whilst younger adolescents were generally accommodated within the new services, those at the older end of the spectrum and particularly with severe mental illness remained within the province of general psychiatry.

The growth of regional adolescent services in Britain in the late 1960s and early 1970s attempted to bridge the gap in services for adolescents, but these developments were generally in association with adult mental hospitals. This split between community provision contained in paediatric and inpatient services, and older adolescent provision within general mental health services has continued in the 1990s, although the more recent development of Community NHS Trusts in Britain has begun to address this dislocation. Chapter 14 reviews the changing function of the 'adolescent unit'.

ISSUES IN ASSESSMENT

In assessing an adolescent with a possible mental health problem there are a number of potential obstacles which should be taken into account.

- *Adolescent as a target of complaint.* In many situations, it is common for someone to be complaining about the adolescent. This is self-evident in forensic cases and with some other conduct problems, but also true of a number of emotional disorders, such as eating disorders and obsessive-compulsive disorder (OCD).
- *Ambivalence about the problem.* Often the adolescent demonstrates ambivalence between the wish to be left alone and the wish to change. This might be because of fear of change or secondary gain from the symptom or behaviour. OCD is an example in which resistance to obsessional ruminations or performance of rituals is very variable. There may be a difference in this respect between the disorder presenting in teenagers and in adulthood, due to the secondary gain of inappropriate power in adolescence. Many adolescents seem able to control family members through an insistence that they comply with obsessional rituals or face the consequences of an outburst of temper or occasionally physical aggression. Eating disorders, phobias and addictive behaviours are also likely to involve similar ambivalences and comparable family dynamics.
- *Stigma of mental illness.* Very few adolescents would wish their friends to know that they had been assessed or treated by a psychiatrist.
- *Articulation.* Many teenagers will lack confidence in their ability to put their ideas into words, particularly when an assessment may appear to recapitulate difficulties encountered in school.
- *Relations with adults or authority figures.* Many teenagers will have had poor relationships with parents, teachers or the police and may see a psychiatrist in the same category. Some will have suffered abuse at the hands of adults.

STEVE

Steve was a 14-year-old boy with OCD who felt compelled to carry out a ritual which involved touching women's hair. This had got him into trouble, after first an adult and then the parents of an 11-year-old girl had complained to the police. Assessment of Steve exemplified many of the above issues. Parental and third-party concern had initiated the assessment, rather than Steve himself. He merely hoped to convince the interviewer that nothing was wrong and be left alone. As is fairly typical in OCD, Steve had taken on a powerful position within the family, in which the parents were fearful of their sons' temper when thwarted in carrying out his rituals, resulting in a situation where they accommodated a range of unreasonable demands. Steve's embarrassment and isolation as a result of this disorder led to a lack of confidence and self-esteem, thus he did not feel able to express the nature of his predicament to an interviewer easily.

The result of these issues is that more than almost any patient group, the adolescent with a mental health problem is, at the outset, very unlikely to fulfil the role of customer.

In any assessment, the interviewer needs to strike a balance between engagement, the need to elicit information and examination. In some cases, there is a conflict between these three, whilst the balance may vary according to whether the assessment is a one-off or the prelude to further treatment. One important consideration is ensuring adequate time for these processes, although account should be taken of the teenager's ability to tolerate a long session.

ENGAGEMENT

Assessment will be facilitated by attention to the setting, outlining the length and remit of the assessment, and the information currently to hand. Thought should be given to the most helpful setting for the interview, in order that one's aims are achieved. Interviews carried out in an adolescent outpatient clinic, in a police station or behind a flimsy screen on a paediatric ward start from rather different positions.

It is usually helpful to explain the stages of the assessment, particularly that the adolescent will have an opportunity to be seen alone. Any unusual equipment, such as video or one-way screen, should be explained and appropriate consent obtained. This, of course, is likely to worry a suspicious or fearful subject particularly, and it may be helpful to let the teenager have a close look at any video equipment and behind a one-way screen.

GATHERING INFORMATION

Included here is the background information contained in the referral, history obtained in various stages of the assessment appointment and other information collected subsequently. This may include reports from school and other third parties. In order that the required information is obtained, thought should be given to who is invited to any appointment, and in what order and combination they are seen. In a straightforward case, an adolescent will attend with parents or other carer. Clearly, different information may be obtained by seeing parents alone, adolescent alone and all together. Usually it is important to ensure that there is an opportunity for each of these, although there are different views on the order of them and some consideration should be given to the age of the subject. Many prefer to start with a joint interview, in order that the remit, the structure of the session and its aims can be discussed and any major misconceptions addressed. It is then often helpful to begin to obtain an account of the problem in general terms. This enables one to begin to see who is the spokesperson, who agrees with who, who is party to what information and each's interpretation of it. Many would advocate that the interview with the adolescent should come next in order not to alienate them and to respect their right to be seen as the customer. I prefer to see parents first for a number of reasons; the patient will usually accept that they will have their opportunity later. It ought to be possible to overcome any disgruntlement then. My main reasons for wishing to see parents first are to do with coherence and confidentiality. Parents are usually in the best position to set the child's difficulties in the context of a developmental and family history. Is this a child whose depressed mood has come on in the context of lifelong peer relationship difficulties or, for example, learning difficulty? It can be frustrating to see a sullen non-communicative adolescent and not understand what is going on, only for the parental interview to clarify a potentially fruitful line of enquiry. An example might be: 'I expect he told you that it started when he was taunted in the school showers. . .'. The boundaries of confidentiality should be clarified at the outset. In general teenagers can expect that information revealed in their individual interview will only be disclosed to others with their consent unless there is a compelling reason. If the individual interview is followed by the parental interview, the adolescent may nevertheless believe that their confidences are being betrayed. If the adolescent is seen second, parents can then be brought in and the adolescent can witness the interviewer's ability to balance the parent's right to know against the adolescents right to privacy. In some cases, the adolescent may not expect to have any privacy from parents. In this situation, demonstrating a contrary expectation may serve to have therapeutic benefit.

Adolescents sometimes wield inappropriate power in the family as outlined above. Here, it can be helpful to model to parents that this can be withstood. Once, when referred a girl with anorexia nervosa, the parents were surprised that they were allowed to give their story before their daughter. 'You've done it now', the father said, 'we only got her here under false pretences, saying that we were going to the seaside. She'll have run off by the time we finish'. In the event, the girl was sitting patiently in the waiting room half an hour later, demonstrating to the parents that they might not need to give in to all her demands and also that there might be a glimmer of motivation in the girl's mind to address her problem.

STRUCTURE OF THE ADOLESCENT PSYCHIATRIC HISTORY

The following are the main elements, which would be included in any general assessment:

- Family composition
- Present complaint
- History of complaint
- Past medical history
- Medication
    Therapeutic effects, unwanted effects
- Drug, alcohol and substance use and abuse
- Personality
- Temperament
- Family history and family psychiatric history
- Developmental history
- Social/peer relationships
- School attendance, attainment, relations

INTERVIEW STYLE

A style, which includes a number of open questions, is more likely to encourage the young person to talk freely, than closed questions which invite brief responses.

Leading questions should not be employed, as suggestible subjects may acquiesce, leaving the interviewer uncertain as to the answers' reliability. Double and multiple questions should also be avoided as they either confuse the subject or leave the interviewer uncertain which part of the question has been answered.

EXAMINATION/INVESTIGATIONS

There are a number of forms of examination of relevance to adolescent psychiatry.

Mental state examination
This comprises an ordered series of observation and enquiry.

Appearance
The young person's facial expression may reveal clues about mood (whether happy, angry, anxious or sad). A number of abnormalities of motor functioning may have psychiatric implications. The most common manifestation is the restlessness and distractibility of hyperactivity, occasionally diagnosed for the first time in adolescence. This must be distinguished from the overactivity with grandiosity or irritability of hypomania. Depression may be accompanied by motor slowness, also seen in OCD, where compulsive ruminations can be

paralysing. Other abnormal movements include tics (usually facial or involving neck and shoulders, sometimes accompanied by vocalisations). Obsessive rituals sometimes include tapping movements of fingers or movements of the legs and feet. Those on medication should be observed for unwanted effects, such as akathisia and dystonias in those on major tranquillisers and the tremor of lithium intoxication.

Speech and language
Articulation defects or stuttering may benefit from specific therapeutic input. Other abnormalities of the form of speech include those of rate and volume. Depression and hypomania may respectively slow or increase the rate of speech, whilst in the former, speech may be reduced to a nearly inaudible mumble. Vocal tics in Tourette syndrome may on occasion be present with motor accompaniment. The content of speech can be difficult to evaluate in adolescence, particularly when discussing beliefs and interests. Sometimes speech content will reveal the flight of ideas of hypomania or in those with developmental disorders, the echolalia or pronoun reversal of autism.

Thoughts
Assessment of mood always requires enquiry about thoughts of hopelessness, that life is not worth living and assessment of suicidality. Where suicidal ideas have been present, one must enquire about plans, such as storing tablets. In those suspected of psychotic disorder, one should explore the presence of delusional ideas. Assessment of unusual beliefs, such as in the activities of aliens or the paranormal, will need to take account of cultural norms in the young person's peer group. Sometimes a young person with a developing psychosis will retain a degree of insight and withhold delusional or overvalued ideas, which may only be revealed by a parent. Adolescents with obsessive ruminations or rituals sometimes express complex abnormal beliefs to explain their expression, which can sometimes be difficult to distinguish from delusional beliefs. Resistance to obsessive rituals is not universal, but enquiry will normally reveal that resistance leads to high anxiety, whilst the magical beliefs of OCD are not usually held with the absolute conviction of delusions.

Abnormal perceptions
It is necessary to distinguish hallucinations from illusions (on the basis of presence or absence of a stimulus). Visual and tactile hallucinations are suggestive of organic (particularly drug-induced) psychoses, whilst in schizophrenia auditory hallucinations often have the same quality as those seen in adults.

Social behaviour
A clinical interview can reveal much about social behaviour, both verbal and non-verbal. The interviewer can note shyness, disinhibition, aggressiveness or

suspiciousness. How easy is it to develop a rapport? Is there normal reciprocal social communication? Is the young person overly friendly or socially inappropriate?

Mood

Shyness or sullenness is quite common at the outset of an interview with an adolescent, but after engagement it is important to determine whether there is suggestion of mood disturbance. As well as looking out for depressed or elated mood, is the young person's mood appropriate to the areas being discussed? Is he or she able to show an appropriate range of affective responses? Is mood unusually labile? Is he or she able to enjoy life and look forward to planned activities? Clearly the assessment in this area may be influenced by pending criminal proceedings. One should enquire about sleep and appetite, noting that the presentation of depression in young people may involve hypersomnia and increased appetite, more commonly than in adulthood. Loss of libido is a rare feature in adolescents.

Cognition

It is usually possible to make a brief assessment of orientation, concentration, attention and memory, whilst comprehensive developmental assessment requires trained standardised testing. A simple evaluation of developmental level can be achieved by testing reading, writing and mathematical ability. However, the subject may be sensitive about lack of academic attainment and the way such information is elicited requires careful attention.

Assessment of family relationships

Much may be gleaned from the initial meeting with all family members or indeed from the waiting room. Parents may be sitting together whilst the adolescent stands apart. Alternatively one parent may be isolated, giving the impression that they have only come to provide the transport. An adolescent sitting between parents may demonstrate the family's support or closeness, or alternatively their power relationships. When members of the family speak, are they critical, empathic or protective? Who agrees with whom and are disagreements expressed or not? Are they accepted or rejected? What are the alliances and identifications in the family? Frequently, assessment of the family requires a more detailed assessment, sometimes as a prelude to family therapy. Assessment instruments are mentioned below.

The physical examination

The importance of a physical examination may vary with the history and the type of presenting problem, but its potential importance should always be considered. A comprehensive assessment should include a physical assessment including measurement of height, weight and pubertal status with completion of appropriate centile charts. A brief general examination should be carried out, with focus on specific systems depending on the nature of the presenting problem. While dressing or undressing, one may note hand preference, any degree of clumsiness, incoordination or unsteadiness. Unusual facial appearance, asymmetrical physical development and pigmented or de-pigmented skin patches should be recorded, along with any bruising or scars. A patient with a psychotic illness or a learning disability will require a comprehensive neurological assessment, whilst one with anorexia nervosa needs assessment of nutrition and haematological function.

A brief neurological assessment should be carried out, though there are few systematic population studies, with attention to accurate neurological assessment. The Isle of Wight study (Rutter *et al.*, 1970) suggested that although there was an association between neurological findings and behavioural abnormality, this was less close than had been previously assumed. The notion of neurological 'soft signs' is controversial and, it has been argued, a subterfuge for unscientific thinking. Soft signs have been described as being over-represented in autism, Tourette syndrome, borderline personality disorder, schizophrenia and anxiety withdrawal (Pincus, 1996). One explanation may be that these disorders do not constitute diseases in themselves, but expressions of a range of biological abnormality. A detailed review of neurological soft signs is provided by Pincus (1996). Asymmetrical physical or neurological findings are reliable indicators of pathology. Assessment should include assessment of coordination by observation of the young persons writing, drawing and copying of figures. Any tremor or abnormal movements should be noted. With the eyes closed, proprioception can be assessed by the finger-nose test. Walking heel to toe, on tip toes, and in turn on the inner and outer edges of the feet (Fog's test; Fog and Fog, 1963) may reveal asymmetry in and the extent of overflow movements, abnormal in post-pubertal children. Any mirroring of foot posture in the hands is also abnormal after the age of 11.

Physical investigations

Investigations are carried out for two main reasons: to examine for organic disorder and to check physical status before prescribing medication. Usually the history and mental state examination provide the main pointers to an organic contribution; a battery of investigations should not be routinely conducted in the hope of uncovering an unexpected condition. When a young person presents with a major change in behaviour or a psychotic illness a remediable physical disorder may be present or it may be important to attempt to assess the contribution of substance misuse. The initial investigation should include full blood count, erythrocyte sedimentation rate (ESR), serum urea and electrolytes, calcium and phosphate, liver function (including aspartate transaminase and albumin), and thyroid function. This latter is of particular importance where lithium therapy is considered. Urine analysis and urine toxicology screen should be conducted as young people may ingest a wider range of drugs than those volunteered. (Hallucinogen's will not be detected by urinalysis, however.)

An acute psychotic presentation merits an EEG and either a computed tomography or magnetic resonance imaging scan, although the pick-up rate is very low. It can be re-assuring to parents, however, that physical causes have been excluded.

INFLUENCES ON THE PRESENTATION OF MENTAL HEALTH PROBLEMS

Abnormal adolescent development has been reviewed along with the various factors which can affect it in Chapter 2. The following, however, are amongst the more important influences to bear in mind in the practical assessment of the mental health of adolescents.

DEVELOPMENT

Given the transitional nature of adolescence, any assessment of mental health will involve a consideration of the presence or absence of illness or disorder, but also an evaluation of various components of development. Assessment of development encompasses personality, social and moral development, including such things as empathy and the ability to form relationships. It also includes physical and intellectual development, both of which have a considerable bearing on psychological development.

Not all aspects of development proceed at an even pace and there are reasons to suppose that a mismatch between the various aspects of development is particularly potent at contributing to disorder. This mismatch may be between two aspects of intellectual functioning or between physical and emotional development. Specific reading retardation (a delay in reading greater than 2 years beyond that which would be predicted by IQ), for example, seems to have a greater association with conduct disorder than a general retardation of equivalent magnitude. Similarly it is probable that a mismatch between physical and emotional development leads to comparable problems. The emotionally immature girl who is physically mature and looks older than her years may find herself involved in demanding relationships which she feels ill-equipped to cope with.

Traditionally, personality is thought of as malleable and in a process of evolution through adolescence, not becoming established until adulthood is reached. This view permits hope for apparent difficulties to be rectified before the door is closed on development and also reduces the potential for the inappropriate use of pejorative labels such as 'sociopath'.

Any judgement about the presence of disorder has to take account of the possibility of different presentations at different stages through development.

Depressive symptoms, for example, may present differently at the age of 12 to those presenting at 18. Later in adolescence, loss of libido may be a feature of depression, not present in pubescence. Where a presentation is abnormal, this may be either in terms of symptoms or behaviours which are within the bounds of normality at an earlier age (developmental delay) or symptoms or behaviours which are abnormal at any age (distorted or deviant development). Bedwetting or fear of the dark provide examples of the former, whilst auditory hallucinations illustrate the latter.

PHYSICAL FACTORS

The relationship between physical development and disorder in adolescence is an important one. Psychological disorder can, on the one hand, influence physical development and, on the other, be influenced by it. Anorexia nervosa is an example of the former case; when it arises before linear growth and pubertal development are completed, it can result in stunting of growth and reversal or retardation of the process of puberty. Some of these physical effects are completely reversible, others only relatively so. Confidence and self-esteem, meanwhile, can be adversely affected by small stature or delayed pubertal development (particularly in boys), leading to anxiety or depression, sometimes mediated through bullying.

Finally, a degree of neuroendocrine maturity appears to be necessary for the development of psychotic illnesses such as bipolar affective disorder and schizophrenia, which become increasingly prevalent during the teenage years.

Genetic predisposition to a range of disorders confers additional risk. Genetic research is resulting in rapid advances. In general polygenic inheritance seems to be more common than single gene effects, with the risk of psychiatric illness increasing with genetic fit to an affected relative (see Chapter 2).

RESILIENCE

The interplay between assessment of development and presence or absence of disorder is highlighted in the assessment of adjustment to a trauma, life event or change of social circumstance. The ability of an adolescent to cope, for example, with placement in a residential home will include presence of depression or anxiety, personality and social adjustment. The concepts of resilience and vulnerability are concerned with the factors that impinge on the ability to cope. Studies of the development of post-traumatic stress disorder in teenagers exposed to a common trauma have attempted to identify features which appear protective, but most are hampered by a lack of comprehensive assessment prior to the given disaster. Family support has long been recognised as one such variable (Garmezy, 1984) and this almost certainly relates to healthy pre-morbid family functioning. The full range of family strengths and difficulties may be represented in a series of children exposed to an 'Act of God' traumatic experience, but family difficulties are likely to be over represented in those experiencing social traumatic experiences such as reception into care or parental divorce.

ILLNESS

Adolescence is a complex stage of development, when considering adjustment to physical disorder and adherence to treatment. Taylor and Eminson (1994) outline the possible ways that children can fail to comply with the expectations of their medical attendants. These include screaming, struggling and vomiting, the demonstration of which may relate amongst other things to their attitudes to compliance with authority and resentment at intrusion on their autonomy. Chronic physical disorders illustrate some of the issues in the interplay between adolescent development and disorder. In diabetes mellitus, metabolic control is dependent on adherence to a dietary and pharmacological routine. This requires a discipline and sense of responsibility, which mirror those being addressed by the adolescent in the rest of his or her life and in relationships with adults. It may be expected to result in some ambivalence. Compliance with any treatment regime is a constraint upon autonomy (Taylor and Eminson, 1994). In childhood, the parents are usually most affected by this constraint, but as responsibility passes to the adolescent they then share the burden with its attendant ambivalence. Each family has to negotiate the appropriate level of protectiveness and supervision. Concern about one's health may be offset by resentment at having to comply overly much, particularly in comparison with peers. Experimentation with alcohol is just one aspect of normal adolescence which is more loaded with meaning in the diabetic, when drinking behind one's parents back involves 'cheating' and putting one's health at risk. Failure of adherence results not only in a greater challenge to authority than that posed by peers, but also may result in being faced with parents own worries about their illness. Frequently teenagers with such a disorder are faced with a choice between being overly protected and relatively lacking in independence or 'super mature' and more responsible than their peers. This responsibility may include a burdensome responsibility for protecting parents from distress, by concealing fears and doubts. There are suggestions that where metabolic control in adolescent diabetes is good, this may be at the expense of vulnerability to depressed mood and also a more rigid style of family functioning (Gowers et al., 1995). Gustafsson et al. (1987) have meanwhile also demonstrated links between family stress and poor diabetic control.

SOCIOCULTURAL FACTORS

Chapter 1 has illustrated that adolescence is a transitional stage of development, between childhood and adulthood. The physical changes of puberty are generally seen as the starting point of adolescence, whilst the end is less clearly delineated.

Adolescence ends with attainment of 'full maturity' and a range of social and cultural factors may influence this. In developed societies these tend to delay progression to adulthood. The extension of compulsory schooling and development of further education, with its economic consequences, generally contributes to a delay in reaching full independence. This may in turn lead to difficulties adjusting to the responsibilities of the next stage of life (Parry-Jones, 1995). In the UK now, it is unusual to be financially self-supporting before one's early 20s.

PSYCHIATRIC DISORDERS OF ADOLESCENCE

A full review of the range of disorders presenting in adolescence and their classification is provided in Chapter 3.

Such disorders tend to fall into three developmental categories, i.e. continuing childhood disorder, mental illnesses typical of adulthood and disorders which although not confined exclusively to adolescence, seem characterised by difficulties surmounting this stage of development. In the first category, a number of presentations, particularly developmental and conduct disorders, will continue from middle childhood into the teens. In the category of adult mental illnesses, schizophrenia and bipolar disorder are both extremely rare before the age of 12. Adolescence is a stage of growing cognitive sophistication and increasing social demand, both of which may play a part in the development of complex psychotic phenomena. It is possible that both are necessary to form, for example, a paranoid delusional belief. Most important though seem to be the neuroendocrine changes in the brain, signalled by puberty, which confer a risk for these disorders, in those genetically at risk. Psychoses precipitated by drugs also become more common as independence offers opportunity.

Disorders in the third category, which are typical of adolescence, can be seen as representing a difficulty in mastering the tasks of this developmental stage. Erikson (1965) identified the development of a personal identity as the main task of adolescence. The Group for Advancement of Psychiatry (1968) considered the following to be crucial supplementary tasks:

- Proficiency in the adult sexual role
- The transition from being nurtured to being able to care for others
- Learning to work and be self-supporting
- Leaving home

As well as arising from task failure, adolescent disorder usually interferes with satisfactory completion of these tasks. A clinical example ('Claire') will illustrate this point.

CLAIRE

Claire was a 15-year-old girl who lived with her parents and elder brother. Claire had experienced bullying at school and suffered poor self-esteem as a consequence of her mild obesity. Her mother suffered from epilepsy. Following an occasion when her mother experienced a partial seizure whilst making a cup of tea and scalded herself, Claire stayed off school for a few days to help her mother with her housework. Very quickly, her school refusal became entrenched, her school non-attendance being attributed by the family to bronchial asthma, which was never very evident at clinical assessment. Claire became, like her mother, socially isolated and the two of them spent little time apart. In this example, individual, family and social elements had come together to result in the presentation of school refusal. One can see that there were difficulties for Claire in achieving an identity for herself separate from that of her mother. In addition, the nurturing roles had become unclear through a mutual dependence of each on the other, in which both was carer and cared for. As social and academic aspirations become limited, the opportunities for Claire to attain further independence or form intimate relationships outside the family were much reduced. In such a situation, the failure to move along a normal developmental trajectory generally results in a widening gulf between the subject's experience and that of her peers, thus compounding the above difficulties.

FORMAL CLASSIFICATION SYSTEMS

A system of classification is, in principal, an invaluable tool for both clinical practice and research. It may help in organising one's thinking about an individual case as well as enabling comparison between clinical series. Classification also provides an aid to case management at a time when clinicians are increasingly encouraged to base decisions on an evidence base. In complex cases where written communication between professionals from a range of discipline features high, a common language of reliable and valid diagnoses would appear to be highly desirable. Graham (1982), however, has drawn attention to some of the problems with existing classification schemes. They tend to be viewed as flawed and many professionals working in adolescent mental health have reservations about a perceived medical bias, the negative consequences of 'labelling', and the lack of association between diagnosis and 'need'. Disciplines outside medicine tend to view adolescents in a different way, e.g. social services tend to view young people as at risk from their social circumstances, whilst educationalists classify pupils by the additional resources required to provide their education and the reason why those resources are necessary.

The formal systems of classification and the epidemiology of adolescent disorder have been reviewed in Chapter 3.

DIAGNOSTIC THRESHOLD

The relationship between symptoms, behaviours and disorders is a complex one. A number of disorders represent quantitative rather than qualitative differences from normality, e.g. *excessive* anxiety for a given situation. In determining caseness, it is usually helpful to consider the degree of associated, secondary difficulties a symptom, such as social avoidance confers. In both the ICD-10 (World Health Organisation, 1992) and DSM-IV (American Psychiatric Association, 1994) systems of classification, an essentially arbitrary issue of threshold must be addressed. ICD-10 offers guidelines to aid diagnostic decision making, whilst DSM-IV operationalises the process by specifying the number and type of symptoms or behaviours required. In conduct disorder for example, three or more behaviours are required from section A, whilst criteria B and C must be satisfied. For most DSM diagnoses, significant impairment of social, academic or occupational function is required.

CHECKLISTS, RATING SCALES, QUESTIONNAIRES AND SEMI-STRUCTURED INTERVIEWS

These have been devised to improve the reliability and validity of information and observation used in diagnostic assessment. They are primarily used for research but can be useful for screening populations or as a diagnostic aid in clinical settings. In general, adolescents report more reliably about feelings and parents about behaviour. These have been developed for a range of different purposes and for use in a specified context. Any interpretation of data yielded from them needs to take account of their original purpose (e.g. research or clinical), whether, for example, they are designed to measure change (or response to treatment) and the intended target population (e.g. cultural context). What degree of training (if any) is required for their use?

SCREENING INSTRUMENTS FOR NORMAL SAMPLES

The recognition that a child's behaviour is abnormal can usually be achieved with sufficient accuracy for routine screening purposes by a brief symptom/behavioural checklist, such as the *Rutter A scale* (Rutter, 1967) or the *Child Behaviour Checklist* (Achenbach and Edelbrock, 1983). The *Strength and Difficulties Questionnaire* (Goodman, 1997) is a newer instrument which has the merit of not focussing on problems alone. The *Conners Parent and Teacher Questionnaires* (Conners, 1971) have shown particular value in evaluating response to pharmacological treatment of children and young adolescents with attention deficit hyperactivity disorder (ADHD).

ASSESSMENT INSTRUMENTS FOR CLINICAL SAMPLES

Highly structured interviews

- *Diagnostic Interview for Children and Adolescents (DICA)* (Herjanic and Reich, 1982). Suitable for children and young people aged 6–17. There are parent and child versions. Takes 60–90 min and requires no clinical judgement by the interviewer. The interview yields information on a wide range of symptoms, their onset and severity. ICD and DSM diagnoses can be yielded. The authors have demonstrated satisfactory inter-rated and test–retest reliability and validity using comparisons of referrals to paediatric and psychiatric clinics.
- *Diagnostic Interview Schedule for Children (DISC)* (Costello *et al.*, 1985). Takes 45–60 min. Suitable for children aged 6–18 years. Symptoms are coded on a three-point (0–2) scale. There are parent and child versions.

Semi-structured instruments

These require greater clinical interpretation and thus greater training to ensure reliability. The most widely used is the *Schedule for Affective Disorders and Schizophrenia for School Age Children (K-SADS)* (Puig-Antich and Chambers), revised by Orvaschel *et al.* (1982). This interview is designed to be administered by clinically experienced interviewers. It starts with identification of all problems and symptoms, followed by a treatment history and observational assessment. Finally, the interviewer rates global functioning on a 1–100 scale – the children's version of the Global Assessment of Functioning. It is designed to be administered to parents first. Inter-rater reliability for individual symptoms of major diagnostic syndromes range from 0.65 to 0.96.

Measurement of family functioning

There are a number of assessment aids for evaluating family functioning, the McMaster model (Epstein *et al.*, 1978) seeming particularly focussed on areas pertinent to the adolescent stage of development. There is a self-rated version the *Family Assessment Device (FAD)* and a clinician-rated version the *McMaster Structured Interview of Family Functioning (McSIFF)* (Epstein *et al.*, 1982, 1983). The ratings of family functioning provided by the McMaster model have been shown to be highly predictive of outcome of adolescent anorexia nervosa (North *et al.*, 1997).

Instruments for rating clinical severity and change over time

- *Health of the Nation Outcome Scales for Children and Adolescents (HoNO-SCA)* (Gowers *et al.*, 1999a). This is a brief outcome scale comprising 13 items rated on a five-point scale from 0 to 4, with a detailed glossary to guide ratings (Gowers *et al.*, 1999b). It was developed as part of the Health of the Nation strategy to improve mental health within the population and is designed as a routine clinical measure. Limited training is required. An adolescent self-rated guided questionnaire is in development.
- *Strength and Difficulties Questionnaire* (Goodman, 1997). This instrument also has self-rating and clinician-rated versions and is suitable for adolescents. The positive attention to areas of strength may make it particularly acceptable to patients and families.

Developmental and psychological tests

The following is a list of the more commonly used psychological and developmental tests used in the field of adolescent mental health, with an indication of their uses. Detailed description of their construction and performance is outwith the scope of this chapter. Full references are not provided, but readers are directed to Racusin and Moss's (1996) overview of this area for further detail.

- *Wechsler Intelligence Scale for Children lll (WISC-lll)*. Age up to 17 years. Yields performance, verbal and full scale IQ.
- *Bruininks-Oseretsky Test of Motor Proficiency.* Age up to 14 years. Measures gross and fine motor performance (eight subtests).
- *Benton Visual Retention Test (BVRT)*. Age to adult. Tests visual perception.
- *Bender Visual Motor Gestalt Test.* Age to adult. Assesses visual–motor deficits and visual memory.
- *Peabody Picture Vocabulary (Revised) (PPVT-R)*. Age to adult. Screening test for language.
- *Peabody Individual Achievement Test- Revised (PIAT-R)*. Age to 18 years. Educational knowledge and skills.
- *Trail Making Test*. Age to adult. Tests attention. Useful in assessment of ADHD in adolescents.
- *Child Behaviour Checklist (CBCL)* (Achenbach and Edelbrock, 1983). School-age children. Parent and teacher rating versions.
- *Conners Teacher Rating Scale.* School-age children. Particularly useful for rating response to treatment in ADHD.
- *Wisconsin Card Sorting Test.* Age to adult. Tests attention.
- *Minnesota Multiphasic Personality Inventory – Adolescent (MMPI-A)*. Age 14–18. Test of personality development.

- *Children's Apperception Test (CAT)*. Age to adult. Test of personality.
- *Vineland Adaptive Behaviour Scales-Survey Form*. Age to adult. Measures social and adaptive behaviour

CONCLUDING REMARKS

The psychiatric assessment of an adolescent may pose a number of difficulties relating to the circumstances of the referral, the adolescent's own views about it and their own developmental status. Assessment is likely to reveal a range of needs and also a number of risks. Health needs can be considered from the perspective of either the individual or a population. In essence, need can be thought of as the best that can be done for an individual in a particular setting (Wallace *et al.*, 1997). Sometimes the need relates directly to a mental health problem, sometimes it is indirect and concerned with the prevention of secondary handicaps, such as through the provision of special education.

Risk is part and parcel of assessment in adolescent psychiatry. It is usually considered in relation to the subject, e.g. risk from self-harm, substance use or anorexia. Sometimes the risk also encompasses others, most commonly through aggressive or other antisocial behaviour, such as fire-setting or from acting on psychotic experiences. Both needs and risks should be considered in planning any intervention. Assessment of risk in forensic settings is discussed in Chapter 16, in relation to self-harm in Chapter 4 and in considering admission to an adolescent unit in Chapter 14.

REFERENCES

Achenbach, T. M. and Edelbrock, C. S. (1983) *Manual for the Child Behaviour Checklist and Revised Child Behaviour Profile*. Burlington, VT: University of Vermont.

American Psychiatric Association (1994) *Diagnostic and statistical Manual of Mental Disorders*, 4th edn (DSM-IV). Washington, DC: American Psychiatric Association.

Conners, C. K. (1971) Recent drug studies with hyperkinetic children. *Journal of Learning Disability*, **4**, 467–483.

Costello, E. J., Edelbrook, C. and Costello, A. J. (1985) Validity of the NIMH Diagnostic Interview Schedule for Children. A comparison between psychiatric and paediatric referrals. *Journal of Abnormal Child Psychology*, **13**, 579–595.

Erikson, E. H. (1965) *Childhood and Society*. London, Penguin.

Epstein, N. B., Bishop, D. S. and, Levin, S. (1978) McMaster model of family functioning. *Journal of Marriage and Family Counselling*, **3**, 19–31.

Epstein, N. B., Baldwin, L. M and Bishop, D. S. (1982) *McMaster Clinical rating Scale*. Providence, RI: Brown University Family Research Programme.

Epstein, N. B., Baldwin, L. M and Bishop, D. S. (1983) The McMaster Family Assessment Device. *Journal of Marital and Family Therapy*, **9**, 171–180.

Fog, E. and Fog, M. (1963) Cerebral Inhibition examined by associated movements. In M. Bax and R. MacKieth (eds), *Minimal Cerebral Dysfunction. Clinics in Developmental Medicine 10*. London: SSMEIU/Heinemann Medical.

Garmezy, N. (1984) Stress resistant children: the search for protective factors. In J. E. Stevenson (ed.), *Recent Research in Developmental Psychopathology*. Oxford: Pergamon, pp. 213–233

Goodman, R. (1997) The Strength and Difficulties Questionnaire: a research note. *Journal of Child Psychology and Psychiatry*, **38**, 581–586.

Gowers, S. G., Harrington, R. C., Whitton, A., Lelliott, P., Wing, J. and Beevor, A. (1999a) A Brief scale for measuring the outcomes of emotional and behavioural disorders in children (HoNOSCA). *British Journal of Psychiatry*, **174**, 413–416.

Gowers, S. G., Harrington, R. C., Whitton, A. , Beevor, A., Lelliott, P., Jezzard, R. and Wing, J. (1999b) Health of the Nation Outcome Scales for Children and Adolescents (HoNOSCA). Glossary for HoNOSCA score sheet. *British Journal of Psychiatry*, **174**, 428–431.

Gowers, S. G., Jones, J. C., Kiana, S., Price, D. A. and North, C. D. (1995) Family functioning; a correlate of diabetic control? *Journal of Child Psychology and Psychiatry*, **36**, 993–1002.

Graham, P. (1982) Child psychiatry in relation to primary health care. *Social Psychiatry*, **17**, 109–116.

Group for the Advancement of Psychiatry (1968) *Normal Adolescence; Its Dynamics and Impact*. New York: GAP.

Gustafsson, P. A., Cederblad, M. and Ludvigsson, J. (1987), Family interaction and metabolic balance in juvenile diabetes mellitus. A prospective study. *Diabetes Research and Clinical Practice*, **4**, 7–14.

Herjanic, B. and Reich, W. (1982) Development of a structured diagnostic interview for children. Agreement between child and parent on individual symptoms. *Journal of Abnormal Child Psychology*, **10**, 307–324.

North, C. D., Gowers, S. G. and Byram, V. (1997) Family functioning and life events in the outcome of adolescent anorexia nervosa. *British Journal of Psychiatry*, **171**, 545–549.

Orvaschel, H., Puig-Antich J., *et al.* (1982) Retrospective assessment of pre-pubertal major depression with the Kiddie-SADS-E. *Journal of the American Academy of Child Psychiatry*, **21**, 695–707.

Parry-Jones, W. (1995) The future of adolescent psychiatry. *British Journal of Psychiatry*, **166**, 299–305.

Parry-Jones, W. (1994) History of child and adolescent psychiatry. In M. Rutter, E. Taylor and L. Hersov (eds), *Child and Adolescent Psychiatry: Modern Approaches*, 3rd edn. Oxford: Blackwell Science, pp. 794–812.

Pincus, J. H. (1996) The neurological meaning of soft signs. In M. Lewis (ed.), *Child and Adolescent Psychiatry: A Comprehensive Textbook*, 2nd edn. Baltimore, MD: Williams & Wilkins, pp. 479–484.

Racusin, G. R. and Moss, N. E. (1996) Psychological assessment of children and adolescents. In M. Lewis (ed.), *Child and Adolescent Psychiatry: A Comprehensive Textbook*, 2nd edn. Baltimore, MD: Williams & Wilkins, pp. 465–478.

Rutter, M. (1967) A children's behaviour questionnaire for completion by teachers: preliminary findings. *Journal of Child Psychology and Psychiatry*, 8, 1–11.

Rutter, M., Tizard, J. and Whitmore, K. (eds) (1970) *Education, Health and Behaviour*. London: Longmans.

Taylor, D. C. and Eminson, D. M. (1994) Psychological aspects of chronic physical sickness. In M. Rutter, E. Taylor and L. Hersov (eds), *Child and Adolescent Psychiatry: Modern Approaches*, 3rd edn. Oxford: Blackwell Science, pp. p737–748.

Wallace, S. A., Crown, S., Cox, A. and Berger, M. (1997) *Health Care Needs Assessment: Child and Adolescent Mental Health*. Oxford: Radcliffe Medical Press.

World Health Organisation (1992) *The ICD-10 Classification of Mental and Behavioural Disorders. Clinical Descriptions and Diagnostic Guidelines*. Geneva: World Health Organisation.

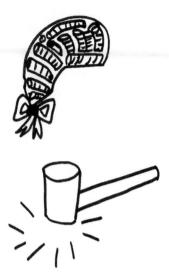

Chapter 12

ETHICAL AND LEGAL ISSUES

David M. Foreman

INTRODUCTION

> A 14-year-old girl confesses to you her bingeing and vomiting, but insists that you do not tell her parents, even though they are worried about her recent loss in weight. What do you do?

Everyone agrees that ethics are essential to ensure good medical practice. However, there is a common belief that ethically correct practice is largely intuitive and needs little tuition or knowledge, beyond an understanding of the practice guidelines of professional associations and a rudimentary grasp of the legal framework governing practice. This is not true (Katz, 1972, pp ix–x). Furthermore, the developmental conditions predicated by adolescence make the ethics of treatment especially vexed in this group. This chapter therefore tries to offer more than a set of guidelines and legal summary. First, it considers the kind of ethical perspective one needs when working with adolescents. Then, it reviews the current legal framework and its relationship to adolescents, emphasising the UK. Next it turns to the development of adolescents from a moral perspective, to help determine the extent to which adolescents of particular ages and abilities can be considered morally autonomous beings. Only then are some guidelines provided, based on the principles previously developed. By understanding the principles on which the guidelines are based, we have a greater chance of adapting them appropriately to contentious circumstances.

ETHICAL PRINCIPLES

No ethical system is perfect. However, there is a lot to be said for defining ethical practice in terms of a few, easily digestible principles. Like diagnoses, principles simplify coping with multifarious circumstances by abstracting common components from them. This allows one to generalise ethical practice consistently across many different situations, by requiring adherence to the principles. Beauchamp and Childress (1994) have developed four such principles in their influential book that are particularly relevant to medical practice. These are respect for autonomy, beneficence, non-maleficence and justice.

RESPECT FOR AUTONOMY

> Do you obtain a 15-year-old's *informed* consent for psychotherapy? What about a 12-year-old?

This principle informs debates over issues of consent, competence and disclosure of professional information. Beauchamp and Childress (1994, p. 123) define it with reference to 'Normal choosers who act (1) intentionally, (2) with understanding and (3) without controlling influences that determine their actions'.

Respect for autonomy is more than an attitude. To show such respect, we must act in such a way that the autonomy of the patient is enabled. As expressed above, the term 'autonomy' itself is synonymous with self-determination. The problem of how to limit self-determination without compromising the principle now arises, as full self-determination will be impaired to some extent in adolescents with (or without) mental health problems. However, there are more restrictive definitions of autonomy that are useful when applying this principle in these circumstances. In its original form, autonomy referred to the individual's ability to follow a freely and rationally adopted moral policy (Kant, 1785, cap. 2). In particular, achievement of autonomy in this sense marks moral maturity. Deciding the extent of an adolescent's 'moral maturity' is the crucial judgement for us, as this marks the ability of an adolescent to rationally decide whether a procedure is good to undergo. For example, consider the seminal Gillick Judgement (Gillick *v* W Norfolk and Wisbech AHA, 1985, p. 422). As Lord Scarman put it 'The parental right yields to the child's right to make his own decisions when he reaches a sufficient understanding and intelligence to be capable of making up his own mind on the matter requiring decision'.

Adolescents may thus over-ride their parents in the judgement of their own good, i.e. achieve autonomy from their parents, immediately they have the capacity to make those judgements. This autonomy is situational and contingent: autonomy in one area does not imply it in all others; and both the topic and the adolescent's ability need consideration.

BENEFICENCE

> How many treatments do we give to teenagers despite knowing there is no evidence for their effect? How do we justify this?

This is what we hope to do when we treat someone. The term refers to our actions as practitioners: so it can refer both to actions that do good or those that prevent harm. However, the benefits that we bring are technical ones, deriving from the application of professional skills (technology). Therefore, the 'good' our technology brings is quite different from the 'good' perceived by the deciding patient. Theirs is a *moral* judgement about the benefit of the treatment in their lives (what is best for me?), while ours is really an offer of improved efficiency in some part of their lives. This non-equivalence between our good and the patient's good defines the problem of medical paternalism – when is it right to over-ride a patient's judgement because we consider it to be in their best interests to do so? The Mental Health Act (1983) is a practical attempt to answer this question for people with mental illness or impairment.

NON-MALEFICENCE

> You are asked to write a report relating to an imprisonable offence committed by a patient with a depressive conduct disorder. How should you relate your report to your treatment plan?

Though famous, the maxim *'primum non nocere'* (first do no harm) is frankly silly. Health services exist to make people better, not to be as harmless as possible. However, the more general idea of avoiding harm wherever possible is of fundamental importance in medicine, including psychiatry. What non-maleficence is really about is distinguishing between effects and side effects of treatment (e.g. Beauchamp and Childress, 1994, pp. 190–191). From the perspective of the intervention, say a drug, there is no such distinction – the drug simply changes the organism's physiology in various ways. The difference between effect and side effect results from the intention expressed in using the drug. Side effects are therefore the *unintended* effects of the treatment. The principle of non-maleficence reminds us that the balance of benefit of intended and unintended effects of an intervention should always be positive. While drug prescription may be the simplest expression of this principle, its most profound implications are seen in decisions about whether to implement entire treatment programs. A particularly poignant example of the significance of this principle is seen in the case of E, a 15-year-old Jehovah's witness with leukaemia. The courts judged that he was not competent to refuse treatment and so he was treated against his will until 18. Once competent to refuse treatment, he did so and died (Alderson and Montgomery, 1996, p. 35). While the courts safe-guarded his life as long as they could (the 'treatment'), his own refusal of treatment later suggests that the quality of existence he was afforded, when his moral position was considered (the 'side effect' of the 'treatment'), was worse than death. The example also illustrates how the principle of non-maleficence is important in justifying harm undertaken for beneficial ends. This is because any harm done in implementing a treatment can be justified by appealing to the greater benefits that a treatment may bring.

JUSTICE

> You can eliminate your waiting list by closing your adolescent unit and redeploying the staff in the community. Is this the right thing to do?

If 'respect for autonomy' is the most individual of the four principles, 'justice' is the most social. It is concerned with how people are treated by each other; in particular, justice embodies the idea that equals should be treated equally and unequals treated unequally. While there are many definitions of justice, Rawls' explication of it as fairness (Rawls, 1985) carries a close correspondence to current British health practice and policy. Many conclusions deriving from a Rawlsian interpretation of health care (Daniels, 1985) can be seen in current plans for the NHS. These include a concentration on preventing, limiting or compensating for reductions in normal functioning, with fair opportunity to access services providing these. Other services, e.g. cosmetic work or luxury hospital rooms, can be available to those able to pay for them. Finally, health investment should be directed at preventing health declining with advancing age (HM Government, 1997). Aside from the benefits to the individual, the costs of health-care in the elderly fall on those younger than they and the sick elderly are in no position to recompense them. As this suggests, the health debates involving justice have been at the level of health policy. In individual cases, while concepts such as 'rights' and 'interests' have frequently been appealed to, 'justice', which regulates such matters, is not extensively discussed.

IMPLEMENTING PRINCIPLES

Knowing the principles does not tell one how to use them. Beauchamp and Childress recommend three inter-related techniques, which they call *specification, dialectic* and *balancing. Specification* (Beauchamp and Childress, 1994, p. 28) describes a process by which the principles are related to norms and practical judgements, leading to guidance towards action. Without this, principles become empty formalism, that allow one to justify any action by appeal to a judicious combination of circumstances (Hegel, 1942, pp. 89–90 and 106–107). *Dialectic* (Beauchamp and Childress, 1994, p. 23) involves comparing our 'considered judgement' on particular situations with the predictions of ethical theories and seeking to maximise the coherence between them. *Balancing* (Beauchamp and Childress, 1994, p. 32) refers to the process of assigning different weights to various norms that may be in conflict with each other, so that an appropriate course of action may be identified. In adolescents, these conflicts typically involve clashes between respect for autonomy and beneficence; and between beneficence and justice. The first clash is better known, as it underpins the arguments surrounding the rights of adolescents with eating disorders to refuse to be force-fed or those with religious beliefs to refuse life-saving treatments that break their principles. The second is reflected in the current debate on the most appropriate approach for managing behaviourally disturbed adolescents (Chesshyre, 1998). It is well known that improving the lot of delinquent adolescents by education and therapy in a caring environment reduces their recidivism (e.g. Pearson, 1987). However, this means that adolescents benefit *twice* from their crimes, immediately from the crime itself, and in the longer term from the therapy and increased support they receive in consequence. Victims, who are frequently unable to recover their loss, are unlikely to see this as just.

Any practitioner must confront two further ethical issues when undertaking a decision about treatment. First, the outcome of any decision is unknown until the decision is enacted. This is the fundamental objection to any ends justifying means. (Non-maleficence is not an ends-means principle, because both effects *and* side effects lie in the future.) Secondly, the practitioner is a participant in the decision, not an observer of the decision. Therefore, the justification of a treatment decision must include more than a claim that the patient will benefit. Practitioners must show that they are entitled to make that decision. This entitlement to decide is discussed in the next section.

RIGHTS AND DUTIES

You are called to a disturbance in a children's home. When you arrive the teenager has barricaded himself in his room. What should you do? What are your powers? When can you exercise them?

Like principles, the importance of rights in both ethics and law is contentious (Dworkin, 1987, p. vii) but one type of right, the claim-right, has direct relevance to clinical decision making. Expressed generally, in a claim-right A has a right to X from B because of Y (Gewirth, 1995, p. 776). Therefore, if A has a claim-right, then B has a duty occasioned by A's right. This leads to a profound conclusion. *Practitioners are required to enact a treatment decision about an adolescent if it fulfils their duty.* So, justifying practitioners' treatment of adolescents begins with a consideration of their duties. If we claim that the duties a practitioner owes an adult are different from those owing to a child, then we have a contradiction, as adolescents may be both adult and child, due to the uneven development of adult abilities during adolescence. Therefore, practitioners must owe the same duties to adults and children. What are they? Respect for autonomy, beneficence, non-maleficence and justice – our four principles specified as duties owed to adolescents by practitioners. Having determined our duties, we now have to work out how to fulfil them. Consideration of the legal framework that governs practitioners is an essential first step to this.

LEGAL FRAMEWORKS

Both the adolescent and the practitioner have a legal framework relating to them. These can be thought of under three main headings: the adolescent in the family, the state as parent and the mentally disordered adolescent.

THE ADOLESCENT IN THE FAMILY

The relationship between adolescents, their families and practitioners in law has focused on consent for treatment. In England and Wales, adolescents may validly consent to treatments on reaching their 16th birthday (Family Law Reform Act, 1969). When younger than 16, parental consent must be sought except in four circumstances: when the treatment has been ordered by a court, when the parents have abandoned the child, when there is a life-threatening emergency and when the Gillick (see above) principle applies (Dewar, 1992, p. 105). However, two cases have separated an adolescent's right to consent from the right to refuse treatment. In Re R (1991, 1992) it was determined that a child's refusal of treatment could be over-ridden by the court, even if the child was Gillick competent. Re W (1992, 1992) further concluded that adolescents were unable to refuse treatment below 18 and could be over-ridden by either doctors or parents. At present, the resultant position needs further clarification. For example, children may not refuse treatments, but can refuse examinations under the Children Act (White et al., 1990, p. 106). The validity of the child's consent is more closely related to agreement with the practitioner, than to the child's developing autonomy. English law may provide children with fewer safeguards against coerced treatments than mentally ill adults (cf. The Mental Health Act, 1983). Perhaps unsurprisingly, there has been blistering academic criticism (e.g. Alderson and Montgomery, 1996, pp. 34–39; Kennedy and Grubb, 1994, pp. 393–396) but the current position can be philosophically justified, using the concept of coherence (Beauchamp and Childress, 1994, p. 27). In the Gillick case, evidence for the child's capacity came from the child agreeing with a decision the doctor already considered rational, i.e. the child's rationality was coherent with the doctor's, and so could be considered equivalent. This additional qualification did not apply in either Re R or Re W, so despite evidence for the intellectual comprehension by R and W of the proposed interventions, it is not clear that either R or W were able to follow a freely and rationally adopted moral policy. This view, that they lacked sufficient autonomy, is consistent both with the mental disorders they suffered from (anorexia and fluctuating psychosis) and, as we shall see below, the developmental status of autonomy in adolescence.

In the US, the position is quite different. Contrary to their English counterparts, American judges have decided that the ability to consent to a treatment implies the ability to refuse it (Sigman and O'Connor, 1991). This has led to the development of the concept of 'assent'. Children are considered to 'assent' (or its alternate, 'dissent') when they have sufficient competence to have some appreciation of a procedure, but not enough competence to give fully informed consent (Anonymous, 1977; Committee on Bioethics, 1995). The age of assent is currently estimated as being about 12.

The most important argument against assent is that it is beside the point. The practitioner controls the delivery of the intervention. Agreement with the intervention is one factor the practitioner has to take into account before proceeding. Therefore, the practitioner needs to know how to respond to agreement or disagreement from the child, the parents or both. Calling the child's agreement 'consent' or 'assent' and the parents 'proxy consent' or 'parental permission' does not tell the practitioner how to respond to them, or how they differ. In fact, guidelines for obtaining assent are equivalent to those for obtaining consent (Committee on Bioethics, 1995; NHS Management Executive, 1990). Therefore, assent disguises rather than resolves the difficulties apparent in English law.

THE STATE AS PARENT

The state involves itself in the parenting of children in three ways. First, there is the ancient concept of *parens patriae*, which is expressed through the inherent jurisdiction of the High Court and, more specifically, through Wardship, where the court reserves to itself the ability to make or prevent important decisions about the child (Dewar, 1992, pp. 487–489). Secondly, there is the 1989 Children Act, which specifically defines a legal framework for the proper care and management of children. Thirdly, the United Nations Convention on the Rights of the Child, ratified in the UK in 1991, seeks to allow children to make claims for good treatment, that are not simply expressions of adult benevolence. As such, it provides a useful set of standards against which to judge provision for children in society. However, it is the first two that bind practitioners.

The Children Act 1989 specifically set out to make child care practice more uniform, effective and accountable (Parton, 1991, cap. 7), as well as reducing the adversarial quality of relationships between parents and local authorities. The protection of children is managed through Area Child Protection Committees, Child Protection Registers and Child Protection Conferences. Accommodation (voluntary residential care) is owed to 'children in need' who:

- have no responsible parent, or
- have been lost or abandoned, or
- cannot be cared for because their usual caretaker cannot provide the resources necessary to do so

It can be seen that the last category could apply because of the special needs of the child, as well as any limitation in the child's caretakers. The authority providing accommodation does not acquire parental rights by doing so. It may not provide accommodation if someone with parental rights can do so and someone with parental rights may remove a child from accommodation at any time. However, these latter limitations do not extend to someone with a residence order, to someone who has been granted care in Wardship or when the child voluntarily accommodated is over 16. Application for any court intervention (including care proceedings) is governed by: a court imposed timetable, an assumption that no order will be made unless it contributes positively to the child's welfare and the following welfare checklist:

- The ascertainable wishes and feelings of the child, considered in the light of the child's age and understanding
- The child's physical, emotional and educational needs
- The likely effect on the child of any change in circumstances
- The child's age, sex, background and any characteristics which the court considers relevant

- Any harm suffered or risk of harm
- The capacity of the relevant adults to meet the child's needs
- The range of powers available to the court under the Act

Apart from statutory proceedings where appropriate, the Local Authority has two more general duties: to offer families support and to prevent the need for court proceedings or admission into care. The matter of children 'in need' is especially relevant in determining who obtains such services, and will be dealt with in more detail in the next section.

Wardship and the inherent jurisdiction (of the High Court) are important to the practitioner as this may be the best legal remedy for regulating the the the child's behaviour or ensuring appropriate treatment (Dewar, 1992, pp. 497–499), especially if the child is subject to a Care Order.

THE MENTALLY DISORDERED ADOLESCENT

The Children Act 1989 defines a child as being 'in need' if:

- the child is unlikely to achieve or maintain, or have the opportunity of achieving or maintaining, a reasonable standard of health and development without the provision for him of services by a local authority under the Act, or
- the child's health or development is likely to be significantly impaired, or further impaired, without the provision for him of such services, or
- the child is disabled

It is easy to see that any child that qualifies for admission under one of the Sections of the Mental Health Act 1983 will also qualify as a child in need under the Children Act 1989, if control over the child needs to be established legally. The traditional view is that child care legislation offers the most appropriate approach (Gelder *et al.*, 1994, pp. 906–907). However, the Children Act permits children to refuse medical or psychiatric examinations, if they are of an age to understand their significance. Also, the contentious cases alluded to above have led to the identification of the Mental Health Act 1983 as a means of securing the rights of mentally disordered adolescents (Alderson and Montgomery, 1996, p. 35). The Mental Health Act does provide useful safeguards for both practitioner and adolescent. First, it requires the practitioner to establish that the presentation reflects some form of mental disturbance, and is not simply unruliness. A multi-professional assessment is required and the intentions of any restriction of liberty, together with the duration of such restriction, are defined. There is an appeals procedure, which can be easily initiated by the patient. In some cases, statutory aftercare procedures must be put in place.

However, there are problems in the application of the Mental Health Act to minors, including adolescents. First, current Approved Social Work courses do not specifically address psychiatric disorder in children, increasing the possibility of inappropriate implementation of the Act. Secondly, under the Children Act the courts must give paramountcy to the interests of the child. This supports the child more strongly than the Mental Health Act, where the interests of the patient are balanced against those of the community. Thirdly, the courts may make Orders that can directly address problems with the child's caretakers, which Mental Health Act Orders cannot do. Fourthly, the appeals procedure seems less effective in practice (Bradley *et al.*, 1995), with those least able to express themselves being least likely to appeal. Fifthly, many of the disorders that present dilemmas in adolescence may be difficult to manage within the Mental Health Act (Elton *et al.*, 1995; Tiller *et al.*, 1993). Thus, while both the Children Act and Mental Health Act are available to the practitioner for mentally disturbed adolescents, there is no clear rule as to which to choose.

The Children Act possesses a framework for adolescent inpatients, even if they are not 'sectioned' under the Mental Health Act. First, any admission that either lasts longer than three months, or is intended to last longer than three months, must be notified to the Local Authority, who have full discretion in what action to take. Secondly, safeguards govern 'restriction of liberty' in section 25 of the Act. Restriction of liberty is 'Any practice or measure that which prevents a child from leaving a room or building of his own free will' (The Children Act 1989 Guidance and Regulations, 1991, p. 120).

A child may have his liberty restricted if:

> he has a history of absconding and if he is likely to abscond from any other description of accommodation
>
> *and*
>
> if he absconds, he is likely to suffer significant harm
>
> *or*
>
> that if he is kept in any other description of accommodation he is likely to injure himself or other persons.

The maximum any child may be kept in secure accommodation with restriction of liberty is 72 h, whether consecutively or in aggregate over 28 consecutive days.

These rules, however, do not apply to a child detained under the Mental Health Act 1983, children detained under the Police and Criminal Evidence Act 1984 or those detained under Section 23 of the Children and Young Persons Act 1969. These last are those who are charged with an imprisonable offence (if over 14 years) or a current or past violent offence.

ETHICS OF TREATMENT AND ADOLESCENT DEVELOPMENT

We have seen above that the existence of the concept of adolescence implies that our duties to children and adults are identical. Therefore, differences between adults and adolescents in how we discharge our duties must relate to characteristics of adolescents that prevent the use of methods that would discharge our duties in adults. Of the four principles, the only one to specifically include a characteristic of the adolescent is 'respect for autonomy'. Therefore, the pivotal question to be addressed in discharging our duties to adolescents is the status of their autonomy. This can be specified (see above) as adolescents' ability to make informed choices about their lives. Failure to establish this has legal consequences as well-informed consent is also the legal justification for undertaking treatment at all (Brazier, 1992, p. 71).

Steinberg and Silverberg (1986) have proposed that adolescent autonomy be considered along three dimensions:

- Emotional autonomy – the adolescent relinquishes childish dependency on parents
- Resistance to peer pressure – the adolescent does not simply seek conformity
- Subjective sense of self-reliance – the adolescent feels in control, able to take the initiative, and is not excessively dependent on others

The simple model, that adolescent autonomy increases with age, does not hold. Instead, increasing emotional autonomy is associated with decreasing resistance to peer pressure (Steinberg and Silverberg, 1986). It seems likely that when family relationships are poor, 'emotional autonomy' in fact represents emotional detachment (Fuhrman and Holmbeck, 1995; Lamborn and Steinberg, 1993; Ryan and Lynch, 1989) from dysfunctional families. Furthermore, while encouraging adolescent autonomy does improve decision making (Turner *et al.*, 1993), optimal adolescent performance is associated with an authoritarian parenting style, combined with acceptance of that style by the adolescent (Shucksmith *et al.*, 1995). However, this authority needs to be flexible, with issues of autonomy raised by the adolescent given priority, in order to resolve issues most effectively (Vuchinich *et al.*, 1996). It is important to distinguish autonomy from the simple capacity for consent, informed or otherwise. To be able to consent meaningfully, an adolescent needs to understand the effect of the intervention; possess the ability to express preferences that consider benefit, as well as like or dislike; and an ability to recognise that a decision leads to consequences. Concepts of personal cause and effect are well-established by 24 months (Koslowski and Bruner, 1972), while behaviour showing understanding acquiescence to everyday requests, and behaviour showing concern for the benefit of others is apparent by 18 months (Kagan, 1981; Nelson and Gruendel, 1981). Thus, children have the basic abilities required for consent by their second birthday. With regard to informed consent, emotional factors are more important than developmental factors in predicting comprehension of medical procedures by the age of seven (Dorn *et al.*, 1995) and the use of appropriate techniques could significantly improve younger children's comprehension of medical procedures (Berryman, 1978). Despite this, a child may lack the cognitive complexity to appreciate all aspects of an intervention at a level allowing a rational response. However, adolescents seem to approach adult levels of understanding. For example, 9-year-olds' ability to understand or reason about treatments is (understandably) limited compared with adults or 14-year-olds (Weithorn and Campbell, 1982), and children between 6 and 12 understand psychiatric hospitalisation in general, rather than individualised terms (Roth and Roth, 1984).

These findings present significant problems to the practitioner trying to assess an adolescent's autonomy. If autonomy is regarded simply as the ability to give informed consent, then there seems little reason to regard adolescents' autonomy as being significantly different from adults. However, Beauchamp and Childress' criteria for self-determination (discussed above) included freedom from external controls. The literature on autonomy just discussed suggests that this criterion is not met – adolescence is more about choosing one's dependencies, than about becoming free of dependency. If one accepts the Kantian definition of autonomy as relating to moral capacity, then one asserts adolescents' lack of autonomy more strongly, as a high proportion of younger adolescents would be considered to demonstrate maturing, rather than fully matured adult moral reasoning, in comparison to adults in their own cultures (Snarey, 1985). This is particularly important in judging acceptable degrees of paternalism under beneficence, because we have already seen that the patient's definition of 'good' is moral and therefore moral competence in the consenting adolescent must be appropriate to the decision being made. Therefore, adolescents' autonomy should be regarded as circumscribed i.e., the adolescent is able to demonstrate full autonomy in a restricted range of circumstances. Those circumstances now need to be defined.

THE FAMILY RULE

One may divide the idea of consent into two broad classes. When practitioners seek consent, they usually want to perform some action. From the point of view of the recipient, if they consent they have agreed to experience an event. Consenting to an event can be contrasted with consenting to a rule. In this latter case, one agrees to follow a set of prescriptions and prohibitions that regulate one's general conduct. Examples might include joining a monastic order or the army. Consideration of these two examples also shows that the two classes are lexically ordered, with consent to a rule taking primacy over consent to an event. Consider a soldier in the army who goes absent without leave. At this point, the soldier has withdrawn consent to follow the instructions that kept the soldier in barracks. However, both the army and the soldier accept the need for punishment in these circumstances and indeed one punishment the army can inflict is to refuse to accept the soldier's continuing commitment to the rule – 'dishonourable discharge.' Thus, consenting to a rule can legitimately circumscribe exercising one's right to consent in ways that break the rule.

With support from the evidence above, we can assert that for adolescents, the most important rule they consent to is that of their family. Acceptance of the family rule implies that parents may inhibit the adolescent's right to consent. However, the family rule, and adolescents' consent to it, differs from that of the examples above. First, consent by adolescents to their family rule is implicit. This is obvious in biological families, but even in adoptive or fosterfamilies, the fit between the child and the family is evaluated before the child–caretaker relationship is formalised. Secondly, the family rule has among its goals the health and welfare of the child. It is this goal that justifies the parents' power over their adolescents, as the inequality benefits both (Barry, 1989; Rawls, 1985). Thirdly, consent to the family rule is not an all-or-nothing affair. Any child's development requires repeated renegotiation of the application of the rule from infancy to adulthood. Thus, consent to events in an adolescent's life may fall within or outside the family rule, dependant on the adolescent's development and the family's situation. As an expression of the adolescent's autonomy, the family rule requires respect. However, in addition to understanding it psychologically, the practitioner also needs to assess it ethically. We can see that the ethical principle most relevant here is *justice* – the adolescent must be dealt with fairly. As practitioners, we must be able to satisfy ourselves that the obedience and consequential loss of autonomy to the family rule by the adolescent is balanced by clear benefit to the adolescent.

GUIDELINES FOR PRACTITIONERS

We have now acquired the tools we need in order to plan ethically and legally safe treatments for adolescents. We have a coherent set of principles, appropriately specified. We have a legal framework to work within. We have identified what differentiates an adult's ethical position from an adolescent's and, using the concept of a family rule, we have been able to appropriately circumscribe adolescent autonomy. It remains to establish some guidelines that can be practically applied.

DISCLOSURE OF INFORMATION

Respect for autonomy and adolescents' developmental status suggests that they are entitled to full information about their condition, its aetiology, proposed treatment and prognosis. Giving this information will help them manage changes in their lives, including those resulting from interventions by professionals (Eiser and Eiser, 1987; Janzen and Love, 1977). The adolescent is not entitled to information given by parents or others in confidence, unless withholding it prevents the practitioner giving a full explanation to the adolescent. Both this, and the converse of needing to break a confidence with an adolescent, is governed by the practitioner's duty of non-maleficence. One can think of supplying the information to the adolescent as the effect, and the breaking of confidence as the side effect. The 'positive' balance to be ensured means that treatment should be facilitated not impeded, by the breach of confidence. In practice, such facilitation is best achieved by careful preparation, i.e. warning parties of the limits to confidence, and detailed explanation if a confidence needs to be broken, together with guarantees to minimise any adverse consequences.

A further important consideration is the language in which information is imparted. For example, there is discussion both of patients 'being consented' (Paul, 1996) and of 'obtaining consent' (Norman, 1996). All of this implies a 'medicalisation' of the process of giving information, with it becoming effectively a medical test, whose result (consent) determines the use of subsequent procedures. The outcome is that the patient's understanding of the information given is paid little attention provided compliance is achieved (Richardson, Jones and Thomas, 1996). Therefore, providing information to the adolescent needs to be separated from any treatment procedure (Draper and Dawson, 1990). Otherwise, there is the risk of appearing indifferent to the adolescent's understanding of the situation, and the chances of a subsequent refusal to cooperate may therefore be increased. It is known that professional-related variables are more important than patient-related variables in determining compliance (Patterson and Forgatch, 1982). Therefore, a careful and sensitive exploration of any resistance to the information, that allows the adolescent to criticise the practitioner, needs to be undertaken before the adolescent can be regarded as unreasonably uncooperative (Bender, 1994). If the language in which consent is sought is excessively extended and formalised, there is also the chance of triggering non-cooperation through anxiety and suspicion. For example, a ponderous discussion about a clearly minor intervention might raise suspicion that there was more to the intervention than was obvious.

CONSENT TO TREATMENT

If a practitioner feels that a treatment is in the best interests of an adolescent, then the practitioner has a duty to persuade the adolescent of this. Persuasion can be distinguished from coercion. In the former, the goal is to bring the child's wants into line with those of the persuader. In the latter, the goal is to change the child's actions, reckless of the child's wants or intentions.

The concept of the family rule creates two partitions in those decisions that constitute consent: decisions that lie inside and outside the rule and decisions that lie either inside or outside the adolescent's competence. Therefore, assessment for consent involves assigning one of four categories to the situation.

- The adolescent can make informed consent within the family rule. This is a 'full family decision' with the child and parents cooperating on the same information to arrive at informed consent. Thus, adolescents and parents are jointly involved in the consenting process.
- The adolescent's competence is limited, e.g. by peer pressure or substance abuse, but the area of consent lies within the family rule. Recall that the family rule means that the adolescent has delegated some autonomy to the parents. In these circumstances, parental views can be given primacy, with the adolescent's position being equivalent of the American concept of assent or dissent, as described above. Thus, assent is to be preferred but dissent should not block the treatment. However, the adolescent is still entitled to full information: giving information to the parents alone in these circumstances is not sufficient, as parents may not convey sufficient information to the child (Chesson et al., 1997).
- The adolescent is judged competent to consent to treatment, and does not consent to the family rule in this area. This is the situation covered by the Gillick judgement.
- The adolescent is not judged to be competent to make a decision about treatment, and also does not consent to the family rule. Here, the best interests of the child (I take this to mean the child's welfare) may require professional coercion.

Assessment of consent involves assessment of the family rule. Therefore this assessment should also include whether the family rule is in the best interests of the child. It is useful to consider the results of such an assessment under four classes. Most of the time, the family rule will be in the best interests of the adolescent. This is the uncontentious result. It may happen that the refusing adolescent is in fact expressing covert concerns in the parents (cf. Smith and Linscheid, 1994). Then, the practitioner must address those concerns and approach the adolescent again. Occasionally, the family rule will clearly be operating against the adolescent's best interests, as in an abusive family. Here, the family rule has been broken, and a necessary justification for the family rule is that it operates in the best interests of the child. Because the family rule has been broken, the circumstances regarding consent are those of Gillick competence, with the adolescent's consent, supported by appropriate professionals, being sufficient to empower an intervention. The fourth possible result is that the family rule and the professional's ethics have differing interpretations of 'the adolescent's best interests'. An example of this might be a Jehovah's Witness family's attitude to blood transfusion, as described above. The professional might profoundly disagree with the family, but there is no question of the family exploiting the adolescent for its own benefit. Instead, the family is interpreting 'best interests' under priorities that differ from the professional's. Deciding who is 'right' in these circumstances is a matter for the courts, whose rule encompasses that of the professional and the family. The example already given illustrates the potentially tragic outcome of these conflicts. Here, Foot's (1970) distinction between mandatory and elective principles may be helpful. Mandatory ethical principles are those that admit no rational disagreement, e.g. opposing murder or torture for pleasure. They may be similar to Hare's (1981) concept of logically based principles. Elective principles are those where convincing ethical arguments may be set up either to support or oppose them. Foot considers the right to abortion to be such an elective principle. To fulfil duties of both respect for autonomy and beneficence in relation to the adolescent, the practitioner (or court) may over-ride the family rule only for mandatory principles, when the practitioner's argument has greater moral force than the family's. This position does not support professional ethical intuition; people on either side of an elective principle will feel that they are 'right'. It follows that the relationship between the family rule relating to the intervention, and the professional's own values will need to be explored concurrently during the assessment procedure. Advice from an ethicist might be sometimes be useful in determining whether there are convincing mandatory principles at stake.

CONTENTIOUS TREATMENTS

Established contentious treatments are prolonged use of medication, electro-convulsive therapy and psychosurgery. Currently, popular culture expresses preferences both between and within physical, psychological and social treatments of adolescents with mental illness. Briefly, physical treatments are unacceptable unless dietary. Expressive or nurturing psychotherapy is acceptable for all children except those suffering from antisocial behaviour disorders. Behavioural psychotherapy is accepted as reward or punishment for good or bad behaviour. Milieu and social therapies are expected to include consensual moral statements, whatever impact this has on their effectiveness. This is in contrast to treatments for children with physical illness, where, prolonged or invasive physical treatments are generally acceptable. This difference is not defensible rationally, if one accepts the conceptual identity of physical and mental illness (cf. Fulford, 1989). In particular, the establishment of additional unnecessary 'safeguards' against effective treatments of serious mental illness is not ethical, as it reduces the availability of such treatments to sufferers. However, such treatments are weighty measures for serious difficulties. Therefore, adolescents and their families must make more difficult judgements in these cases than for more routine interventions, as the risks and benefits to be judged are both more extreme. The model proposed above is valid independent of the seriousness of the decision to be made. However, in these more serious cases, especial care needs to be taken that it is adhered to closely.

Innovative treatments are contentious in that they have less evidential support, making the benefit to the adolescent less easy to judge rationally by the innovating practitioner. The practitioner may therefore be more likely to take an inappropriately positive bias in recommending such treatments, which the adolescent or parents would find hard to challenge. The need to separate provision of information from provision of treatment is especially important here. First, the practitioner must make clear that the treatment is innovative, so that the family may judge it in that light. If the treatment involves significant risk to the child, a second opinion should *always* be sought before presenting the treatment to the family, so that the professional may be confident that the information has been presented without inappropriate positive bias. With no significant risk, a warning that the treatment is unusual is probably all that needs to be added. Unfortunately, and despite the existence of guidelines, no generally applicable categorisation of 'risk' has yet been achieved (Ethics Advisory Committee, 1992; Nicholson, 1986), although such guidelines may be used to express an intent (Glantz, 1996). Therefore, the question of significant risk will need to be decided on a case-by-case basis. It seems that allowing some risk after careful consideration would be acceptable generally (Berglund, 1994). Unusual treatments may of course be researched, as in cancer research trials. Here, consent to the treatment should be separated from consent to researching the treatment. This is because the pattern of benefits is different in research trials, as discussed below. However, if the research simply involves the recording of monitoring information that would be collected anyway during the treatment, then the research is effectively audit and should be treated as such.

PARTICIPATION IN RESEARCH

The concept of a 'family rule' offers a different approach to the conventional debate in this area, which sets the reduced autonomy and increased risks to adolescents (Hiller, 1981) against their right and duty to contribute to the common good (Gaylin, 1982; McCormick, 1974). Instead, adolescents are seen as actively participating in the consent process with the support of their families. The family rule determines the balance between adolescent and family as discussed above. This is similar to the developmental approach recommended by the Working Group of the 1993 NIMH Conference on Ethical Issues in Mental Health Research (Arnold *et al.*, 1995).

Medical research differs from treatment in that goal of the intervention is to obtain information about a disorder (or disorders), rather than improve any individual child's condition. This has three implications. First, children participating in comparison groups as 'normal controls' are unlikely to benefit from the main research results, even indirectly. Secondly, children should not be exposed to significant risk solely for the purposes of research (Medical Research Council, 1992; Ramsey, 1970). Thirdly, the relationship between the researcher and the participants is quite different. All work together to obtain the information, but differ both in the roles each takes and the benefits each receives. Therefore, the researcher has a duty to ensure that all the participants should benefit and undertaking research with patients should be based round this relationship, which continues for the duration of the study. Glantz (1996) has pointed out that parents and researchers alone are not sufficient safeguard for adolescents, and has stressed the importance of oversight from the State. This shows the importance of the Research Ethics Committee structure, which performs this role in the UK. Because of the differences in benefit applying to cases and controls, these groups will be dealt with separately.

Cases

Cases experience several benefits from participating in research. They stand to learn more about their condition. Others perceive their contribution as valuable. They increase the probability of an improvement in the prognosis of their disorder. These goals are broadly in line with the researcher and so the relationship is as between colleagues. Because of this, the researcher cannot claim the practitioner's duty to persuade the child (or family). Nonetheless, the practitioner should make the benefits of participation clear, as deciding participation includes balancing benefits against inconveniences. Despite this, the imbalance of knowledge between researcher and subject makes the risk of unfair persuasion greater than between *professional* colleagues. Prior approval by an Ethical Committee ensures that at least some of these benefits are confirmed by the researcher's peers, as a safeguard against this. Aside from the duty to persuade and overcome resistance if it is in the child's best interests, the researcher's duties are similar to the practitioner's. Therefore, the process of obtaining cooperation should broadly be as already discussed, although without adverse consequences for refusing to take part. The information gained is one of the benefits to the participants. Therefore, it should be made available to them, when the study is completed, in a form they can understand.

Controls

Controls have only one benefit – their contribution may be perceived as valuable by others. They are therefore in a similar position to donors to charity, donating time and effort instead of money. Benefit deriving from charity is unlikely to outweigh the adverse consequences of a child being involved against the wishes of the parents, whatever the family rule. Therefore, while there may be circumstances in research on cases (e.g. abused children), where it may be appropriate to accept the child's consent without parental agreement, this cannot be so for controls or comparison groups. To allow them to evaluate the benefit of their participation, controls should also have real (i.e. comprehensible) access to the results of the study.

For both cases and controls, the relationship each is in with the researcher makes it ethical to provide remuneration as an additional benefit, if the inconvenience seems to justify it. However, care needs to be taken to offer remuneration as a benefit, rather than an inducement, as then the child or family's ability to consent rationally may be distorted by the inducement. Therefore, research protocols that include remuneration should be subject to close scrutiny by Research Ethics Committees.

CLAIMS OF MALPRACTICE

Mistakes happen – in ethics as much as any other branch of medicine. Knowledge of the principles of malpractice can therefore help the practitioner identify situations in which especial care is needed. In law, good practice requires the fulfilment of two basic principles (Brazier, 1992, p. 71):

- The patient must consent to treatment.
- Treatment must be carried out with proper skill and care on the part of all the practitioners involved

A practitioner must be shown to be at fault in one of those two principles and, if the patient is suing for negligence, the fault must have harmed the patient.

The first principle, that of consent, has been dealt with above, while the purpose of this book is to ensure that adolescents are treated with proper skill and care. One final question remains – who is one's patient? Essentially, to be a patient there needs to be an agreement (usually implicit) that the patient has requested medical services and the doctor consequentially agrees to provide them (Kennedy and Grubb, 1994, p. 64). Thus, in working with a family, one must be clear about who is requesting services for themselves, as an equivalent duty will be owed to *all* the practitioner's patients. For example, a family therapist might be working with a bereavement reaction that involves both the adolescent and a caretaker. Furthermore, a duty of care may also have been incurred by the practitioner because the family member has attended the practitioner's institution seeking care (Barnett *v* Chelsea and Kensington Hospital Management Committee, 1968/9).

LOOKING TO THE FUTURE

This chapter goes to press amidst a flurry of new developments in Mental Health legislation. There is to be a new legal test of incapacity (Lord Chancellor, 1999). There is to be a major reform of the Mental Health Act, the framework of which has been broadly set out (Richardson *et al.*, 1999). From 2 October 2000 the new Human Rights Act will affect the legality of treatment decisions in Mental Health both directly and via European law (Steering Committee on Bioethics, 2000). Adolescent care will be profoundly influenced by these changes. First, it is proposed to de-couple compulsion for treatment from restriction of liberty. This will make the Mental Health Act immediately relevant to those adolescents whose treatment does not require such restriction, but who are refusing the treatment offered. Secondly, in the new Act children will be assessed using the new incapacity criteria, with a concept of 'rebuttable capacity' for children between, possibly, the age of 10 and 16 years. This is, of course, equivalent to 'assent', and is necessary because, as in America, capacity does not distinguish between consent and refusal of a treatment. However, it is not clear whether this will supplant 'Gillick competence' more generally, and it appears to contradict the latest European approach which emphasises developmental continuity and individualised assessment. Finally, the thrust of this legislative initiative is concerned with issues of autonomy and justice, rather than beneficence and non-maleficence. As these principles are of equal ethical importance, it suggests that the impact of the new legislation on the kind of care delivered will require close examination.

REFERENCES

Alderson, P. and Montgomery, J. (1996) *Health Care Choices: Making Decisions about Children*. London: Institute for Public Policy Research.

Anonymous (1977) *Report and Recommendations: Research Involving Children* (DHEW publ. OS 77–0004). Washington, D.C.: National Commission for the Protection of Human Subjects of Biomedical and Behavioral Research.

Arnold, E., Stoff, D., Cook, E., Cohen, D. J., Kruesi, M., Wright, C. *et al.* (1995) Ethical issues in biological psychiatric research with children and adolescents. *Journal of the American Academy of Child and Adolescent Psychiatry*, **34**, 929–939.

Barnett *v* Chelsea and Kensington Hospital Management Committee (1968/9) *1969 1 QB 428, 1968 1 All ER 1068*.

Barry, B. (1989) *Theories of Justice, Vol. 1*. London: Harvester-Wheatsheaf.

Beauchamp, T. and Childress, J. (1994) *Principles of Biomedical Ethics*, 4th edn. Oxford: Oxford University Press.

Bender, S. (1994) Remarks of a paediatrician on informed consent in children. *Acta Paediatrica Supplement*, **83**, 58–61.

Berglund, C. (1994) A survey of Sydney adults about the conduct of medical research. *Australian Health Review*, **17**, 135–144.

Berryman, J. (1978) Discussing the ethics of research on children. In J. van Eys (ed.), *Research on Children: Medical Imperative, Ethical Quandaries, and Legal Constraints*. Baltimore, MD: University Park Press, pp. 85–104.

Bradley, C., Marshall, M. and Gath, D. (1995) Why do so few patients appeal against detention under Section 2 of the Mental Health Act? [see comments]. *British Medical Journal*, **310** (6976), 364–367.

Brazier, M. (1992) *Medicine, Patients and the Law*. London: Penguin.

Chesshyre, R. (1998) Catching them young. *Daily Telegraph*, 24th January.

Chesson, R., Harding, L., Hart, C. and O'Loughlan, V. (1997) Do parents and children have common perceptions of admission, treatment and outcome in a child psychiatric unit? *Clinical Child Psychology and Psychiatry*, **2**, 251–270.

Children Act 1989 Guidance and Regulations (1991) *Volume 4: Residential Care.* London: HMSO.

Committee on Bioethics (1995) Informed consent, parental permission, and assent in pediatric practice. *Pediatrics*, **95**, 314–317.

Daniels, N. (1985) *Just Health Care*. New York: Cambridge University Press.

Dewar, J. (1992) *Law and the Family*. London: Butterwoths.

Dorn, L., Susman, E. and Fletcher, J. (1995) Informed consent in children and adolescents: age, maturation and psychological state. *Journal of Adolescent Health*, **16**, 185–90.

Draper, R. and Dawson, D. (1990) Competence to consent to treatment: a guide for the psychiatrist. *Canadian Journal of Psychiatry*, **35**, 285–289.

Dworkin, R. (1987) *Taking Rights Seriously*. London: Duckworth.

Eiser, C. and Eiser, J. (1987) Explaining illness to children. *Communication and Cognition*, **20**, 277–290.

Elton, A., Honig, P., Bentovim, A. and Simons, J. (1995) Withholding consent to lifesaving treatment: three cases. *British Medical Journal*, **310**, 373–377.

Ethics Advisory Committee, British Paediatric Association (1992) *Guidelines for the Ethical Conduct of Medical Research Involving Children*. London: British Paediatric Association.

Family Law Reform Act (1969) s8.

Foot, P. (1970) Morality and art (Henrietta Herz Lecture). *Proceedings of the British Academy*, **LVI**.

Fuhrman, T. and Holmbeck, G. (1995) Contextual-moderator analysis of emotional autonomy and adjustment in adolescence. *Child Development*, **66**, 793–811.

Fulford, K. (1989) *Moral Theory and Medical Practice*. Cambridge: Cambridge University Press.

Gaylin, W. (1982) Competence: no longer all or none. In W. Gaylin and R. Mackie (eds), *Who Speaks for the Child*. New York: Plenum, pp. 27–54.

Gelder, M., Gath, D. and Mayou, R. (1994) *Oxford Textbook of Psychiatry*, 2nd edn. Oxford: Oxford : University Press.

Gewirth, A. (1995) Rights. In T. Honderich (ed.), *The Oxford Companion to Philosophy*. Oxford: Oxford University Press, p. 776.

Gillick *v* W Norfolk and Wisbech AHA (1985) *All England Law Reports*, **402**.

Glantz, J. (1996) Conducting research with children: legal and ethical issues. *Journal of the American Academy of Child and Adolescent Psychiatry*, **34**, 1283–1291.

Hare, R. M. (1981) *Moral Thinking: Its Levels, Method and Point*. Oxford: Clarendon Press.

Hegel, G. (1942) *Philosophy of Right*. Oxford: Clarendon Press.

Hiller, M. (1981) *Medical Ethics and the Law*. Boston, MA: Ballinger.

HM Government (1997) *The New NHS: Modern, Dependable*. London: HMSO.

Janzen, W. and Love, W. (1977) Involving adolescents as active participants in their own treatment plans. *Psychological Reports*, **41**, 931–934.

Kagan, J. (1981) *The Second Year: The Emergence of Self-Awareness*. Cambridge, MA: Harvard University Press.

Kant, I. (1785) *Groundwork to the Metaphysic of Morals*. Translated by Paton, H. J. (1964). New York: Harper.

Katz, J. (1972) *Experimentation with human beings*. New York: Russell Sage Foundation.

Kennedy, I. and Grubb, A. (1994) *Medical Law: Text with Materials*. London: Butterworth.

Koslowski, B. and Bruner, J. (1972) Learning to use a lever. *Child Development*, **43**, 790–799.

Lamborn, S. and Steinberg, L. (1993) Emotional autonomy redux – revisiting Ryan and Lynch. *Child Development*, **64**, 483–99.

Lord Chancellor (1999) *Making Decisions* (Report to Parliament Cm 4465). London: HMG.

McCormick, R. (1974) Proxy consent in the experimental situation. *Perspectives in Biology and Medicine*, **18**, 2–20.

Medical Research Council (1992) The ethical conduct of research on children. *Bulletin of Medical Ethics*, **96**, 8–9.

Mental Health Act (1983) London: HMSO.

Nelson, K. and Gruendel, J. (1981) Generalised event representation: Basic building blocks of cognitive development. In A. Brown and M. Lamb (eds), *Advances in Developmental Psychology*. Hillsdale, NJ: Erlbaum, pp. 131–158.

NHS Management Executive (1990) *A Guide to Consent for Examination or Treatment*. London: Department of Health.

Nicholson, H. E. (1986) *Medical Research with Children: Ethics, Law and Practice*. Oxford: Oxford University Press.

Norman, J. (1996) Should house officers obtain consent for operation and anaesthesia? (Letter). *Health Trends*, **28**, 147.

Parton, N. (1991) *Governing the Family: Child Care, Child Protection and the State*. Basingstoke: Macmillan.

Patterson, G. and Forgatch, M. (1982) Therapist behaviour as a determinant for client non-compliance: a paradox for the behavior modifier. *Journal of Consulting and Clinical Psychology*, **53**, 846–851.

Paul, M. (1996) Should house officers obtain consent for operation and anaesthesia? (Letter). *Health Trends*, **28**, 147–148.

Pearson, G. (1987) Long-term treatment needs of hospitalised adolescents. *Adolescent Psychiatry*, **14**, 342–357.

Ramsey, P. (1970) *The patient as person*. New Haven, CT: Yale University Press.

Rawls, J. (1985) *A Theory of Justice*. Oxford: Oxford University Press.

Re R (1991, 1992) (a minor) (wardship: medical treatment). *7 BLMR 147, Fam 11 (CA)*.

Re W (1992, 1992) (a minor) (medical treatment). *4 All ER 627, 9 BMLR 22 (CA)*.

Richardson, G., Alstead, R., Bingley, W., Bird, A., Goodall, G., Lind, R. *et al.* (1999) *Review of the Mental Health Act 1983* (Report of the Expert Committee). London: HMG.

Richardson, N., Jones, P. and Thomas, M. (1996) Should house officers obtain consent for operation and anaesthesia? *Health Trends*, **28**, 56–59.

Roth, E. and Roth, L. (1984) Children's understanding of psychiatric hospital-isation. *Americal Journal of Psychiatry*, **141**, 1066–1070.

Ryan, R. and Lynch, J. (1989) Emotional autonomy versus detachment: revisiting the vicissitudes of adolescence and young adulthood. *Child Development*, **60**, 340–356.

Shucksmith, J., Hendry, L. and Glendinning, A. (1995) Models of parenting – implications for adolescent well-being within different types of family contexts. *Journal of Adolescence*, **18**, 253–270.

Sigman, G. and O'Connor, C. (1991) Exploration for physicians of the mature minor doctrine. *Journal of Pediatrics*, **119**, 520–525.

Smith, F. and Linscheid, T. (1994) Effect of parental acceptance or rejection of a proposed aversive intervention on treatment acceptability. *American Journal of Mental Retardation*, **99**, 262–269.

Snarey, J. (1985) Cross-cultural universaility of social–moral development: a critical review of Kohlbergian research. *Psychological Bulletin*, **97**, 202–232.

Steering Committee on Bioethics (2000) *White Paper on the Protection of the Human Rights and Dignity of People Suffering from Mental Disorder* (CM Documents Addendum CM (2000)23). Brussels: Council of Europe.

Steinberg, L. and Silverberg, S. (1986) The vicissitudes of autonomy in early adolescence. *Child Development*, **57**, 841–851.

Tiller, J., Schmidt, U. and Treasure, J. (1993) Compulsory treatment for anorexia nervosa: compassion or coercion? *British Journal of Psychiatry*, **162**, 679–680.

Turner, R., Irwin, C., Tschann, J. and Millstein, S. G. (1993) Autonomy, relatedness, and the initiation of health risk behaviors in early adolescence. *Health Psychology*, **12**, 200–208.

Vuchinich, S., Angelelli, J. and Gatherum, A. (1996) Context and development in family problem-solving with preadolescent children. *Child Development*, **67**, 1276–1288.

Weithorn, L. and Campbell, S. (1982) The competency of children and adolescents to make informed treatment decisions. *Child Development*, **53**, 1589–1599.

White, R., Carr, P. and Lowe, N. (1990) *A Guide to the Children Act 1989*. London: Butterworth.

Chapter 13

PRIMARY CARE AND COMMUNITY ADOLESCENT MENTAL HEALTH SERVICES

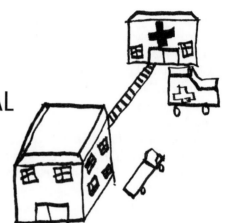

Clive North

INTRODUCTION

Comparison of the epidemiology of psychiatric disorder in adolescents (see Chapter 3) and the provision of inpatient beds in the UK (see Chapter 14) leads to the inevitable conclusion that the overwhelming majority of adolescents requiring treatment for a mental health problem must be managed in non-residential settings. This is entirely appropriate in most cases, although there are times when clinicians and families have to manage unacceptably high levels of risk in the community (Anonymous, 1997). The provision of adolescent mental health services has been regularly reviewed and discussed in the last 20 years.

Adolescent psychiatry is a relatively new speciality, community-based treatment even more so. Outpatient services for children and adolescents, either hospital based or in child guidance clinics, were not offered before 1920–1950. Little is known about the non-institutional management of disturbed young people before that time. Services, including outpatient clinics, exclusively for adolescents were substantially developed in the 1960s (Parry-Jones, 1984). They were very diverse in terms of theoretical orientation and operational policy.

Perhaps as a result of this rather haphazard process, many of the reviews of child and adolescent mental health services (CAMHS) have reported that services are often incomplete and uncoordinated as well as being patchy across the country (Kurtz et al., 1994; NHS Health Advisory Service, 1986; Parry-Jones, 1984). In particular, comment is made that services are not provided to meet local need, excluding those who do not meet the criteria for the particular treatment(s) offered by the local service. Lack of planning is criticised, especially insufficient liaison among the three statutory agencies (education, health and social services), and between these and the voluntary sector. Other identified deficiencies of adolescent mental health services have included poor or ineffective relationships with adult psychiatry and medical services; resorting to the use of adult services, especially inpatient beds; and the adoption of fixed exclusion criteria, e.g. upper age limit of 16 years or presence of learning difficulties.

The criticisms levelled against CAMHS are important and must be considered in further developments. However, there are a number of challenges to be addressed when establishing or refining adolescent mental health services. Adolescence as a developmental phase has been recognised for many centuries but the boundaries are vague and depend on a number of factors (Parry-Jones, 1995), any one of which may be of more relevance to one agency than another, e.g. whether a teenager is still in full-time education. Establishing the age range for adolescent services is therefore difficult. The nature of problems that should be addressed by mental health services is also controversial. Goodman (1997a, p. 11) has argued that mental health professionals have viewed too many of the problems of young people to be within their remit and that for some presentations alternative management strategies should be developed with colleagues from education and social services. Facing some of these challenges in the context of the history and criticism of CAMHS a number of new models of service delivery have been developed.

MODELS OF CHILD AND ADOLESCENT MENTAL HEALTH SERVICES

New arrangements for delivering CAMHS (Bickman, 1996a; NHS Health Advisory Service, 1995; Sawyer and Kosky, 1995) have all emphasised a continuum of care, whereby the aim is to offer a range of treatments in a variety of settings, non-residential, intermediate (i.e. day care) and residential. A graded response may then be offered to adolescents presenting with mental health problems, achieving a smooth (ideally seamless) transition from one level of care to the next. In the UK, the Department of Health has been recommended to encourage adoption of a tiered service (Health Committee, House of Commons, 1997). This is shown in Figure 13.1. As presented, the model centralises the role of CAMHS. It is of course the case that each area of service provision will have its own tiers (see Figure 13.2). There will be many different relationships: between tiers of one service (e.g. social services), between different services as a whole (e.g. CAMHS and the voluntary sector) and between different tiers of different services (e.g. liaison between an adolescent inpatient unit and the adolescent's mainstream school), illustrated as (a), (b) and (c) in Figure 13.2. Adolescents may follow a great variety of routes through this complex system. Case examples will demonstrate two very different pathways to care.

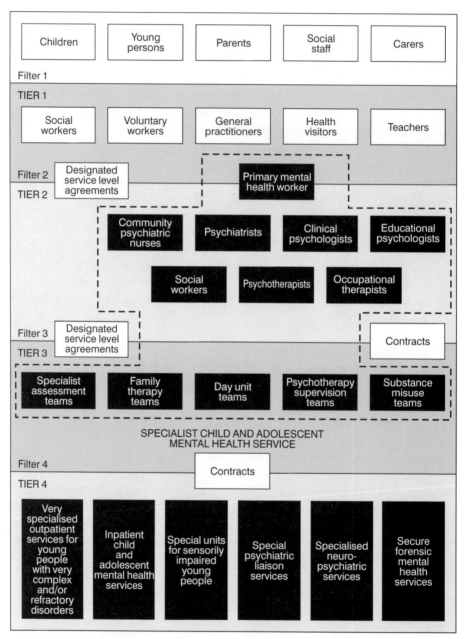

Figure 13.1 A strategic approach to commissioning and delivering a comprehensive CAMHS.

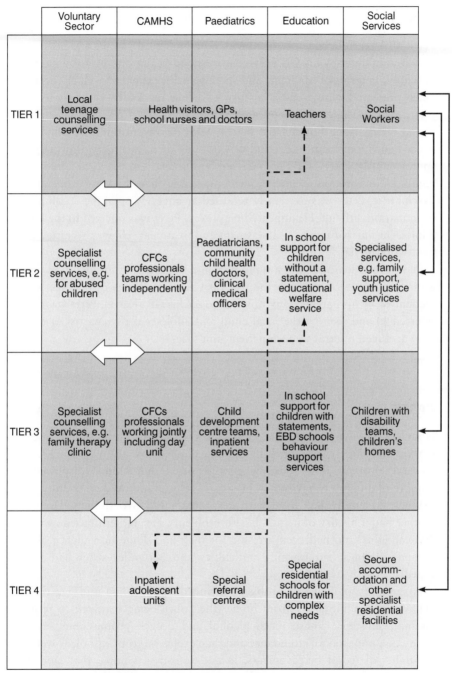

Figure 13.2 Relationships between different tiers and services.

CASE 1

Peter, a 14-year-old boy, who lived with both biological parents and his sister, was seen initially by his GP. Previously of good health and performing well at school, in terms of academic and sporting achievement as well as socially, Peter presented with a 24-h history of being markedly withdrawn and retarded. Physical examination and routine blood tests revealed no abnormality. Forty-eight hours later Peter's self-care deteriorated notably. He needed encouragement to eat and was not talking to members of his family spontaneously. Peter's GP then referred him urgently to the local Child and Family Consultation Service. Seen the same day by the Consultant Psychiatrist, Peter was extremely retarded at interview, making a complete examination difficult. He appeared perplexed. Peter was referred to the local adolescent unit for intensive assessment and treatment. He was admitted the next working day.

Peter's case demonstrates a rapid response to an urgent presentation with a quick progression through the tiers of CAMHS. Peter's difficulties were recognised by his parents who took him to see his GP (Tier 1). Peter was then referred to and seen by the local child and adolescent psychiatrist (Tier 2) who arranged referral to an inpatient unit (Tier 4).

CASE 2

Donna, a 14-year-old girl, was referred to CAMHS by the local duty social worker and shortly afterwards by the on-call paediatric team at the District General Hospital. The social worker reported that Donna displayed a number of difficult behaviours. The second referral followed an overdose of sleeping tablets. Donna lived with her parents and two siblings. Donna's mother had a history of mental health problems. Her father abused alcohol and cannabis, and had been arrested for theft and domestic violence. Both Donna's siblings had learning difficulties and her older sister had been raped.

A summary of Donna's problems included oppositional and aggressive behaviour, running away from home (the police being involved to return Donna), substance abuse (both alcohol and drugs), promiscuous sexual behaviour, poor school attendance and then exclusion from school, as well as a number of recent bereavements. In addition, it was noted that Donna's parents were finding it very hard to control her and that there were other difficulties in family relationships. The assessing CAMHS clinician concluded that a multiagency approach would be most helpful. Accordingly, a meeting was planned to coordinate work with Donna and her family.

Professionals invited included representatives from CAMHS, Social Services, Donna's school and the Education Welfare Service. It was noted at the CAMHS assessment that Donna was unwilling to attend the local clinic for further sessions. However, she agreed to consider attending a therapy group for adolescents. It was hoped that this might give Donna the opportunity to work on issues that were important to her, e.g. the bereavements. If Donna found this intervention helpful then further work to address other problems, including substance abuse and risk-taking behaviour, could possibly follow which, at the time of presentation, she would not contemplate. The local CAMHS also planned to offer family work to address some of the difficulties in relationships in the family and to work with Donna's parents on their parenting of Donna.

Prior to referral, Donna was putting herself at considerable risk. Her behaviours came to the attention of a variety of services. In the end she was referred to CAMHS by a social worker (Tier 1) and from the paediatric ward (Tier 3). However, she could equally have been referred from her school or by her GP. Donna was then seen by a clinician in the local CAMHS (Tier 2). A meeting was planned with Tier 2 representatives from health, education and social services. For Donna's needs to be met each agency will have to work with Donna and her family. CAMHS will offer appropriate pieces of work but will probably be limited what it can achieve, Donna being unwilling to attend.

The path each adolescent takes through health, education and social services should be designed to meet the needs of that individual. In some cases, e.g. Case 1 (Peter), CAMHS will take a strong lead. Nevertheless, it will still be essential to work closely with other services, e.g. education. In other cases, e.g. Case 2 (Donna), CAMHS need not take the lead role, only doing pieces of work that may be best undertaken by a member of a CAMHS. In each case though an initial intervention should be offered at the appropriate level, its effect reviewed and a decision made as to future management. If the problem is not resolved, this may include referral to a higher tier or to a different service.

The tiered model of CAMHS has been adopted as a blueprint for service provision in a number of areas [e.g. Essex (North Essex Health Authority *et al.*, 1998)]. Whilst widely accepted, the model has been criticised too. Goodman (1997a, p. 10) has argued that undue weight is given to mental health services in the management of the problems of disturbed adolescents. The model does not give adequate recognition to the importance of pastoral care as an educational task and working with abused adolescents as a social work task, for example. He also proposes (Goodman, 1997a, p. 36) that the division of secondary mental health services into Tiers 2 and 3 is unhelpful. He suggests that the multidisciplinary CAMHS clinic should be retained and a flexible approach to uni- or multiprofessional working maintained. Whatever the model of service adopted it is important that it be adequately evaluated. This point is reinforced by the Fort Bragg project, a 5-year study designed to evaluate a full continuum of mental health services for children and adolescents. The project was implemented at much greater cost to comparison CAMHS at other sites in the US (Foster *et al.*, 1996). Despite

- more systematic and comprehensive assessment and treatment planning approach,
- more parent involvement,
- better case management,
- more individualised services,
- fewer treatment dropouts,
- a greater range of services,
- enhanced continuity of care,
- increased length of treatment, and
- better match of treatment and needs as judged by parents,

no better clinical outcomes were reported (Bickman, 1996b).

ADOLESCENTS' MENTAL HEALTH PROBLEMS AT HOME

Unless disturbed adolescents are admitted to an inpatient unit or other residential facility, they are bound to spend most of their time outside mental health services, i.e. with parents, other carers, or family, friends or at school. Visits to professionals in Tier 1 or 2 are for but small periods of time. In many Tier 2/3 mental health units today, an hour per week is the maximum that any worker can offer adolescents and their families and often appointment time is less than that. Even when adolescents are admitted to a Day Unit they are still likely to spend the majority of their time outside it. This means that there is a large potential role for informal helping agents in supporting adolescents with mental health problems. This point was well demonstrated in a study by Offer *et al.* (1991). Adolescents reported that they frequently sought help for emotional problems from friends or parents. Disturbed adolescents chose to speak to their friends more often than non-disturbed adolescents did. Non-disturbed adolescents, in turn, opted to talk to their parents more frequently than disturbed adolescents did. Non-disturbed adolescents found their parents more helpful than adolescents in the disturbed group.

Parents will also often have a key role in referring adolescents to CAMHS, especially those who are younger. They may be the first to recognise the presence of psychiatric disorder. However, the relationship between adolescent psychiatric disorder and referral to CAMHS is not straightforward. The likelihood of a young person with a psychiatric disorder receiving mental health services is increased if school performance is poor, parents have been treated for a nervous condition or there is high parental burden resulting from the young person's psychiatric disorder (Angold *et al.*, 1998; John *et al.*, 1995).

Once taken on for treatment, parents, especially of younger patients, still have a vital role to play. They may need to make sure that adolescents attend appointments. They may also have a crucial role in managing the adolescent's difficulties at home. For example, parents of adolescents with eating disorders need to be actively involved in the treatment in many ways, not least managing meal times. Even ensuring compliance with a medication regime can be demanding. Not surprisingly, therefore, parents of children and adolescents with psychological difficulties report greater levels of burden [defined as 'the presence of problems, difficulties or adverse events which affect the life (lives) of the psychiatric patients' significant others (Platt, 1985)] than carers of those without (Angold *et al.*, 1998). A number of studies, which have included older adolescents as well as adult patients, have also demonstrated the considerable impact of schizophrenia and other major psychiatric disorders on patients' families (Platt, 1985).

TIER 1: GENERALISTS WORKING WITH ADOLESCENTS WITH MENTAL HEALTH PROBLEMS

Only a minority of adolescents with psychiatric disorder will be seen by specialist services. More adolescents with mental health problems are seen in Tier 1 than in Tiers 2–4. Furthermore, studies of both children and adults (including older adolescents) indicate that the frequency of psychiatric disorder amongst GP attendees is greater than in the general population (Garralda and Bailey, 1986b; Goldberg *et al.*, 1976). Similarly, children with physical illness or special educational needs, who have committed an offence or are victims of abuse are also at increased risk of developing a psychiatric disorder, reviewed in *Together We Stand* (The NHS Health Advisory Service, 1995). The role of GPs, paediatricians, social workers, teachers and voluntary staff in the management of psychologically disturbed adolescents is a vital one.

THE ROLE OF WORKERS IN TIER 1

The mental health problems of adolescents will only ever be part of the remit of any Tier 1 professional involved in their care. The local social worker or general practitioner has to keep many factors in mind at any one time. The degree to which Tier 1 professionals take on mental health work with adolescents will vary greatly between professionals, reflecting different interests, training, experience and access to supervision of mental health work. There will also be variation between cases held by the same professional, depending on the worker's other commitments to each adolescent.

All Tier 1 professionals should be alert to the presence of psychiatric disorder in the adolescents they meet. However, it has been found that GPs do not recognise psychiatric disorder when present in 50% or more children (Garralda and Bailey, 1986a) or adults (Goldberg and Bridges, 1987) attending surgery. Whilst teachers may readily notice adolescents displaying oppositional or aggressive behaviour, depressed, withdrawn or thin adolescents are less likely to be noticed and their problems overlooked. Following recognition of mental health problems the Tier 1 professional may then be able to offer an intervention – a brief discussion of the roles of some Tier 1 professionals follows. For some adolescents though, referral to CAMHS will be indicated. A referral is more likely to be successful if the Tier 1 professional has information about the service (s)he is suggesting the adolescent and family attend, if the CAMHS is easily accessible, sees the adolescent quickly and the referrer supplies sufficient information to assist the CAMHS in deciding the optimum response.

GENERAL PRACTITIONERS

GPs occupy a key position in the Health Service of the UK, being gatekeepers between primary (Tier 1) and secondary care (Tiers 2/3). Whilst with respect to mental health services others share the role, GPs make more referrals to CAMHS than any other agency (NHS Health Advisory Service, 1995). GPs will continue to be involved throughout an adolescent's period of involvement with CAMHS and after discharge will continue to support the young person.

Despite this important position in the structure of adolescent mental health services, there is little knowledge of how GPs actually manage teenagers' mental health problems (Garralda, 1994). Twenty years ago, Bailey et al. (1978) found that 6.9% of consultations with children and adolescents, under 18 years of age, were for mainly psychological reasons. On over half these occasions an opportunity was given to ventilate the problem. Reassurance, advice or comments designed to promote insight were also offered. Around 46% of children and 6% of mothers were prescribed drugs. Only 3.8% were referred to child psychiatry services. A more recent study (Adams, 1991) demonstrated that about 70% of GPs and consultant child psychiatrists prescribed medication to children under the age of 17 years in a three month period. In the group including younger adolescents (8–13 years), GPs most commonly prescribed antidepressants for enuresis and, in the older group (14–17 years), antidepressants for depression (not always with the recommendation of a consultant) and hypnotics. In over 20% of consultations in the study by Bailey et al. (1978) a mixture of physical and psychological problems were noted. GPs have a very important role in the management of these disorders. Many minor psychosomatic presentations will resolve with reassurance but more specific techniques, e.g. reattribution, may be used if necessary (Goldberg *et al.*, 1989). In more severe cases, it is often the GP that the adolescent and family will consult first with many and varied physical symptoms. The GP will have to decide on each occasion whether referral to specialist services is warranted. Close liaison between primary and secondary services including CAMHS is required.

SOCIAL SERVICES

It is apparent from the discussion above that many adolescents seen by social services staff will have mental health problems. Social workers will therefore need to frame all their interventions bearing that in mind, being alert not only to the presence of such difficulties but what effect that they may have on the issue currently being worked on. Many of the issues that social workers are obliged to address with adolescents are major events in themselves often provoking anxiety or reawakening painful memories, e.g. entering or leaving care. Social workers' guidance is that young people's views should be sought prior to a care placement and well before leaving, enabling an appropriate care plan to be developed (Department of Health, 1991, pp. 48 and 101). Considerable skills are required to negotiate these matters in a sensitive manner that really allows the young person's voice to be heard in the proceedings. In addition local team social workers may also offer supportive psychotherapy or counselling to their clients as well as family work, not directly related to their statutory obligations but which may facilitate that work.

EDUCATION SERVICES

Schools often need to respond to adolescents with emotional and behavioural problems. A Code of Practice (Department of Education, 1994) gives practical guidance on the identification and assessment of special educational needs which can include emotional and behavioural difficulties. There are five stages to this process.

- *Stage 1.* The young person's class teacher notes any special educational needs and works with the school's special educational needs coordinator to develop and implement an initial intervention.
- *Stage 2.* The school's special educational needs coordinator now directs the gathering of further information and organises the child's special educational provision, working with the child's teachers.
- *Stage 3.* Specialist support from outside the school is sought, e.g. from an educational psychologist or, in appropriate cases, CAMHS.
- *Stage 4.* The Local Education Authority (LEA) considers whether a statutory assessment of educational needs is indicated. If so, a multidisciplinary

assessment is arranged. Advice from professionals involved with the child being assessed (including those working in CAMHS) will be sought.

- *Stage 5.* The LEA considers the results of the assessment. If appropriate, a statement of special educational needs is produced. The LEA arranges the child's special educational provision. This may include further help in the child's mainstream school or in extreme cases, placement in a special school, e.g. for children with emotional and behavioural difficulties.

In addition to the formal role teachers have they may also be used by adolescents to talk over difficult issues in an informal way. This may amount to a considerable piece of work at times, especially if the adolescent is unwilling to accept a specialist mental health service intervention. Links between schools and Tier 2/3 CAMHS are important but not always well established. Detailed information about adolescents in the school setting is sometimes vital in the assessment process. Schools and associated services, e.g. the Education Welfare Service and the Educational Psychology Service, can also play a key role in the management of young people's psychological difficulties. Referrals may be made to CAMHS from the education system via the over-stretched Educational Psychology Service or directly from school staff.

VOLUNTARY SERVICES

The role of the voluntary sector in the prevention and management of adolescents' mental health problems has been increasingly recognised over recent years. Malek (1997) has provided a timely review. The full extent of the services offered by the voluntary sector is not known. Whilst some of the larger organisations are nationally recognised (e.g. Save the Children, Barnardo's, National Society for the Prevention of Cruelty to Children, etc.), much work is done at a very local level, meeting a local need with locally derived funding, lasting only as long as the local population wishes. Projects may therefore be set up and closed down much more quickly than health, education or social services facilities. Voluntary organisations offer a wide range of interventions from counselling for minor worries or mild upset to the more specialist therapy that may be required after sexual abuse. In or near the author's place of work, the voluntary sector provides a very valuable contribution to the overall provision for adolescents with mental health problems, e.g. a local drop-in counselling service and therapy for children who have been physically or sexually abused as well those who have abused others.

PRIMARY MENTAL HEALTH WORKERS

One of the important recommendations of *Together We Stand* is the development of a new role within CAMHS, i.e. the primary mental health worker (PMHW).

Persons in this post would attempt to bridge the gap between professionals in Tier 1 and those in Tier 2, and support Tier 1 professionals in their work with disturbed adolescents. The exact way that this would be achieved would probably depend on local factors. Certainly close links with CAMHS would be essential if the PMHW was actually based elsewhere with frequent discussion of cases of concern, perhaps even formal supervision with a member of the CAMHS team. A PMHW could be linked to a particular service, e.g. local social service teams, or all services, i.e. schools, social services and primary medical care, within a particular geographical area. The main tasks of the primary mental health worker would include:

- Establishing and keeping contacts with the professionals in the Tier 1 services to which they are linked
- Establishing and keeping contacts with the local Tier 2/3 CAMHS
- Developing and maintaining a network of contacts amongst all other relevant agencies and voluntary organisations in the area
- Consulting to Tier 1 professionals regularly about cases the Tier 1 professionals are managing
- Offering short-term pieces of work to adolescents and their families
- Referring adolescents on to Tier 2/3 services as indicated
- Organising multiagency meetings regarding adolescents where appropriate.

If successful the PMHW role could be very valuable. Coordination of local Tier 1 services should be to the advantage of the adolescent. Support for Tier 1 professionals, with the aims of increasing their knowledge base and their skills in managing adolescents with mental health problems, could reduce the numbers of professional involved with any one adolescent and perhaps reduce the numbers of referrals to local CAMHS. Many clients referred to mental health services only need or accept a very brief intervention (Talmon, 1990). Providing this in an ultra-local, non-threatening environment, e.g. GP clinic or school, may facilitate and enhance it. Like all other innovations, adequate evaluation of the PMHW role is required.

TIER 2: MENTAL HEALTH SPECIALISTS WORKING INDEPENDENTLY

A proportion of adolescents with mental health problems will be referred to Tier 2/3 CAMHS. Referrals may come from a wide variety of sources, not only from parents and Tier 1 professionals, but also other Tier 2/3 services, e.g. paediatric clinics, specialist social service teams, youth justice workers and educational psychologists. The percentage of disturbed adolescents seen in specialist mental health services has been found to vary from 10 to 20% (Burns et al., 1995; Offord *et al.*, 1987; Rutter *et al.*, 1970), but always reflects a large degree of unmet need. This poses a challenge to CAMHS providers, i.e. how they may be useful both to the adolescents who are referred and, in the absence of PMHWs, to those who are not. Although the tiered model divides local specialist CAMHS into Tiers 2 and 3, this is often not a physical segregation but rather reflects different ways of working in the local CAMHS clinic, i.e. clinicians working on their own or together. This section will briefly consider what treatments should reasonably be offered by Tier 2/3 professionals acting independently to adolescents and their families, and then other ways in which they may work to facilitate adolescent mental health. A consideration of ways in which Tier 2/3 professional may work together will follow.

DIRECT WORK AT TIER 2

Given the limited resources available, care is needed in planning adolescent mental health services. Tier 2/3 CAMHS in general should offer effective treatments that meet identified needs of the adolescent population. Any particular clinic should vary the therapies offered according to the profile of adolescent mental health problems in the local area. Unfortunately, this is a counsel of perfection. Progress is being made in the epidemiology of adolescent psychiatric disorder but some adolescents identified as being in need of mental health services do not fit neatly into the psychiatric classification system. Even if they did, achieving a consensus as to what that means in terms of treatments required and who should provide it appears a long way off (Goodman, 1997b, and subsequent commentaries). In the local clinic service planning is even more difficult. It is likely that the needs of the local population are not known in sufficient detail and it may not be possible to recruit staff who would be able to provide the treatments identified as being most valuable.

Considering the nature of psychiatric disorder in adolescence, it would seem desirable for a service to be offered to teenagers with a wide range of problems. These include following the classification given in *Child and Adolescent Mental Health Services: Together We Stand* (NHS Health Advisory Service, 1995): emotional disorders, conduct disorders, hyperkinetic disorder, developmental disorders, eating disorders, habit disorders, post-traumatic syndromes, somatic disorders and psychotic disorders. The effectiveness of treatment has been more adequately demonstrated for some of these disorders than others. The extent of CAMHS involvement will vary. In the management of some disorders, CAMHS should take a lead, e.g. depression and obsessive-compulsive disorder, but not necessarily others, e.g. conduct disorder. In these cases CAMHS might only need to be involved for specific work, social services coordinating care.

However, the workload is divided between health, education and social services, the local CAMHS is still faced with attempting to provide a broad range of interventions. Psychotherapy may be offered to adolescents alone or in groups, to adolescents and their families, or to their parents alone. The theoretical framework of the psychotherapy may be behavioural, cognitive-behavioural, interpersonal, systemic, psychodynamic or psychoeducational. Non-verbal therapies may also be used. The aim of the treatment may be to achieve symptom reduction or to support an individual or family during the course of a long-term disorder. Therapy offered may be short or long term. Medication may be used including antidepressants, antipsychotics, mood stabilisers and stimulants. Social skills training and rehabilitation work are also important. Indications for the various therapies are given in the relevant chapters. However, there is a further complication in deciding what local CAMHS should provide. It appears that the results of treatment trials conducted in academic centres do not equate to the results of therapy offered in CAMHS clinics. Weisz and Weiss (1993) report much smaller effect sizes for treatment in the outpatient mental health clinic setting compared to the results of meta-analyses of child and adolescent psychotherapy outcome studies. Weisz and Weiss later propose a number of reasons why this may be so and include differences between settings and therapists, clients recruited, therapies offered, focus of outcomes measured and goodness-of-fit between client and therapy. Further work is evidently required to establish the important differences between research treatment studies and clinic interventions. It is also important to know which of the current therapies are effective in CAMHS clinics and to develop therapies that may be applied in that setting to the benefit of clients and their families.

This summary of the interventions that an adolescent mental health service should provide has implications for the staff required to make up a local Tier 2 service. All members of a Tier 2 team will have to be able to assess clients adequately. The assessment offered might vary with the profession of the assessing clinician but the results should include an understanding of the client's presentation, an evaluation of the risk the client poses (to self and others) and an indication of the treatment required. As to how a CAMHS team should be formed, a psychologist, psychiatrist and family therapist would appear to constitute the core. Other professionals trained in the relevant treatment modalities could then be added. Clinical nurse specialists often make a very valuable contribution by working with patients in their homes, providing practical programmes for teenagers with, for example, agoraphobia. The role of the psychoanalytically trained psychotherapist is still controversial, particularly in regard to long-term intensive treatment, provision varying in different clinics.

CONSULTATION AND LIAISON

Given that the majority of adolescents with mental health problems will not be attending CAMHS and that clinical experience suggests that a fair proportion of those adolescents who professionals would like to refer to CAMHS will not attend, alternative interventions are also required. In hospital practice, there are a number of possibilities for liaison between psychiatrists and paediatricians or physicians. These include an easy referral route for the assessment and psychological management of adolescents presenting after deliberate self-harm or other urgent presentations, joint working on a case, or offering opportunities to discuss cases (North and Eminson, 1998). The last of these is especially valuable in the management of adolescents and families who will not attend CAMHS. It also has the advantage that principles discussed may then be applied to other cases, perhaps decreasing the numbers of adolescents referred for direct work and increasing the appropriateness of cases which are referred. Whilst liaison of this type is between services at Tier 2/3 level, CAMHS professionals may just as well as offer consultation to Tier 1 professionals in health, education and social sectors. This aspect of the work of a CAMHS professional will be further discussed in Chapter 15.

TIER 3: MENTAL HEALTH SPECIALISTS WORKING TOGETHER

Members of a CAMHS team may work jointly in a number of different ways, with referred adolescents and their families, other agencies, themselves and most intensively in a Day Unit.

WORKING WITH REFERRED ADOLESCENTS AND THEIR FAMILIES

A great many of the young people referred to CAMHS can be managed by one clinician working independently. Many local child and family clinics now have so many referrals that mental health specialists working together on a case appears to be becoming less common, and to be reserved for the assessment and treatment of particularly complex and/or severe cases when considerable advantages may be noted.

The understanding of a case may be greatly enhanced by conducting a multidisciplinary assessment. This may be carried out with each professional seeing the family on their own or perhaps more effectively with all professionals working together, one or two clinicians interviewing the family and the others observing.

Cases may be assigned to ongoing joint work as need arises. For example, in the case of an adolescent with a depressive disorder one worker may see the adolescent for cognitive-behavioural therapy (CBT) and another the family as a whole for family work. In the case of an adolescent with schizophrenia, the psychiatrist may supervise the medication regime, a clinical nurse specialist implement a rehabilitation programme and the family as a whole attend a psychoeducational group. Alternatively, multidisciplinary working may be established more formally in clinics dedicated to particular treatment approaches or disorders, e.g. eating disorder clinics, family therapy clinics, neurodevelopmental disorder clinics.

WORKING WITH OTHER AGENCIES

As discussed before the majority of adolescents with mental health problems will not be seen by the CAMHS and consultation to other professionals can be useful. On occasions it may be most appropriate for the consultation to be offered by more than one mental health worker. This may be the case if the work to be reviewed is particularly difficult or challenging or if the consultation is to be offered to a group of other professionals or is to continue over a long period. It is then likely that two CAMHS workers will be more able to monitor the process of the group as well as focus on the clinical work presented. An example where all three factors might come together might be long-term consultation to the staff group of a local authority children's home.

THE CAMHS WORKING TOGETHER

Just as it is valuable for CAMHS staff to work together on more complex cases so it is useful for them to consult with each other on their work more generally. This allows each worker to hold cases that might not be possible without the input of colleagues and can add to the clinical approach of each member of the multidisciplinary team. It provides a useful forum for review of casework on a regular basis. It is also important for the CAMHS team members to offer each other support and maintain an attitude of development both clinically and as a team.

THE ADOLESCENT DAY UNIT

Some adolescents require more intensive treatment than can be achieved as an outpatient. Tier 3 CAMHS have an important role in making appropriate referrals for such interventions. If an inpatient unit is to be used there are major consequences for the adolescent and his/her family in terms of removal from the family unit, removal from the local community and interruption to the adolescent's education. These effects will be less apparent with use of a Day Unit. Adolescents as a whole may use any of a number of different types of day unit, those for children and younger adolescents, those more particularly for adolescents and those for adults, which will include some older adolescents. Space does not permit a detailed description of the working of a Day Unit here but many of the therapeutic opportunities found in an inpatient unit (see Chapter 14) will be offered. A study of a day treatment for adults found there to be no absolute contraindications against day treatment (Kluiter et al., 1992). Units for children and adolescents and adults have been found to be clinically effective (Kiser et al.,

1996; Nienhuis *et al.*, 1994). In a randomised trial of the use of a day unit and inpatient services by adult patients (Nienhuis *et al.*, 1994) similar outcomes were noted regarding psychopathology but greater improvement in self-care was reported in the day unit group.

ADOLESCENT MENTAL HEALTH PROVISION – A SPECIAL CASE?

So far in this discussion non-residential mental health services for adolescents have often been referred to as part of an overall CAMHS. This is indeed how the service is usually delivered across the UK at least as far as younger adolescents are concerned – older adolescents often being seen in adult psychiatry clinics. However, whether this is the most helpful way to organise mental health services for this age group has been questioned. The *Bridges over Troubled Waters* report (NHS Health Advisory Service, 1986) advises that young people aged 12–19 years require 'special separate consideration and provision' (p. 57). Patton (1996) argues that many adult mental disorders often have their onset during adolescence and, furthermore, that the needs of young people with adolescent-onset mental disorders are inadequately provided for by existing CAMHS which focus on the needs of children and younger adolescents. Birleson and Luk (1997) respond, however, that just as there are many disorders which arise *de novo* in adolescence, so there are many continuities between child and adult psychiatric disorder. Further division of service provision for young people with a long-term, perhaps lifelong, disorder may not be in their best interest. Birleson and Luk also question exactly which age range should be catered for by a separate adolescent service and find no research evidence to suggest that separate adolescent services currently in existence result in improved outcomes.

The development of separate adolescent mental health services has considerable resource implications. It is therefore important that those services that are currently being established are carefully evaluated and compared to existing provision. It may be especially important to develop new ways of delivering services to particular groups of disturbed adolescents, e.g. offenders with mental health problems and adolescents with substance misuse disorders. In areas without specific adolescent services, other ways of working are required.

Adolescent psychiatry incorporates aspects both of adult and child psychiatry. There is no natural age cut-off between the two areas of work. The opinion of adult psychiatrists as to the age of majority has been sought though. Watts *et al.* (1989) reported that adult psychiatrists working in Yorkshire believed most adolescents to reach maturity shortly before their 18th birthday. The same doctors were content to manage younger psychotic patients but wished adolescent services to deal with teenagers with behavioural, emotional and developmental disorders, and anorexia nervosa. Exactly how the handover from child psychiatry to adult services is managed is likely to depend on local factors including services available from all agencies in any one locality. There are also special considerations, which apply to inpatient provision (see Chapter 15). However, Health Authorities have to ensure that there is no gap in community service provision between the ages of 16 and 18 years and that the professionals, from either CAMHS or adult services, treating late adolescents have the necessary training. Important areas of knowledge will include, for example, an appreciation of developmental and educational issues, a potential area of weakness for members of an adult mental health service team, and being up to date with advances in psychopharmacology, an area that may be more challenging for members of CAMHS teams. A reasonable approach is perhaps that CAMHS deal with all referrals up to the age of 16 years or school leaving age. Adult psychiatry services should then begin to accept referrals of older adolescents. It is important, if such an arrangement is to work to the benefit of young people, that there be good relationships between CAMHS and adult psychiatry without rigid adherence to age related divisions between services. This will allow a flexible response, the team with the most relevant skills responding to the young person presenting for help. It would also be helpful for members of both CAMHS and adult services to consult with each other regularly about cases in the 16–18 years age range and particularly about difficult cases. On occasions it may be appropriate to manage cases jointly. The approach outlined above may represent an extension of the service offered by CAMHS in some areas. If it is to be adopted CAMHS need to be sufficiently well resourced to be able to span the extended age range.

REFERENCES

Adams, S. (1991) Prescribing of psychotropic drugs to children and adolescents. *British Medical Journal*, **302**, 217.

Angold, A., Messer, S. C., Stangl, D. K., Farmer, E. M. Z., Costello, E. J. and Burns, B. J. (1998) Perceived parental burden and service use for child and adolescent psychiatric disorders. *American Journal of Public Health*, **88**, 75–80.

Anonymous (1997) Emergency admissions: an open letter. *Young Minds Magazine*, **31**, 6–8.

Bailey, V., Graham, P. and Boniface, D. (1978) How much child psychiatry does the general practitioner do? *Journal of the Royal College of General Practitioners*, **28**, 621–626.

Bickman, L. (1996a) The evaluation of a children's mental health managed care demonstration. *Journal of Mental Health Administration*, **23**, 7–15.

Bickman, L. (1996b) Implications of a children's mental health managed care demonstration evaluation. *Journal of Mental Health Administration*, **23**, 107–117.

Birleson, P. and Luk, E. L. S. (1997) Continuing the debate on a separate adolescent psychiatry. *Australian and New Zealand Journal of Psychiatry*, **31**, 447–451.

Burns, B. J., Costello, E. J., Angold, A., Tweed, D., Stangl, D., Farmer, E. M. Z. *et al.* (1995) Children's mental health service use across service sectors. *Health Affairs*, **14**, 147–159.

Department of Education (1994) *Code of practice on the identification and assessment of special educational needs.* London: Department of Education.

Department of Health (1991) *The Children Act, Guidance and Regulations: Residential Care, Vol. 4.* London: HMSO.

Foster, E. M., Summerfelt, W. T. and Saunders, R. C. (1996) The costs of mental health service under the Fort Bragg demonstration. *Journal of Mental Health Administration*, **23**, 92–106.

Garralda, M. E. (1994) Primary care psychiatry. In M. Rutter, E. Taylor and L. Hersov (eds), *Child and Adolescent Psychiatry: Modern Approaches*, 3rd edn. Oxford: Blackwell Science, pp. 1055–1070.

Garralda, M. E. and Bailey, D. (1986a) Children with psychiatric disorders in primary care. *Journal of Child Psychology and Psychiatry*, **27**, 611–624.

Garralda, M. E. and Bailey, D. (1986b) Psychological deviance in children attending general practice. *Psychological Medicine*, **16**, 423–429.

Goldberg, D. and Bridges, K. (1987) Screening for psychiatric illness in general practice: the general practitioner versus the screening questionnaire. *Journal of the Royal College of General Practitioners*, **37**, 15–18.

Goldberg, D., Kay, C. and Thompson, L. (1976) Psychiatric morbidity in general practice and the community. *Psychological Medicine*, **6**, 565–569.

Goldberg, D., Gask, L. and O'Dowd, T. (1989) The treatment of somatization: teaching techniques of reattribution. *Journal of Psychosomatic Research*, **33**, 689–695.

Goodman, R. (1997a) *Maudsley Discussion Paper 4: Child and Adolescent Mental Health Services: Reasoned Advice to Commissioners and Providers.* London: Institute of Psychiatry.

Goodman, R. (1997b) Child mental health: who is responsible? *British Medical Journal*, **314**, 314–315.

Health Committee, House of Commons (1997) Session 1996–97, Fourth Report: *Child and Adolescent Mental Health Services.* London: The Stationery Office.

John, L. H., Offord, D. R., Boyle, M. H. and Racine, Y. A. (1995) Factors predicting use of mental health and social services by children 6–16 years old: findings from the Ontario Child Health Study. *American Journal of Orthopsychiatry*, **65**, 76–86.

Kiser, L. J., Millsap, P. A., Hickerson, S., Heston, J. D., Nunn, W., Pruitt, D. B. *et al.* (1996) Results of treatment one year later: child and adolescent partial hospitalization. *Journal of the American Academy of Child and Adolescent Psychiatry*, **35**, 81–90.

Kluiter, H., Giel, R., Nienhuis, F. J., Ruphan, M. and Wiersma, D. (1992) Predicting feasibility of day treatment for unselected patients referred for psychiatric treatment: results of a randomized trial. *American Journal of Psychiatry*, **149**, 1199–1205.

Kurtz, Z., Thornes, R. and Wolkind, S. (1994) *Services for the Mental Health of Children and Young People in England: A National Review.* Report to the Department of Health, South West Thames R.H.A.

Malek, M. (1997) *Nurturing Healthy Minds: The Importance of the Voluntary Sector in Promoting Young People's Mental Health.* London: National Children's Bureau.

NHS Health Advisory Service (1986) *Bridges over Troubled Waters: A Report on Services for Disturbed Adolescents.* London: Department of Health.

NHS Health Advisory Service (1995) *Child and Adolescent Mental Health Services: Together We Stand.* London: HMSO.

Nienhuis, F. J., Giel, R., Kluiter, H., Ruphan, M. and Wiersma, D. (1994) Efficacy of psychiatric day treatment. Course and outcome of psychiatric disorder in a randomised trial. *European Archives of Psychiatry and Clinical Neurosciences*, **244**, 73–80.

North, C. and Eminson, M. (1998) A review of a psychiatry–nephrology liaison service. *European Child and Adolescent Psychiatry*, **7**, 235–245.

North Essex Health Authority, South Essex Health Authority, Essex County Council – Social Services/Learning Services, Southend Borough Council – Social Services/Education and Thurrock Borough Council – Social Services/ Education (1998) *Promoting Positive Mental Health for Children and Adolescents in Essex – A Joint Strategy.* Essex Social Services, Communications Department.

Offer, D., Howard, K. I., Schonert, K. A. and Ostrov, E. (1991) To whom do adolescents turn for help? Differences between disturbed and nondisturbed adolescents. *Journal of the American Academy of Child and Adolescent Psychiatry*, **30**, 623–630.

Offord, D. R., Boyle, M. H., Szatmari, P., Rae-Grant, N. I., Links, P. S., Cadman, D. T. *et al.* (1987) Ontario child health study. II. Six-month prevalence of disorder and rates of service utilization. *Archives of General Psychiatry*, **44**, 832–836.

Parry-Jones, W. L. (1984) Adolescent psychiatry in Britain: a personal view of its development and present position. *Bulletin of the Royal College of Psychiatrists*, **8**, 230–233.

Parry-Jones, W. L. (1995) The future of adolescent psychiatry. *British Journal of Psychiatry*, **166**, 299–305.

Patton, G. (1996) An epidemiological case for a separate adolescent psychiatry? *Australian and New Zealand Journal of Psychiatry*, **30**, 563–566.

Platt, S. (1985) Measuring the burden of psychiatric illness on the family: an evaluation of some rating scales. *Psychological Medicine*, **15**, 383–393.

Rutter, M., Tizard, J. and Whitmore, K. (1970) *Education, Health and Behaviour.* New York: Longman.

Sawyer, M. G. and Kosky, R. J. (1995) Approaches to delivering child and adolescent mental health services: the South Australian experience. *Australian and New Zealand Journal of Psychiatry,* **29**, 230–237.

Talmon, M. (1990) *Single-Session Therapy. Maximizing the Effect of the First (and often Only) Therapeutic Encounter.* San Francisco, CA: Josey-Bass.

Watts, E. L., Jenkins, M. E. and Richardson, G. J. R. (1989) Who cares for the older adolescent? *Psychiatric Bulletin,* **13**, 345–346.

Weisz, J. R. and Weiss, B. (1993) *Developmental Clinical Psychology and Psychiatry. Vol. 27. Effects of Psychotherapy with Children and Adolescents.* London: Sage.

Chapter 14

THE ADOLESCENT UNIT

Andrew J. Cotgrove

INTRODUCTION AND BACKGROUND

The concept of the 'adolescent unit' covers a multitude of different services and therapeutic philosophies. The service provided by an adolescent unit may focus on inpatient work or it can provide a range of other services including, day patient, outreach and outpatient work. Therapeutic philosophies may be narrow, such as working with therapeutic community principles, or broad, offering an eclectic service. Historically, in the absence of clear evidence for good practice, the chosen philosophy often depended on the beliefs and experience of a charismatic leader (Parry-Jones, 1995). Nowadays, services still vary widely from the highly specialised, such as those treating eating disorders or offering forensic secure facilities, to those offering assessment and management for a wide range of mental health problems. The adolescent unit may relate in a range of different ways with other services for adolescents such as community child and adolescent mental health services (CAMHS), education, social service departments, general practitioners and paediatricians to name but a few. Hence the adolescent unit is not a single entity, but more a broad concept that differs considerably around the country.

In this chapter, I will attempt to describe the functioning of the 'General Purpose Adolescent Unit' as it is in the UK, with an inpatient service at its core. However, I will also expand and develop the difficult and sometimes controversial dilemmas faced in providing such a service when so many different demands are placed upon it.

THE GENERAL PURPOSE ADOLESCENT UNIT

Adolescent units are unusual within the NHS as they tend to specialise in an age range rather than a clinical area. This inevitably leads to problems when trying to provide treatment for the diverse range of disorders referred. Nevertheless, the majority of adolescent units, within their limited resources, attempt to address the needs of those adolescents with the most severe mental health problems. This can result in adolescents with wide-ranging difficulties and different treatment needs being managed under the same roof.

Attempts to provide therapeutic stability in the inpatient or day patient environment can be further jeopardised by requests for immediate admission. Such requests can be a source of significant disagreement between adolescent unit staff and referrers (see section on 'Assessment procedure'). Despite this wide range of pressures placed on the adolescent unit, or perhaps because of them, the diversity of philosophies and operational policies in adolescent units around the country is reducing. Units which previously might have provided a single therapeutic philosophy, or units which treated a narrow range of disorder, are fast disappearing. In their place are emerging, for better or worse, less idiosyncratic and more eclectic services which have commonly come to be known as General Purpose Adolescent Units.

SCALE OF THE PROBLEM

Approximately 15–21% of adolescents have mental health problems in any one year (Offord *et al.*, 1987; Rutter *et al.*, 1976) Conservatively, this would result in approximately 50 000 adolescents per annum having significant mental health problems in a region such as Merseyside, with a total population of 2.4 million. Only a small proportion of these adolescents will be seen by CAMHS, and a smaller proportion again, approximately 0.1% of the total with problems, receive treatment in an adolescent unit. The 'referral iceberg' (Figure 14.1) illustrates that adolescent units only see the tip of the tip of the iceberg!

HEALTH ADVISORY SERVICE RECOMMENDATIONS

In 1995 the Health Advisory Service published a document (*Together We Stand*) outlining their recommendations for the future of CAMHS. Three main themes come out of this document:

- Recognition of the need for improved cooperation, collaboration and integration between existing services and disciplines
- The need for the further development of services for older adolescents and young adults

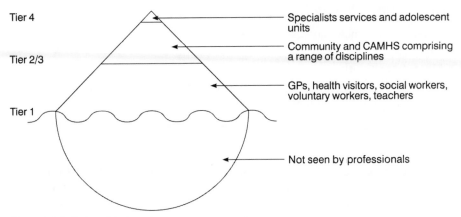

Tier 4 — Specialists services and adolescent units

Tier 2/3 — Community and CAMHS comprising a range of disciplines

— GPs, health visitors, social workers, voluntary workers, teachers

Tier 1

— Not seen by professionals

Figure 14.1 'Referral iceberg'.

- Development of a four tier CAMHS, with an emphasis on developing the role of a primary mental health care worker (PMHW)

The four tiers described are summarised in Figure 14.1, with adolescent units and other specialist services placed in Tier 4.

THE PROCESS OF REFERRAL, ASSESSMENT AND ADMISSION

PATHWAYS OF REFERRAL

There are far more adolescents in need of help with mental health problems than receiving it from specialist services. Many have problems which remain unidentified by professionals, whilst others receive support in Tier 1 services from GPs, teachers, school nurses, educational welfare officers, social services departments, voluntary services, etc. Those that have come into contact with Tier 1 services but whose needs are not being met, may then be referred on to community CAMHS in Tiers 2/3. Adolescent units generally act as tertiary referral centres (or Tier 4), accepting referrals primarily from other specialist services, such as community CAMHS. Some units provide a service directly to primary care referrers, reducing unnecessary delays for urgent referrals, but this can result in duplication of services and a lack of clarity around pathways of referral.

Together We Stand (Health Advisory Service, 1995) suggested that pathways of referral can be hindered by a lack of coordination between existing services. Ideally, social services departments, education, voluntary services and health, should be collaborating and communicating in their work with troubled adolescents. Unfortunately, these services have different approaches to assessment and treatment, which may result in less than ideal management of an individual's difficulties.

On a more positive note, there is now clearly an emphasis coming from the highest level within government departments on increased cooperation and collaboration on the planning, commission and delivery of services.

ASSESSMENT PROCEDURE

The question that needs to be answered in any assessment should be 'is admission desirable?'. This simple question is often quite complex to answer. Table 14.1 summarises the main issues which need to be taken into account.

In order to ascertain whether an adolescent's difficulties are likely to improve with an admission to an adolescent unit, a full psychiatric and systemic assessment is necessary. This can be done in a number of ways and does not necessarily require that professionals from the adolescent unit gather all this information first hand. To avoid too much duplication, much of this information can be gathered from the referrer. In some cases it is useful to suggest a professionals meeting, where all the professionals who have been involved in the case can meet to share information. This can also facilitate consideration of alternatives to a possible admission to an adolescent unit, as well as help planning an admission if this is considered the best option. Whilst information from the referrer and other professionals can be extremely useful and save duplication, it is not a substitute for a direct assessment with the adolescent and their family. This can help develop a systemic understanding of how the family view the problem, what ideas they have about who or what needs to change and how they think an adolescent unit may or may not be helpful. Such information is vital in planning possible treatment approaches with the adolescent and their families. It also allows you to start engaging with the adolescent and their family, and exploring motivations for change.

There are various aspects to and different parties involved in the motivation for the referral to an adolescent unit. It is desirable, but not essential, to have motivation and cooperation from the adolescent, their family and the referrer. This motivation needs to be based on informed consent, and it is important that the adolescent and usually their family have a clear idea about what is on offer

Table 14.1 Assessment procedure

Is admission desirable?
- Are the presenting problems likely to be helped by admission?
- Is there motivation to change? (clear aims and objectives can help clarify this)
- Are there any suitable alternatives?
- Could admission cause more harm than good?

and know something about how the adolescent unit works. In some cases, such as in the treatment of anorexia nervosa, an admission is far more likely to be successful when there is a clear motivation to change on the part of the adolescent and their family. In others, such as with psychotic illnesses, inpatient treatment may still be indicated without it. Referrer support and cooperation with the treatment package is also desirable, particularly when negotiating admission and follow-up after discharge. Conversely, it may be that the adolescent and their family have no motivation for change or to receive treatment, and the customer for the service is the referrer or another professional. In such cases admission is only likely to follow if it is supported by legislation such as the Mental Health Act 1983, the Children Act 1989 or by the granting of a Wardship Order. This area is explored further in the section on 'Issues of consent'.

Clear aims and objectives for the admission need to be identified with the adolescent, the family and sometimes the referrer. These can be helpful in clarifying motivation for change, but also to gauge progress during an admission. Such aims can range from quite small, quantifiable changes, such as reducing excessive hand-washing, to grander aims, like improving self-esteem. However, even with grander aims it can be helpful to clarify examples of how these might be measured and attempt to monitor improvement by, for example, using a rating scale. Whatever the aims, even if they are difficult to measure, they need to be realistic. It is not possible to repair all the damage done to an individual who, for example, has faced years of deprivation and abuse in a short admission to an adolescent unit.

The issue of whether an admission could cause more harm than good is one which clinicians, in their enthusiasm to be helpful, can sometimes overlook, but which should always be considered. As a general rule of thumb, when a voluntary admission is agreed by the adolescent, their family, the referrer and the assessing professionals from the adolescent unit, and there are clear achievable aims for that admission, it is unlikely to be harmful. Even in these cases there are possible risks, including increased dependence and institutionalisation. More concerning is when an adolescent is forced into an admission against their will. It can be a major step, particularly for the younger and less mature adolescents, to be removed from their families and other support networks, and even with the best intentions such a step should not be taken lightly. It is possible, on occasion, this experience could be quite traumatic and compound problems which already exist. Generally, such a step should only be considered when admission is needed to ensure the adolescent's safety, where there is evidence of abuse or neglect in the home and/or there is good evidence that inpatient treatment will improve the youngsters mental health.

Consideration should be given to the location of the initial assessment. Once invited to an adolescent unit, a family will have some degree of expectation that an offer of admission will follow. In some cases, such expectations may be followed by disappointment or a sense of rejection if admission is not offered.

It can be helpful then to make a judgement from the information passed on by the referrer and other professionals as to the likelihood that an admission will follow. If it seems likely that alternatives to admission will be recommended, then it may be helpful to carry out the initial assessment at the referrers base or in the family home. This can also help give the message that responsibility for the case remains with the referrer at the time of the initial assessment.

The age of the adolescent, both chronological and developmental, needs to be taken into account as part of the assessment. For example, a pre-pubertal child with some educational difficulties, even if their chronological age fits the admission criteria for an adolescent unit, may be better off receiving treatment in a specialist children's unit. Similarly, an older adolescent with an enduring mental illness, such as schizophrenia, may have their inpatient treatment needs better served by an adult service, which is likely to be involved in their longer-term follow-up. Working with an age range which overlaps with both children's inpatient services and adult services allows for flexibility in this respect.

Adolescent service staff may be asked to offer an assessment in order to provide a second opinion or a consultation to facilitate planning future management. As community-based adolescent services are, as yet, poorly developed nationwide, adolescent units often provide the main source of expertise in adolescent mental health issues for large geographical areas. Some units, such as the Bethlem Adolescent Unit (Steinberg, 1994), provide a specialist outreach service, which can offer assessments, consultations and second opinions to local CAMHS, whilst also working as part of the integrated team within the inpatient unit.

AIMS OF ADMISSION

There are a number of ways in which an admission to an adolescent unit may be helpful. The most obvious of these is to help with the difficulties which have been identified at referral and during the assessment procedure. These can include problems identified by the adolescent and their family, such as to reduce self-harming behaviour or to improve relationships within the family, or may be defined by professionals, e.g. to treat a psychotic illness.

There are other aims or benefits from an admission which can be achieved that may not be identified during the assessment. Firstly, an admission may facilitate positive changes in an adolescent's lifestyle. For example, supportive feedback can result in improvements in self-care. Admission to an adolescent unit may be the first significant period the youngster has spent away from home; this then can be an opportunity for them to increase their sense of self-responsibility, their feelings of independence and reduce dependency on their parents.

Secondly, an inpatient admission can provide an opportunity for a positive peer group experience, where previously an adolescent may have felt isolated or been bullied by their peers. This positive experience can improve their ability to make friends and form relationships with others, which, along with other achievements during an inpatient's stay, can improve the adolescent's self-esteem and feelings of self-worth.

Finally, an aim for any admission should be to reduce the risk or severity of long-term psychopathology. An intensive inpatient experience has the potential to impact significantly on the personality development of an adolescent. This can then impact on the trajectory the adolescent may embark on through life, shifting it from one of repeated recourse to psychiatric or psychological services, to one where the individual acquires the personal resources to be more effective in resolving future difficulties, enabling them to find personal fulfilment and happiness in life.

Questions regarding the possible mechanisms for the above benefits are addressed in the section 'Theories and models of change'.

INDICATIONS FOR ADMISSION

Previous sections have addressed the assessment procedure, and the aims and benefits from an admission. This section deals with the indications and contraindications for admission. These are summarised in Table 14.2.

An inpatient adolescent unit can offer 24 h a day assessment and supervision by a multidisciplinary team to gather information to guide further management. This may involve observing the adolescent's behaviour and their interaction with others, observing the effects of a specific intervention, such as the use of medication, or allowing time for a range of investigations to be carried out, such as cognitive assessments or neurological tests such as magnetic resonance imaging or EEGs. Inpatient or day patient admission can also allow for an assessment of the adolescents difficulties out of the context of their home or school. For example, an adolescent may appear severely depressed in the home environment or at school, but their mood may lift significantly when admitted. This information can be helpful in guiding future management, whether or not further inpatient treatment is indicated.

Table 14.2 Indications and possible contraindications for admission

Indication for admission

- Intensive assessment
- Safety
- Treatment of complex disorders when outpatient treatment is insufficient

Possible contraindications for admission

- Treatment unlikely to be effective
- Extreme risk of violence/dangerousness (which cannot be contained)
- Specific expertise/treatments not available
- Problems with case mix

Safety of the adolescent or others is the second main indication for an admission. Concerns about safety may be due to a psychotic process associated with disturbed and aggressive behaviour, putting others at risk; or confused and chaotic behaviour which could put the adolescent themselves at risk. Suicidal and self-harming behaviour raises obvious safety issues. This may be as a result of depression or an acting out of distress for other reasons. Caution is needed when considering admission for reasons of safety with those who are self-harming, as very often, unless there are other clear indications for admission, other interventions are preferable (Hawton *et al*, 1998) (see also Chapter 4). Occasionally extremes of self-neglect may warrant an admission. This may include conditions such as pervasive refusal syndrome, where the adolescent may be neglecting basic levels of hygiene and nutrition.

Thirdly, admission may be indicated for complex problems where outpatient work has been tried and failed or the intensity of treatment needed is not available elsewhere. Such adolescents may present with problems which pervade all aspects of their life, e.g. they may have difficulties at home, educationally at school and with their peers. Admissions for complex difficulties, such as these, often warrant an extended pre-admission assessment. It is particularly important with this group to be clear about the aims of an admission, as often their difficulties are such that only limited objectives are likely to be achievable.

It is worth noting that there are no particular conditions that give rise to an absolute indication for admission, as even quite severe mental health problems, such as an acute schizophreniform psychosis, can sometimes be managed effectively by community services. Conversely, adolescents with problems such as emotional disorders or mild to moderate depression, which would normally be managed in the community, may require admission due to a range of compounding family, social and personal difficulties.

However, to give an indication of the diagnoses made on admission to an adolescent unit, Table 14.3 summarises the main diagnoses made and their relative frequencies based on admissions to 'Pine Lodge' Young People's Centre over a 3-year period.

Table 14.3 combines the commonest diagnostic categories of 'Mixed disorder of conduct and emotions' (F92) and 'Borderline personality disorder' (F60.31). Because these are ICD-10 diagnoses (World Health Organisation, 1992) the term 'Personality disorder' has only been applied to those over the age of 16. A diagnosis of 'Mixed disorder of conduct and emotion' (F92) has been applied to those youngsters under the age of 16 years who commonly present with: maladaptive coping strategies such as deliberate self-harm; difficulties relating to peers often forming intense, brief and destructive relationships; low self-esteem; labile moods which can be overwhelming; an intolerance of being alone with chronic feelings of boredom; impulsiveness; substance misuse; and commonly a history of sexual abuse. Strictly speaking, these features have more in common with borderline personality disorder, particularly as defined by the

Table 14.3 The range of psychiatric disorders treated in a General Purpose Adolescent Unit

Disorder	%
Mixed disorder of conduct and emotions (F92) and borderline personality disorder (F60.31)	36
Psychotic disorders (including affective psychosis) (F20, F23 and F30–32)	23
Non-affective emotional disorders including obsessive-compulsive disorder (F42), phobias (F40) and anxiety states (F41)	13
Depression (without psychosis) (F32)	11
Eating disorders (F50)	10
Psychosomatic and dissociative disorders (F44 and F45)	4
Others	3

DSM-IV (American Psychiatric Association, 1994) classification, but ICD-10 does not offer a satisfactory category for this group when presenting under the age of 16.

The other Axis I diagnoses shown in Table 14.3 are more straight forward and self-explanatory, but still only give part of the picture. ICD-10 Axis V codes, such as a history of abuse, history of deliberate self-harm and family problems, can help to make sense of why some individuals with a particular diagnosis require admission, whilst others do not.

Possible contraindications for admission are quite variable and often depend on local factors such as the structure of the building (when security is needed) or the availability of a specific expertise. However, it will be a universal point that if an admission will not be helpful, or possibly even harmful, then alternatives need to be found.

Occasionally, a referral may be made for an assessment for inpatient treatment when further outpatient treatment might be considered sufficient. The referrer may be happy to pursue this or alternatively the adolescent unit staff may take it on.

Some units may develop a particular expertise in the management of specific conditions such as neuro-developmental disorders or learning disabilities. Where this expertise is not available, admission to an adolescent unit for assessment or treatment is unlikely to be helpful and so adolescents with these difficulties may be excluded.

As a General Purpose Adolescent Unit has to deal with such a wide range of difficulties and disorders, there may be occasions when the admission of a particular patient is undesirable because of the particular case mix at the time. That might mean delaying the admission of a particularly sensitive, vulnerable and impressionable adolescent, when there is a high level of disturbance in the unit. It could mean avoiding another admission where the problem, such as anorexia nervosa or self-harming behaviour, is already prevalent in the unit and there are fears that another similar case could undermine progress for those already admitted.

ISSUES OF CONSENT

As previously discussed in the section on the 'Assessment procedure', it is desirable to only admit adolescents with both their informed consent and that of their parents. For the majority of admissions this will be the case; however, there may be times when professionals involved in the case believe admission is desirable, but one of the other parties do not consent. The combinations of this are: (1) the adolescent themselves refuses treatment, although the parents wish for it, (2) the adolescent wants treatment but the parents refuse, and (3) both the parents and the adolescent are refusing treatment. For the purposes of this section I am including any legal guardian or whoever has parental responsibility under the term 'parent'.

If an adolescent refuses treatment but the parent and the professionals involved feel strongly enough that treatment is desirable, then the adolescent's wishes can be over-ruled. From a legal point of view this is fairly straightforward up until the youngster's 18th birthday, before which parents have a right to consent to treatment for their child against their will. There is a commonly held view that after their 16th birthday, an adolescent has the right to refuse treatment; however, this is not the case and if the doctors and parents agree an adolescent can be treated against their will until their 18th birthday. For example, in 1992, a 16-year-old anorexic girl (Re W) had her appeal against treatment over-ruled by Lord Donaldson, in favour of the wishes and views of her parents and the doctors involved. The legal rights of the parents with regard to medical treatment end on the child's 18th birthday (Lord Denning).

The rather vague and difficult concept of 'competence' comes into play with adolescents under the age of 16 who wish to receive treatment without their parents knowledge or against their wishes. The 'Gillick Ruling' (House of Lords, 1985) ruled that a 14-year-old should be allowed to receive contraception from her GP without her parents' consent or knowledge as long as the GP thought she was competent to make an informed decision on the matter. This ruling has since been generalised so that adolescents under the age of 16 are entitled to make a decision regarding any form of medical treatment, as long as the medical practitioners involved consider they are competent to make such a decision and the treatment is in their best interests. '. . . parental rights yield to the child's right to make his own decisions when he reaches a sufficient understanding and intelligence to be capable of making up his own mind on the matter requiring a decision.' (House of Lords, 1986). Hence an adolescent deemed 'Gillick competent' wishing to receive treatment in an adolescent unit, is entitled to do so against their parent's wishes.

It is extremely rare that professionals will wish to pursue an admission against both the parents and the adolescent's wishes. This would normally only happen if the professionals consider the adolescent's safety to be severely compromised without admission, either due to the severity of their mental illness or if there is evidence that they will come to significant harm if they were to remain with their parents. In the former circumstances a range of options are available. These include using legislation under the Children Act 1989 such as a Care Order (Section 31) or a Specific Issue Order (Section 8). Both of these options would normally involve Social Services and could be time consuming. A rapid alternative available to mental health professionals is to apply for a Wardship Order which, in an emergency, can be done by a phone call to the appropriate judge. However, this can become costly if the Wardship is contested and I am not aware of this option being used. Lord Donaldson in his ruling Re W (1992) stated that all the above options are preferable to the use of the Mental Health Act 1989 when treating minors (under 18 years old) as the Mental Health Act can lead to stigma and restrictions later in life for the person that it has been applied to. In practice, many psychiatrists feel more comfortable using the Mental Health Act as it includes safeguards such as the involvement of other professionals, a time limit, a straightforward procedure for appeals and regular reviews.

In the latter case, where the treatment of an adolescent is indicated but there is also evidence of significant harm whilst the adolescent remains at home, then the use of the Children Act 1989 or Wardship proceedings would be more universally accepted. The Local Authority or a guardian *ad litem* would then take on the role of parenting. The issues then regarding treating the adolescent against their will apply as above as determined by the Donaldson ruling (1992).

I have assumed to this point that both parents will share the same view, but of course there will be occasions when parents do not agree. In addition, re-constituted families can add a further complexity, particularly when parental responsibility is shared between parents living apart. Despite these circumstances adding complexity to the issue of consent, the same basic principles outlined above apply. If in doubt, it is always worth consulting a solicitor specialising in family law.

SERVICE CONFIGURATION AND COMMISSIONING

EMERGENCY OR PLANNED ADMISSIONS

Most adolescent units prefer to plan their admissions. This allows time to clarify the problem, to set shared aims and objectives, to allow the adolescent and their family to gain an understanding of what is on offer, and thereby allow for informed consent for treatment. There are a number of possible problems associated with unplanned emergency admissions including:

- Disruption to the therapeutic programme, reducing treatment efficacy
- The potential loss of a safe and secure environment

- A longer waiting list for treatment places if beds have to be kept open for possible emergencies
- The possibility that emergency referrals could be made to queue-jump a waiting list for planned admissions
- The loss of the advantages of planning prior to admission outlined above.

Given the quite significant problems associated with emergency admissions, are they ever justified? In 1995, 'Pine Lodge' Young People's Centre in Chester piloted an emergency admission service (Cotgrove, 1997). The majority of requests for emergency admission were on the grounds of safety due to risk of deliberate self-harm. There is no evidence that admission following self-harm is effective in reducing suicide risk, although there is an absence of good studies in this area (Cotgrove et al., 1995; Hawton et al., 1998). A common scenario of such a referral might be of a youngster living in an unstable home situation, either with their family or in social services care, but where there is a risk of the placement breaking down. Often there is repeated absconding and self-harming behaviour and emergency inpatient psychiatric treatment is requested to treat their self-harming behaviour, which has raised the anxiety of the referrer. However, what is probably needed is a safe, containing, consistent and caring environment that would accept the youngster for a long-term placement rather than risk another rejection which would follow after a short-term admission to an adolescent unit.

Psychotic or severely depressed adolescents, although less common, still featured prominently amongst the emergency referrals. The use of adult psychiatric beds is often considered in such cases, but such a suggestion frequently provokes strongly negative feelings. However, the reasons given why a particular adult psychiatric ward is unsuitable for young people, often amount to it being unsuitable for anybody! (Steinberg, 1994).

Initially, the staff at the Chester Adolescent Unit and the referrers disagreed about the appropriateness of many of the emergency referrals. Over time, differences in assessment have reduced. In addition to being able to admit genuine emergencies, there are other positive aspects to the service which had not been fully anticipated. The emergency team is able to provide rapid second opinions which can be supportive to professionals working in community services who might, at times, feel isolated, without access to an experienced clinician for an urgent second opinion. Perhaps most importantly, the community CAMHS teams within Merseyside know that there is an emergency service available, which can be perceived as an insurance policy, hopefully rarely called upon, but reassuring to have.

DAY UNIT OR INPATIENT UNIT?

Ideally the decision as to whether an adolescent needs an inpatient admission or Day Unit admission should be on clinical grounds; however, the choice is often limited by the resources available. In many parts of the country there are no specialist Day Units. Conversely, geographically there are some areas where only Day Units are available locally with no easy access to a specialist inpatient unit. Obviously in either of these circumstances the choice of where to admit is going to be largely influenced by what is available.

Where they are available the configuration of adolescent Day Units varies considerably. A recent survey revealed approximately 30 'stand alone' Day Units in the UK and a further 28 Day Units or day services attached to an existing inpatient service for both children and adolescents (Bester and Bailey, 1998). Only about two thirds of these are available for the adolescent age range. Education can often form a key component to a day service, particularly when provided for younger adolescents where problems have at least in part been associated with school.

When there is a genuine choice available between Day Unit and inpatient admission, there are two key factors in determining which will be more appropriate. Firstly, the degree of severity with an associated need for supervision. If a risk assessment suggests that an adolescent is in need of 24 h a day supervision for reasons of safety, then clearly inpatient admission is preferable. Secondly, inpatient admission can also provide a useful separation from a home environment where patterns of interaction appear stuck, inhibiting the psychological development of the adolescent. Admission can then facilitate the individuation and growth of independence needed at this stage of life. However, it is important not to replace an unhelpful dependence on the home environment with a dependence on the institution of the adolescent unit. For this reason, even when inpatient admission is indicated it is usually useful to maintain links with the home by, for example, incorporating weekend leave as part of the programme and having regular family meetings. Occasionally a return home may not be the preferred outcome in which case alternatives need to be considered on discharge.

Where there is a lesser need for an intensive therapeutic input and no need for separation from the home environment, then admission to a Day Unit would be preferable. This might, for example, allow for a specific psychological therapeutic programme to be implemented or allow a school refusing adolescent a chance to receive some education away from the home maintaining contact with a peer group.

COMMISSIONING ADOLESCENT UNITS

Adolescent units have been going through unstable times. After the burgeoning of services during the 1960s and 1970s the last two decades have seen a retraction in both inpatient and day patient provision. The purchaser–provider split and devolvement of funding from Regional Health Authorities to District Health Authorities provided a particular challenge over the last decade. Previously Regional Health Authorities would commonly oversee the provision of adolescent services for large catchment area populations and often fund them directly. However, with the devolvement of funding to the District Health Authorities in the early 1990s these arrangements have been revised. This has resulted in different local solutions to the problem of purchasing a service which usually provides for a population larger than a single district. 'Pine Lodge' Young People's Centre in Chester has been quite fortunate in that it has negotiated an arrangement whereby the funding from the six districts that used to make up the old Region have agreed a 'top slicing' arrangement which is reviewed every 3 years. Such an arrangement has given some security and allowed for a degree of long-term planning. Other adolescent units have negotiated a more piecemeal contract with their purchasers, sometimes accepting funding based on estimated activity and sometimes on a cost-per-case basis. Whilst such arrangements can reduce the long-term security of a unit and add to administrative complexity they have allowed for some entrepreneurial activity enabling any extra money earned to be ploughed into service developments.

Unfortunately, in some parts of the country services have been cut for local financial reasons without clear consideration being given to the psychiatric needs of the population.

The commissioning of adolescent units is now set to change again. A recent consultation document produced by the NHS Executive, *The New NHS: Commissioning Specialised Services* (1998), has suggested the setting up of 'Regional Specialist Commissioning Groups'. These will comprise representatives from all Health Authorities and set about reviewing planning and commissioning specialist services as defined by a 'longlist' set out in the Audit Commission's 1997 report *Higher Purchase*. Inpatient psychiatric services for children and adolescents are included which is a very positive step. The result should be a considered and coherent approach to commissioning adolescent services which will take into account the large population catchment areas normally involved.

THE WORK WITHIN AN ADOLESCENT INPATIENT UNIT

THEORIES AND MODELS OF CHANGE

Adolescent units can provide a unique opportunity for intensive treatment, often over an extended time period. This allows for a range of different therapeutic interventions to be used, but also for a sustained experience for an adolescent which has the potential to have a profound affect on their personality development. The next section 'Therapeutic interventions', will outline the range of treatments commonly used in an adolescent unit. Firstly, however, in this section a theoretical model based on attachment theory is used to describe how a non-specific, intense and extensive therapeutic experience for an adolescent in an adolescent unit could significantly and positively change the trajectory of their personality development, thus reducing the risk of severe and crippling life-long psychopathology. This model is not intended to represent the 'truth' about what happens in adolescent units, but more a helpful way to think about it.

Attachment theory emphasizes the importance and biological function of intimate relationships between individuals, the central role of care givers on a child's development and the persistence of attachment styles (ways of relating to others) throughout life. For the development of a secure attachment, a child needs to be sure that should he encounter any frightening or adverse situations, his parents will respond in a predictable and helpful fashion. When this occurs the child is able to use the attachment figure as a secure base from which to explore the world and play returning for comfort should the need arise (Bowlby, 1969/82). As the child develops he becomes able to internalise and generalise the pattern of attachment. When a child's care is disrupted by inconsistent or abusive parenting a helpful secure attachment style is unlikely to develop. Instead the child is likely to become ambivalent to the care givers, seeking but then rejecting comfort. This may have a profound effect on their ability to form relationships throughout their life. Ambivalent attachment patterns have been shown to be strongly associated with poor personality development and the acquisition of personality disorders such as borderline personality (Patrick *et al.*, 1994). Conversely, an experience of consistent, sensitive and responsive parenting in childhood will improve the individuals resilience to adversity. Whilst there are no studies classifying the attachment patterns of adolescents admitted to adolescent units, it is clear that many have suffered extremes of adversity in terms of neglect and abuse in childhood and display many of the features of borderline personality functioning.

Negotiating a contract for admission with clear aims and objectives can provide material for the content of the therapeutic work carried out during an admission; however, the adolescent unit also has the opportunity to provide a safe, caring and containing environment, in which this work can be carried out. For some the experience of consistent and responsive care giving as provided by the staff group may be new, and over a period of time could be internalised. Such an internalised 'secure base' can give the adolescent a new repertoire for relating to people in a positive way, which may then have positive spin-offs in other aspects of their personality functioning such as self-esteem. Thus overall there is the potential, through a change in internalised attachment constructs, to profoundly affect the trajectory of the adolescent's personality development.

THERAPEUTIC INTERVENTIONS AND PHILOSOPHIES

Attachment theory has been used as an example to illustrate how a consistent approach to caring for adolescents in a residential setting could have significant benefits in their personality development, particularly for those who have had inadequate or abusive care giving early in life. Other developmental models could equally have been used to justify the value of such an approach, including psychoanalytic or cognitive psychological models.

Whilst a particular theory, model or philosophy may underpin the thinking or therapeutic structure of an adolescent unit, the day to day treatments involved tend to be varied and multiple to reflect the individual needs of adolescents with a wide range of disorders. Hence, in practice, the therapeutic milieu of an average general purpose adolescent unit tends to be eclectic. Programmes are designed to treat specific disorders and alleviate symptomatic disturbance, as well as promoting self-esteem, consolidating a stable sense of identity, improving confidence to manage independent living and the formation of realistic vocational goals.

The range of therapeutic interventions used in an adolescent unit are summarised below.

General therapeutic benefits

- Therapeutic milieu
- Safe, containing and responsive environment, i.e. 'secure base'

Specific therapies

- Group work including:
  - group psychotherapy
  - art and drama therapy
  - outward bound activities
  - social skills
- Family Therapy
- Individual work including:
  - psychodynamic therapy
  - cognitive and behaviour therapy
  - daily living skills
- Psychopharmacology

Details of the theories and practice of some of the specific treatments and therapies listed above are described in Chapters 19–22. In what follows a description of these interventions is limited to how each treatment or therapy can fit in within the overall therapeutic milieu of an adolescent unit.

Generally, adolescent units have a core of communal activities which involve most or all of the adolescents. This usually includes regular community meetings, when staff and residents can discuss day to day practical issues arising from the adolescent's living together. Sometimes such meetings also include the discussion of individual emotional difficulties or difficulties the adolescents may have in their relationships with each other. Schooling or other educational activities also often form part of the core life of an adolescent unit and in some units most of the 'working day' will be taken up in schooling.

Beyond these core activities, the ratio of communal therapeutic activity to specific individual therapy is quite variable. Historically, many adolescent units drew on therapeutic community principles whereby little or no specific individual work took place. Whilst this mode of working is no longer viable for the general purpose adolescent unit which has to treat a wide range of disorders, some principles involved are still used. Therapeutic programmes can be designed to try and make all the activities throughout the day in some way therapeutic. This model of working can have some significant advantages in terms of using the peer group to facilitate positive change and to encourage the taking on of responsibilities. Practical activities, such as planning, shopping for and cooking meals together, can have a range of benefits, such as developing cooperative and relationship skills, improving basic living skills as well as benefiting self-esteem by providing a meal which others will eat and compliment.

At 'Pine Lodge' Young People's Centre in Chester, we run a fully self-catering programme. The residents plan the meal and shop together for the ingredients a week in advance, and draw up a rota for two of them and a member of staff to cook each meal. Not only is the quality of the meals higher than that previously provided by the hospital canteen, but we can also see the other benefits listed above.

Other group activities can include group psychotherapy, creative therapies, such as art and drama and outward bound activity. Many of the therapeutic benefits of this type of work are described in Chapter 20. However, group work in an inpatient or day patient setting can have the added power of working with a group of adolescents who are also spending a great deal of the rest of their day to day lives together. This can enable them to work on relationship skills by looking at their relationships with each other in an intensity that would not normally be available in outpatient group work. Creative therapies such as art and drama therapy and outward bound activities can provide an opportunity for adolescent's to work on their emotional difficulties as well as relationship issues in ways that do not rely as heavily as some on verbal communication skills. For example, an adolescent may be able to express feelings of hopelessness and despair in a painting, in a way they could never express verbally. Similarly, outward bound activities sometimes allow adolescents to excel in their physical abilities or cooperative group abilities when otherwise they may see themselves as low achievers.

Whilst such a 'therapeutic milieu' of group activities can have significant benefits for most adolescents, occasionally it can be in an individuals best interest to be excluded from some aspects of the programme. The overall effect of participating in the group activities can be quite stimulating and arousing, and for some, such as those in an acute psychotic episode, it is better to follow a lower stimulus programme. Even with such cases, the structure of a clear timetable for the day can have an important containing effect.

Family work is generally considered an essential part of the work of most adolescent units. Chapter 21 describes the indications for family therapy, the therapeutic styles appropriate for working with the families of adolescents and the potential benefits. In an inpatient setting work carried out in family therapy will often parallel that which is provided in an outpatient setting, however, there are some additional benefits. Family work allows there to be a formal, regular exchange of views regarding the adolescent's progress. The parents can find out about their child's progress and any difficulties at the unit and the family workers have an opportunity to gain information about the adolescent's progress in their parents' eyes, e.g. when they are home on weekend leave. This information can be useful both in direct therapeutic work with the family and also to guide further work within the adolescent unit.

The amount of individual work carried out within an adolescent unit is perhaps the most variable of all the therapeutic modalities. Some units develop specific individual therapeutic programmes, which may include individual cognitive or behaviour therapy, individual psychodynamic psychotherapy and individual task setting. The indications and benefits of such treatments are described elsewhere in the book. Apart from the intensity with which they may be used, their benefits are much the same in an inpatient as outpatient setting. However, some units offer little or no individual work, on the basis this can distract from the other therapeutic activities which take place. For example, an adolescent may save up discussing their emotional difficulties or past traumatic experiences for the privacy and seclusion of an individual session with 'their' therapist, then not wishing to continue this work with anyone else or in any other setting. If this happens, it may negate some of the benefits of inpatient treatment, with (in the extreme case) the adolescent unit perhaps offering no more than accommodation for the adolescent, whilst they receive individual therapy which could be provided as an outpatient. There is no generally agreed satisfactory resolution to this dilemma, but sometimes compromise solutions such as offering limited individual work with specific aims, may avoid the problems associated with either excluding individual work or undermining the opportunity for group work with peers. Examples where specific therapies are indicated include exposure and response prevention programmes for the treatment of obsessive-compulsive symptoms, a behavioural programme to help with agoraphobia, or some supportive counselling to discuss in private some particularly traumatic or abusive experiences.

Finally, the place for the use of psychopharmacology with some disorders is well recognised. Whilst individual practice remains variable these differences are not specific to inpatient work. However, it is likely that when working with the severe end of the spectrum in terms of psychopathology, that the use of psychopharmacology will be higher in inpatient practice than in outpatient practice. This is particularly true for the use of neuroleptics, as many adolescents with early onset psychosis will be admitted to an adolescent unit for assessment and treatment. On the other hand, occasionally admission to an adolescent unit can enable assessment and containment of quite worrying symptomatology without recourse to medication in the first instance. This can be particularly helpful when assessing adolescents presenting with a depressive disorder, where the evidence for the efficacy of medication is weak and when admission may result in a resolution of many of the symptoms suggesting a large environmental component to that individual's difficulties.

STAFFING

Multidisciplinary teams will contain representatives from some or all of the following professions: psychiatrists, psychiatric nurses, social workers, psychologists and teachers. There will usually be administrative, secretarial staff and caretakers. Other specialist input may be provided by psychotherapists, creative therapists such as art, drama or music therapists, occupational therapists and research and academic staff. Each of these disciplines may also have trainees passing through the unit for limited periods. In addition, some units will employ unqualified staff, such as psychology graduates wishing to gain clinical experience.

All adolescent units will have their own unique mix of the above staff, both in proportions and in absolute numbers. Although there are no guidelines as to how many staff are needed for a typical adolescent unit, in the US the American Academy of Child and Adolescent Psychiatry (1990) has drawn up some recommendations for ratios of staff to patients depending on the levels of therapy being employed, the need for observation, the time of day, etc. Whilst no such guidance is available from any professional body in the UK, work is currently underway to provide this (Green et al., 1998).

Most adolescent units will have enough nursing staff to provide care and therapeutic input 24 h a day. This will inevitably result in nurses out-numbering most other disciplines, and perhaps being seen, and seeing themselves, as the core of the unit. Although smaller in numbers, psychiatrists and teachers are commonly the other key professionals. Whilst the doctors and nurses share some medical training and experience within the Health Service, a teacher's professional background is quite separate. In terms of their roles, it generally falls upon the nursing staff to provide day to day care and containment for the adolescents, as well as, to a greater or lesser extent, specific therapeutic activities. Psychiatrists tend to take on the role of assessing the more disturbed mental health problems, including mental state assessments. They may also take on a leadership role, with clinical responsibility resting with a consultant psychiatrist. However, leadership is sometimes shared by senior professionals of different disciplines.

The roles of teachers and the importance of schooling varies quite considerably between adolescent units. In some units the schooling may be set up quite separately by a team of teachers who are solely involved in the educational side of the service. In other units, schooling takes on a smaller role and the teachers are involved in a range of activities around the unit.

Social workers can have a particular role in liasing with social services departments over accommodation issues for 'looked after' adolescents and should have expertise in child protection matters. Psychologists can provide psychometric assessments and often have particular therapeutic skills, such as in cognitive-behaviour therapy or cognitive-analytic therapy. The primary role of other staff such as psychotherapists, art and drama therapists, administrative and secretarial staff is clearly suggested by their professional title.

The way the rest of the work, including assessments, second opinions, general milieu therapy and specific therapies, such as individual, group and family therapy is allocated, depends partly on the philosophy of the unit and partly on the skills of the individuals involved. In some units this work may be divided up irrespective of profession or discipline, whereas in others professions such as psychiatrists, psychologists and social workers may take the lead in carrying out assessments and specific therapies.

A particular danger can be to give too much of the responsibility for the general milieu therapy to the untrained or least-skilled members of staff without adequate supervision. Such staff can sometimes befriend residents, becoming the preferred therapist, but as the least skilled and experienced there is a risk of them transgressing boundaries. It is, therefore, vital that such staff are given training and a high level of supervision early in their employment.

STAFF GROUP DYNAMICS IN THE MULTIDISCIPLINARY TEAM

'In the broad field of adolescent psychiatry, there is work, multidisciplinary work and team work' (Steinberg, 1986). In the preface to his book *The Adolescent Unit*, Steinberg goes on to point out that whilst there is sometimes a belief that these terms should be considered synonymously, there are significant risks in doing so. For example, the 'tyranny of the team' or the wish for a united approach at all costs, can sometimes result in a individual professional's skills or talents being suppressed. On the other hand, a group of professionals in an adolescent unit all 'doing their own thing' may lead to chaos and loss of any sense of safety or security. So is there a middle path or compromise between these two extremes? Well, probably there is, but nonetheless, this issue often exercises a considerable amount of staff time within many adolescent units.

Multidisciplinary working raises other issues and dilemmas. How can different professional philosophies and theoretical models be reconciled, for example viewing problems as social dysfunction or 'illness'? Are all team members entitled to an equal say, from the unqualified health care assistant to the consultant psychiatrist? If not, how are 'team decisions' made? Do some professions have 'special' expertise in some areas, and can this be accepted by others?

In practice there is no easy answer to these questions and no single pattern of teamwork or multidisciplinary working which is universally applicable, acceptable or desirable. So, just as it can be helpful to draw on both social dysfunction and illness models to help understand an adolescent's difficulties, it can be helpful to bring the skills of different professions to bear on the problem. Hence, inter-professional respect for different ways of thinking and working, and a collaborative ethos has to be an ideal worth striving for and preferable to a solely generic or egalitarian approach.

A key component to good multidisciplinary team functioning is clear and open communication. Regular and frequent meetings are needed involving as many of the staff team as possible, or at least representatives of the different disciplines, to discuss all aspects of the work from management issues and unit philosophy, to the day to day clinical work in the therapeutic milieu. Such practice gives a good opportunity for disagreements to be aired and hopefully resolved, and reduces the risk of splits in the staff team. Whilst this may all sound obvious, because of its time-consuming nature, it is not surprising how easy it is to neglect.

An important factor in team functioning is how the staff deal with the primitive ego defence mechanisms of the adolescent group, in particular projections and splitting. Staff group dynamics can sometimes reflect those of the resident group. It can be helpful to consider this, particularly when a tension or disagreement emerges in the staff group that has no more obvious explanation. In addition, individual adolescents may evoke feelings or patterns of interacting between staff that replicate their experiences from within their own family. An extreme, but not uncommon, example may be an adolescent who has been abused within their family evoking feelings of anger or uncomfortable sexual feelings in some staff. This may be confusing and difficult to deal with, particularly for the untrained and least experienced staff and it is, therefore, essential that opportunities are given for such feelings to be talked about openly or in supervision.

A forum which many adolescent units use to address some of the issues arising out of multidisciplinary team working and staff dynamics is the 'staff group'. Sometimes referred to as the 'staff support group' or 'sensitivity group', it can provide an opportunity for the staff to pause and reflect on their work, and the effect it has had on them. It also gives a chance to think about how people are getting on working as a team or individually and reflect on whether the balance seems right. Such a group can give a message to all in the unit, both staff and residents, that group work is important and valued, and not just something 'done to' the adolescents!

ISSUES OF LEADERSHIP

Any organisation requires leadership. This may be provided by an individual or shared, elected or appointed. It is hard to avoid and even if leadership appears to be shared, it is usually because an individual with the authority chooses for it to be so. Leadership encompasses many roles including:

- Dealing with the interface between the outside world and the unit
- Facilitating team and multidisciplinary working
- Providing a vision for the service
- Offering theories and models for working
- Containing staff anxiety

All of these roles are important and some are touched on elsewhere in this chapter, but it is worth commenting further on the issue of containing staff anxiety. Often anxiety focuses on a dilemma faced when making a difficult decision – such as whether or not to use restraint with a disturbed adolescent. This process has to be a balance between providing clarity (of philosophy, structure and hierarchy), which if too extreme can be stifling, and space to think creatively, but not without some boundaries. Ideally, staff should feel that they will be supported in making some decisions, feel able to share responsibility for others, and ultimately expect their leader to help make or take responsibility for the most difficult.

There are different styles of leadership, each of which has implications for the roles described above. The style favoured here broadly agrees with that described by Lampen (1986). An individual leader who encourages autonomy and initiative taking by staff internally, but taking a high degree of personal responsibility with regards to the outside world. Internal decision making can also include a degree of client participation. Good communication is important to facilitate such a style.

Alternatives include a more directive style of leadership, leadership from the front. Such a style runs the danger of being demotivating for the staff, whilst the leader bears the pressures of the staffs projections. At the other end of the spectrum is leadership by committee or by democracy. Whilst this may seem ideal, interpersonal relationships can interfere with such a system making the decision process time consuming and unclear. It also runs the risk that no one person attends to the boundaries between internal and external pressures.

EVIDENCE-BASED PRACTICE AND OUTCOMES

GENERAL

Adolescent units have not, at least until recently, been good examples of evidence-based practice. Assessment of the quality of treatment in adolescent units have been addressed through measures of referrer satisfaction (Gowers *et al.*, 1991) and reviews of general outcomes of series of admissions. A study of consumer views of an adolescent service suggested that the factors which determine parents' and patients' satisfaction may vary with the nature of their difficulties and, in particular, their agreement with the referral (Gowers and Kushlick, 1992). Green *et al.* (1998), when looking for predictors of outcome in a children's psychiatric unit, found that a good therapeutic alliance with the child and positive ratings of engagement with the parents at follow-up correlated with a good outcome. It is likely that such a finding would also apply to adolescent units.

The development of routine clinical outcome measures, such as the Health of the Nation Outcome Scales for Child and Adolescents (HoNOSCA) (Gowers *et al.*, 1999), will potentially add to the outcome data available and help inform decisions on issues such as length of stay, and enable some degree of comparison between services. However, as yet there has been no randomised controlled trial comparing inpatient and outpatient treatment, and there is little good evidence about who can benefit most from inpatient treatment. In addition, further work is needed to disentangle which aspects of inpatient treatment are most useful.

SPECIFIC DISORDERS

A number of services have reported follow-up data on specific syndromes such as psychotic illness (Cawthron *et al.* 1994), obsessive-compulsive disorder (Bolton *et al*, 1996), eating disorders (North *et al*, 1997), and conduct and emotional disorder (Wells and Farragher, 1993). Although the outcome of these has often been quite good, particularly in comparison with the same presentations in adults, it is difficult to separate the effects of admission per se from other aspects of treatment.

CONCLUSIONS

Adolescent units find themselves in a demanding position. They are a scarce resource and a highly specialised one, expected to meet a huge range of needs. They generally cover an age range, e.g. 13–18 years, which includes youngsters at quite different developmental stages. They are usually expected to treat adolescents with the full range of psychiatric disorders. Sometimes they are called upon to support other agencies, such as social services and education, in containing a disturbed young person while other provision is obtained. Finally, they are expected to admit immediately when there is a crisis in the community, but at the same time provide an environment which is safe, containing and secure for those who need longer-term treatment.

Despite these challenges adolescent units are usually able to meet the vast majority of the varied demands made upon them. Often, the greatest criticism concerns an insufficiency of beds, with many adolescent units having to operate a waiting list for admission.

REFERENCES

American Academy of Child and Adolescent Psychiatry (1990) *Task Force on Adolescent Hospitalisation. Model for Minimum Staffing Patterns for Hospital Providing Acute Inpatient Treatment for Children and Adolescents with Psychiatric Illness*. Washington, DC: American Academy of Child and Adolescent Psychiatry.

American Psychiatric Association (1994) *Diagnostic and Statistical Manual of Mental Disorders*, 4th edn (DSM-IV). Washington, DC: American Psychiatric Association.

Bolton, J., Luckie, M. and Steinberg, D. (1996) Obsessive-compulsive disorder treated in adolescence: 14 long-term case histories. *Clinical Child Psychology and Psychiatry*, **1**, 409–430.

Bowlby, J. (1969/82) *Attachment and Loss*, vol. 1. London: Hogarth.

Bester, P. and Bailey, V. (1998) Child and adolescent psychiatric day units survey. Poster presentation at the *Royal College of Psychiatrists Child and Adolescent Section Annual Residential Meeting*, Bristol.

Cawthron, P., James, A., Dell, J. and Seegroatt, V. (1994) Adolescent onset psychosis. A clinical and outcome study. *Journal of Child Psychology and Psychiatry*, **35**, 1321–1332.

Cotgrove, A. (1997) Emergency admissions to a regional adolescent unit: piloting a new service. *Psychiatric Bulletin*, **21**, 604–608.

Cotgrove, A., Zirinsky, L., Black, D. and Weston, D. (1995) Secondary prevention of attempted suicide in adolescence. *Journal of Adolescence*, **18**, 569–577

Gowers, S. and Kushlick, A. (1992) Customer satisfaction in adolescent psychiatry. *Journal of Mental Health*, **1**, 353–362

Gowers, S., Symington, R. and Entwistle, K. (1991) Who needs an adolescent unit? A referrer satisfaction study. *Psychiatric Bulletin*, **15**, 537–540.

Gowers, S., Harrington, R. C., Whitton, A., Lelliot, P., Wing, J., Beevor, A. *et al.* (1999) Brief scale for measuring the outcomes of emotional and behavioural disorders in children. Health of the Nation Outcome Scales for Children and Adolescents. *British Journal of Psychiatry*, **174**, 413–416.

Green, J., Jacobs, B. and Jaffa, T. (1998) *Guidance for the Staffing of Child and Adolescent Inpatient Units*. Draft proposal submitted to the Royal College of Psychiatrists.

Green, J., Kroll, L., Imrie, D., Francis, F. M., Begun, K., Gannon, L. *et al.* (1998) Health gain and predictors of outcome in in-patient and day-patient child psychiatric treatment. Poster presentation at the *Royal College of Psychiatrists Child and Adolescent Section Annual Residential Meeting*, Bristol.

Hawton, K., Arensman, E., Townsend, E., Breminer, S., Feldman, E. and Goldney, R. (1998) Deliberate self-harm: a systematic review of efficacy of psychosocial and pharmacological treatments in preventing repetition. *British Medical Journal*, **317**, 441–447.

Health Advisory Service (1986) *Bridges over Troubled Water.* London: DHSS

Health Advisory Service (1995) *Together We Stand.* London: HMSO

Lampen, J. (1986) Aspects of Leadership. In D. Steinberg (ed.), *The Adolescent Unit.* Chichester: Wiley, pp. 179–191.

North, C., Gowers, S. and Byram, V. (1997) Family functioning and life events in the outcome of adolescent anorexia nervosa. *British Journal of Psychiatry*, **171**, 545–549

Offord, D. R., Boyle, M. H., Szatmari, P., Rae-Grout, N., Links, P. S. and Cadman, D. T. (1987) Ontario child Health Study II: six month prevalence of disorder and rates of service utilisation. *Archives of General Psychiatry*, **44**, 832–834.

Parry-Jones, W. (1995) The future of adolescent psychiatry, *British Journal of Psychiatry*, **166**, 299–305.

Patrick, M., Hobson, R. P. and Castle, D. (1994) Personality disorder and mental representation. *Journal of Development and Psychopathology*, **6**, 375–388.

Rutter, M., Graham, P., Chadwick, O. and Yule, W. (1976) Adolescent turmoil: fact or fiction? *Journal of Child Psychology and Psychiatry*, **17**, 35–56.

Steinberg, D. (1994) Adolescent Services. In M. Rutter, E. Taylor and L. Hersov (eds), *Child and Adolescent Psychiatry.* Oxford: Blackwell Science, pp 1006–1022.

Steinberg, D. (1986) *The Adolescent Unit.* Chichester: Wiley.

Wells, P. and Farragher, B. (1993) In-patient treatment of 165 adolescents with emotional and conduct disorder. A study of outcome. *British Journal of Psychiatry*, **162**, 345–352

World Health Organisation (1992). *The ICD-10 Classification of Mental and Behaviour Disorders. Clinical Descriptions and Diagnostic Guidelines.* Geneva: World Health Organisation.

Chapter 15

TREATMENT IN NON-PSYCHIATRIC SETTINGS

Mary Eminson

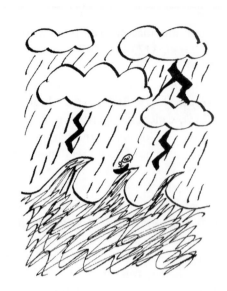

INTRODUCTION

Other chapters in this book have addressed the way in which adolescents with various problems use health services and the implication that this has for clinical practice with different client groups. Thus the chapters on substance abuse (Chapter 6), forensic services (Chapter 16), adolescents and health care (Chapter 11), and treatment in primary and secondary services (Chapter 13) refer to a range of non-psychiatric settings in which mental health inputs (assessment and treatments) may be delivered. Several other chapters deal with specific conditions (e.g. depression) which are also relevant in the groups of patients discussed here. The focus of this chapter is in describing the needs of adolescents who are found in three further non-psychiatric arenas: in secondary and tertiary medical settings (especially hospitals) in both paediatric and adult medical services ('paediatric' will be used for simplicity here), in specialist educational provision of various kinds, including residential schools, and those in the care of the local authority.

GENERAL CONSIDERATIONS

These special circumstances, of work in non-psychiatric settings, require child and adolescent mental health service (CAMHS) professionals to adapt their thinking and approach if they are truly to provide a service to these adolescents; and this means more than sometimes offering appointments away from a clinic base. Although 'treatment' is used in the title, the work in these settings is not confined to face to face contact with young people: the other important elements are various forms of input with groups of professionals. 'Liaison-consultation' and 'consultative work' are the overall terms used for this: terms that are used in broad and quite different ways by different authors. 'Liaison-consultation' describes a range of working relationships and practices between CAMHS and non-CAMHS services, for the explicit benefit of the latter. Liaison contacts may include senior management and junior workers, and direct and indirect work with the client groups of the non-CAMHS professionals, as well as direct work with staff.

'Consultation' here is used to refer to one aspect of liaison work, summarised by Steinberg and Yule (1985) as 'the activity undertaken when one professional worker (the consultant) helps another (the consultee) with a problem or an issue in the consultee's work. The approach has a number of special characteristics. First, the emphasis is on helping the consultee make the most effective use of his own experience, skills and resources. The consultant does not take over responsibility for the child. Second, the consultee remains autonomous in deciding on whether or not to use what emerges from the consultation. Third, the consultant has no formal authority over the consultee, and their relationship is one of mutual and equal collaboration. . .'.

'These three features of consultation reflect a number of fundamental assumptions. In the first place, although both the consultant and consultee may have some training and experience in common, say of child development, it is the *consultee's* knowledge and skills that are mobilised to help the child. Thus, a psychiatrist or psychologist acting as a consultant to a school or children's home does not presume to have expertise in classroom management or residential child care. Rather, the consultant emphasises that these skills are rightly those of the consultee, although they may be enhanced by discussions of children's behaviour or of group dynamics. A second assumption is that by helping the consultee clarify problems and formulate possible solutions, the consultant is helping the consultee to be more effective in dealing with similar problems in the future. In other words, consultation is not only a problem-solving approach, but one which contributes to prevention through a process of professional development and education.' (Steinberg and Yule, 1985).

The issue of responsibility for any decisions or actions taken following discussion with the 'consultant' may require further clarification and should always be explored thoroughly before liaison-consultation arrangements are set up. Obviously, if a mental health professional is undertaking face to face work, they have professional responsibility for this. Equally clearly, if a non-CAMHS professional uses a 'consultant' to reflect and gain understanding, the consultee is responsible for their own learning. An area of greater uncertainty exists when a consultee asks a consultant's advice about undertaking specific interventions (some forms of counselling of a young person, perhaps) or about specific behaviours (sexual interest or the assessment of self-harming behaviour, for example). In these circumstances all parties must be clear about the training and skills of the consultee, and their clinical and managerial arrangements; this includes such issues as whether the young person concerned and their family are aware that they are being discussed with a professional outside the organisation (or part of the organisation) to which they usually relate. The limits of the consultee's confidence, qualification for the task, level of skill and responsibility may need careful analysis in individual circumstances – time well spent to ensure good practice and to protect the client/patient, consultee and consultant.

ADOLESCENTS IN SECONDARY AND TERTIARY MEDICAL CARE SETTINGS: PAEDIATRIC LIAISON

'Paediatric liaison', which is how hospital paediatric work is usually described, has a long and honourable tradition in child and adolescent psychiatry, in part because of the medical links between paediatricians and psychiatrists, but also because the psychological needs of physically sick children have in the past been afforded high priority. It is a term which may be used very broadly. '. . .Paediatric liaison work is used to mean all consultations, diagnostic, therapeutic, teaching, support and research activities carried out by psychiatrists and other mental health professionals in paediatric clinics or on paediatric wards.' (Lask, 1994). Here it is restricted to clinical work carried out directly with medical patients or inputs from clinicians to paediatric health service staff which are to assist them in coping with patients, rather than research or formal teaching.

DISTRICT PAEDIATRIC SERVICES

Recently, the focus of new CAMHS development has shifted to unmet need in other groups of young people and being in 'the community' is seen as ideologically more sound than working in hospital. Even generic district paediatric services are, however, likely to see higher rates of psychiatric disorder than are seen in the general population; in general paediatric outpatients, rates of psychiatric disorder are 30–40% (Garralda and Bailey, 1989). There are also good clinical reasons why the need for paediatric liaison inputs continues to rise: factors which are likely to be increasing the prevalence of psychiatric illness in all hospital attendees. Rates of deliberate self-harm in teenagers have been rising (albeit less so recently). Rates of substance misuse in early adolescents continue to rise. Poverty and socioeconomic deprivation are associated with increased rates of hospital admission (Ryan et al., 1995) and with increased risk taking, amongst other health risks (McKee, 1999).

As a result, the district paediatric ward and outpatient clinics are where many common psychiatric disorders present. The main groups include:

- Physical presentations of psychiatric illnesses: psychosomatic disorders, depression and anxiety presenting with physical symptoms, losses of function in dissociative disorders; adolescents with eating disorders: all may first come to attention through paediatricians.
- A variety of adjustment, mood, conduct and relationship difficulties may present with self-harm, most commonly 'overdoses' of analgesics or other medication, but also through intoxication with drink or drugs.
- Common chronic childhood illnesses such as diabetes and asthma, usually managed at a district level, provide extra stress upon both individual and family functioning which may increase the risk of adjustment and emotional disorder in vulnerable adolescents: the need to adhere to a regular treatment regime may provide the focus for adolescent 'acting out', with consequent problems in medical management. Furthermore, these common illnesses which constrain adolescent autonomy in the way diabetes and epilepsy may do can occur in any family. When such conditions develop in a young person who has a pre-existing severe conduct or attachment disorder, or autistic spectrum difficulties (or, indeed, any pre-existing psychiatric disorder), or in a family with other significant difficulties, problems in managing the illness can be expected.
- Hyperkinetic, conduct and attachment disorders are associated with risk taking in adolescence so that amongst young people who have accidents, including those with drug and alcohol intoxication, head injuries, and broken bones, one can expect an excess of boys particularly with these diagnoses; which may not necessarily have been recognised previously.

The roles of mental health professionals in medical non-psychiatric settings can be very substantial, depending on resources, relationships with the ward team (nurses, paediatricians and others) and mutual respect. Cottrell and Worrall (1995) identified five types of clinical work: an emergency service, psychosocial ward rounds, consultation on individual cases and groups of cases, joint work with paediatricians and others, in addition to direct referrals. In a district service, many of the paediatric presentations of psychiatric disorders require simple recognition and a transfer of care to the appropriate CAMHS professional, so that there may be little that is special about the setting. However, for most of those whose psychiatric disorder presents medically this represents some form of difficulty with a more direct verbal expression of psychological problems; this is the case for many more extensive psychosomatic presentations (see Chapter 10). In these cases, particularly, paediatric staff are crucial intermediaries in the negotiation of a psychiatric assessment. Their attitude, both to the patients and to the mental health team, will affect the likelihood of psychiatric referral being accepted and welcomed, and may also subtly affect the treatment the young person receives on the ward and the sympathy or otherwise with which they are managed. Working with paediatric staff themselves, as well as jointly clinically, is likely to continue in many cases both in the ward and through various forms of treatment/follow-up. Throughout, the paediatric team must maintain an understanding of psychosomatic and other psychiatric 'presentations', so that both teams can facilitate each others' work. Even for the most common and straightforward parts of the emergency service (risk assessments following self-harm), the quality and integration of patient care improves if there is good understanding of the issues in such behaviour, the pressures on each service and the skills of the different health service professionals.

Another taxing CAMHS role is in those cases, such as the uncontrolled diabetic or adolescent with a combination of severe epilepsy with factitious seizures, where the mental health problem is having a profound effect on the management of the organic illness. The physical illness and its treatment may have become the focus for enacting relationship difficulties and displaying individual psycho-pathology: so some diabetics use their insulin as a way to lose weight, or repeatedly fail to control diet or blood sugar with life threatening results. These cases call for the most skilled continuing input from both teams and demand the most trusting working relationships. Sometimes the adolescent and their family are unable or unwilling to engage with psychiatric help, or the psychological problem itself (severe relationship and conduct problems perhaps) is very difficult to treat. In these circumstances the CAMHS team role may become that of offering direct help which is repeatedly unsuccessful or refused, leaving only the role of supporting the paediatric team and offering understanding of the difficulties. Frustrations from the case itself sometimes attach to the 'useless' psychiatrist in these circumstances. Beyond these three roles, the extent to which more extensive liaison services, such as joint clinics or psychosocial ward rounds, exist in district paediatric settings is very varied and depends on resources and often on personalities. This is an area with clear potential for development which may include joint community paediatric and mental health services, e.g. to provide an integrated response to adolescents with attention deficit hyperactivity disorder (ADHD) or autistic spectrum and other learning disabilities.

SPECIALIST AND TERTIARY PAEDIATRIC SERVICES

Specialist paediatric services have a population with needs over and above those identified in district services (Mrazek, 1985). It has long been established that rates of disorder are increased amongst the chronically physically sick as a group (Pless *et al.*, 1989) and that such risks may be particularly high when the brain is involved (Breslau, 1985). Thus the adolescent age group contains many young people who have severe and sometimes disfiguring conditions: epilepsy, neurofibromatosis, chronic orthopaedic and rheumatology problems affecting the skeleton and limbs, dwarfing syndromes, to name but a few. As survival rates of children with major life-threatening illnesses [cancer, cardiac, respiratory (including cystic fibrosis), gastrointestinal, renal and hepatic conditions, burns, head injuries, extreme prematurity, brain tumours] continue to improve, the population of young people entering adolescence with potential psychological handicaps also increases. A multiplicity of health and other professionals are likely to be involved in their care (27 non-CAMHS professionals were listed in one review by Cottrell and Worrell, 1995). Adolescence is itself a stage when rates of psychological disorders tend to rise, quite apart from the extra vulnerability caused by physical disease processes, their treatment or their emotional impact. Studies of psychological difficulties in the severely chronically sick reflect the way in which paediatric services are organised (i.e. around particular diseases and organ systems) and even the most rigorous studies (Garralda *et al.*, 1988) may quickly become out of date if medical practice changes in that field. The psychosocial support services provided for these specialist teams are often determined on the basis of historical working relationships and sometimes charitable funding rather than from a more scientific analysis of mental health needs in that group of children.

This chapter is not the place for a comprehensive review of the sources of adolescent and family psychiatric disorder arising in all chronic illnesses, which must be inferred from an analysis of the studies of psychological disorders in the various disease groups, and from audit of the physical and cognitive handicaps of children seen within services (Goodman and Graham, 1996; North and Eminson, 1998) combined with a knowledge of vulnerability factors for psychiatric disorders in the age group. These studies suggest the chronically sick may benefit from the specific skills of *many* members of the CAMHS team (psychiatrist, psychologist, psychotherapist, including expertise in psychopharmacology, and those with therapeutic skills in family, cognitive, behavioural and psychodynamic approaches), although such needs may not always be recognised.

Of course, some conditions will be common to all the disease groups which receive substantial medical interventions: specific phobias of needles, anxiety about other procedures, adjustment reactions following stressful illness phases and procedures such as major surgery, fears of sickness and death, failure to adhere to the increasingly complex treatment regimes, and learning and school problems consequent upon interruption of schooling. Equally, research into common coping and resilience factors will also generalise across disease groups (Eiser, 1993). These issues are often addressed most effectively by a combination of nursing and psychologist inputs.

As an example of liaison work, the range of problems faced by a paediatric nephrology service are explored here, to illustrate the interplay of staff and patient issues and how service delivery may be effected.

A SPECIALIST SERVICE EXAMPLE: PAEDIATRIC LIAISON NEEDS IN PAEDIATRIC NEPHROLOGY

Paediatric nephrology services now contain many adolescents who would not, in the past, have survived into the age group and who if in 'end-stage' renal failure (ESRF) are constrained, not only by an exacting dietary and medication regime, but sometimes by the requirements of dialysis several times a week. The increasing trend to identify renal disease in pregnancy, which facilitates early intervention, has resulted in life-saving treatment being offered to those who may have very substantial physical and cognitive difficulties, sometimes very unusual ones. This in turn may have a profound effect upon attachments, consequent upon an understanding of the child's difficulties, from disruption of early relationships through illness, hospitalisation and threat of loss including the loss of the healthy baby for which the parents hoped. A proportion of children in ESRF will have substantial short stature as a result of their illness (and sometimes its treatment with steroids), requiring daily injection treatment with growth hormone and some also have congenital physical abnormalities in the urogenital area or have acquired urinary diversions of various kinds. The combination of these various inherited and acquired disabilities is a profound challenge to any adolescent and their family. Simultaneously, they must attempt to negotiate the developmental tasks of this age group in the areas of self-esteem, peer group relationship skills, academic attainments, sexual development and acquisition of independence. In addition, many face the possibilities of increasing problems with venous access, multiple operations, transplant loss, deterioration and death which may follow failed treatment, or worsening of the underlying disease. Premature death remains a real possibility. Such illnesses and treatments place enormous pressures and demands upon the family, who may find times of change between different sorts of treatment (starting dialysis or receiving a transplant) particularly stressful, and likely to have an impact on parental mental health (Garralda *et al.*, 1988) and on the marital relationship. In the functioning of parents at these times there may be difficulties in ordinary boundary and limit setting when faced with an adolescent with a life-threatening illness.

Finally, a new sort of family stress has arisen for some from the possibility of donation of a kidney by family members (living related donation) which has increased the pressure on parents and siblings to donate an organ. This includes a need for the accompanying surgery, potential long-term risk to the donor's health and an added sense of 'owing' in the recipient – especially burdensome in those with poor treatment adherence if for any reason the transplant fails.

Some of the 'psychiatric' or mental health difficulties in association with ESRF at this developmental stage are summarised in Table 15.1.

ORGANISATION OF SERVICES

DIRECT WORK WITH ADOLESCENTS AND FAMILIES

It is a challenge to combine all the usual skills of a CAMHS team with a method of service delivery which respects the demands and priorities of patients and families, and with a knowledge of the physical difficulties of the speciality – the

Table 15.1 Psychological conditions and reactions in a paediatric nephrology service

- Attachment disorders
- Adjustment reactions of many kinds: responses to changes in intensity of treatment demands, anxiety about treatment, mood changes in response to awareness of the impact and meaning of the illness, including concern about survival
- Anxiety and depressive disorders – to which there may be inherited vulnerability
- Conduct problems usually expressed as oppositionality and acting out through the illness, rather than as antisocial behaviour
- Threats to self-esteem; concerns about size, appearance and function as an adolescent both generally and sexually
- Eating disorders, usually of a non-specific kind
- Self-harming urges (acted upon through manipulation of medication or dialysis equipment)
- Difficulties in peer group relations as a consequence of differences in size, appearance, ability, consistency of school attendance and physical frailty (a particular issue for boys)
- Increased risk of organic psychosis
- Cognitive functioning may be affected acutely and/or chronically leading to failure to achieve academically

Family and parental issues
- Disturbance of early relationships contributing to attachment problems
- Parental mood and other problems in response to the burden of illness, its emotional impact and the effect on relationships
- Illness demands overwhelm parental competence resulting in poor treatment adherence, resulting in further parental guilt and sometimes rejection of the child
- Difficulties in managing sibling relationships and demands
- Over-protectiveness may make it difficult to allow the development of autonomy
- Stress upon marital relationships

tension between input from an 'expert' or a 'familiar' member of the CAMHS team may sometimes be present. The setting in which the patients find themselves, of a very demanding illness with many appointments with different paediatric team members, reviews, blood tests and numerous admissions, mitigate against many adolescents and families being able to undertake extensively demanding conventional psychiatric treatment – the existing illness burdens are just too great. As a result, service delivery may be achieved at least in part by a number of other routes and depending how far away the family lives:

- Direct mental health contact with the adolescent may have to be curtailed to fit in with other times when they are visiting the hospital base: not always ideal psychologically but at least practical.
- Arrangements of convenience may need to be found, such as carrying out a group for adolescents which fits around their hospital visits for dialysis, or a holiday where adolescents are away together.
- The mental health professional may have to accept that assessment on one or two occasions only may be possible, and that further direct intervention may be curtailed or undertaken in a different way by a member of the paediatric team. This increases the importance of input to the paediatric staff.

GROUP WORK

Group work with adolescents has considerable potential and may be carried out by professionals from the paediatric team, the mental health team or a mixture of the two depending on the therapeutic skills and focus. Siblings and parents' groups too, with a variety of educational, self-help and general supportive roles, can be useful for dealing with many issues: again, the CAMHS team may share in running these or may perhaps offer help in setting up and supervision.

LIAISON-CONSULTATION TO ASSIST PAEDIATRIC STAFF TO WORK DIRECTLY WITH ADOLESCENTS

A key function of paediatric liaison work is to assist the paediatric team in a very demanding and difficult job with chronically and acutely sick young people in order to carry out what are, in the broadest terms, mental health interventions with specific patients and problems. For example, nursing staff may ask for help in carrying out treatment programmes to reduce fears about procedures, manage pain, explore mood states and help the family routines so that the young person can cope with their difficulties and adhere to the treatment regime – in adolescents, especially, the issues of autonomy and treatment adherence will probably be entwined. Sometimes these interventions will follow some initial direct assessment by a mental health specialist. Direct monitoring of mood swings and of psychotropic medication can be carried out in the same way. The social worker attached to a specialist team may be assisted to work in a more focused way on specific psychological issues with parents, siblings and families if an initial joint appointment with a mental health professional has helped with the formulation of the individual or systemic issues. Medical staff in outpatients may need to explore in a neutral way the extent of suicidal thoughts and poor treatment adherence. Working through the paediatric team in this way requires a careful assessment of their existing strengths and time to appraise circumstances where it would be more appropriate for a mental health specialist to undertake the work instead. Such input may also shade into formal education. Increasingly, many members of the multidisciplinary paediatric team are taking on many of these roles themselves and specialist teams, e.g. in pain management, are increasing in number.

OTHER ROLES WITH PAEDIATRIC STAFF

The second aspect of staff working in paediatric liaison is when it is the staff group themselves who are asking directly for help – either help to work out how, as a group, to respond to and manage particular behaviours of a patient (distress and acting out, refusal to accept treatment offered, threats to act dangerously to themselves or others) or help to cope with a decision or a family which is producing tension and discord in the staff group. This is an example of consultation which aims to help the staff group function better generally. All staff need to feel comfortable with helping families make difficult decisions and allowing them to display their grief and disappointment about the adolescent's burdensome illness, sometimes in angry and hostile ways.

Examples of other situations which polarise the staff group are when young patients with long and close contact with the team reach a crisis in their illness, necessitating decisions about whether and to what extent further medical intervention should be undertaken or whether palliative care should be considered. At such times, differences of opinion between parents and angry projections of their despair result in blaming particular members of staff, and may threaten to create severe splits in the staff team, who themselves have understandable differences of opinion about how active they should be. Discussion of the family's predicament and staff members' feelings helps to separate the two, to give a 'breathing space' where the staff can acknowledge the difficulties of their work and finds ways to support each other *and* the family. Often the staff are so closely involved with the family that maintenance of professional boundaries is difficult, especially when a child is dying. At these times the professional offering help to the staff team must be respected by all team members or the systemic work to assist them in negotiating these difficult times is impossible and splits are perpetuated. Specially convened liaison meetings of the most involved staff members may be necessary at such times.

Essentially, staff working closely, physically, intensely and over a long period with a group of severely sick children and families are assisted by having breathing space to reflect, absorb and make sense of the enormous emotional burden which results for the workers as well as the families themselves – CAMHS professionals standing outside these intense dynamics but with sufficient knowledge to understand them can help the team to function better by acknowledging the struggles. Building up trust between professionals is crucial and this usually means the paediatric team relates best to a small team of mental health professionals. Regular meetings away from the bedside and including different disciplines are often key ingredients – in some circumstances these are focused on individual patients ('psychosocial ward rounds') and sometimes on more general issues. Such meetings may not meet the needs of all staff at all levels and of seniority at the same time (North and Eminson, 1998) but they may provide a model which encourages the paediatric staff themselves to organise similar groups for other staff members, e.g. junior nurses.

The following case example includes direct and indirect work with a patient and staff in a complex situation where the liaison psychiatrist was in touch with the young person and the staff team over several years.

VIGNETTE: TARNIA

Tarnia was discussed with the liaison consultant on many occasions and formally referred by the paediatric nephrology team twice. The first time, when Tarnia was 12 years of age, was because of worries about her failure to achieve academically, causing concerns that this might be because she was depressed. There was also worry and concern about the timing of, and preparation of Tarnia for, genital surgery. The second referral, when Tarnia was 15, was because of increasing concerns about her withdrawal and unusual eating habits with weight loss.

Born with normal chromosomes (XX) but an abnormal renal and genital tract, Tarnia developed renal failure in early childhood and then suffered aluminium encephalopathy following dialysis, thus she also acquired moderate learning difficulties. Tarnia had many investigations and operations in early childhood. Her mother, a single parent, died when Tarnia was 10; she had no siblings and was taken in by her mother's partner. Relationships with the extended family network became increasingly strained with hostility and criticism towards Tarnia as her adolescence progressed. At school Tarnia made few friendships and achieved little, although her teachers were convinced she could achieve more. Although she had a ureterostomy and colostomy, in early adolescence Tarnia was relatively stable physically, but medical problems increased throughout her teens. A multi-axial classification system makes the complexity obvious; in addition to a diagnosis of depression and non-specific eating disorders on Axis I, codings on all the other axes were appropriate for Tarnia.

Involvement of the CAMHS team was different at various times in Tarnia's illness. A direct face to face diagnostic assessment was made when she was first referred at the age of 12, specifically to try and understand her withdrawal, and the inter-relationship of her various physical problems with her learning difficulties, her mood state and personality, all of course in the context of her unusual family setting. Direct contact with Tarnia as well as liaison with her school, educational psychologist, nurses both locally and in the paediatric nephrology team, and with her family was required. The initial face to face work involved understanding Tarnia's functioning, including helping her to understand the way her body worked. It was concluded that her rather passive approach to both school and her family had led staff to a greater concern about her having a low mood than was justified when talking to Tarnia herself, although she had a number of questions about her physical functioning and some very ordinary dissatisfactions about family life.

Following the assessments, direct work was undertaken by the liaison psychiatrist by coordinating meetings with family and with education staff from Tarnia's home area. More formal psychometric testing was arranged (which enlightened all concerned about her level of abilities) and two sessions were used to explore concerns with Tarnia and her 'father'. These two sessions allowed the consultant to help both the professional network and the family subsequently by direct discussion and explanation of Tarnia's moods and concerns, and how these were displayed.

A second key area for the nephrology team arose because there were tensions between ward-based and community nursing staff about whether and when Tarnia should receive reconstructive genital surgery. Ward staff were acutely aware of Tarnia's shyness and sensitivity about her body, and thought that she should have surgery soon. Community staff saw Tarnia as having adjusted relatively well to her substantial problems and thought intervention was unnecessary. This left the medical staff caught between the different views, attempting to talk about a sensitive issue, in which they had little or no training, with Tarnia and her step-father who were both reluctant to discuss it.

This conflict was addressed in one of the regular liaison meetings with the whole staff group, leading to increased understanding of two issues: the way in which each group's perspective inevitably led to different conclusions and the way in which their differences of opinion left medical staff feeling under great pressure to resolve them, yet also incompetent to do so. At the end of the meeting it was possible to make a plan for the staff team to allow Tarnia's thoughts and feelings to be explored separately from her stepfather's, in a way which respected her level of ability and understanding. This in turn led to a discussion of the difficulties that professionals have when trying to make decisions about areas where they have little knowledge, but strongly held opinions. The team decided they needed to seek advice from people with experience of learning disabled teenagers' responses to genital surgery.

Following these interventions, both psychological and physical care of Tarnia proceeded relatively smoothly for about 2 years. Then, when Tarnia was 15 she started eating less, became more withdrawn again and there was a report that family relationships were more strained. Tarnia's stepfather had in the intervening years acquired a new partner and relationship difficulties seemed to have gradually developed from this point; in addition Tarnia's physical health was declining.

During the course of a long admission to the specialist centre, Tarnia's eating had gradually become less. Assessing her again directly it was evident that she had become quite severely depressed as a combination of family, academic and physical difficulties had come together. Whilst in hospital Tarnia was seen by the CAMHS team members. Liaison work was to assist both ward and subsequently community nursing staff to monitor Tarnia's eating and her mood, and help her family with a sensible eating plan, to ensure that her school made opportunities available for eating

lunch with her peers and to assist Tarnia's support at school by intervention from the school nurse.

Sessions of formal family therapy were undertaken to address the
relationship issues that seemed to be so troubling. Discussion and consultation was also held with the team social worker to consider the impact that
the family difficulties and relationships were having upon Tarnia and the
resulting level of harm. The possibility was considered that Tarnia needed
time away from her 'family', perhaps with a substitute or foster family on
occasion. Again this reappraisal of the difficulties, with active intervention to
try and support Tarnia in school and at home, seemed to improve matters to
some extent.

Quite apart from the direct work with Tarnia and her family, and also the
interventions to involve paediatric nephrology staff in forms of monitoring
and other intervention, this case involved a strong sense of sharing with a
nephrology team over several years their distress and difficulty in decision
making for a teenager whose lot in life was so unfair. Tarnia never underwent
the genital surgery which had provoked so much concern and dissension; she
died in late adolescence as a result of her renal disease.

ROLES WITH OTHER PAEDIATRIC SPECIALITIES

The examples given within the paediatric nephrology service are by no means
exhaustive – each specialised area of paediatrics will provide particular sources of
psychological and psychiatric vulnerability consequent upon the specific conditions and their treatment. In general, services for young people with the most
extensive brain involvement in their illness (paediatric neurology and neurosurgery most obviously) will also provide the most complex neuropsychiatric
problems, e.g. organic psychoses, together with adolescents suffering the
behavioural and attentional problems consequent upon brain disorders or injuries
– many of these will be chronic problems. Other services such as haematology and
oncology will provide a greater component of bereavement work. Finally, it
should not be forgotten that tertiary paediatric services, especially surgical ones,
are also the places where the most extreme forms of factitious illness by proxy
(parentally fabricated, invented or induced illness) will be found. These forms of
family dysfunction and abuse tend to be referred on to tertiary centres when local
paediatric services have failed to clarify the presentation and complaints – the
CAMHS liaison team is important here as a sounding board and psychological
'second opinion' whilst full appraisal of such cases is made (see Chapter 10), and
may also be used after recognition of abuse, to support staff (especially nursing
staff) whose trust in parents' good intentions has been damaged (Lloyd and
MacDonald, 2000).

LIAISON AND CONSULTATION WITH SOCIAL SERVICES

Although the analogy between paediatric liaison work and mental health input in social services settings may not seem obvious, the similarities are greater than they initially appear. Indeed the general considerations at the beginning of this chapter with issues of responsibility and role are of equal, if not greater relevance than in health service settings.

In health service settings, however, there is usually general understanding about the training and backgrounds of the various professionals, and sometimes a level of shared experience; the lines of responsibility and accountability are usually clear, the rules about how information is recorded and exchanged, and about patient confidentiality, are part of agreed and understood systems, and often the management is a shared one. This is quite different when working with non-health professionals and the room for misunderstandings of all kinds is correspondingly increased. An acute and difficult situation with a disturbed young person is the most likely scenario to reveal failures or gaps in the managerial and operational policies between agencies – time and patience in setting up crystal clear arrangements between agencies is never wasted.

The local authority's key task with children and adolescents is to secure their well-being and protect them from all types of harm. The child clients generally are 'children in need', usually defined at a number of levels of risk. The clients of social services have substantial levels of psychiatric disorder (McCann *et al.*, 1996), are particularly difficult to reach through direct, face to face contact with mental health services, and, as with paediatric liaison, the role of the mental health professionals includes helping staff groups to use interventions directly as well as working better as a team in response to the difficulties of a young person. The range of psychological difficulties of adolescents accommodated outside the family home ('looked after' by the local authority in current terminology) is also somewhat different to that found in paediatric liaison, although a similarity is the increase in the severity and complexity of difficulties seen in the young people, by comparison with a generation ago.

THE CONTEXT

The primary efforts of social workers are to keep families together, and as a result only those from the most dysfunctional and abusive backgrounds, and those containing the most disturbed young people will be 'looked after'. Whilst in some areas there remain children's homes containing quite large groups of adolescents and staff; in other places small homes with perhaps three or four children and a similarly pared down staff team have become the norm. In all areas there is substantially greater use of foster families, who may have several fostered children and some of their own. Those whose substitute placements in foster homes or with other family members have failed will of course also be found in specialised children's homes (sometimes in the independent sector or in special individual arrangements). These different arrangements each produces their own different institutional dynamics, stresses and tensions.

Young people 'looked after' are at the heart of what is meant by 'treatment in non-psychiatric settings' for local authorities. A recent review of needs and services to meet them is a useful starting point when planning new approaches (Richardson and Jonghin, 2000). Numerically small (probably 100–200 adolescents in any one district), they are extremely costly in terms of their care and the impact that they have on services – neglected, and emotionally, physically and sexually abused to the extent that intervention to keep the family together has failed. The cardinal issue which dominates mental health services to adolescents who are the responsibility of the local authority is that the prior experiences of these young people have generally, over a long period, damaged their capacity for relationships. This damage interferes, of course, with their ability to use mental health interventions of all kinds directly (including psychopharmacology, although perhaps less than other approaches) but this impact is relatively trivial in most cases compared with the effects for all other relationships, especially in key settings such as the home/substitute home and with the substitute family or professional carer who is fulfilling this role. As a direct result of these damaged capacities, the young people may go on to create further difficulties and more instability and rejection in new situations. Thus the main thrust of CAMHS interventions to improve the mental well-being of these adolescents, can only be through improving the quality and stability of relationships around them. This perspective is not one which is shared by all who work in the field. Within local authorities there is often an almost religious belief in the value of individual dynamic and behavioural approaches with children and young people ('anger management', 'grief work'), and within child and adolescent psychiatry there have been recent efforts to withdraw from providing services except in a limited neuropsychiatric arena (Goodman, 1997). There are some arguments in favour of both of these points of view and limited resources in the past have perhaps understandably led CAMHS professionals to prioritise direct work with those with more easily measurable outcomes. Certainly there are no 'hard and fast' rules about which professions are best placed to provide help to the carers of 'looked after' young people in order to improve their lot. However, if the task of improving relationships in order to improve mental health is taken seriously, this dictates that core aspects of services must be focused around the groups of staff (foster carers or residential workers) who attempt to maintain relationships with young people day to day and must be with CAMHS professionals who are consistent and familiar. Thus, as in paediatric liaison, the nature of the client group has a profound effect on the way the service is organised and delivered.

RANGE OF DISORDERS

Attachment disorders are commonplace and by the time these young people reach adolescence, such early and severe difficulties will often be expressed through conduct disorders, including risk taking and excitement seeking in various forms, e.g. substance abuse and prostitution. Because of the disturbed and untrusting relationships formed by the adolescents, they are particularly difficult to help and their emotional reactions are also sudden and extreme at times: resulting in much self-harm and many distressed changes of mood. Some have extensive physical presentations with somatoform disorders and self-harm such as 'cutting' or overdoses. Many abused adolescents may have forms of mood and eating disorders, and some will have post-traumatic and other dissociative disorders.

TYPES OF INPUT WITH LOCAL AUTHORITY STAFF

STAFF LIAISON

It has been argued that the core provision must be through regular liaison between key CAMHS individuals and groups of local authority staff, most particularly around children's homes or foster homes, and that the key aim is to increase understanding and empathy together with skills in managing the relationship between the responsible adults and the individual clients.

Staff members are acting in the role of parent in relation to the adolescent: having to be an authority figure in terms of rules and boundaries, whilst also attempting to befriend and support, but without the depth and length of relationship which a biological parent has with their adolescent son or daughter. This quasi-parental role is also made more complex when carried out by young and inexperienced members of staff who have no experience of adolescent children of their own. Exploration of specific responses may involve searching out the client's background and experience: understanding the behaviours of groups of young people requires integration of thinking about adolescent developmental issues, and how these are affected both by family background and current interactions with peer group, school and authority figures.

Staff group liaison probably requires skills in formulating and sharing an understanding of individual psychodynamic and group processes, a systemic perspective, problem-solving and cognitive approaches – it is a task for a senior and extensively trained CAMHS professional. The sources of relevant literature on such consultation to institutions are correspondingly widely spread (Campbell et al., 1991; Mawson, 1994; Rifkind, 1995).

DIRECT SERVICE PROVISION TO YOUNG PEOPLE 'LOOKED AFTER'

Out of the core staff liaison may come opportunities for the liaison consultant to see individual adolescents with a variety of disorders and difficulties (see above) in various settings. An alternative is to facilitate referral of the young person (usually, with their carer) to another specific aspect of the CAMHS service – for consideration of medication for their ADHD, for more formal individual therapy or a problem-solving group for self-harming teenagers perhaps. As with paediatric liaison, no one CAMHS professional is sufficiently trained and expert to provide all these inputs, but the 'liaison' professional may be tempted to try to do so because of their acceptability to the staff and the difficulty of getting young people to services. These tensions are genuine and should not be ignored.

It is not necessary to assume that young people *cannot* use conventional adolescent mental health services provided in hospital or community clinics, although they may need quite a lot of support to do so (as do many adolescents living in their families of origin). Anecdotal experience suggests that for some young people with a long history of contact with the local authority, skilled and thoughtful input in a setting and from a professional who is clearly independent of any decisions about their placement, behaviour or family gives them a welcome opportunity to make a fresh start in therapeutic relationships. Both group and individual interventions may be helpful in a CAMHS setting, either by the liaison consultant or another team member.

Many other services (substance abuse, youth justice, 'drop-in' and counselling services including contraceptive and sexual health clinics) and settings (in primary care, youth facilities, schools and colleges) also have a role in providing information, assessment and treatment relevant to 'looked after' young people's mental health needs. Good communication between all these services is essential if input is not to become fragmentary and confusing for the young person.

FORMAL EDUCATION

In addition to regular liaison-consultation meetings with a staff team, which have both clinical and educational purposes regularly combined, more formal and systematic staff education by the liaison consultant and others is a further way to improve the quality of young people's relationships. Courses in cognitive-behavioural approaches and in systemic and psychodynamic formulation, with an understanding of the nature and effects of attachment disorders, all tailored to the particular client group, have been delivered with positive responses and measured effectiveness. Foster parents may also be included in developments of this kind as well as in more general educational courses about adolescent development, mental health difficulties, and their treatment and prevention. Youth offending teams' needs for 'parenting' courses (essentially understanding adolescents' emotional and behavioural difficulties and their management) may also have an overlap with the needs of some local authority staff and foster parents, and there is much potential for development and systematic evaluation of such inputs.

OTHER LOCAL AUTHORITY TEAMS

Social work fieldwork, child protection, and learning and physical 'disability' teams are organised differently in various parts of the country but will also be working with a client group of adolescents with substantial difficulties, often in their own homes. Many of these young people are known to numerous agencies, and it is the coordination and integration of multi-disciplinary work between professionals from education, health and local authority which is a key issue. These young people are in families which are often struggling to use existing conventional services in routine ways and may be 'hard to reach' for all agencies. The adolescents are often out of school (truant or excluded), delinquent and making erratic use of a variety of services. Roles for CAMHS professionals may be diagnostic and therapeutic, offering both risk assessment and direct and indirect intervention often in conjunction with other professionals (Department of Health, 2000).

Local authorities are also involved with young people going through the courts because of family breakdown and parental inadequacies (although most of these are younger children of course) and provision of reports to assist the local authority and courts in relation to these children, and those involved with Juvenile Justice and Youth Offender Teams is an important role which is considered further in Chapter 16. An increasing role for coordination of advice between child mental health and local authority personnel is envisaged in the latest guidance under the 'Quality Protects' initiative (Department of Health, 1998). Not only is more systematic use of well-validated instruments of child and family functioning proposed, but resources to permit joint collaboration may be more available in future.

EDUCATIONAL SETTINGS

Residential schools and other special educational establishments have also been an area in which psychiatrists have traditionally had an active role, many such schools having in the past had formal sessional input. As trends in education have altered to place a greater emphasis upon inclusivity, and maintaining young people within their community and within a less disturbed peer group educationally, the number of young people in residential and special schooling has fallen. Residential provision is deemed appropriate for a group of children who have correspondingly more serious and extreme difficulties. This parallels the experience of local authority residential provision.

Specialisation has occurred within residential schooling and such establishments (e.g. those for autistic children or those with sensory handicaps such as deafness) will require psychiatric input from those who have special expertise in the area. Nevertheless, 'ordinary' special schools, both day and residential, such as those for adolescents with learning difficulties and emotional and behavioural difficulties (EBD), may provide opportunities for mental health treatment. The more specialised and highly staffed schools, especially those which provide year-round placements, contain a population of young people with significant neuropsychiatric difficulties as well as many who have experienced severe psychosocial adversity and, often, a combination of the two.

The models of working outlined earlier are equally applicable in this area, with different considerations applying to direct work with children and families from that undertaken with the staff group themselves. There is a similar need for clarity in roles and responsibilities.

The training of professionals who work within these schools is extremely varied and may contain a mixture of skills and experience in health and educational settings: a range which is perhaps wider than is found in local authority staff. Some special schools contain highly trained and very specialised staff, e.g. music therapists. However, as when working with any staff group, it is important to establish the extent to which practices and assumptions are shared, including the extent to which staff and the consultant share beliefs about the aetiology of difficulties and models of change in children's behaviour. Whilst a pragmatic and flexible approach is essential in all consultative work, this is obviously more likely to be successful if core beliefs are held in common to some degree.

The range of roles for the liaison consultant and the types of disorder found in the young people will be heavily affected by the clientele. However, all such establishments are likely to contain children whose current handicaps have been affected by family relationship issues. 'Challenging behaviour' is likely to feature frequently, and both behavioural and psychodynamically informed understandings may be helpful in addition to practical advice. In settings such as these it may be easy for common conventional mental health difficulties such as depression to be hard to recognise because conduct problems are so prominent. Furthermore, the inter-relation of psychiatric, cognitive and psychosocial issues may require a mixture of pharmacological and psychological inputs with careful monitoring and review. Some of the young people may live far from their families of origin, making work in these domains difficult and also making it hard for staff to know what issues may have been disturbing young people during holiday periods. This is especially true if direct verbal expression of feelings is difficult, e.g. for autistic children.

CONCLUSIONS

A range of inputs to adolescents and staff of non-psychiatric settings has been described, ranging from the most direct face to face psychiatric work to much more indirect support of approaches to encourage mental health. Work in these settings is often with the most disturbed young people with extremely extensive mental and physical health difficulties and, sometimes, mental illnesses – often the most resistant to treatment initiatives. Approaches have been described which include treatment and secondary prevention, together with inputs to support staff groups working together and also separately in formal educational approaches. Evaluating the services and effectiveness of these services remains a challenge which merits a comprehensive answer.

REFERENCES

Breslau, N. (1985) Psychiatric disorder in children with physical disabilities. *Journal of the American Academy of Child Psychiatry*, **24**, 87–94.

Campbell, D., Draper, R. and Huffington, C. (1991) *A Systematic Approach to Consultation*. London: Karnac.

Cottrell, D. and Worrell, A. (1995) Liaison child and adolescent psychiatry. *Advances in Psychiatric Treatment*, **1**, 78–85.

Department of Health (1998) *The Quality Projects Programme: Transforming Children's Services*. Local Authority Circular (L.A.C. (98) 22). London: Department of Health.

Department of Health (2000) *Framework for the Assessment of Children in Need and their Families*. London: HMSO.

Eiser, C. (1993) *Growing up with a Chronic Disease*. London: Jessica Kingsley.

Goodman, R. and Graham, P. (1996) Psychiatric problems in children with hemiplegia: cross sectional epidemiological survey. *British Medical Journal*, **314**, 813–820.

Goodman, R. (1997) Child mental health: who is responsible? *British Medical Journal*, **314**, 813–820.

Garralda, E. and Bailey, D. (1989) Psychiatric disorders in general paediatric referrals. *Archives of Disease in Childhood*, **64**, 1727–1733.

Garralda, M. E., Jameson, R. A., Reynolds J. M. and Postlethwaite, R. J. (1988) Psychiatric adjustment in children with chronic renal failure. *Journal of Child Psychology and Psychiatry*, **29**, 79–90.

Lask, B. (1994) Paediatric liaison work. In M. Rutter, E. Taylor and L. Hersov (eds), *Child and Adolescent Psychiatry: Modern Approaches*, 3rd edn. Oxford: Blackwell Science, p. 997.

Lloyd, H. and MacDonald, A. (2000) Picking up the pieces. In D. M. Eminson and R. J. Postlethwaite (eds), *Munchausen Syndrome by Proxy Abuse: A Practical Approach*. Oxford: Butterworth-Heinemann, pp. 295–314.

McCann, J. B., James, A., Wilson, S. and Dunn, G. (1996) Prevalence of psychiatric disorder in young people in the care system. *British Medical Journal*, **313**, 1529–30.

McKee, M. (1999) Sex and drugs and rock and roll. *British Medical Journal*, **318**, 1300–1301.

Mawson, C. (1994) Containing anxiety in work with damaged children. In A. Obholzer, and V. Z. Roberts (eds), *The Unconscious at Work*. London: Routledge.

Mrazek, D. (1985) Child psychiatry consultation and liaison to paediatrics. In M. Rutter and L. Hersov (eds), *Child and Adolescent Psychiatry: Modern Approaches, 2nd edn*. Oxford: Blackwell Science, pp. 888–899.

North, C. and Eminson, D. M. (1998) A review of psychiatry–nephrology liaison service. *European Child Adolescent Psychiatry*, **7**, 235–245

Pless, I. B., Cripps, H. A., Davis, J. M. C. and Wadsworth, M. E. J. (1989) Chronic physical illness in childhood; psychological and social effects in adolescence and adult life. *Developmental Medicine and Child Neurology*, **311**, 746–755.

Richardson, J. and Jonghin, C. (2000) *The Mental Health Needs of Looked-after Children*. London: Gaskell.

Rifkind, G. (1995) Containing the containers. *Group Analysis*, **28**, 209–222.

Ryan, M., Barret, G. and Lessof, L. (1995) Monitoring effects of deprivation on health. *British Medical Journal*, **310**, 398.

Steinberg, D. and Yule, W. (1985) Consultative work. In M. Rutter and L. Hersov (eds), *Child and Adolescent Psychiatry: Modern Approaches, 2nd edn*. Oxford: Blackwell, pp. 914–926.

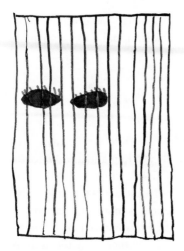

Chapter 16

RESPONDING TO THE NEEDS AND RISKS OF YOUNG OFFENDERS

Sue Bailey

INTRODUCTION

Throughout Europe and the US, the nature and level of juvenile offending has long absorbed the attention of the public, politicians, practitioners and researchers. The terms delinquency and crime imply at least the possibility of conviction but the majority of crimes do not result in an individual appearing in court. The term juvenile usually relates to a lower age limit set by the age of criminal responsibility and an upper age when a young person can be dealt with by courts for adult offenders. However, these ages vary between countries, can and do change over time, and are not the same for all offences (Justice, 1996).

In describing young offenders the terms 'frequent', 'persistent', 'serious' and 'chronic' have all been used to indicate a perceived extreme end of a continuum of juvenile offending. In addition to unclear criteria as to when offending becomes 'frequent' and 'frequent offending' becomes 'persistent', there is often a conflation of 'frequency' and 'seriousness' of offending. Some young offenders who commit the most serious crimes will not have an extensive criminal history and many frequent offenders will not commit the most serious of crimes (Bullock and Milham, 1988).

Studies that have looked at persistent offenders reveal they are broadly similar to other offenders, but display their characteristics to a much greater degree (Farrington and West, 1993). Hagell and Newburn (1994) reported that approximately one in 250 young people aged between 10 and 16 (male and female) were arrested three times or more. A picture is emerging of young people with more educational problems, lower levels of social integration, more disrupted family backgrounds and experience of institutional care, and more developmental difficulty including hyperactivity.

HISTORICAL

Approaches to the issue of how best to respond to juvenile crime have been dominated by the perceived need to punish the offender. In England and Wales (as mirrored in other European countries) during the 1970s and early 1980s there was a move away from a 'nothing works' to a 'what works' philosophy. Strenuous and partially successful efforts were made across many agencies to de-escalate the juvenile justice process. Many young offenders entered community-based treatment and diversionary programmes. This, together with the welfare principles enshrined in the Children Act 1989, meant that increasingly restrictive criteria had to be satisfied before the imposition of custodial sentences for juveniles. The Crime and Disorder Act 1998, England and Wales, has at its heart a stated purpose for the Youth Justice System to cut offending by young people, and a mandate within it that all jurisdictions of justice, education, care and health will be involved in this process. Core to this major overhaul of the Youth Justice System is involvement, responsibility and accountability of parents and youth as reflected in Antisocial Behaviour Orders and Parenting Orders.

RATES AND PATTERNS OF JUVENILE CRIME

Accepting that the vast majority of antisocial acts do not become recorded crime statistics, best information can be obtained both over time and between countries by combining sources of information, such as official statistics, self report data and victimisation studies. For example, the main source of data on offences committed in England and Wales is *Criminal Statistics*, an annual publication from the Home Office. In the US these are published by the Federal Bureau of Investigation as the *Uniform Crime Report (UCR)* and there is a United Nations Crime Survey sent out every 5 years to member states. Victim surveys include the US National Crime Victimisation Survey and the British Crime Survey (BCS) (Mirrlees-Black *et al.*, 1996). Self-report studies, despite major methodological difficulties (Junger-Tas *et al.*, 1994), do concur in their findings in terms of frequency of delinquent acts and differences between delinquents and non-delinquents.

Between countries and systems the processing of criminal behaviour remains similar (Rutter *et al.*, 1998) with respect to the legal definition of the behaviour as criminal, recognition that a criminal act has been committed, decision to report to the authorities, police handling of a report, identification of a suspect, decision on how to deal with the suspect and sentencing decisions.

Under 18s account for between a quarter to a third of offences in England and Wales and the US. Of those cautioned or convicted of indictable offences in 1995 (England and Wales), 26% were aged 10–17. Criminal Statistics for England and Wales (1995) show that 48% of males between 14 and 17, and 74% of females in the same age group were cautioned or prosecuted for theft related offences (in the main shoplifting). If burglary is included in this category, the rates increase to 64 and 78%, respectively. This finding is in keeping with other countries (Smith, 1995). Violent crimes form a relatively small proportion of known offending by young people – 10% in England and Wales.

Crimes involving a weapon vary greatly, but those involving a gun are 15 times greater in the US than in Europe (Synder *et al.*, 1996). Of those cautioned or found guilty of weapon-related offences (England and Wales, 1995), 80% were males.

The peak age of offending is usually in the late teens, with considerable international variation. In the UK, it is 18 for young men and 15 for young women. Adolescent self-report studies reveal higher levels of delinquency than official statistics, this is particularly so for young females. On self-report data over a third of all offenders have committed one violent offence at some time in their criminal career.

To understand the origins of delinquency, it is necessary to understand the nature and variety of antisocial behaviours displayed by young people. Adolescents with antisocial behaviour present the key dilemma of where and how to set the boundary between normal and pathological, between health and illness. It is important not only to establish the prevalence of antisocial behaviour but also key stages of antisocial careers, age of onset, the probability of persistence after onset, the duration of antisocial behaviour and the age of desistance. More is known about criminal than about antisocial careers. The difficulties surrounding the complexity of antisocial behaviour, identifying successful interventions and predicting which individuals will engage in more versus less serious behaviour remains very apparent in both the recent literature on adolescent offenders and psychosocial disorders in young people (Farrington, 1996; Smith, 1995).

Thus as is the case with adult mentally disordered offenders, young people at the interface of the criminal justice system and mental health service risk double jeopardy for social exclusion, alienation and stigmatisation.

Definitions of antisocial behaviour have arisen largely out of the adult literature. The cluster of antisocial symptoms is classified differently in different countries, dissocial personality disorder in ICD-10 (World Health Organisation, 1992), antisocial personality disorder in DSM-IV (American Psychiatric Association, 1994) with the added complexity of legal classifications such as psycho-pathic disorder, Mental Health Act 1983, England and Wales. For adults with severe personality disorder the disturbance in inner experience, relationships and behaviour manifests itself by wide-ranging and diffuse interference of all areas of functioning. This invariably extends from individual relationships to society in the widest sense. Using the conventional classifications of personality disorder

(ICD-10 and DSM-IV) this is shown by co-occurrence (co-morbidity) from two or more domains (clusters) of personality function. These domains are commonly divided into three groups: flamboyant/dramatic, odd/eccentric and anxious/fearful groups. The flamboyant/dramatic group of personality disorders includes those who have the most impact on society [antisocial, (dissocial) impulsive, borderline, histrionic, and narcissistic disorder]. One of these is invariably present in severe personality disorder together with one or more disorders from other groups (Tyrer and Stein, 1993).

The diagnosis, classification, assessment and treatment of young people with conduct disorder is dealt with elsewhere in this book. Extrapolating from the established literature in addressing young offenders, Kazdin (1997) has described serious antisocial behaviour as a chronic long-lasting disease that requires continuous monitoring and intervention over the life course. Thus in bridging our understanding of the gap between the known literature on adult definitions of antisocial behaviour and the Childhood Classifications of Conduct Disorder and Oppositional Defiant Disorder what emerges for those adolescents who display serious antisocial behaviour is heterogeneity related to pervasiveness, persistence, severity and pattern of behaviour. The main possible groupings that emerge include:

- Antisocial behaviour that overlaps with genetic influences, e.g. hyperactivity with its associated cognitive and social problems, its possible persistence into adulthood
- Antisocial behaviour with very early onset and life course persistence
- Violent and antisocial behaviour associated with altered biochemical activity in the brain, e.g. possible low serotonin turnover
- Antisocial behaviours resonant with adult 'psychopathic disorder' with lack of remorse, absence of close relationships, and apparent emotional detachment and antisocial behaviour
- Serious mental disorder where the behaviour is intrinsically part of the mental disorder

Less certain is the validity of subgroups of offending, e.g. juvenile sexual offenders, young arsonists, and the complex relationship between offending and substance abuse (see later).

In the UK the challenge to public safety presented by the minority of adults with severe personality disorder, who because of their disorder pose a risk of serious offending, has been recognised by successive administrations. Dealing with this problem has brought together criminal justice, health and social policy, and has raised complex and sensitive ethical questions.

It is increasingly recognised that the most dangerous, severely personality disordered adults have a lifelong history of profound difficulties from an early age; many are the children of violent, abusive or inadequate parents and some may have been removed into care (Rutter et al., 1998). Many are poorly educated and have a history of difficulty in finding work and housing. In adult life they have difficulty forming meaningful relationships, frequently become involved in substance misuse and suffer from depression or other mental illness (Royal College of Psychiatrists CR71, 1999).

The UK government has launched a series of preventative initiatives targeting the family and parenting, named 'Supporting Families', using multisystemic family approaches (Henggeler, 1999) together with Sure Start, based on the Perry Pre-school Projects (Schweinhart *et al.*, 1993). An action plan for 'Meeting Special Educational Needs', together with a 'National Literacy Strategy' and a 'Healthy Schools Programme' is being added to antibullying strategies, 'Excellence in Schools' together with a Social Inclusion Pupil Support Scheme. In September 1998 the Secretary of State for Health launched 'Quality Protects', a 3-year programme designed to improve the management and delivery of children's social services.

The Crime and Disorder Act 1998 provides for Youth Offending Teams in which Police, Probation, Health and Social Services are working together to address all factors associated with offending by young people. Major resource allocation is being made to tackle the problem of substance misuse by children, and to improve service provision within child and adolescent mental health services (CAMHS) to improve outcomes for those young people at high risk. Over half of the personality disordered adults admitted to maximum secure psychiatric hospitals in the UK had had contact with child psychiatric services from a young age.

For those children who display the criminal behaviours of interpersonal violence including juvenile homicide (Bailey, 1996), arson and in particular sexual offending (Dolan *et al.*, 1996; Vizard *et al.*, 1996), there is an increased drive in the UK to approach the assessment, risk management and treatment of young perpetrators as a specific entity, with a focus on developmental issues rather than past tendencies to apply 'adult' treatment models to young people.

The 'disadvantage' of gender is now being recognised, whether this refers to self-harming girls who are displaying increased levels of externalised aggression and violence or violent boys in whom the risk of serious self-harm and past abuse is poorly recognised (Jasper *et al.*, 1998; Widom and White, 1997; Zoccolillo *et al.*, 1996). Both carry with them the risk in adult life for the development of severe personality disorder.

MORAL DEVELOPMENT, ADOLESCENCE AND CRIMINAL RESPONSIBILITIES

If we cannot escape from the use of some sort of concept of personality and more particularly personality disorder in adulthood, we cannot avoid the need to ask how it develops. The greatest gap in knowledge lies in the understanding of personality development during adolescence, and how different factors and influences interact over time to set a fixed trajectory into serious antisocial behaviour in adulthood (Bailey, 1992).

Theorists have described adolescent personality development from the perspectives of psychosexual development, ego development and defensive operations, identity formation, cognitive development, object relations, and more latterly self-psychology. The developmental tasks of adolescence centre on autonomy and connection with others, rebellion and development of independence, development of identity, and distinction from and continuity with childhood. We need to know what is and how to define normal functioning and development before we can safely intervene with those who have been designated 'abnormal'. In dealing with self-image, major bodily changes, impulse control, emotional tone, social relationships, morals, sexual attitudes, family relationships and educational or vocational goals, 'normal' adolescents are characterised more by their similarities than their differences, although they hold diverse views of their psychological world and themselves. Adolescence needs to be seen as both a context and a phenomenon, thereby laying the foundation for an understanding of the unique developmental issues for the individual adolescent who displays serious antisocial behaviour.

Criminal justice is based on the premise that blame can and should be attributed. Stephenson (1992) described the attribution of blame as the 'originating and vindicating activity' in the whole criminal justice process. The age of criminal responsibility varies widely between countries from 7 in Switzerland, 10 in England and Wales, 12 in Canada, 14 in Germany, 15 in Sweden, 16 in Spain up to 18 in Belgium (Pease and Tseloni,, 1996).

In many countries, within these age bandings in order to secure a conviction the prosecution has to prove not only that a child has committed the offence but that the child knew the act they committed was seriously wrong. In practice, below the age of criminal responsibility, official intervention can and does occur using civil law and the social welfare system.

During early adolescence, thinking processes become more abstract, multidimensional and self-aware. Young people can start to hold several different viewpoints of any subject at the same time and so can produce more alternatives when making decisions. They can check their own thought processes for inconsistencies and missing information. In adolescence young people have a framework from which to look back and to consider the future. Critically, in the context of criminal justice, they start to think about the consequences of their actions beyond the immediate and short term, they start to take on a sense of responsibility for their own actions, in particular the effect these may have on others. Two parallel developments of importance in the field of juvenile offenders are a young person's increased capacity to remember events and their ability to feel guilt and shame (Bailey, 1996; Hagell and Newburn, 1994). Adolescents not only gradually increase in their ability to recall events and in particular the sequencing of events but also become less likely to be influenced by adults when being interviewed, particularly in the context of police interviews (Gudjonnsson and Clark, 1986; Mirrlees-Black *et al.*, 1996).

At its simplest, guilt involves the appreciation of responsibility for negative outcomes, arising from acts of omission or commission. Shame is associated with negative feelings about oneself on the basis of a self-perception of being bad or unworthy. With an evolving capacity for self-evaluation comes a recognition that there is personal choice over antisocial acts, and an increasing awareness of the harm these acts can and do cause to others. Linked with the developmental tasks of adolescence and the considerable biological transition of puberty, a strong case can be made for a different approach to criminal responsibility when those who have committed antisocial acts are still only young.

This whole subject poses considerable ethical and practical dilemmas when balancing the rights of children, e.g. 1989 United Nations Convention on the Rights of the Child, and the constant and understandable pressure to reduce the rates of youth crime. The tension between crime prevention and the welfare of children who offend is ever present, and should be set in the context of developmental capacity and the inter-relationship between the sequence of systems, family and peers, school, welfare systems, and the criminal justice system that act as the main arenas for social control as a child makes the transition through adolescence into adulthood. This issue has been highlighted by the judgement of V versus UK (Application No. 2, 4888–94) and the right under Article 6 of the Human Rights Act to a fair trial and effective participation of a child in Criminal Court proceedings (Ashford and Chard, 2000).

RISK AND RESILIENCE

Surveys of the general population show that 90% of boys admit to acts that could have led to appearance in court; however, most are minor in their nature. Delinquent acts by young children are less frequent but more likely to be associated with psychological abnormalities that are persistent and reflect both social dysfunction and individual psychopathology.

Although more is known about criminal careers and chronic juvenile offending than antisocial careers *per se*, the research literature reveals that there are three major risk areas in children and adolescents with persistent antisocial behaviour: child centred, family centred and contextual. They have an interactive effect on antisocial behaviour, providing support for a proposed cumulative protection model of prevention of both antisocial behaviour and offending.

Antisocial behaviour is heterogeneous and for many still a normal phenomenon, a deliberate principled act of protest of transient adolescent onset and course. Those with early onset are at far higher risk in the adult life course for development of antisocial personality disorder and importantly also for affective disturbance. For those who go on from childhood to display serious antisocial behaviour in adulthood the risk factors remain.

Broad child-centred factors
- Genetic vulnerability
- Perinatal risk
- Male gender
- Cognitive impairment
- School underachievement
- Hyperactivity/inattention
- Temperament

Family factors
- Criminality in parents and siblings
- Family discord
- Lack of supervision
- Lack of emotional support
- Abuse
- Scapegoating
- Rejection
- Neglect

Influential contextual factors
- Drug and alcohol abuse
- Unemployment
- Crime opportunity
- Peer group interaction

Important perpetuating factors include continued substance abuse and unemployment. Significant turning points include the establishment and maintenance of a harmonious stable relationship, and the continuing potential for growth and developmental change in the individual. These risk and resilience factors are fully described in Chapter 5.

GENDER

SERIOUS ANTISOCIAL BEHAVIOUR IN GIRLS

In the past there were always more boys than girls in care, now in England there are approximately 15 000 adolescent girls in care, either accommodated by the local authority or the subject of an order from court (Coleman, 1997). The peak age of offending is 15, one in five young offenders are female and offences of violence are the second most common crime committed by female offenders. With no current specific provision for young female offenders under 17 within the prison system it is likely that the majority remain within social services provision and supervision. Of the adult female prison population, 30–50% have been in care as compared with 2% of the general population (Calouste Gulbenkian Foundation, 1995). From the literature, girls and women commit different crimes from their male counterparts and receive differential treatment for similar crimes.

In the past girls have received harsher treatments than boys from the courts for the same crimes (Armstrong, 1977). In the US it remains not uncommon for girls to have had fewer recorded offences before being imprisoned in older adolescence.

Drug and alcohol misuse by females is reported to be influenced by different factors (Bodinger-Deuriate, 1991). A study of adult female offenders in British prisons (Maden et al., 1994) reveals a higher rate of psychiatric disturbance, personality disorder and substance misuse than in adult male prisoners.

Research in the US shows that adolescent female offenders have experienced more sexual abuse at a higher frequency than their male counterparts (Chesney-Lind, 1987). Smith and Thornberry (1995) found significant relationships between child abuse before the age of 11 and later delinquency. Zingraff et al. (1993) found that maltreated boys and girls had higher rates of delinquency than non-maltreated, impoverished children.

Widom and White (1997), in a recent prospective design cohort study, report that among abused and neglected children, females but not males are at significantly higher risk for a diagnosis of drug dependence and arrests for violent crimes in adulthood than control groups.

In the UK there is a paucity of literature relating to adolescent females who offend and who have mental health problems. In a study of 100 consecutive referrals of girls aged 11–17 (Jasper et al., 1998) to an Adolescent Forensic Mental Health Service referrers, only correctly documented violent and aggressive behaviour in 54% of cases. Over 70% had been the subject of abuse (emotional, sexual, or physical), the majority having been multiply abused. Half of the violent girls had misused substances, more abused girls had been violent to objects (50%) or set fires (20%). A high number of deliberately self-harming girls had a mental illness, and a significantly high number of deliberately self-harming girls misused substances (50%) and had been sexually abused (54%).

BOYS AND GIRLS

Most crime is committed by boys and there remains a large difference between the number of boys held in both Secure Care local authority units and Young Offender Institutions and the number of girls of similar age. Understanding both the changing trend for violent behaviour in girls and the protective factors which still operate for girls should help inform preventative measures for both boys and girls. The link between childhood abuse and adult substance abuse and violent behaviour is emerging for women, but not as yet for men. Substance misuse and drug dependency feature as a considerable problem for adult women in prison (Mohan *et al.*, 1997). Widom and White (1997) suggest that male control groups may be complicated by undisclosed childhood abuse, obscuring a link for males. It may be that currently girls are more able to disclose abuse than boys. Girls who engage in violent behaviour therefore present as a useful study group in trying to understand the pathway from experiences in childhood to adult serious antisocial behaviour.

PSYCHIATRIC DISORDERS

SCHIZOPHRENIA

The prodromal phase of non-psychotic behavioural disturbance occurs in about half of early-onset cases of schizophrenia and can last 1–7 years (Maziade *et al.*, 1996). Non-psychotic behavioural disturbance can include obsessive-compulsive disorder, avoidant personality, anxiety states and, significantly in considering all possible causes for antisocial behaviour in adolescents, externalising behaviours, attention deficit disorder and conduct disorder. This adds to the importance of the early detection of 'at-risk' or prodromal mental states. Adolescents may experience multiple periods of 'at-risk mental states' influenced by life events and family stress. In making the differential diagnosis between an adolescent with late-onset or escalating serious antisocial behaviour and ensuring that the young person is not developing a major mental illness, the following should be looked for: a clear change in social functioning from a baseline level and presence of an 'at-risk' mental state (perceptual change, ideas of reference and delusional mood).

As with adults, the great majority of young people who have a major mental illness such as schizophrenia present no increased risk factors for offending, violence and antisocial behaviour. The best predictors of future offending in mentally disordered young people remain the same as for the whole population. Young people suffering from severe mental illness may present an increased risk to others when they have active symptoms especially when they also abuse drugs or alcohol. Mental states in the young person that would give rise to particular concern about possible violent acts are subjective feelings of tension, ideas of violence, delusional systems that incorporate those currently close to the young person, persecutory delusions with fear of imminent attack, feelings of sustained anger and fear, passivity experiences reducing their sense of self-control, and command hallucinations. Protective factors against carrying out serious antisocial behaviour are responding to and compliance with medical treatment, good social networks, a valued home environment, no interest in or knowledge of weapons or the means of violence, and good insight into the psychiatric illness. Also important are a lack of any previous aggressive behaviour and, critically, a fear of their own potential for violence.

The interconnections between homelessness, mental disorder, substance misuse and offending are complex and remain poorly understood. A flexible approach from psychiatric services working in court diversion schemes is required, with innovative partnerships with the voluntary sector agencies working with young people.

The Joint Prison Service/NHS Executive Working Group (H.M. Prison Service, 1999) has recently recommended a partnership to improve the health care provided to prisoners. Nowhere is this a greater priority than in Young Offender Institutions where young people with early onset psychosis await long periods before transfer to secure adolescent forensic inpatient beds. This report also underpins the importance of regimen and social conditions, and helps promote of the health of young people in prison. Particularly vulnerable are girls and young people from ethnic minority groups.

AFFECTIVE DISORDERS

A series of studies (Harrington *et al.*, 1991) based on clinic samples has shown that among those with conduct disorders risks of affective disorder are elevated or that among those with affective disorders risk of conduct disorder is increased.

Fergusson *et al.* (1996) explored the origins of co-morbidity between conduct disorder and affective disorders during the analysis of a 16-year longitudinal study of a birth cohort of New Zealand children. At age 15 and 16, of the shared variance between conduct disorder and affective disorders, more than two-thirds was explained by common risk factors. A substantial amount of the correlation arises because the risk factors and life pathways that predispose adolescents to one outcome are associated with the risk factors and life pathways that predispose them to the other. Nonetheless even after control for common causal factors there remained evidence of unexplained co-morbidity between the two disorders.

'PRODROMAL' PERSONALITY DISORDER

The two-factor model used in the literature to describe severe personality disorder in adults may be important for furthering understanding of those young people whose personality development through adolescence gives rise to most concern. Hare (1993) describes a psychopathic personality as having an unemotional and callous interpersonal style which is less strongly associated with a conduct problem diagnosis, in contrast with the poor impulse control and antisocial behaviour and lifestyles of adults with antisocial personality disorder. O'Brien and Frick (1996) argue that these two groups have a diversant aetiology. Christian *et al.* (1997) described a subgroup of children with conduct disorder who also exhibit high levels of callous unemotional (CU) interpersonal style, lacking guilt, who do not show empathy and do not show emotions. They have a greater variety and number of conduct problems, higher rates of police contact and a stronger parental history of antisocial personality disorder despite being of higher intelligence than other children with significant conduct disorder. The critical pathway to their serious antisocial behaviour, in particular directed interpersonal violence, lies within the family, their evolving personality features and situational context.

Family features
- Parental antisocial personality disorder
- Violence witnessed
- Abuse, neglect, rejection

Personality features
- Callous unemotional interpersonal style
- Evolution of violent and sadistic fantasy
- Viewing people as objects
- Morbid identity
- Paranoid ideation
- Hostile attribution

Situational features
- Repeated loss and rejection in relationships.
- Threats to self-esteem
- Crescendo of hopelessness and helplessness
- Social disinhibition
- Group processes
- Changes in mental state over time

SUBSTANCE MISUSE

Drug abuse among young people has increased rapidly over the past 10 years. The importance of an integrated health service response to substance misuse by young people was clearly stated in the NHS Health Advisory Service report of 1996. The complex interaction between offending and high-risk behaviours to self and others is still poorly understood. However, an important starting point for dealing with high-risk substance misusers with or without associated mental illness is to review the DSM-IV substance use disorder criteria for adolescent persons. This is in order to understand better the progression from conduct disorder to antisocial personality disorder after treatment for adolescent substance misuse, and to explore the possible connections between substance use disorder and its relationship to executive cognitive functioning, aggressivity and impulsivity. If service responses are to include any secure provision, this raises difficult ethical and moral issues. The Standing Conference on Drug Abuse and the Children's Legal Centre (1998) recognised that very specialised and intensive forms of intervention for young drug users with complex care needs would involve specialist residential services and mental health teams, including child and adolescent forensic psychiatrists.

LEARNING DISABILITY

Within the field of adolescent forensic learning disability, a number of issues have to be considered in the assessment and subsequent treatment programmes. The latter needs to be carried out over a longer time period that is matched to the pace at which the adolescent person who has a learning disability can cope and demonstrate change, balancing inherent vulnerability with risk to others.

These include:

- Factors influencing the assessment and treatment of young offenders
- General issues of offending among adults with learning disability
- Role of severity of the learning disability in offending behaviour among adolescent persons
- Relevance of the cause/aetiology of learning disability to the individual's offending behaviour (particularly in autism)
- Impact of the nature of the individual's cognitive profile in offending
- Importance of super-added psychiatric disorder among learning disabled adolescent persons
- Role of life experience and personal history in the offending behaviour

PREVENTION AND INTERVENTION

There are four major types of prevention which relate to reduction of serious antisocial behaviour and juvenile offending (Tonry and Farrington, 1995).

(1) *Criminal justice prevention.* Deterrence, incapacitation and rehabilitation strategies operated by law enforcement and criminal justice agencies.
(2) *Situational prevention.* Designed to reduce the opportunities for antisocial behaviour and to increase the risk and difficulty of committing antisocial acts.
(3) *Community prevention.* Interventions designed to change the social conditions and social institutions that influence antisocial behaviour in communities.
(4) *Developmental prevention.* Interventions designed to inhibit the development of antisocial behaviour in individuals, by targeting risk and protective factors that influence human development. Successful early preventative interventions for juvenile offending and related antisocial behaviour depend on the efficacy of parent training, and pre-school programmes that enable young

children to understand more readily the consequences of their behaviour for self and peers, critically helping them to make safe choices and reach safe autonomy in adolescence. Lipsey (1995) in a review of outcome studies of education and psychotherapeutic intervention and Kazdin (1997) in a major review of the effectiveness of psychotherapy in reducing problem behaviour in young people, suggest the importance of three strategies:

- Primary population-based preventative intervention
- Secondary interventions focused on high-risk groups
- Tertiary treatment centred programmes

Prevention and early intervention programmes are described in Chapter 5. When reviewing the prevention and intervention programmes it should be noted that with respect to serious antisocial behaviour, outcomes are related to delinquency and adult crime more than antisocial behaviour *per se*.

Prevention and intervention programmes are geared to the full variation of antisocial behaviour rather than serious antisocial behaviour.

They are still largely orientated towards males and utilise techniques that are primarily risk focused rather than taking an holistic approach.

Overall approaches are those of tackling social aspects of crimes and psychological criminology. These do not always encompass individual development and psychopathology. The process of personality development in adolescence remains poorly understood.

For that group with serious antisocial behaviour there remains a need for specialist treatment and care.

RESPONDING TO YOUNG PEOPLE WITH SERIOUS ANTISOCIAL BEHAVIOUR

SYSTEMS ISSUES

In England and Wales, the Youth Justice Board are commissioned to purchase secure accommodation for all those young people under 18 sentenced or remanded by the Courts.

	Approximate bed numbers 2000
Young Offender Institutions (YOI) < 18	2800
Local Authority Secure Accommodation	300
Independent Sector Secure Training Centres (STCs)	120
Secure Psychiatric Adolescent beds, NHS and independent sector	70

In the community at anyone time it is likely there are between 2500 and 5000 young people being dealt with by Youth Justice Services and the Probation Service who present with a similar level of risk, need and antisocial behaviour.

There is currently clinical information about young people in each part of this system, but still a lack of systematically collected data about this total needy population, nor is there seamless, planned transition of care as serious young offenders serving long sentences (S53 1933 Children and Young Persons Act) move through the system from secure care, YOI, adult prison and back into the community.

The new Detention Training Orders for the 12–14-year-olds being admitted to the new Secure Training Centres with their heavy emphasis on education, avocation and rehabilitation contains within it an automatic follow-up and supervision as half the order is served back in the community. Although such establishments raise major ethical issues and are viewed by many as child prisons, the statutory introduction of aftercare and sentence planning potentially allows care and treatment to be implemented with family and local community initiatives via the Youth Offending Teams (YOTS).

The research evidence is accumulating that shows clearly that the rate of mental health disorder is high in young offenders, particularly persistent offenders and those that are convicted. Gunn *et al.* (1991) found that a diagnosis of primary mental disorder can be made in a third of young men aged between 16 and 18 years who have been sentenced by a court. The prevalence of mental disorder in male remand prisoners aged 21 years and over was found to be 26% (excluding substance misuse) (Birmingham *et al.*, 1996) and a third of those supervised by a large probation service had a history of deliberate self-harm (Wessely *et al.*, 1996). Prevalence of mental health problems is increased amongst young offenders before during and following incarceration. The most obvious and serious example of this is demonstrated by the high rates of suicide or attempted suicide amongst young offenders (Liebling, 1991).

In the only UK psychiatric screening of 10–17 year olds attending a city centre Youth Court showed high levels of both psychiatric and physical morbidity, including learning difficulties, mood disorder, epilepsy, frequent use of alcohol and illicit drugs, and frank mental illness (Dolan *et al.*, 1999). In the then specialist secure care provision of the Youth Treatment Service, reported mental health problems that justified specialist clinical assessment were found in 50% of the population.

Factors strongly associated with mental health problems such as childhood trauma in the form of abuse and/or loss were found in 91% of Section 53 offenders (1933 Children and Young Person's Act) – those young people who have committed serious crimes of violence, arson or rape (Bailey, 1996; Boswell, 1995). There is now good evidence of a high rate of disorder among groups of young people who have a high risk of delinquency. McCann *et al.* (1996) reported a 67% prevalence of psychiatric disorder in adolescents in the Oxfordshire care system, compared with those living with their own families. A national study of the demand and need for adolescent forensic mental health services for children (under 18s) in the criminal justice and secure care systems (Kurtz *et al.*, 1997) confirmed the view of practitioners in the field that the mental health needs of young people who display high levels of antisocial behaviour, who are psychologically disturbed, and who present a danger to themselves and others, are not well recognised, widely understood or have their needs safely met.

A major survey by the Audit Commission (1996) of Youth Justice Services in England and Wales reported that the seven or eight agencies in Youth Justice have different objectives, pursuing their own key targets, thus decreasing cooperation. Most resources are invested in the investigative process and few in changing behaviour. The Crime and Disorder Act (1998) is now overhauling what was viewed as a failing youth justice system (Statement by the Home Secretary, June, 1997). Although it is always stressed that community interventions work better than residential, good residential interventions in both care and custody have to deal with more seriously disturbed young people, and both those in secure care and custody are hampered by lack of coordination of aftercare and family support. With the setting up of Young Offender Teams (YOTS) to which all agencies have a statutory duty to be involved, and with a National Youth Justice Board to review and monitor the functioning of YOTS, there is an opportunity for young offenders at least to be dealt with as a whole rather than in part.

RISK ASSESSMENT

The general priorities of risk assessment, arising from the adult forensic literature combined with a developmental perspective are useful in providing a context for risk assessment of specific forms of behaviour.

VIOLENCE

Grave acts of violence carried out by adolescents are seen as one of the most important problems facing both European countries and the US, not least because of the costs – economically, socially and emotionally.

In the US the arrest rate of those under 18 years of age for murder and manslaughter rose by 60% between 1981 and 1991 compared with a 5% rise for those over 18 (Federal Bureau of Investigation, 1992). However these figures are greatly influenced by the ready availability of firearms in the US and the concentration of juvenile homicide within the African-American subpopulation (Synder and Sickmund, 1995). The rate of grave offences committed by children and young adolescents in Britain, particularly juvenile homicide, has not risen to any significant extent (McNally, 1995). Fear of violent crime at the hands of young people is an important and debilitating problem (Shepherd and Farrington, 1993).

Common disorders that may result in displays of violent aggressive sadistic or destructive behaviour inevitably involve serious malfunction of individuals in their social setting. To understand how this arises there is a need to understand the process of individual development and social conditions. Violent offenders commit offences of many types and nearly all chronic offenders have committed a violent offence. Delinquent young people are as much at risk of injury and other victimisation as they are of committing offences. Important preventative strategies include understanding of early predictors, availability of early family support and pre-school education. Violence as a public health issue has the advantage that it focuses on injury rather than crime. A focus on revictimisation suggests that rapid but short-term prevention initiatives are most likely to prevent further domestic violence. Juvenile violence, in particular, leads to increased morbidity and draining of health resources.

TRANSITION OF AGGRESSION INTO VIOLENCE

Violence is particularly subject to rhetoric, which is born largely out of factual ignorance and understandable fear. Sadistic violent acts carried out by adolescents bring with them both in the UK and in Europe and the US a surfeit of public and media interest which at times becomes voyeuristic in its nature. Violence occurs in the context of a system and in the context of individual differences. The development of violent behaviour often involves a loss of sense of personal uniqueness and a loss of sense of personal value; the adolescent engages in their actions without concern for future consequences or past commitments.

Loeber (1990) lays out a convincing argument that a developmental approach to violence in children and adolescents 'can open many avenues to knowledge'. The onset of boys' aggression is often in the pre-school period. Throughout childhood and into adolescence increasing numbers of boys experience the onset of aggression (Hacipasalo and Tremblay, 1994). More serious violence tends to increase with age, especially during adolescence. Loeber and Hay (1994) argue that growing rates of aggression and violence from pre-school age to young adulthood actually represent diverse groups of youth that can be classified into four broad groups:

- Young people who desist from aggression
- Young people whose aggression is stable and continues at the same level
- Youth who escalate in the severity of their aggression and make the transition to violence
- Youth who experience the onset of aggression stability

SEXUALLY INAPPROPRIATE BEHAVIOUR IN ADOLESCENTS

Juvenile sexual offending constitutes a substantial health and social problem. It represents an important mental health issue, first because abusers often come from disadvantaged backgrounds with a history of victimisation and many suffer from psychiatric disorders, and second because victims of abuse suffer high rates of psychiatric disorder. Child mental health services are increasingly being asked to assess and provide treatment not only for victims but also for perpetrators (especially as young abusers are now also considered under the child protection framework).

Official prevalence rates for sexual offending in the UK are remarkably similar to those in the US, at 1.5/1000 12–17 year olds (James and Neil, 1996). The majority of abusers are male, with a history of neglect, physical and/or sexual abuse, with below average ability and high rates of behavioural and psychological problems. In a series of 121 male juvenile sex offenders, their sexual acts were not isolated incidents in normally developing adolescents (Dolan et al., 1996). Many had a previous record of similar or less serious offences but multiagency and indeed previous psychiatric assessment had not explored the presence or evolution of rape fantasies. The authors stressed the need in psychiatric interview to enquire into the presence of rape fantasies and other concurrent violent behaviours in addition to the paraphilias. Vizard et al. (1996) highlight the need to balance the assumptions of the UK Children Act 1989, 'taking into account the wishes and feelings of the child', with the need to challenge this assumption when the young person has 'wishes and feelings' directed towards abusing others. A model is suggested that places emphasis on a multidisciplinary team that can create a full interagency systemic context around each referred case of a young sexual abuser, following the child protection procedure and the need for early preventative input. The majority of adult sexual abusers of children started their abuse in their own adolescence and yet there is as yet no diagnostic category for paedophilia for those under the age of 16, either within DSM-IV or ICD-10. The authors suggest the creation of a new disorder 'Sexual arousal disorder of childhood' to help identify this vulnerable group who can in turn place vulnerable others at risk. There is currently a lack of epidemiological surveys in the UK, using standardised instruments and interviews. Prospective studies using good baseline data should inform the planning of treatment programmes that should be tailored to adolescents and not just be taken from existing adult programmes.

YOUNG ARSONISTS

Fire-setting and arson are devastating behaviours impacting on the victim and wider society. There is a paucity of literature that facilitates a consistent view regarding the emergence, maintenance or promotion of fire-setting behaviour.

Classification of fire-setting traditionally focuses on the individuals underlying motivation to engage in such acts.

Fineman (1980) stressed the interaction between personal and familial factors predisposing the young person to the behaviour. Vreeland and Levin (1990) suggested fire-setting is the culmination of difficulty/fear of direct expression of aggression, Patterson (1982) suggested that it occurs at the end of a continuum of antisocial behaviours but the major authors in the field, Kolko and Kazdin (1992) highlight the key features of attraction to fire, heightened arousal, impulsivity and limited social competence.

Above and beyond the global assessment, child mental health services would make in considering the domains of development, social/family problems, educational history, personal/family history, health history and offence history, the specific domains to be explored are:

- History of fireplay
- History of hoax telephone calls
- Nature of behaviour – fires set alone, with peers or combination
- Setting – open/green space, occupied/unoccupied dwelling
- Previous threats/targets
- Type of fire – single, multiple seats of fire, ritualistic
- Motivation – anger resolution, boredom rejection, cry for help, thrill seeking, fire fighting, crime concealment, no motivation, curiosity, peer pressure

Treatment of recidivistic fire-setters who fall outside the norms of delinquency and/or conduct disorder include:

- Psychotherapy to promote the adolescent's understanding of the behaviour including antecedents, defining the problem behaviour and establishing what are the reinforcers of the behaviour
- Skills training – promoting the adolescent's ability to use adaptive coping mechanisms as an alternative to fire
- Understanding of environmental factors to provide strategies to manage or avoid trigger situations such as alcohol use and stressful social situations
- Counselling to reduce the adolescent's psychological distress
- Behavioural techniques to extinguish the behaviour
- Supervision and support to be provided to all concerned – therapist, individual, carers and all involved staff
- Fire education – to promote the adolescent's understanding of cause and effect of their behaviour, and to establish acceptance of responsibility for their actions

Treatment resistance is most likely to occur in adolescents whose life experiences have included :

- Early modelling (vicarious) experiences
- Early exposure to related phenomena
- Enduring antisocial behaviours and aggressive response patterns
- Limited judgement skills
- Low academic achievement
- Clusters of confrontative acts
- Personality traits of callousness
- Jealousness and revenge
- Limited parental/carer supervision
- Erratic punishment schedules
- Absent, neglecting or abusive parenting
- Parental psychopathology

As with serious property offending, adolescent arsonists are not a homogenous group, demonstrating a wide range of familial, developmental, social, inter-personal clinical and 'legal' needs. Thus no one standard treatment approach will be appropriate for all individuals (Repo and Virkkunen, 1997).

JUVENILE HOMICIDE

In a UK study of 50 juvenile murderers (aged 10–17) (Bailey et al., in press) assessed and given long-term treatment (Bailey, 1997b) by an adolescent forensic service, many had pre-existing conduct disorder and emotional difficulties with adverse family and social circumstances, a smaller group had learning difficulties and neuropsychological problems, but no one of 76 variables studied stood alone as causing the young person to act as they did. Alcohol was a significant contributory factor in older adolescents. These findings mirror those in the US (Myers and Kemph, 1990) when use of firearms in the US has been studied. The characteristics of this group also mirrored those of young people referred to the service with less serious, antisocial behaviour, and highlights the need for individual health needs assessment for all delinquent young people by social services and probation, before being offered cognitive behavioural treatment programmes (Heide, 1999).

Realistically, psychodynamic therapy with young people who have committed sadistic acts of violence, has to be tailored to the demands of the external environment and approached cautiously. Motivational dynamics are complex.

Given the frequent distortion of perception of self and others, the emergence of a true sense of guilt and shame can be and often is a slow, difficult, painful and angry process. Within the UK this group is liable to periods of lengthy incarceration. Irrespective of the treatment model provided the parallel process of education, vocation, provision of consistent role models and continued family contact are of critical importance. This is best facilitated in a milieu of warmth and harmony, with clear organisation, practicality and high expectations allowing for the establishment of positive staff–adolescent, staff–staff and adolescent–adolescent relations (Harris *et al.*, 1987).

Against the inevitable waxing and waning of the outside pressures of the still public and adversarial pre-trial, trial and post-trial process current in the UK, the adolescent has to move safely through the process of disbelief, denial, loss grief anger and blame. Post-traumatic stress disorder, arising from the participation in the sadistic act, has to be treated, as does trauma arising from their own past personal emotional, physical and/or sexual abuse. Qualities such as previous frequent and severe aggression, low intelligence and a poor capacity for insight weigh heavily against a safe long-term outcome and raise the possibility of emerging formal mental illness, in particular depression. Adolescents with sadistic behaviour have a depth of sensitivity and reaction to perceived threat not seen in other young people. They may see threat and ridicule in many ordinary day to day events. A related theme is saving face. As the young person starts to discuss their sadistic act, they may have to confront past loss, trauma and abuse. This disclosure leads to the fear of being vulnerable. Therapy may bring about change they neither like nor above all that they can control. Their past sadistic acts have been attempts at maladaptive control over the outside world that they are reluctant to relinquish. A combination of verbal and non-verbal therapies, in particular art, has much to offer this group of adolescents. With disclosure and understanding comes victim empathy, saying sorry and reattribution of blame which is often accompanied by expression of anger and distress within sessions which often may be sexualised in form and content. Emotions engendered can spill outside sessions leading to disruptive behaviour in the closed institution. This is difficult not only for the adolescent but for his carers, and can in turn lead to both becoming collusively rejecting and dismissive of the therapists. Combining a consistent cognitive behaviourally driven positive regime within the institution with individual psychotherapy offers the best chance of safe resolution and a halting of a trajectory into adult antisocial personality disorder.

MODELS OF SERVICE DELIVERY

Core to service provision for young offenders is a strategic, comprehensive and integrated intra-agency and interagency approach to their mental well-being. Any model of delivery has to recognise the high mobility of this group, associated poor planning and continuity of care, and the changing and diverse nature of their needs. This also needs to recognise how the latter is understood, comprehensively assessed, and addressed by different agencies. Any strategy devised by policy makers that is taken forward by commissioners and implemented by providers must ensure that resourcing of specialist forensic services is not at the direct expense of local CAMHS services and that any extra work undertaken by CAMHS is accompanied by adequate additional resources. Building on the recommendations of Kurtz *et al.* (1997) to the Department of Health in 1997, regionally based specialist services should include outreach services in the community, other agencies and secure units; inpatient services; development of specialisation within other services; expertise in the needs of the homeless; evaluation and research; evidence-based practice; training; and preventive measures. Multidimensional concepts of problems encountered by these young people have to subsume problem behaviours; diagnostic category; associated problems; reasons for seeking entry into services, for assessment, treatment or admission; cost utility; and user and carer opinion.

Improved triage of patients to treatments that are likely to work will continue to require understanding of children, parents and families that will make them more or less amenable to current treatments. Any new models of treatment delivery have to face the difficulties of retaining cases in treatment, the problems of co-morbidity and the relative paucity of long-term follow-up evidence for the clinical significance of change in the individual. Multisystemic therapy (Borduin *et al.*, 1995) has been shown to give long-term benefits most importantly in high-risk juveniles who have already carried out antisocial acts of violence.

From, recent demand and needs surveys, commissioning exercises, clinical experience in this field and current strategic thinking about both development of child mental health services and fulfilling the mandates of the Crime and Disorder Act of 1998, a framework for services should encompass the following:

- CAMHS, the goals of which should be (a) proper recognition of the current role of these services in the prevention and early intervention of antisocial behaviour in young children, with enhancement and enrichment of such services; and (b) the development within the current multidisciplinary team of special interest in forensic child and adolescent psychiatry, building on both the skills in (a) and on the developmental approach and expertise in the field of child protection, and management and treatment of high-risk complex cases within a medico-legal framework.
- Clarification of the role, purpose, accountability and clinical supervision of child and adolescent health and mental health staff, in particular nursing staff, currently being appointed to YOTs. How will they link into, work with or be part of local CAMHS and specialist forensic services to act as affective facilitators between and within services?
- Specialist workers within CAMHS and YOTs should be augmented by advice, training and consultation by a peripatetic multidisciplinary forensic outreach team.

- Regional forensic child and adolescent consultant assessment and treatment teams – multidisciplinary teams serving the 'community' in its widest sense, including court diversion, local authority secure care provision, young offender institutions and secure training centres.

Could and should services offer intensive 'home'-based service delivery that could allow for intensive services to young persons, carers and family; defined limited durations of treatment; and 24 h a day, 7 days a week availability of therapists? Such an intensive 'home'-based service might enable a young offender with mental health problems to be maintained in the community without the need to admit to a specialist psychiatric inpatient provision.

All community services and provision must work in close collaboration with specialist inpatient provision if we are not to re-enact some of the current dilemmas facing the commissioners of services for the care and treatment of adult mentally disordered offenders, in particular services for adults with personality disorder who offend, whom we know had childhood needs and risks that were poorly addressed.

Inpatient services could well be shared by more than one geographical health region and each inpatient unit may develop a focused range of expertise, while reorganising the principles enshrined in the Children Act of 1989, of providing services for children and young people as close to home and family as possible. Any individual young person presenting with particular problem profiles over time may require one or more of the following levels of inpatient services:

- 'Intensive care' adolescent inpatient services
- Habilitation/rehabilitation psychiatric secure and structured open inpatient services
- Maximum secure inpatient services

In developing services and interventions to meet needs and reduce the risk to mental health and risk of offending, commissioners and providers should avoid causing gaps in provision for one group while providing services for another.

Forensic mental health services could well learn from models of health care from the American Academy of Paediatrics 'managed care' proposals for children with special health care needs. These involve creating variable systems and care monitoring that is capable of producing process and outcome data from which appropriate adjustments are made to refine care in order to benefit children and families.

In describing programmes of public health care for children in Asia, the authors note that several child health care programmes, although well conceived, are poorly implemented, focusing on quantitative achievement but neglecting quality of care. Components and indicators of quality of care for an overall programme perspective include the following:

- Balance between short-term and long-term goals
- Effective management of services
- Coverage
- Health service provider–client partnership
- Reduction of symptoms/maladaptive behaviour

Recruitment, training and retention of multidisciplinary teams from across agencies in developing adolescent forensic services whether locally, regionally or nationally must as a first step understand the level of competency that has been reached when any professional has completed their respective training. Both understanding and valuing the skills acquired by each professional discipline is an important first step from which to develop a set of core and advanced skills in child and adolescent mental health.

Traditional research concentrates on either individual differences or developmental pathways. In order to understand both individual developmental processes and to specify the causal mechanisms that account for change in the frequency of disorders in the community at large, it is necessary to appreciate historical trends over time and to integrate causal explanations. To date concepts of causation have focused in the main on individual differences. Rutter *et al.* (1997) stress the need to draw distinctions between the processes involved in:

- Individual differences in the liability to engage in antisocial behaviour
- The translation of that liability into performance of an illegal act
- Differences over time, between places and in overall levels of crime
- Situational variations in delinquent activities
- Persistence or non-persistence of antisocial behaviours as the individual grows older

Cicchelti and Newcombe (1997) challenge researchers and clinicians to examine the implicit and explicit assumptions that guide their work and to devise constructive solutions to those potential impediments. Developmental psychopathology is put forward as the bridge across fields of study which span the life cycle and aid in the discovery of important new truths about the process underlying adaption and maladaption, as well as the best means of preventing or ameliorating psychopathology. Nowhere is this more needed than in the field of serious antisocial behaviour. There is evidence that, independently of socioeconomic variables, injury in violent crime is associated with a spectrum of disease in young adults comprising drug abuse, assault, elective surgery and trauma which can be explained by impulsivity.

Meanwhile the debate no doubt will continue as to whether it is the genetic alphabet rather than cultural differences that are the key determinants in the evolution, pattern and act of serious antisocial behaviour. Whatever the balance, policies that follow social explanation will require money and political will. Any underlying risk status, however it has arisen, is ultimately expressed in the social context. It is increasingly being recognised that local communities should play a pivotal role in helping young people to make pro-social choices. It takes a village to raise a child (Heide, 1995). There will have to be acceptance at a national level that programmes aimed at prevention and early intervention may take a minimum of ten years to demonstrate direct results. Denying mental health and social services benefits to children and adolescents today to save money will ensure that in future the prison population will grow. Above all, there needs to be a recognition of the importance of the power of any one individual adult to influence the life of any young person. Adults, who as children and adolescents, were exposed to many of the risk factors for serious antisocial behaviour, but proved to be resilient, frequently acknowledge the importance of an adult, who communicated intentionally or inadvertently that they believed in the adolescent, and cared for him or her.

REFERENCES

American Psychiatric Association (1994) *Diagnostic and Statistical Manual of Mental Disorders*, 4th edn (DSM-IV). Washington, DC: American Psychiatric Association.

Armstrong, G. (1997) Females under the law: 'protected' but inequal. *Crime and Delinquency*, **29**, 109–120.

Ashford, M. and Chard, A. (2000) *Defending Young People in the Criminal Justice System*. London: Legal Action Group (LAG).

Audit Commission (1996) *Misspent Youth. Young People and Crime*. London: Audit Commission.

Bailey, S. (1996) Adolescents who murder. *Journal of Adolescence*, **19**, 19–39.

Bailey, S. (1997a) Adolescent offenders. *Current Opinion in Psychiatry*, **10**, 445–453.

Bailey, S. (1997b) Review: sadistic and violent acts in the young. *Child Psychology and Psychiatry Review*, **2**, 92–102.

Bailey, S. (1992) Personality development in adolescents. *Journal of Forensic Psychiatry*, **4**, 413–319.

Bailey, S., Smith, C. and Dolan, M. (In press) The social background and nature of children who perpetrate violent crimes: a UK perspective. *Journal of Community Psychology*.

Birmingham, L., Mason, D. and Grubin, D. (1996) Prevalence of mental disorder in remand prisoners consecutive case study. *British Medical Journal*, **313**, 1521–1524.

Bodinger-Deuriate, C. (1991) Female adolescents: what prevention programmes need to know (update 9). *The Northwest Report*, September.

Borduin, C. M., Marin, B. J., Core, L. T., Henggeler, S. W., Fucci, B. R., Blaske, D. M. *et al.* (1995) Multisystemic treatment of services for juvenile offenders. Long term prevention of criminality and violence. *Journal of Consulting and Clinical Psychology*, **63**, 569–578.

Boswell, G. (1995) *Violent Victims. The Prevalence of Abuse and Loss in the Lives of Section 53 Offenders*. London: The Prince's Trust.

Bullock, R. and Milham, S. (1998) *Secure Treatment Outcomes: The Care Careers of Very Difficult Adolescents*. Dartington: Ashgale.

Calouste Gulbenkian Foundation (1995) *Children and Violence. Report of the Commission on Children and Violence*. London: Calouste Gulbenkian Foundation.

Chesney-Lind, M. (1987) Girls and violence: an exploration of the gender gap in serious delinquent behaviour. In D. Cromwell, I. Evansand and R. O'Donnell (eds), *Childhood Aggression and Violence: Sources of Influence, Prevention and Control*. Plenum: New York, pp. 207–229.

Christian, R. E., Frick, P. J., Hill, N. L., Tyler, L. and Frazer, D. R. (1997) Psychopathy and conduct problems in children. Implications for subtyping children with conduct problems. *Journal of the American Academy of Child and Adolescent Psychiatry*, **36**, 233–241.

Cicchelti, D. and Newcombe, B. (1997) Special issue. Conceptual and scientific underpinnings of research in developmental psychopathology. *Developmental Psychopathology*, **9**, 189–472.

Coleman, J. (1997) *Key Data on Adolescence 10–12*. Brighton: Trust for the Study of Adolescence.

Communities that Care (UK) (1997) *A New Kind Of Prevention Programme. A Guide – 1997*. London: Rowntree Foundation.

Criminal Statistics, England and Wales (1994). London: HMSO.

Criminal Statistics, England and Wales (1995) London: HMSO.

Dodge, K. A., Bates, J. E. and Petit, G. S. (1990) Mechanisms in the cycle of violence. *Science*, **250**, 1678–1683.

Dolan, M., Holloway, J., Bailey, S. and Kroll, L. (1996) The psychosocial characteristics of juvenile sex offenders referred to an Adolescent Forensic Service in the UK. *Medicine, Science and the Law*, **36**, 343–352.

Dolan, M., Holloway, J., Bailey, S. and Smith, C. (1999) Health status of juvenile offenders. A survey of young offenders appearing before the juvenile courts. *Journal of Adolescence*, **22**, 137–144.

Farrington, D. P (1995) The development of offending and antisocial behaviour from childhood. Key findings from the Cambridge Study in Delinquent Development. *Journal of Child Psychology and Psychiatry*, **36**, 929–964.

Farrington, D. P. (1996) *Understanding and Preventing Youth Crime*. York: Joseph Rowntree Foundation.

Farrington, D. P. and West, D. J. (1993) Criminal, penal and life histories of chronic offenders. Risk and protective factors and early identification. *Criminal Behaviour and Mental Health*, 3, 492–523.

Farrington, D. P., Barnes, G. and Lamberst, S. (1996) The concentration of offending in families. *Legal and Criminological Psychology*, 1, 47–63.

Federal Bureau of Investigation (1992) *Uniform Crime Reports for the United States 1991*. Washington, DC: US Government Printing Office.

Fergusson, D. M., Lynskey, M. T. and Harwood, J. L. (19??) Origins of comorbidity between conduct and affective disorders. *Journal of the American Academy of Child and Adolescent Psychiatry*, 35, 451–460. [Year??].

Fineman, K. R. (1980) Firesetting in childhood and adolescence. *Psychiatric Clinics of North America*, 3, 483–500.

Gunn, J., Maden, A. and Swinton, M. (1991) Treatment needs of prisoners with psychiatric disorders. *British Medical Journal*, 303, 338–341.

Goodman, R. (1997) *Child and Adolescent Mental Health Services: Reasoned Advise to Commissioners and Providers. Maudsley Discussion Paper 4*. London: Maudsley Publications.

Gudjonnsson, G. and Clark, N. (1986) Suggestibility in police interrogation. A social psychological model. *Social Behaviour*, 1, 88–104.

Hacipasalo, J. and Tremblay, R. E. (1994) Physically aggressive boys from age 6 to 12. Family background, parenting behaviour and prediction of delinquency. *Journal of Consulting Clinical Psychology*, 62, 1044–1052.

Hagell, A. and Newburn, T. (1994) *Persistent Young Offenders*. London: Policy Studies Institute.

Hare, R. D. (1993) *With our Conscience: The Disturbing World of the Psychopaths among Us*. New York: Pocket.

Harrington, R., Fudge, H., Rutter, M., Pickles, A. and Hill, J. (1991) Adult outcome of childhood and adolescent depression. Links with antisocial disorders. *Journal of the American Academy of Child and Adolescent Psychiatry*, 30, 434–439.

Harris, D. P., Cole, J. E. and Vipond, E. M. (1987) Residential treatment of disturbed delinquents. Description of centre and identification of therapeutic factors. *Canadian Journal of Psychiatry*, 32, 579–583.

Hawkins, J. D. and Catalano, R. F. (1992) *Communities that Care*. San Francisco, CA: Jossey-Bass.

Heide, K. M. (1995) Violence in America. How can we save our children? *Stanford Law and Policy Review*, 7, 43–49.

Heide, K. M. (1999) *Young Killers: The Challenge of Juvenile Homicide*. New York: Sage Publications.

Henggeler, S. W. (1999) Multi-systemic therapy: an overview of clinical procedures, outcomes and policy implications. *Child Psychology Review*, 4, 2–10.

H.M. Prison Service (1999) *Joint Prison Service and National Health Service Executive Working Group on the Future Organisation of Prison Health Care.* London: H.M. Prison Service.

James, A. C. and Neil, P. (1996) Juvenile sexual offending. One year period prevalence study within Oxfordshire. *Child Abuse and Neglect,* **13,** 477–485.

Jasper, A., Smith, C. and Bailey, S. (1998) One hundred girls in care referred to an Adolescent Forensic Service. *Journal of Adolescence,* **21,** 555–568.

Junger-Tas, J. *et al.* (1994) *Delinquent Behaviour among Young People in the Western World: First Results of the International Self-report Delinquency Study.* Amsterdam: Kugler.

Justice (1996) *Children and Homicide. Appropriate Procedures for Juveniles in Murder and Manslaughter Cases.* London: Justice.

Kazdin, A. E. (1997) Practitioner review. Psychosocial treatments for conduct disorder in children. *Journal of Child Psychology and Psychiatry,* **38,** 161–178.

Kurtz, Z., Thornes, R. and Bailey, S. (1997) *A Study of the Demand and Needs for Forensic Child and Adolescent Mental Health Services in England and Wales.* London: Department of Health.

Kolko, D. J. and Kazdin, A. E. (1992) The emergence and re-occurrence of child firesetting. A one year prospective study. *Journal of Abnormal Child Psychology,* **201,** 17–37.

Liebling, A. (1991) Suicide and self injury amongst young offenders in custody. *Dissertation.* Cambridge University.

Lipsey, M. (1995) What do we learn from 400 research studies on the effectiveness of treatment with juvenile delinquents? In J. McGuire (ed.), *What Works: Reducing Reoffending Guidelines from Research and Practice.* Chichester: Wiley, pp. 66–78.

Loeber, R. (1990) Development and risk factors of juvenile antisocial behaviour and delinquency. *Clinical Psychological Revue,* **10,** 1–41.

Loeber, R. and Hay, D. F. (1994) Developmental approaches to aggression and conduct problems. In M. Rutter and D. Hay (eds), *Development Through Life: A Handbook for Clinicians.* Oxford: Blackwell Science, pp. 488–516.

Maden, A., Swinton, M. and Gunn, J. (1994) Psychiatric disorder in women serving a prison sentence. *British Journal of Psychiatry,* **164,** 44–54.

Maziade, M., Bouchard, S., Gingras, N. and Charron, L. (1996) Long term stability of diagnosis and symptom dimensions in a systematic sample of patients with onset of schizophrenia in childhood and early adolescence II. Positive/Negative distinction and childhood predictors of adult outcome. *British Journal of Psychiatry,* **169,** 371–378.

McCann, J., James, A., Wilson, S. and Dunn, G. (1996) Prevalence of psychiatric disorders in young people in the care system. *British Medical Journal,* **313,** 1529–1533.

McNally, R. B. (1995) Homicidal youth in England and Wales 1982–1992. Profile and Policy. *Psychology Crime and the Law*, I, 333–342.

Mirrlees-Black, C., Mayhew, P. and Percy, A. (1996) *The 1996 British Crime Survey England and Wales*. London: Home Office Research and Statistics Directorate.

Mohan, D., Scully, P., Collins, C. and Smith, C. (1997) Psychiatric disorder in an Irish female prison. *Criminal Behaviour and Mental Health*, 7, 229–235.

Myers, W. C., Kemph, J. P. (1990) DSM-III-R – classification of homicidal youth – help or hindrance? *Journal of Clinical Psychiatry*, 5, 239–42.

O'Brien, B. S. and Frick, P. J. (1996) Reward dominance associations with anxiety conduct problems and psychopathy in children. *Journal of Abnormal Child Psychology*, 24, 223–240.

Patterson, G. R. (1982) *Coercive Family Process*. Eugene, OR: Castilla.

Patterson, G. R., Capaldi, D. and Bank, L. (1991) An early starter model for predicting delinquency. In D. J. Pepler and K. H. Rubin (eds), *The Development and Treatment of Childhood Aggression*. Hillsdale, NJ: Erlbaum, pp. 139–168.

Pease, K. and Tseloni, A. (1996) Adult differences in criminal Justice. Evidence from the United Nations Crime Survey. *The Howard Journal*, 35, 40–60.

Pope, A. W., Bierman, K. L. and Mumma, G. H (1989) Relations between hyperactive and aggressive behaviours and peer relations at three elementary grade levels. *Journal of Abnormal Child Psychology*, 17, 253–267.

Rowe-Grant, N., Thomas, B. H., Offord, D. R. and Boyle, M. H. (1989) Risk, protective factors, and the prevalence of behavioural and emotional disorders in children and adolescents. *Journal of the American Academy of Child and Adolescent Psychiatry*, 28, 262–268.

Royal College of Psychiatrists' Council Report CR71 (1999) *Offenders with Personality Disorder*. London: Gaskell Publications.

Rutter, M. (1981) The city and the child. *American Journal of Orthopsychiatry*, 51, 610–625.

Rutter, M., Maughan, B., Meyer, J., Pickles, A., Silberg, J., Simonoff, E. *et al.* (1997) Heterogeneity of antisocial behaviour. Causes, continuities and consequences. In R. Dienstbier and D. W. Osgood (eds), *Nebraska Symposium on Motivation. Vol. 44. Motivation and Delinquency*. Lincoln, NE: University of Nebraska Press.

Rutter, M., Giller, H. and Hagell, A. (1998) *Antisocial Behaviour by Young People*. Cambridge: Cambridge University Press.

Schweinhart, L. J., Barnes, H. O. and Weikart, D. P. (1993) *Significant Benefits*. Ypsilanti, MI: High/Scope Press.

Shepherd, J. P. and Farrington, D. P. (1993) Assault as a public health problem. *Journal of the Royal Society of Medicine*, 6, 89–92.

Smith, D. J. (1995) Youth crime and conduct disorders. Trends, patterns and causal explanations. In M. Rutter and D. J. Smith (eds), *Psychosocial Disorders in Young People: Time Trends and their Causes*. Chichester: Wiley, pp. 389–489.

Smith, S. and Thornberry, T. P. (1995) The relationship between childhood maltreatment and adolescent involvement in delinquency. *Criminology*, **33**, 451–481.

Stephenson, G. (1992) *The Psychology of Criminal Justice*. Oxford: Blackwell.

Synder, H. N. and Sickmund, M. (1995) *Juvenile Offenders and Victims. A National Report*. Washington, DC: Office of Juvenile Justice Delinquency Prevention.

Synder, H. N., Poe-Yamagata, E. and Sickmund, M. (1996) *Juvenile Offenders and Victims. 1996 Update on Violence*. Washington, DC: Office of Juvenile Justice and Delinquency Prevention.

Tonry, M. and Farrington, D. P. (1995) Strategic approaches to crime prevention. In M. Tonry, and D. P. Farrington (eds), *Building a Safer Society: Strategic Approaches to Crime Prevention*. Chicago, IL: University of Chicago Press, pp. 1–20.

Tyrer, P. and Stein, G. (1993) *Personality Disorder. Reviewed*. London: Royal College of Psychiatrists/Gaskell.

Virkunnen, M., Goldman, D. and Linnoila, L. (1995) Serotonin in alcoholic violent offenders. *Genetics of Criminal and Antisocial Behaviour*. Chichester: Wiley, pp. 168–182.

Vizard, E., Wynick, S., Hawkes, C., Woods, J. and Jenkins, J. (1996) Juvenile sexual offenders. Assessment issues. *British Journal of Psychiatry*, **168**, 259–262.

Vreeland, R. G. and Levin, B. M. (1980) Psychological aspects of firesetting. In D. Canter (ed.), *Fires and Human Behaviour*. New York: Wiley.

Wessely, S., Akhurst, A., Brown, I. and Moss, L. (1996) Deliberate self-harm and the probation services: an overlooked public health problem? *Journal of Public Health Medicine*, **18**, 129–132.

Widom, C. S. and White, H. R. (1997) Problem behaviours in abused and neglected children grown up: prevalence and co-occurence of substance abuse, crime and violence. *Criminal Behaviour and Mental Health*, **7**, 287–310.

World Health Organisation (1992) *The ICD-10 Classification of Mental and Behavioural Disorders. Clinical Descriptions and Diagnostic Guidelines*. Geneva: World Health Organisation.

Zingraff, M. T., Leifer, J., Myers, K. A. and Johnson, M. L. (1993) Childhood maltreatment and youthful problem behaviour. *Criminology*, **31**, 173–202.

Zoccolillo, M., Tremblay, R. and Vitaro, F. (1996) DSM-III-R and DSM-III criteria for conduct disorder in pre-adolescent girls: specific but insensitive. *Journal of the American Academy Child and Adolescent Psychiatry*, **35**, 461–471.

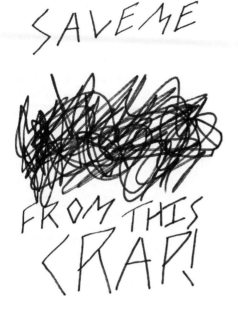

Chapter 17

PREVENTION

Robin Glaze

INTRODUCTION

Since 1995 we have seen a terrific growth in the academic literature base on preventive strategies for psychiatric disorders, and the availability of both easily accessible and digestible information on psychiatric health issues for adolescents. This chapter describes the scope of psychiatric preventive work, illustrates the spread of responsibility for its execution, describes the role of poverty, employment and housing, illuminates the work of health promotion bodies, and provides a taste of current thinking on prevention in depression, disaster management, eating disorders and schizophrenia.

PREVENTION IN CONTEXT

In the post-war years, mortality rates for physical illness have dropped to historically low levels in most Western countries as new medical treatments and improved standards of nutrition and housing have reduced the occurrence of acute infectious illness (Patton, 1998). Similarly, treatments are now available for a number of non-infectious diseases that previously would have resulted in death, like childhood malignancy and cystic fibrosis. These factors have led to a general perception of adolescence being an age of good health and so it has been perceived in mental health too. Coupled with an absence of evidence for later emotional or social difficulties arising out of, what was seen as, the normal adolescent turmoil, ambivalent attitudes led to poorly coordinated provision of adolescent mental health services.

Specialist adolescent services in most countries have tended to have an inpatient focus, with a mandate for treating the most severe behavioural disturbances. Severe mental illness in older adolescents would often be dealt with in an adult ward setting and younger adolescents were treated in child guidance or child psychiatric clinics. In this way the opportunities for specialist intervention with the commoner, less severe, disorders were limited by poor accessibility to, and limited availability of, adolescent mental health services. There is little doubt that the future of adolescent psychiatry will be greatly influenced by the recognition of rising incidence rates for many common psychiatric disorders, and the changes in pattern of disorders and problem behaviours post puberty. In particular:

- Hazard rates for depression and substance abuse are highest in the teens and early 20s (Kessler *et al.*, 1994)
- Rising rates of depression and suicide, delinquency, eating disorders, and drug and alcohol abuse (Fombonne, 1998)
- Downward age trend in tobacco use, sexual activity, and alcohol and illicit substance use (Fergusson, 1998)
- Depressive symptoms increase, anxiety syndromes become more adult like, and behavioural syndromes such as eating disorders, substance abuse and suicide, which are uncommon in childhood, rise in frequency in adolescence (Patton, 1998)

Finally, it is worth remembering that problems like the conduct and attention deficit disorders (externalising) have strong continuity between childhood and adolescence. The early behaviour difficulties are complicated by resultant school problems with educational under-achievement, mixing with disaffected peers, and often an increasing pattern of antisocial and other health risk behaviours. Preventive strategies for these disorders must therefore aim to minimise this developmental sequence, and are likely to require multifaceted interventions involving school, and youngsters' families and peers, alongside a notion of important turning points such as leaving school and marriage (Fergusson, 1998).

DEFINITIONS

Prevention includes the overlapping areas of health promotion, health education and disease prevention. Health promotion has been defined by the World Health Organisation as the process of enabling people to increase control over, and to improve, their health. This process usually involves a combination of health education, specific preventive services such as immunisation and screening, and policies and regulations (health protection). The key goal of health promotion is to enhance positive health (well-being and fitness) whilst preventing ill-health. Health promotion also acknowledges that physical, social and mental components are interlinked. The Department of Health in the UK now recommends that this should be one of the major activities of child mental health services (Department of Health, 1995), a position endorsed by a parliamentary select committee (Parliamentary Select Committee, 1997), and the Child and Adolescent Faculty of the Royal College of Psychiatrists (1990).

Health education can be viewed as the liaison arm of health promotion. It is concerned with both the fostering of motivation and skills that promote health, along-side the actual giving of information. It aims to influence the broad context of health and not just the individual's behaviour. Health education has to influence not just the general public, but also those organisations and bodies in a position to formulate health protection policies and regulations.

Disease prevention involves decreasing (or eliminating) risk, or aetiological factors, that contribute to or cause disease. Preventive strategies have traditionally been thought of as occurring prior to (prevention), during (treatment) and after (maintenance) index episodes of illness (Harrington and Clark, 1998).

PRIMARY PREVENTION

Primary prevention involves activities that act to reduce the incidence of disorder in those that have not yet developed it. An example of this in physical medicine would be aseptic technique in the operating theatre acting to prevent wound infection post-procedure or immunisation to eradicate smallpox. In adolescent psychiatric practice, primary prevention is necessarily targeted on risk factors and risk mechanisms, which is not without difficulty. Taking depression as an example, the key risk factors can be summarised as personal disposition, social disposition and current adversities.

SECONDARY PREVENTION

This involves the early detection of illness and its standard treatment. Again borrowing examples from physical medicine, the Papanicolaou smear test for pre-cancerous change in the cervix and post-operative antibiotic treatment both represent secondary prevention. Psychiatric disorders are rarely amenable to early detection at a point when no symptoms are present, because their diagnosis largely depends upon the report of symptoms (Greenfield and Shore, 1995). Thus the focus must be on detection at an early stage when only a few symptoms are present, or when they have existed for only a short time.

Secondary prevention thus relies on screening tests for treatable disorders being implemented in appropriate populations. To be economic, the following criteria must be applied:

- The disorder screened for must have a treatment intervention
- Early detection and treatment must reduce morbidity (and/or mortality)
- The screening test must be of high sensitivity (to avoid false negatives)
- The screening test must have high specificity (to avoid false positives)
- The prevalence of the disorder in the target population must be high

TERTIARY PREVENTION

This involves maintenance, treatment or rehabilitation to reduce the debilitating impact, discomfort or severity of a disorder once experienced. It might also involve the reduction of the acute and chronic complications of the disorder. An example from physical medicine might be regular exercises following a shoulder or back injury. In psychiatric practice examples include maintenance treatment with lithium to prevent relapse in paediatric bipolar illness, educational or vocational rehabilitation of adolescents with chronic psychotic disorders to reduce social impairment, and sometimes the usage of psychotropic medications and psychotherapy.

TYPES OF PREVENTIVE ACTIVITY

Preventive activities may be universal or selective. Universal preventive strategies are applied to everyone, without any attempt to target groups at risk of a disorder. Childhood immunisation for smallpox or tetanus is a good example of this approach. Universal prevention has the following advantages:

- It is less stigmatising
- It can dramatically reduce incidence (as in the complete eradication of smallpox)
- Where the burden of care affects whole families (as in depression or schizophrenia) or where morbidity is associated with symptoms rather than a full-blown disorder (as in depression), everyone benefits a little

Selective prevention aims to target high-risk groups. These may be vulnerability, event focused (Newton, 1988) or indicated (Mrazek and Haggerty, 1994). Vulnerability-focused interventions seek to improve the resilience of adolescents at risk of mental illness, perhaps by working with the individual or their family. Event-centred interventions aim to impact on happenings that may be linked to mental illness. Thus the effects of bereavement, sexual abuse and other traumas can be ameliorated using debriefing, and other techniques aimed at externalising the traumatic experience. Finally, indicated interventions are those targeted towards high-risk individuals who have minimal, but discernible, symptoms known to be consistent with the later onset of a mental disorder. Selective interventions have the following advantages:

- They are more cost-effective
- They minimise the risk of harm to non-affected individuals
- The interventions can be tailored to particular circumstances

THE ROLE OF POVERTY, EMPLOYMENT AND HOUSING

Intellectual development and educational achievement are much more strongly related to social class (a proxy measure of income) than the majority of child psychiatric disorders (Rutter and Madge, 1976), so that the reduction of serious poverty *per se* may have more of an effect on intellectual development than on rates of adolescent disorder. One in three children in Britain currently live in poverty, a rise from 1.3 million in 1979 to over 4 million today (Smith, 1999). Two of every five children are born in poverty, whilst one in six families are pushed into poverty by the birth of another child. Children are more likely to be poor if they live in large families, have lone parents or are from ethnic minorities (especially Pakistani and Bangladeshi families).

Longitudinal studies of teenagers in and out of employment have shown that they are more likely to offend whilst unemployed, indicating the possibility of poverty as a mediating factor (Farrington *et al.*, 1986). Similarly, older teenagers failing to find a job post leaving school have more psychiatric symptoms (Banks and Jackson, 1982), which also holds true for adults. Equally, mothers of young children in work feel better supported and experience fewer anxiety states or depression (Bebbington, 1984). Graham (1994) has described homelessness amongst families in the UK as a scandal, pointing out the high rates of vandalism and delinquency in teenagers, and high rates of developmental delay, emotional and behavioural problems, and parental depression amongst children living in homeless families' accommodation.

AGENCIES RESPONSIBLE FOR PREVENTION

GOVERNMENTS

The role of the legislature in adolescent mental health issues impacts directly and indirectly at many levels. The new NHS reforms include:

- Primary care groups (PCGs) and trusts (PCTs) to replace existing commissioning and funding arrangements

- The slimming down of health authorities with stronger powers to oversee the health of local residents
- A duty of partnership between health authorities, local authorities, primary care groups and NHS Trusts
- Three-year health improvement programmes
- Longer term service agreements between Trusts and PCGs, usually focused around a particular group or disease, for example children or eating disorders
- National Service Frameworks

The notion of preventive policy was further strengthened by the subsequent Green Paper, *Our Healthier Nation*, whose themes were explicit:

- Tackling the root causes of illness, lifestyle and inequalities (poverty, low wages, unemployment, poor housing, and crime and disorder)
- A 'contract for health'
- Improvement of the health of the population as a whole
- To narrow the 'health gap' between the best and worst off in society
- To set targets for major killer diseases such as reduction of death by suicide and undetermined injury by a sixth

The following wide ranging actions were proposed:

- *Wired for Health*, a computerised link to the National Grid for Learning, for all schools and colleges in the country
- An advisory group on personal, social and health education by the Department for Education and Employment
- An integrated national transport policy
- Tough measures on crime
- Health improvement programmes
- Health outcomes of NHS care
- Health Action Zones (HAZ)
- Healthy schools initiative
- Healthy workplace projects

In an effort to formulate a linking concept, the government has coined the phrase 'social exclusion'. This is used as a shorthand label for what can happen when individuals or areas suffer from the combination of the linked problems of unemployment, poor skills, low income, poor housing, high crime environments, bad health and family breakdown. The Social Exclusion Unit (SEU) is a Cabinet Office department which reports directly to the Prime Minister, along with a network of ministerial champions, to draw together exclusion issues in their own departments. The membership of the department is taken from the civil service, people from local government, business, the voluntary sector, police and probation services. Amongst its key initial work tasks are:

- Truancy and school exclusions
- Rough sleeping
- Worst estates
- Improving mechanisms for integrating the work of departments, local authorities and other agencies
- Linking with the comprehensive spending reviews
- Drawing up key indicators of social exclusion

A relevant and illustrative example of the need for substantial inter-connectedness of policy and services, arises in the preventive management of teenage pregnancy, drug and alcohol abuse, and smoking. The UK has the highest rates of teenage pregnancy in western Europe, British teenagers are more likely to have used all categories of illicit drugs than their counterparts in any other European Union country, 15-year-old boys in Wales and Northern Ireland are likely to drink alcohol at least weekly, and a quarter of Welsh girls smoke at least once a week (McKee, 1999). A good general education is a major factor in delaying pregnancy and education level is important in determining smoking rates. The UK vies with the US for bottom place among major industrialised nations on a range of measures of literacy, numeracy and basic skills (Department for Education and Employment, 1996). Increasingly since the 1980s, many more UK families live in poverty than in the rest of the European Union. Being below the poverty line has an effect on both smoking and the ability to stop. British parents work the longest hours in Europe, thus being less available to supervise their children, an important factor in truancy. Truancy and exclusion are major risk factors for teenage pregnancy, unemployment and homelessness or ending up in prison (Social Exclusion Unit, 1998a). The poorest neighbourhoods have tended to become more rundown, more prone to crime and more cut off from the labour market, with weakening family structures, more divorce and more children born outside of marriage (Social Exclusion Unit, 1998b).

HEALTH AUTHORITIES/BOARDS

The Health Education Authority in England is supported by the NHS. Regional Health Authorities work in partnership with them to provide funding, and in return receive advice on health promotion issues. A similar arrangement exists in Scotland for the Health Education Board for Scotland.

OTHER AGENCIES

Child and adolescent mental health services

In the author's experience of district-based practice, the current climate of chronic under-funding and rising referral rates makes it difficult for clinics to focus on primary preventive work, although necessarily routine opportunities for second-ary and tertiary prevention do arise (see 'Clinical practice points').

Paediatric services

Yager's (1989) survey of 316 paediatricians' attitudes toward mental illness prevention for high-risk children in routine paediatric practice showed that although most had a generally positive attitude they were also wary of serious financial, educational and time barriers to its implementation.

Health Education Authority

Based in London, the Health Education Authority (HEA) is England's lead body for health promotion. It aims to help people nationally and internationally, to make a sustainable improvement in health and reduce health inequalities. The HEA advises the government on health promotion strategy, works with professionals on practical projects designed to improve health, maintains a substantial knowledge base and undertakes research in key areas of health promotion like the usefulness of the Internet as a vehicle for health promotion. The HEA was founded in 1987 as a Special Health Authority and is largely funded by the UK government's Department of Health. Approximately 250 people with a wide range of professional skills in research, health, health promotion policy, education and communications are employed to:

• Work with decision makers and opinion formers on health strategy
• Work with, and for, professionals involved in health and health improvement
• Work with, and for, members of the public

The HEA provide publications such as leaflets for GP surgeries and all new mothers receive a free copy of their pregnancy book. The HEA also publishes articles in the press, consumer magazines, specialist and professional publications, and programmes on TV and radio. They are involved in advertising campaigns like the recent TV campaign on smoking. Finally there are a series of excellent websites (see Table 17.1) and CD-ROMs such as 'D-Code' which presents information on drugs.

Similarly, Scotland has the Health Education Board for Scotland (HEBS). HEBS was established on 1 April 1991, replacing the Scottish Health Education Group as the national agency for health education in Scotland. As with the HEA, HEBS is a Special Health Board within the NHS in Scotland. The responsibility for ensuring appropriate health promotion at local levels rests with the 15 Scottish health boards who are HEBS's principal partners.

Compared with the HEA, HEBS stated goals are to:

• Ensure that people have adequate information on health and the factors influencing it
• To help people to acquire the motivation and skills to enable them to safeguard their own health and other people's health
• To promote commitment to, and participation in, health promotion in all levels of society

Table 17.1 HEA websites

Website	Description
www.thinkfast.co.uk	An interactive website for young people on fast food
www.active.org.uk	Information on becoming more active
www.trashed.co.uk	A website giving straightforward information about drugs, the risks and what the law says
www.d-code.co.uk	Gives information on the HEA's award-winning CD-Rom, trailers sections of it and has on-line ordering via E-mail
www.wrecked.co.uk	An interactive website for young people exploring alcohol usage
www.lifesaver.co.uk	Support, advice and motivation to give up smoking
www.wad.hea.org.uk	An annual website explaining the World Aids Day
www.lovelife.hea.org.uk	HEA's sexual health website for young people – it provides up to date information on sexual health issues, including how to avoid HIV, other sexually transmitted infections and unwanted pregnancy
www.hea.org.uk/locate	Provides free information for professionals on out-of-school drug education and prevention activities for 11–25 year olds in England; the aim of this site is to put local providers, purchasers and planners in touch with others around the country
www.interact.hea.liv.ac.uk/hipp	A website for health professionals interested in the commissioning process

- To encourage and enable policy makers at all levels to recognise possible health consequences of their activities and to make policies which promote health

HEBS is funded by the NHS in Scotland, through the sale of publications, and through charging for education and training events. Besides working in partnership with the 15 Health Boards of Scotland, HEBS has contact with a broad spectrum of national organisations and educational institutions, as well as liaison with the HEA, Health Promotion Wales and the Health Promotion Agency for Northern Ireland. Finally, HEBS too has an excellent Internet site called HEBSWeb (at http://www.hebs.scot.nhs.uk/) with good information on the main psychiatric disorders, with advice on where to go for help, useful addresses and suggestions for further reading, both for adults, children and people with learning difficulties. Drugs and alcohol are well covered, and all major areas have journal articles listed for further information.

PREVENTION IN PRACTICE

Most psychosocial disorders involve multiple causes and, even though many risk factors have been identified, there has not always been a clear way to eliminate them or ameliorate their effects. This led Rutter (1982) to the notion that primary prevention strategies should be targeted at known risk factors by implementing policies that improve general health measures such as:

- Reduce the incidence of organic brain dysfunction
- Prevent unwanted births
- Promote the continuity of good quality parenting (reduce multiple foster placements)
- Improve and enrich children's environments (day care, pre-school, school)
- Decrease the availability of drugs and alcohol

However, over the last 5 years there has been a significant growth in the literature on preventive approaches to a number of adolescent and adult disorders. So much so in fact that it is not possible, within the space available, to attempt anything other than brief coverage. With this in mind, examples from a selection of disorders are presented to illustrate primary, secondary and tertiary preventive approaches.

DEPRESSION

Harrington and Clark (1998) present a scheme of possible interventions. They argue that the difficulties in defining depression and identifying risk factors that can be easily remedied make it unlikely that primary prevention programmes will prove to be more effective than treatment and rehabilitation in the foreseeable future. A balanced preventive programme for depression should give a higher priority to treatment services than to those focused on early intervention. Selective interventions (see Table 17.2) can be usefully targeted on the following risk factors:

- Family history of depression
- Traumatic experiences (e.g. bereavement and sexual abuse)
- Depressive symptoms (predict depressive disorder)

Clinical practice points

Once a clinical diagnosis has been made it is important to carefully plan the treatment process with the family. It is important to be up-beat with the youngster, who may be despairing and feeling hopeless, and their family, who may be experiencing guilt feelings at not having recognised their child's depression. The author finds it helpful to use a series of ritual statements along the following line:

Table 17.2 Prevention levels and selective interventions

Prevention level	Strategy	Intervention
Primary	Universal preventive	Permanency planning to reduce multiple foster placements Reduction of unwanted pregnancies by better contraceptive advice and birth control strategies Improving self-esteem and individual's competence to buffer against the effects of later trauma
	Vulnerability-focused selective	Clinician-administered educational programme for depressed parents (Beardslee, 1993); found to be better than a lecture intervention Befriending schemes like Newpin and Homestart Genetic counselling Treatment of co-morbid disorders such as conduct disorder
	Event-centred selective	Psychological debriefing for the sexually abused and bereaved; with an attributable risk of 14% for depression amongst the sexually abused (Fergusson et al., 1996), they would be a more efficient target than the bereaved
Secondary	Vulnerability-focused selective	12 school-based treatment sessions for children with depressive symptoms or maternal conflict (Jaycox, 1994) Group cognitive intervention for children with depressive symptoms; lowers the risk for later depressive syndrome (Clarke et al., 1995)
Tertiary	Vulnerability-focused selective	Continuation of cognitive-behaviour therapy (CBT) post depression may be effective at preventing relapse (Kroll et al., 1996) Global functioning improves more after treatment with CBT than with relaxation training, whereas treatment of co-morbid anxiety and conduct problems has no effect (Wood et al., 1996) Use of safer treatments to reduce the risk of suicide
Vigorous treatment	Vulnerability-focused selective	Treatment in early adolescence could in theory reduce the risk of later depressive episodes by up to 10% (Harrington and Clark, 1998)

- Indicate the diagnosis
- Indicate the frequency of depressive disorders – many youngsters are relieved to be told that they are not unique, and benefit from being told the prevalence rate and approximately how many others will also be suffering, for example, in their year at school
- Emphasise that an excellent range of modern treatments for depression are available and an optimistic prognosis
- Outline the range of treatments (conversational and physical) and link them to the severity of the patients own depression

Sometimes during this process, a parent will indicate that they too have suffered from depression. A brief exploration of this, making links to the youngster's own depressive illness, also helps to reduce the patient's isolation. At this stage the initial treatment regime and any medication can be discussed. Many parents and some adolescents have substantial worries about the use of medication. It is an investment to spend considerable time dealing with these worries and, provided you are open, realistic and honest, the majority will be persuaded to give it a try. The following points should be covered:

- The type of medication proposed
- Its likely common side effects and potential risks and benefits
- The timescale involved for improvement in mood
- The possibility of having to increase the dosage to achieve optimum effect
- What to do in the event of side effects
- What would happen if the drug did not work
- The benefits of maintenance treatment and its duration, e.g. 4–6 months further treatment at the dose that brought about initial response roughly halves the rate of relapse (Kupfer and Frank, 1992; Reimherr et al., 1998)
- When to stop continuation therapy – incomplete recovery is the most important risk factor for relapse within 1 year of treatment withdrawal (Kupfer and Frank, 1992)
- The risk of dependence
- Any specific points the youngster or family raise

A frequent question is what to do about school attendance. This really depends on the adolescent's individual circumstances, their wishes and the effects of their depression on school performance. There is a balance to be struck between the helpful effects of continued peer contact, and the general levels of stress engendered by the school environment and study pressures. As a general principle, the youngster should be encouraged back into increasing socialisation as the depression improves. Cognitive-behavioural techniques are useful in countering loss of confidence, and dealing with peers' questions and other issues arising out of their mental illness, in addition to dealing with social stresses contributory to the depressive episode (e.g. bullying) or resulting from it (e.g. depressive irritability).

Future sessions should focus on enabling the youngster to manage their own depression. This involves:

- General education on depressive illness
- Information on prognosis, e.g. the mean length of major depressive disorder is 7–9 months, 90% have remitted by 1.5–2 years, 6–10% become protracted, there is a high relapse rate with a cumulative probability of recurrence of 40% by 2 years and 70% by 5 years, and 20–40% of adolescents develop periods of

major depressive disorder and mania (bipolar I disorder) within 5 years of the onset of depression (Birmaher *et al.*, 1996)
- Help to recognise their own depressive symptoms (relapse signature)
- Advice on seeking early treatment during further episodes

DISASTER MANAGEMENT

Partial symptomatology and co-morbidity are common in post-traumatic stress disorder (Pfefferbaum, 1997). Since, by definition, the condition is likely to occur after disaster situations, much of the literature describes the child's response, which will vary with the exact nature of the trauma, the child's age, developmental stage and the reactions of trusted adults. Child witnesses respond to violent events in two stages. First, there is an immediate reaction to the trauma, then secondly a further response to the trauma and grief. Secondary prevention in the first phase focuses on protection and advocacy, whilst in the second phase interventions help the child to acknowledge (recall and re-tell) and tolerate the violent event (Rollins, 1997). Schools and communities are common venues for such interventions.

Common symptoms amongst children following the Aberfan disaster, in which a coal tip slid down a mountainside killing 116 children and 28 adults, included sleep difficulties, nervousness, lack of friends, reluctance to go out to play, instability and enuresis (Lacey, 1972). Some anxious parents became over-protective. Fears of the dark and nightmares caused sleep problems, and bad weather (which had occurred prior to the accident) upset the children. The children rarely spoke of their experiences spontaneously. The children who had prior difficulties were at greater risk of symptoms. Yule (1994), reporting on the symptoms of children and adolescent survivors of the capsize of the *Herald of Free Enterprise* car ferry and those from the sinking of the cruise ship *Jupiter*, notes similar reactions. Most children suffered repetitive and intrusive thoughts about the accident, particularly at quiet times or whilst waiting to sleep. Vivid recollections were triggered by reminders in their environment. Vivid flashbacks were common. Sleep problems were very common, particularly in the first few weeks, with fears of the dark, bad dreams and nightmares, and waking through the night. For the first few days children did not want to let parents out of their sight, often reverting to sleeping in the parental bed, and even teenagers had problems separating.

Children reported difficulties in concentration, especially in school. Others reported problems, both in mastering new material and in remembering old skills such as reading music. Survivors learned that life is fragile and became alert to danger in their environment. Many developed fears associated with specific aspects of their trauma and avoided situations associated with the disaster. 'Survivor guilt' occurred where there were concerns about having survived when others died, about thinking they should have done more for others and about what they themselves had done to survive. Adolescent survivors often developed depression, having clinical symptoms, suicidal thoughts and taking overdoses in the year after the disaster. Other children were bereaved and needed bereavement counselling. Many children found it difficult to talk to their parents and peers. Often they would fear upsetting adults and peers often avoided asking about the incidents in case they upset the child further. As a result parents were often unaware of the full extent of the child's trauma and the child felt rejected by its peers.

Clinical practice points

- Stress inoculation techniques have been proposed (Meichenbaum and Cameron, 1983), in order that children could be taught coping strategies in advance of having to deal with common life stressors. These focus on the analysis of problems, monitoring for maladaptive thoughts, monitoring behaviours, and practising coping strategies such as problem solving, relaxation and behavioural reversal. These methods have been used successfully to prepare children for hospital admission and have been suggested as a method of preparation for terrorist attacks on Israeli children. The practicality of more general usage, however, must remain in doubt due to the inherent difficulties of predicting when a disaster will strike.
- Depending on the nature and severity of the stressor, initial attention focuses on physical needs which might involve rescue efforts, and medical care in a disaster. Shelter, relocation, assistance with physical needs and finances, and education about the potential effects of the experience may be needed (Pfefferbaum, 1997).
- Children separated from family members during a disaster should be re-united as soon as possible (Gillis, 1993).
- Debriefing, although popular, is under-researched in terms of its effectiveness, the likely beneficiaries, and the most appropriate timing in the treatment of adolescents (Yule, 1993). It does provide a systematic mechanism for discussing the traumatic event and responses to it, clarifying misconceptions about the experience, exploring feelings, identifying coping strategies, promoting support for others with similar experiences, and providing referrals for more intensive evaluation and treatment (Gillis, 1993).
- Avoidance, and sometimes shame, can conceal the presence of post-traumatic stress disorder unless its symptoms are systematically assessed. Equally, untreated or under-treated reactions can evolve in ways that can become, or at least be labelled with, another diagnosis. This is especially the case for adolescents repeatedly exposed to severe trauma (Davies and Flannery, 1998). These children may be diagnosed with attention deficit disorder, depression, dissociative disorders, separation or attachment problems, substance abuse and personality disorders.

- A number of studies have shown that parents do not accurately estimate the distress of their children. This may represent denial on the part of the parents, although children may also be especially compliant during traumatic events and not fully display their distress or adults may collude in the avoidance to escape discomfort.
- There is little comparative information on the various treatment modalities. Individual, family, group, behavioural and pharmacological interventions have been tried.
- Individual work begins with a sensitive clinical interview. Pynoos and Eth (1986) have described a three-stage method for conducting this interview with traumatized children aged 3–16. The interview begins with projective drawing and storytelling, which usually will contain reference to the traumatic event. Next there is a discussion of the event, the child's perception of the threat, the consequences, and the child's feelings of fear, self-blame and revenge. The interview ends with a review of the session and the anticipated course.
- The difficulty for the therapist is to help the survivor re-experience the event and the feelings aroused, so that the distress can be mastered rather than amplified. Exposure sessions that are too short may sensitise, rather than ameliorate (Rachman, 1980).
- Sleep disturbance should be analysed and managed according to whether the main problem is one of getting off to sleep or waking following nightmare.
- Group treatments and support groups are appropriate where larger numbers of children have been exposed to the same event. Parallel parent groups provide a way of dealing with parental distress, and to discuss effective support and management of their children. Group work also provides an efficient means of identifying children in need of more intensive help (Gillis, 1993). Groups provide space to give age appropriate information about post traumatic stress reactions, for survivors to recount and share their experiences, to reassure hesitant children that their experiences are not unique, to view a variety of coping strategies, to see others in various stages of resolution and to gain pleasure from helping others.
- Be aware that group experiences may re-traumatise (Pfefferbaum, 1997). Not all children feel comfortable sharing emotional content in a group. Children may adopt others' coping strategies prematurely, before they have fully examined their own responses.
- It is important to contain extreme expressions of anger and aggression which may create anxiety in peers (Gillis, 1993).
- Issues such as sensitive reminders, anniversaries, common reactions to trauma and coping mechanisms should be raised on behalf of the group if they do not occur spontaneously.
- Family therapy and social support have a key protective effect against the adverse effects of trauma on children (Garmezy, 1985). The presence of, and ability to use, social networks assists progress in adults and should be

facilitated where possible. The goals of family work include educating the child and parents about post-traumatic stress disorder, its symptoms and its course. The child needs to be helped to regain a sense of security, to have their feelings validated instead of dismissed and sensitive situations identified in order that additional support can be given.

- Pulsed interventions are advocated by some authors. The principle is based on a recognition that new issues related to trauma commonly emerge as the child matures. Interventions at strategic points following the acute trauma should anticipate and address the course of recovery, and reflect the child's developmental stage (Pynoos and Nader, 1993; Terr, 1989).

- School-based treatments offer opportunities for direct preventive work, and later treatment strategies. School-based programmes may include curricular interventions addressing the traumatising events and stress responses, opportunities for disclosure and discussion, small group activities, projective techniques like storytelling, artwork and play, and other formal and informal opportunities for assessing psychological responses, correcting misconceptions and fears, and encouraging normalisation and recovery (Pfefferbaum, 1997). It is important that the goals of school-based interventions are appropriate for the setting (Pynoos and Nader, 1993).

- Few studies have investigated pharmacotherapy. When used, it is as an adjunctive therapy for severe symptoms, where these are disabling (Marmar *et al.*, 1994). Positive symptoms (e.g. autonomic symptoms from re-experiencing the trauma) are more responsive than negative symptoms (e.g. avoidance). Co-morbid conditions should guide the selection of agent, and patients may not respond to standard doses of medication. The literature is unclear about the role of polypharmacy in the treatment of post-traumatic stress disorder, but combinations are used in refractory cases in adults (Marmar *et al.*, 1994).

- Clonidine has been used for severely abused and neglected pre-school children not responsive to day hospital management (Harmon and Riggs, 1996). It has also been used for persistent arousal in shooting incidents, especially exaggerated startle response and sleep disturbance (Pynoos and Nader, 1993). Finally, propranolol has been used in 6–12 year olds, though placebo effect was not ruled out (Famularo *et al.*, 1988).

EATING DISORDERS

The prevention of anorexia nervosa first received attention in the literature at the end of the 1970s (Huon *et al.*, 1998). Interventions will be difficult because of the lack of any physical disability, though they may be preventive (Crisp, 1979), so special attention should be paid to the early recognition of so-called 'pre'-anorectics (Vandereycken and Meerman, 1984). Some authors have focused on the enumeration of salient risk factors within the constitution, personality structure, family dynamics and social class (primary preventive approach), whilst others have concentrated on the outcomes of interventions aimed at reducing those risk factors in female adolescents (secondary preventive approach). Since the causative factors are multivariate and multidetermined, it is difficult to make meaningful inferences about the predisposing characteristics of dieting induced disorders beyond their age and sex distributions (Huon, 1996). We know little about the way in which an initial, and common, concern about weight in the pubertal female, through the vessel of dieting, turns into a clinically diagnosable eating disorder. Proponents of the sociocultural point-of-view feel that dieters who internalise values emphasising thinness are more likely to develop eating disorders, whilst others emphasize the prerequisite for psychiatric disorder to also be present. Thus, from a preventive standpoint, dieting should be seen as a necessary, but not sufficient, condition for the development of anorexia or bulimia nervosa (Huon *et al.*, 1998).

Huon argues that interventions for dieting-induced disorders ought to be generic and particularly target transitional risk-taking behaviours. Programmes for healthy dieting are advocated within the health and social curricula of schools, employing open discussion and cognitive (Socratic dialogue) techniques. This strategy aims to avoid the difficulties in simple information-giving sessions, where youngsters may be trained to diet in more effective, or damaging ways. Other workers have also focused on school based intervention programmes, emphasising models using multilevel intervention (Neumark-Sztainer, 1996; Schwitzer *et al.*, 1998). Key components include staff training, classroom interventions, curriculum work, individual and small group work with high-risk students, referral systems, opportunities for healthy eating, modifications to the physical education programme, and outreach activities.

Preventive programmes for eating disorders simultaneously attempt to prevent new cases arising (primary prevention), whilst also encouraging symptomatic students into early treatment (secondary prevention). Supporters argue that simply providing students with information will achieve both aims (Crisp, 1988), yet these goals may be incompatible within a single intervention (Mann *et al.*, 1997). For example, to prevent abnormal eating patterns, it might be useful to stress the abnormality of the behaviours, their rarity and how difficult they are to treat. However, the opposite message would be required to encourage people with early disorders into treatment. The assumption within this model is that information leads to knowledge, which then leads to a change of attitudes and that this leads to behaviour change. This is not necessarily sound and this type of programme may backfire, paradoxically increasing the likelihood of students engaging in disordered eating (Garner, 1985). Other evidence comes from a comparison with substance abuse prevention programmes and suicide prevention programmes. The majority of interventions in general student populations had no preventive effect and some seemed to increase substance abuse. Similarly firm conclusions cannot yet be drawn about the usefulness of information-giving strategies in the secondary prevention of suicide.

Clinical practice points

There are now several good models for school-based preventive programmes (e.g. Neumark-Sztainer, 1996; Schwitzer *et al.*, 1998), the interested reader is commended particularly to the very practical Neumark-Sztainer model of primary and secondary prevention. The high cost and relatively low success rates of treatment certainly justify the investment in preventive efforts, though untargeted preventive intervention is equally unlikely to be cost-effective (Killen *et al.*, 1993).

- Preventive programmes need to focus on a wider spectrum of eating disorders than strictly defined anorexia and bulimia nervosa. This is because even whilst anorectic, bulimic or unhealthy dieting (e.g. extreme calorie restriction) may not be frequent or intense enough to meet formal criteria, these behaviours may still have short-term harmful consequences and may prelude more severe eating disorders (Neumark-Sztainer, 1996). Based on this principle it is reasonable to include eating disorders, anorexic or bulimic behaviours, unhealthy dieting, unhealthy eating behaviours (e.g. high-fat consumption or skipping meals), and obesity. Schwitzer *et al.* (1998) advocate the use of the DSM-IV 'Eating disorder not otherwise specified' framework as a suitable tool with which to identify this wider range of eating concerns.
- Although eating disorders and obesity appear opposite in nature, they tend to share features such as excessive weight preoccupation, skipping meals and binge–diet cycles (Brownell and Fairburn, 1995). Thus primary prevention probably needs to address both within the same programme, although this will make evaluation more difficult.
- The beneficiaries of any school-based preventive programme must be identified according to their risk of developing an eating disturbance, their interest and motivation, and the available time and resources present.
- Although the preventive benefits of addressing pre-school through to college-age children may seem self evident, it may be better to target middle school adolescents. In determining which year to approach, a balance must be struck between having enough students interested in the material, but not so many already engaging in the unwanted behaviours, since preventive programmes may be more effective at prevention than treatment (Neumark-Sztainer *et al.*, 1995).
- Males also develop body and eating worries, and are certainly part of the wider culture emphasising thinness. Their inclusion has the potential to positively influence female peers, though some boys may not be interested in the material and disturb the intimacy of the discussion.
- Age, gender, level of body dissatisfaction, body weight, weight loss behaviours, eating and exercise behaviours, other health concerns and family history should be considered in the assessment of risk.
- Methods for assessing those in need of secondary or tertiary prevention include the observation of weight changes, excessive exercise, eating rituals, reduced

academic performance, style of dress and overall appearance, discussion with the youngster's peer group and family, and formal assessment with suitable tools.

- Issues to be addressed by school-based preventive programmes should be those which play an aetiological role, are possible to change and are suitable for addressing within a school setting.

- Body dissatisfaction is a strong predictor of both mild and severe eating disturbances (Emmons, 1994). Preventive work should try to increase adolescents' understanding of the role of sociocultural issues on body image and should help them to critically examine social norms, e.g. by helping girls to view bodily changes in a more positive and normal way, despite values which emphasize small hips and breasts.

- Programmes should promote increased understanding of general nutritional issues such as appropriate healthy eating and exercise behaviour, healthy methods of weight control, the consequences of morbid weight loss, eating disorders, and obesity. Staff and students should be helped to have better attitudes towards overweight individuals and an understanding of genetic contribution.

- Psychological and family issues contributing to eating disorders may be suitable for classroom or small group discussion.

- Approaches to prevention may range from a simple one-off classroom lecture on eating disorders, through to a wide-ranging programme involving a number of within-school teaching venues and formats, and full community linkages. Topics may be approached through a nutritional, health, gender equality or life skills focus.

- One-off sessions with students should aim at increased awareness of the dangers of eating disorders, surveillance of and seeking help for students with weight and eating concerns.

- Comprehensive programmes can address wider objectives, such as the improvement of body image, encouragement of less maladaptive eating behaviours, improvements in the physical and social school environments, and outreach.

- Staff training for teachers, school nurses, counsellors and catering staff can assist in generating a more health-promoting school environment.

- Wherever possible use the existing infrastructure, both within and outside of the school, and use a multidisciplinary planning model.

- Evaluation. Process evaluation should focus on the implementation itself, looking particularly at barriers, and participant and provider satisfaction. Outcome evaluation looks at the specific goals of the individual project.

SCHIZOPHRENIA

Therapeutic pessimism and despair have been prevalent amongst clinicians working with schizophrenia since Kraepelin's time, not least because of the very selected (and usually very severe) nature of the cases routinely dealt with.

Equally, cases having only one episode are only seen the first time, and many milder cases may not present at all. Cohen and Cohen (1984) coined the phrase 'the clinician's illusion', highlighting these difficulties. However, in recent years there has been a renaissance in research and thinking around preventive work for this challenging group of patients. The logic for this rests on four pillars (McGorry, 1996):

- Delays in initiating treatment are often prolonged, and the duration of untreated psychosis is associated with substantial functional decline, treatment resistance and higher subsequent rates of relapse.
- Intensive and sophisticated intervention following detection during the early phase of the illness could minimise iatrogenic damage and more effectively promote recovery (McGorry *et al.*, 1996), which frequently occurs later anyway. Late recoveries are often seriously incomplete and seem to occur despite treatment. Much of the damage is to the person's personal development, social environment and lifestyle.
- Targeting failure of initial remission, or early treatment resistance, with recently enhanced drug treatments and psychosocial interventions could result in a lower rate of prolonged treatment resistance, relapse and disability (Edwards *et al.*, 1998).
- Maintaining remission and preventing or limiting relapse, by reducing the total duration of active psychosis, is a post-psychotic analogue of reducing the duration of untreated psychosis.

The hope in all this is that, as well as improving outcomes of first episode patients and those moving through the first 2–3 years after onset, it may be possible to offer interventions to those who are in the pre-psychotic stages of illness. Unfortunately, the clinical features identified retrospectively in first-episode samples are mostly non-specific (Yung and McGorry, 1996) and have only limited predictive power. In recent ground breaking work, Yung *et al.* (1998) have combined state and trait risk factors for psychosis to define a high-risk group, and found that 40% of these cases convert to frank psychosis over a 6-month period. This type of prediction opens the door to the possibility of indicated preventive interventions using low-dose neuroleptics and general stress reduction, lifestyle restructure, and enhanced coping using modern cognitive behavioural treatments (McGorry, 1996). These interventions will need to be carefully trialed to discover optimum regimes, avoid iatrogenic damage and maximise the risk/benefit ratio.

Finally, no discussion of prevention in schizophrenia would be complete without mention of tertiary strategies for tackling high expressed emotion (EE) in families of schizophrenic patients. The social relations within 59% of patients' families are strained, often to the limit of what would ordinarily be regarded as tolerable (Wing *et al.*, 1964). Brown *et al.* (1972), and later Vaughn and Leff

(1976), pointed to the damaging effects of 'expressed critical emotion', both in terms of relapse rates and the need for higher dose medication. This work has been robustly replicated in schizophrenia, even across cultures, and been found to be applicable in mood and eating disorders too. There are now a variety of standard assessments for EE, including a relatives version of the Cardinal Needs Assessment, the Camberwell Family Interview, the Five-Minute Speech Sample and the 30-item Family Attitude Scale.

The effects of psychosocial interventions have thus far met with mixed results, however. Nugter *et al.* (1997) examined the effect of behavioural family therapy on 52 families of recent-onset schizophrenic patients. The intervention did not have a significant positive effect on EE level, a finding comparable with prior EE research. Psycho-educational family groups, however, may be beneficial as an opportunity to discuss and exchange experiences positively, offer relief and support, and receive information (Klank *et al.*, 1998). Educational training for staff has also been investigated. On long-stay wards it gave measurable benefits to patients, despite no measurable effect on nurses' EE (Finema *et al.*, 1996). A similar finding emerged from a staff training programme in five community care facilities (Willetts and Leff, 1997).

Clinical practice points

- The majority of adolescent, first episode, psychotic patients have a schizo-affective presentation. It is thus rarely possible to be dogmatic about diagnosis or prognosis initially. Many families will ask outright 'doctor, is this schizophrenia?'. In the absence of a clear presentation it is usually helpful to discuss the diagnostic difficulties and prognostic factors up front. This allows a realistic picture to be given, whilst avoiding the overwhelming distress of a schizophrenia diagnosis. This said, the initial discussions with the patient and their family can be biased towards the management principles of schizophrenia, rather than towards those of affective disorder. In years to come, when the true nature of the diagnosis becomes clear, nothing really changes but the name. In this way, parents and adolescents have access to the maximum amount of information about their own and related disorders.
- Behavioural abnormalities, like social withdrawal and socially embarrassing behaviour, are not intrinsic or inevitable results of the schizophrenic process, but much more the product of a monotonous and unstimulating environment (Wing and Brown, 1961). Too much stimulation, either pleasant or unpleasant, can often precipitate schizophrenia where the subject's normal lifestyle has been disrupted as a result (Brown and Birley, 1968). Returning to live with a critical or hostile relative also greatly increases the relapse rate over the next year (Brown *et al.*, 1972; Vaughn and Leff, 1976).
- The management of the adolescent schizophrenic thus involves attempting to provide a domestic setting in which the daily routine includes order and

predictability, without being too boring, avoiding high EE and critical comments, whilst retaining some level of meaningful responsibility. A carefully chosen educational setting, or occupation, may provide an additional way of giving an otherwise under-stimulating environment extra variety and structure, and perhaps reducing face to face contact with critical parents and siblings too.

- Parents and youngsters will need information on their drug treatments. Alongside information on the neuroleptics themselves, there are important issues arising from the need for good compliance, and relapse prevention. The efficacy of drug treatment in postponing (rather than preventing) relapse is well established, with the interval prolonged at least two-fold, although in the long run most patients relapse (Lader, 1998).

- Relapse is reduced by maintenance neuroleptic treatment over a period of 1–2 years (Leff and Wing, 1971; Goldberg *et al.*, 1977) for schizophrenic patients with moderate risk of relapse, e.g. from 80 to 35%. Conversely, good prognosis patients may remain well without medication (27% relapse) and high-risk patients relapse despite it (67% relapse) (Leff and Wing, 1971).

- Neuroleptic discontinuation, even in patients well for as long as 5 years, results in a relapse rate similar to that seen in patients given placebo (Kinon, 1998). Around 50% of schizophrenic patients, under normal treatment conditions, relapse within 1 year after their latest episode and may spend 15–20% of their time in psychiatric institutions (Ayuso-Gutierrez and del Rio Vega, 1997). Indeed, non-compliance with medication is the most important factor in relapse requiring hospitalisation (73%), although pharmacological factors, psycho-social factors, alcohol and drug abuse also contribute to new psychotic episodes.

- Depot medication is more convenient for the less well, less compliant patients, though side effects may be more marked than with oral medication. Depot medication also leads to more regular patient contact, which is also beneficial for supervision. Low-dose and intermittent medication has also been tried, although results have not been as successful as hoped because of difficulties in identifying prodromata or where prodromata do not precede relapse (Lader, 1998). Psycho-educational treatment studies also confirm that the major influence on the rate of rehospitalisation is the dose of conventional maintenance medication.

- The case for giving neuroleptics in perpetuity is much less compelling. Side effects include movement disorders and subjective dysphoria, weight gain, and endocrine changes. With conventional neuroleptics, the risk of tarditive dyskinesia rises at 5% per year for patients with up to 10 years of neuroleptic exposure. Findings suggest that atypical agents are at least as effective and may be better tolerated. Olanzapine has demonstrated efficacy in maintenance treatment and is less likely to cause tarditive dyskinesia than haloperidol (Kinon, 1998).

REFERENCES

Ayuso-Gutierrez, J. L. and del Rio Vega, J. M. (1997) Factors influencing relapse in the long-term course of schizophrenia. *Schizophrenia Research*, **28**, 199–206.

Banks, M. and Jackson, P. (1982) Unemployment and risk of minor psychiatric disorder in young people: cross-sectional and longitudinal evidence. *Psychological Medicine*, **12**, 786–798.

Beardslee W. R., Salt, P., Porterfield, K., Rothberg, P. C., van de Velde, P., Swatling, S. *et al.* (1993) Comparison of preventive interventions for families with parental affective disorder. *Journal of the American Academy of Child and Adolescent Psychiatry*, **32**, 254–263.

Bebbington, P., Sturt, E., Tennant, C. and Hurry, J. (1984) Misfortune and resilience: a community study of women. *Psychological Medicine*, **14**, 346–364.

Birmaher, B., Ryan, N. D., Williamson, D. E., Brent, D. A., Kaufman, J., Dahl, R. E. *et al.* (1996) Childhood and adolescent depression: a review of the past 10 years. Part I. *Journal of the American Academy of Child and Adolescent Psychiatry*, **35**, 1427–1439.

Brown, G. W. and Birley, J. T. (1968) Crises and life changes and the onset of schizophrenia. *Journal of Health and Social Behaviour*, **9**, 203–214.

Brown, G. W., Birley, J. T. and Wing, J. K. (1972) The influence of family life on the course of schizophrenia: a replication. *British Journal of Psychiatry*, **121**, 241–258.

Brownell, K. D. and Fairburn, C. G. (1995) Preface. In K. D. Brownell and C. G. Fairburn (eds), *Eating Disorders and Obesity: A Comprehensive Handbook*. New York: Guilford Press, pp. ix–xii.

Child and Adolescent Section of the Royal College of Psychiatrists (1990) Roles, responsibilities and work of a child and adolescent psychiatrist. In J. Harris Hendricks and M. Black (eds), *Child and Adolescent Psychiatry: Into the 1990s*. London: Royal College of Psychiatrists, pp. 83–89.

Clarke, G. N., Hawkins, W., Murphy, M., Sheeber, L. B., Lewinsohn, P. M. and Seeley, J. R. (1995) Targeted prevention of unipolar depressive disorder in an at-risk sample of high school adolescents: a randomized trial of a group cognitive intervention. *Journal of the American Academy of Child and Adolescent Psychiatry*, **34**, 312–321.

Cohen, P. and Cohen, J. (1984) The clinician's illusion. *Archives of General Psychiatry*, **42**, 1178–1182.

Crisp, A. H. (1979) Early recognition and prevention of anorexia nervosa. *Developmental Medicine and Child Neurology*, **21**, 393–395.

Crisp, A. H. (1988) Some possible approaches to prevention of eating and body weight/shape disorders, with particular reference to anorexia nervosa. *International Journal of Eating Disorders*, **7**, 1–17.

Davies, W. H. and Flannery, D. J. (1998) Post-traumatic stress disorder in children and adolescents exposed to violence. *Pediatric Clinics of North America*, **45**, 341–353.

Department for Education and Employment (1996) *The Skills Audit: A Report from an Interdepartmental Group*. London: HMSO.

Department of Health (1995) *A Handbook on Child and Adolescent Mental Health*. London: HMSO.

Department of Health (1997) *The New NHS Modern Dependable*. London: The Stationary Office.

Edwards, J., Maude, D., McGorry, P. D., Harrigan, S. M. and Cocks, J. T. (1998) Prolonged recovery in first-episode psychosis. *British Journal of Psychiatry*, **172** (Suppl.), 107–116.

Emmons, L. (1994) Predisposing factors differentiating adolescent dieters and nondieters. *Journal of the American Dietetic Association*, **94**, 725–731.

Famularo, R., Kinscherff, R. and Fenton, T. (1988) Propranolol treatment for childhood posttraumatic stress disorder, acute type. *American Journal of Diseases of Children*, **142**, 1244–1247.

Farrington, D. P., Gallagher, B., Morley, L., Ledger, R. J. and West, D. J. (1986) Unemployment, school leaving and crime. *British Journal of Criminology*, **26**, 335–356.

Fergusson, D. M. (1998) Stability and change in externalising behaviours. *European Archives of Psychiatry and Clinical Neuroscience*, **248**, 4–13.

Fergusson, D. M., Horwood, L. J. and Lynskey, M. T. (1996) Childhood sexual abuse and psychiatric disorder in young adulthood: II. Psychiatric outcomes of childhood sexual abuse. *Journal of the American Academy of Child and Adolescent Psychiatry*, **35**, 1365–1374.

Finema, E. J., Louwerens, J. W., Slooff, C. J. and van den Bosch, R. J. (1996) Expressed emotion on long-stay wards. *Journal of Advanced Nursing*, **24**, 473–478.

Fombonne, E. (1998) Increased rates of psychosocial disorders in youth. *European Archives of Psychiatry and Clinical Neuroscience*, **248**, 14–21.

Garmezy, N. (1985) Stress resistant children: the search for protective factors. In J. E. Stevenson (ed.), Recent Research in Developmental Psychopathology. *Journal of Child Psychology and Psychiatry*, **4** (Suppl.), 213–233.

Garner, D. (1985) Iatrogenesis in anorexia nervosa and bulimia nervosa. *International Journal of Eating Disorders*, **4**, 701–726.

Gillis, H. M. (1993) Individual and small group psychotherapy for children involved in trauma and disaster. In C. F. Saylor (ed.), *Children and Disasters*. New York: Plenum, pp, 165–186.

Goldberg, S. C., Schooler, N. R., Hogarty, G. E. and Roper, M. (1977) Prediction of relapse in schizophrenic outpatients treated by drug and sociotherapy. *Archives of General Psychiatry*, **34**, 171–184.

Graham, P. (1994) Prevention. In M. Rutter, E. A. Taylor and L. A. Hersov (eds), *Child and Adolescent Psychiatry: Modern Approaches*, 3rd edn. Oxford: Blackwell Science, pp. 815–828.

Greenfield, S. F. and Shore, M. F. (1995) Prevention of psychiatric disorders. *Harvard Review of Psychiatry*, **3**, 115–129.

Harmon, R. J. and Riggs, P. D. (1996) Clonidine for posttraumatic stress disorder in preschool children. *Journal of the American Academy of Child and Adolescent Psychiatry*, **35**, 1247–1249.

Harrington, R. and Clark, A. (1998) Prevention and early intervention for depression in adolescence and early adult life. *European Archives of Psychiatry and Clinical Neuroscience*, **248**, 32–45.

Huon, G. F. (1996) Health promotion and the prevention of dieting-induced disorders. *Eating Disorders: The Journal of Treatment and Prevention*, **4**, 27–32.

Huon, G. F., Braganza, C., Brown, L. B., Ritchie, J. E. and Roncolato, W. G. (1998) Reflections on prevention in dieting-induced disorders. *International Journal of Eating Disorders*, **23**, 455–458.

Jaycox, L. H., Reivich, K. J., Gillham, J. and Seligman, M. E. (1994) Prevention of depressive symptoms in school children. *Behaviour Research and Therapy*, **32**, 801–816.

Kessler, R. C., McGonagle, K. A., Zhao, S., Nelson, C. B., Hughes, M., Eshleman, S. *et al.* (1994) Lifetime and 12-month prevalence of DSM-III-R psychiatric disorders in the United States. Results from the National Comorbidity Survey. *Archives of General Psychiatry*, **51**, 8–19.

Killen, J. D., Taylor, C. B., Hammer, L. D., Litt, I., Wilson, D. M., Rich, T. *et al.* (1993) An attempt to modify unhealthful eating attitudes and weight regulation practices of young adolescent grils. *International Journal of Eating Disorders*, **13**, 369–384.

Kinon, B. J. (1998) The routine use of atypical antipsychotic agents: maintenance treatment. *Journal of Clinical Psychiatry*, **59** (Suppl. 19), 18–22.

Klank, I., Rost, W. D. and Olbrich, R. (1998) Family therapy as a component of routine management of schizophrenic patients. A report of experiences. *Psychiatrische Praxis*, **25**, 29–32.

Kroll, L., Harrington, R., Jayson, D., Fraser J. and Gowers, S. (1996) Pilot study of continuation cognitive-behavioral therapy for major depression in adolescent psychiatric patients. *Journal of the American Academy of Child and Adolescent Psychiatry*, **35**, 1156–1161.

Kupfer, D. J. and Frank, E. (1992) The minimum length of treatment for recovery. In S. A. Montgomery and F. Rouillon (eds), *Long-term Treatment of Depression*. Chichester: Wiley, pp. 102–131.

Lacey, G. N. (1972) Observations of Aberfan. *Journal of Psychosomatic Research*, **16**, 257–260.

Lader, M. (1998) Pharmacological prevention of relapse. *Kaohsiung Journal of Medical Sciences*, **14**, 448–457.

Leff J. P. and Wing, J. K. (1971) Trial of maintenance therapy in schizophrenia. *British Medical Journal*, **3**, 599–604.

Mann, T., Nolen-Hoeksema, S., Huang, K., Burgard, D., Wright, A. and Hanson, K. (1997) Are two interventions worse than none? Joint primary and secondary prevention of eating disorders in college females. *Health Psychology*, **16**, 215–225.

McGorry, P. D., Edwards, J., Mihalopoulos, C., Harrigan, S. M. and Jackson, H. J. (1996) EPPIC: an evolving system of early detection and optimal management. *Schizophrenia Bulletin*, **22**, 305–226.

McKee, M. (1999) Sex and drugs and rock and roll: Britain can learn lessons from Europe on the health of adolescents. *British Medical Journal*, **318**, 1300–1301.

Marmar, C. R., Foy, D., Kagan, B. and Pynoos, R. S. (1994) An integrated approach for treating posttraumatic stress. In R. S. Pynoos (ed.), *Posttraumatic Stress Disorder: A Clinical Review*. Lutherville, MD: Sidran Press, pp. 99–132.

Meichenbaum, D. and Cameron, R. (1983) Stress inoculation training: toward a general paradigm for training coping skills. In D. Meichenbaum and M. E. Jaremko (eds), *Stress Reduction and Prevention*. New York: Plenum, pp. 115–154.

Mrazek, P. J. and Haggerty, R. J. (eds) (1994) *Reducing Risks for Mental Disorders: Frontiers for Preventive Intervention Research*. Washington, DC: National Academy Press.

Neumark-Sztainer, D. (1996) School-based programs for preventing eating disturbances. *Journal of School Health*, **66**, 64–71.

Neumark-Sztainer, D., Butler, R. and Palti, H. (1995) Eating disturbances among adolescent girls: evaluation of a school-based primary prevention program. *Journal of Nutrition Education*, **27**, 24–31.

Newton, J. (1988) *Preventing Mental Illness*. London: Routledge.

Nugter, A., Dingemans, P., Van der Does, J. W., Linszen, D. and Gersons, B. (1997) Family treatment, expressed emotion and relapse in recent onset schizophrenia. *Psychiatry Research*, **72**, 23–31.

Parliamentary Select Committee, Number 4 (1997) *Mental Health Services for Children*. London: HMSO.

Patton, G. (1998) Adolescent psychiatry: its potential to reduce the burden of mental disorder. *European Archives of Psychiatry and Clinical Neuroscience*, **248**, 1–3.

Pfefferbaum, B. (1997) Posttraumatic stress disorder in children: a review of the past 10 years. *Journal of the American Academy of Child and Adolescent Psychiatry*, **36**, 1503–1511.

Pynoos, R. S. and Eth, S. (1986) Witness to violence: the child interview. *Journal of the American Academy of Child Psychiatry*, **25**, 306–319.

Pynoos R. S. and Nader K. (1993) Issues in the treatment of posttraumatic stress in children and adolescents. In J. P. Wilson and B. Raphael (eds), *International*

Handbook of Traumatic Stress Syndromes. New York: Plenum, pp. 535–549.

Rachman, S. (1980) Emotional processing. *Behaviour Research and Therapy*, **18**, 51–60.

Reimherr, F. W., Amsterdam, J. D., Quitkin, F. M., Rosenbaum, J. F., Fava, M., Zajecka, J. *et al.* (1998) Optimal length of continuation therapy in depression: a prospective assessment during long-term fluoxetine treatment. *American Journal of Psychiatry*, **155**, 1247–1253.

Rollins, J. A. (1997) Minimizing the impact of community violence on child witnesses. *Critical Care Nursing Clinics of North America*, **9**, 211–220.

Rutter, M. (1982) Prevention of children's psychosocial disorders: myth and substance. *Paediatrics*, **70**, 883–894.

Rutter, M. and Madge, N. (1976) *Cycles of Disadvantage*. London: Heinemann, pp, 110–117.

Schwitzer, A. M., Bergholz, K., Dore, T. and Salimi, L. (1998) Eating disorders among college women: prevention, education, and treatment responses. *Journal of American College Health*, **46**, 199–207.

Secretary of State for Health (1998) *Our Healthier Nation: A Contract for Health*. London: The Stationary Office.

Smith, R. (1999) Eradicating child poverty. *British Medical Journal*, **319**, 203–204.

Social Exclusion Unit (1998a) *Truancy and School Exclusion Report by the Social Exclusion Unit*. London: Social Exclusion Unit.

Social Exclusion Unit (1998b) *Bringing Britain Together: A National Strategy for Neighbourhood Renewal*. London: Social Exclusion Unit.

Terr, L. C. (1989) Treating psychic trauma in children: a preliminary discussion. *Journal of Traumatic Stress*, **2**, 3–20.

Vandereycken, W. and Meerman, R. (1984) Anorexia nervosa: Is prevention possible? *International Journal of Psychiatry in Medicine*, **14**, 191–205.

Vaughn C. E. and Leff J. P. (1976) The influence of family and social factors on the course of psychiatric illness. *British Journal of Psychiatry*, **129**, 125–137.

Willetts, L. E. and Leff, J. (1997) Expressed emotion and schizophrenia: the efficacy of a staff training programme. *Journal of Advanced Nursing*, **26**, 1125–1133.

Wing, J. K. and Brown, G. W. (1961) Social treatment of chronic schizophrenia: a comparative survey of three mental hospitals. *Journal of Mental Science*, **107**, 847–861.

Wing, J. K., Monck, A. M., Brown, G. W. and Carstairs, G. M. (1964) Morbidity in the community of schizophrenics discharged from London mental hospitals in 1959. *British Journal of Psychiatry*, **110**, 10–21.

Wood, A., Harrington, R. and Moore, A. (1996) Controlled trial of a brief cognitive-behavioural intervention in adolescent patients with depressive disorders. *Journal of Child Psychology and Psychiatry and Allied Disciplines*, **37**, 737–746.

Yager, J., Linn, L. S., Leake, B., Goldston, S., Heinicke, C. and Pynoos, R. (1989) Attitudes toward mental illness prevention in routine pediatric practice. *American Journal of Diseases of Children*, **143**, 1087–1090.

Yule, W. (1993) Technology-related disasters. In C. F. Saylor (ed.), *Children and Disasters*. New York: Plenum, pp. 105–121.

Yule, W. (1994) Posttraumatic stress disorders. In M. Rutter, E. A. Taylor and L. A. Hersov (eds), *Child and Adolescent Psychiatry: Modern Approaches*, 3rd edn. Oxford: Blackwell Science, pp. 392–406.

Yung, A. R. and McGorry, P. D. (1996) The prodromal phase of first episode psychosis: past and current conceptualisations. *Schizophrenia Bulletin*, **22**, 353–370.

Yung, A. R., Phillips, L. J., McGorry, P. D., McFarlane, C. A., Francey, S., Harrigan, S. *et al.* (1998) Prediction of psychosis: a step towards indicated prevention of schizophrenia. *British Journal of Psychiatry*, **172** (Suppl.), 14–20.

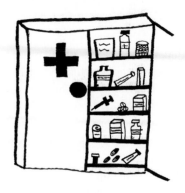

Chapter 18

ADOLESCENT PSYCHOPHARMACOLOGY

Paul Cawthron

Drugs are part of adolescent subculture. Use of powerful mind altering substances, of an illicit kind, is widespread amongst young people in the community (Weinberg *et al.*, 1998). It is an interesting parallel that in recent years there has also been a renaissance of interest in the use of psychotropic medication for the treatment of mental disorders in the child and adolescent clinic population. This has led, during the last decade, to an increase in the prescription of psychotropic medication in general child and adolescent mental health services (Safer, 1997).

Child and adolescent psychiatry in Britain encompasses a multidisciplinary practice. The re-evaluation of a medical model, in which medication plays an important role in the treatment of mental disorders in young people, represents a sea change for many practitioners of child and adolescent psychiatry. Within the profession, this group, who have an ideological opposition to the prescription of psychotropic medication for children and young people, interpret its use as a vehicle for the social control of behaviour rather than as part of a treatment package for mental disorders. However, this developing interest in medication has not only been driven from within the specialism of child and adolescent psychiatry. General practitioners, in the management of adolescent depression, and community paediatricians, in the treatment of attention deficit hyperactivity disorder (ADHD) in children, have often taken the lead in prescribing. It is of concern that physicians initiating such treatments are not mental health specialists and therefore unlikely to be skilled in, and have access to, the therapeutic options available in a child and adolescent mental health service (CAMHS) team.

In a multidisciplinary context it is essential that a wide range of treatment approaches are available. Medication is one option and the psychiatrist in the team will be expected to have 'expert knowledge of the theory and practice of psychotropic drug use' (Royal College of Psychiatrists, 1998). Re-emphasis on medication is not to re-polarise the debate between biological or social models of understanding, but to recognise the benefits and the associated risks medication brings as one part of a comprehensive treatment plan.

There are many differences between the health care systems on each side of the Atlantic. One marked difference is in the rate of drug prescription by child and adolescent psychiatrists. This is very low in Britain compared to the USA. A survey of an American child psychiatric clinic (Storch, 1998) revealed that 44.5% of the patients were prescribed psychotropic medication. The three most common types of medication, in descending order of frequency, were (1) the anti-depressants, (2) the psychostimulants and (3) the mood stabilisers. While not strictly comparable, Bramble (1995) surveyed British child psychiatrists to study the pattern of prescribing of antidepressant medication. The large majority (85%) of the psychiatrists who replied to the postal questionnaire had prescribed antidepressants. However, the rate of prescribing was low with, on average, only one or two new prescriptions each year.

Before considering using psychotropic medication, the psychiatrist undertakes a full clinical examination and reaches a diagnosis. A treatment plan must then be formulated. This plan will usually involve individual, group or family inter-ventions concurrent with, or at times as potential alternatives to, medication. For each treatment considered the psychiatrist must weigh up the research evidence, evaluate it in the context of the individual presentation and balance issues of risk, such as side effects, against the potential effectiveness of the treatment. Such information is essential in order that appropriate informed consent for the treatment plan can be obtained in discussion with the individual patient (and their parents/carers).

Informed consent is an essential component of the therapeutic alliance that is necessary to establish compliance with the treatment plan. Non-compliance is a general problem of adolescent health care (Lloyd et al., 1998). The general stigma that is still attached to mental disorders and attending psychiatric services may well compound the problem. Another factor, when the young person is reluctantly bought to clinic by their parents, is that issues of control between parents and offspring may influence any treatment plan. It is important to recognise and address these issues in developing the management plan and in working out how to facilitate compliance with medication. The role of parents versus young person in taking responsibility for the safe-keeping and safe administration of the prescribed drug also necessitates balancing the risks, which in turn can influence the choice of medication.

The research basis for adolescent psychopharmacology, which has grown substantially in recent years, is still not extensive. It appears rare for drug companies to sponsor research in this age group, leading to the current situation where many of the medicines used in clinical practice are not licensed and therefore 'not recommended' for use in children (*British National Formulary*, 1999). Using drugs outside the licensed indication places added responsibility on the prescribing practitioner to ensure best practice.

Clinical empiricism based on adult research and clinical practice has guided the adolescent psychiatrist in the use of medication. In adolescence consideration must be given to the diagnostic equivalence to adult mental disorders, possible differing patterns of co-morbidity, as well as issues of developmental processes that may significantly effect the clinical response to medication. The clinician has to make a judgement as to the weighting given to the evidence from adult psychiatry, to compare it with any age relevant research and to translate this into general clinical practice with adolescents.

The 'gold standard' of clinical trials, the double-blind placebo controlled study, is still so rare in treatment trials for adolescent mental disorders that Walkup *et al.* (1998) have made the case for continuing the publication of 'open and uncontrolled pharmacological trials'. The authors reflect on the need for clarity of both the presentation and the assessment of the information published leading them to propose a set of guidelines for the public reporting of such studies.

Clinicians, as well as assessing the research evidence, should also be evaluating the effectiveness of their clinical interventions. It is no longer acceptable to measure outcome on the basis of a subjective 'improved' or 'not improved'. There are many rating scales, which can be utilised, in everyday clinical practice. This seems of particular importance when evaluating the effectiveness of medication given the balance of risks versus benefits. Many of the ADHD clinics have developed models of good practice by including evaluation in their clinical protocol (Hill and Cameron, undated). Through the processes of clinical audit, opportunities exist for more collaboration amongst clinicians to further evaluate the effectiveness of different treatments for the various clinical disorders.

CLINICAL DISORDERS

DEPRESSIVE DISORDERS

It is now accepted that depression, as an illness, can occur in adolescence and can be diagnosed using ICD-10 (World Health Organisation, 1992). The symptom profile in young people is, in general, similar to that in adults (Ryan *et al.*, 1987). However, by comparison to adult research, in which is demonstrated the significant benefit of antidepressant medication over placebo, this finding has not been consistently replicated in the adolescent age group.

In the biological model of depression the importance of the biogenic amines remain as the central theme for psychopharmacological research. The focus has, in recent years, concentrated on serotonin [5-hydroxytryptamine (5-HT)], leading to the development of the class of antidepressant medication known as the selective serotonin reuptake inhibitors (SSRIs).

The availability of these drugs, with reported clinical advantages over traditional antidepressants, has, it would seem likely, contributed to the increased prescription of such medication. As a group, the SSRIs have a different side effect profile to the previous standard treatment of tricyclic antidepressants (TCA). The most common side effects contrast with the anticholinergic action (dry mouth, constipation and visual impairment) of the TCAs. Young people prescribed fluoxetine were found instead to have greater irritability of mood, symptoms of gastrointestinal disturbance, sleep disorder and occasional hypomanic like disturbance (Jain et al., 1992). Of possibly greater importance, especially for outpatient prescribing, is the increased safety given the reduced lethality of the SSRIs in overdose (Leonard et al., 1997).

In the adolescent clinic population there are studies showing the effectiveness of these medications. Rey-Sanchez and Gutierrez-Casares (1997) found, in an open study of outpatient young people with a diagnosis of major depressive disorder treated with paroxetine, that, at the end of treatment, all the patients had complete remission of their symptoms. Rodriguez-Ramos et al. (1996) using the same medication to treat a group of adolescents, who had displayed various depressive symptomatology for a period of 6 weeks, found a positive outcome for 76% of the patients.

Fluoxetine was studied in another open trial with a group of young people diagnosed with major depression (Colle et al., 1994). Seven out of eight patients (88%) were improved after 24 weeks of treatment. Similarly, again in an open trial with adolescents, sertraline has been shown to have a positive effect on depressive symptomatology (Alderman et al., 1998).

In adult populations the SSRIs have been shown to be as effective as the TCAs in a large number of double-blind, controlled studies. However, the balance of research evidence does not clearly support the use of medication for the treatment of depressive disorder in the adolescent age group. Generally the published data, describing beneficial effects of antidepressant medication in young people, is in the form of reports of open clinical trials. The evidence for the superiority of medication in controlled studies is less strong. Simeon et al. (1990), in a placebo-controlled, double-blind study of fluoxetine, found no statistically significant differences, although the active medication scored better on all clinical measures except sleep disorder.

Reports such as this have led to a number of review articles and meta-analyses to collate the results of the studies in the field. Hazell et al. (1995) undertook a meta-analysis of trials comparing TCAs to placebo in the treatment of depression in children and adolescents. The conclusion reached, by the authors, is that there is no evidence supporting the effectiveness of the TCAs in this population. Others argue for the use of antidepressant medication. DeVane and Sallee (1996) in a review of the SSRIs in this age group reached an opinion that depression was the clearest indication for the use of such medication. Kutcher (1997) reviewing the pharmacotherapy of depression in adolescents argues that the SSRIs should be considered the 'first-line medications'.

The lack of convincing evidence, from large controlled studies, for the effectiveness of antidepressants has led to debate as to whether clinicians should continue to prescribe such medication. Eisenberg (1996) and Pellegrino (1996), in the same journal, argue that without scientific support it is not ethical to continue to prescribe antidepressants for children and adolescents. The dilemma, for the practicing clinician, is in trying to reconcile the clear evidence from adult studies together with the variation of the findings in adolescent populations. This is especially the case in the treatment of young people, around the developmental transition into adulthood, who have a significant depressive illness.

This suggests that in clinical practice, with young people, only a medical psychiatric specialist in a CAMHS service should undertake the prescription of antidepressant medication. Such a model will ensure that there is a full diagnostic assessment of the mental state of the young person, together with consideration being given to their developmental, social and educational circumstances, in order that an individual treatment package can be designed for the management of the patient. This will include the possible use of alternative psychological methods of treatment of depression, such as cognitive-behavioural therapy (Reineche et al., 1998).

The use of medication, as a first option in treatment, should be limited to those young people with diagnosed major depressive disorder. The clinical knowledge base now supports an initial choice from the group of SSRIs in preference to a TCA antidepressant. In general, it is preferable to begin with a low starting dose of antidepressant, and to ensure that the prescription is regularly reviewed and increased to a clinically adequate dose. This level should then be maintained at the therapeutic level for a period of at least 4 weeks. If there is no response the dose of antidepressant can be increased, within dosage guidelines (*British National Formulary*, 1999), for a further similar period. Medication non-response at that time requires reconsideration of the management plan. Within the range of physical treatments there is the potential for changing the class of antidepressant or for adding in another compound such as lithium (Ryan *et al.*, 1988) or if the clinical situation is extreme recourse may be made to electroconvulsive therapy (ECT) (Kutcher and Robertson, 1995; Walter and Rey, 1997).

OBSESSIVE-COMPULSIVE DISORDER

In the treatment of obsessive-compulsive disorder (OCD) in young people first line management techniques should involve psychological therapies using cognitive-behavioural techniques (March *et al.*, 1994). It is often necessary to engage the parents/carers in such therapy, in particular, if they have become involved in the ritualistic behaviours. Unfortunately, in young people, the long-term prognosis for severe OCD is poor. Leonard *et al.* (1993), in a 2–7 year follow-up, found complete remission in only 6% of patients. In the management of patients with this disorder, if non-pharmacological interventions are unsuccessful, it is then appropriate to commence a trial of medication. In the group of traditional TCAs, clomipramine appears to be the most efficacious in the treatment of OCD (Leonard *et al.*, 1989). This is probably related to the serotonergic properties of clomipramine vis-à-vis the other TCAs. However, the SSRIs with their more specific pharmacological action on the 5-HT systems, and, for reasons similar to the rationale for their preferred use in depression, they have become the first choice medication in the treatment of OCD. Fluoxetine, fluvoxamine and paroxetine are licensed (in adults) for the treatment of OCD.

Although many of the research trials for this disorder have used adult subjects, evidence for the effectiveness of the SSRIs in the treatment of OCD in the adolescent age group is available. Riddle *et al.* (1992) reported a double-blind trial of fluoxetine versus placebo in which the active treatment was superior over an 8-week period as shown by a decrease in symptom severity. Alderman *et al.* (1998) report, in the open study previously mentioned, that sertraline is also effective in the treatment of OCD in young people. A similar open treatment study of paroxetine found a reduction of symptom scores, in the majority (55%) of young people, in the 12 weeks of the trial (Rosenberg *et al.*, 1999).

When the decision to use medication is progressed, the indicated first-line treatment is a trial from the group of SSRIs. It is important that the dose is at a therapeutic level and the medication should be given for at least 8 weeks to determine if there is a clinical improvement. If there is no response, or the medication is not tolerated, the next psychopharmacological option is trial of clomipramine, at a therapeutic level, for a similar duration.

ANXIETY DISORDERS

In young people anxiety disorders take the form both of the childhood types continuing into adolescence as well as the emergence of adult-type pathology. Treatment using non-pharmacological approaches is usually attempted. When the disorder is having a significant effect or is not responding to the primary intervention, medication should be considered. Surprisingly, there are few treatment studies in this area.

School phobia has been subject to a series of double-blind, placebo controlled studies, by a variety of authors, assessing the effectiveness of the TCAs. In the last of these the results contradicted the group's earlier findings and did not demonstrate any benefits of medication over placebo (Klein *et al.*, 1992). On balance, there is no clear research support for the use of this group of drugs for the disorder.

The benzodiazepines can be considered for short-term use, with the assumption that, as in adults, there is a risk of tolerance and dependence. Kutcher and Mackenzie (1988) reported the successful use of clonazepam in four adolescents with panic disorder. Developing on from this a double-blind study the researchers confirmed the benefits on both the frequency and the severity of symptoms (Kutcher et al., 1992). In this area the SSRI paroxetine has been licensed for use, in adults, for panic disorder and also for social phobia. The age of onset for this latter disorder is reported to occur frequently in adolescence (Schneier et al., 1992). These two disorders may well be the next growth area of interest in the field of psychopharmacology in young people.

Another SSRI, fluoxetine, was used in an open study of 21 11–17 year olds diagnosed with an anxiety disorder and importantly, who had not responded to earlier treatment interventions including in two-thirds (67%) a trial of a TCA (Birmaher et al., 1994). In this non-responding group the results are positive with 81% showing moderate or better improvement in anxiety symptoms on a global assessment scale. This group was careful in excluding young people who had a co-morbid disorder. As with many of the disorders of adolescence, co-morbidity is an important consideration. Kashani and Orvaschel (1988), in a community sample, found high rates of co-morbid major depression. This recognition is important in planning the treatment intervention and can guide the choice of medication.

THE PSYCHOSES

Adolescence is the beginning of the period of greatest risk for the onset of psychotic disorders. For those with a lifetime risk of a continuous or relapsing major mental disorder, the initial management of such an illness is of great importance. The use of medication, as part of a comprehensive treatment package, is a key component in the early intervention phase (Power et al., 1998).

In a situation that is similar to the introduction of the newer antidepressants, there have also been significant developments in the choice of antipsychotic medication in recent years. The 'novel' or atypical antipsychotics have been released and marketed on the basis of a reduction in side effects compared to the traditional groups. One of the atypical antipsychotics, clozapine, has a specific indication for treatment-resistant schizophrenia.

While the antipsychotic action of this group of drugs is mediated in the dopaminergic system in the brain, the drugs also affect a wide range of other receptor sites. These combined effects lead to a range of common side effects which, in broad terms, can group the traditional antipsychotics. One group, that includes chlorpromazine, has a significant sedative action, which can be used to clinical effect. This contrasts with another group, which includes trifluoperazine and haloperidol, that are less sedating but with a more pronounced risk of extrapyramidal side effects. Choices can therefore be made based on the clinical presentation of the patient. If sedation is required in the initial management this will guide the choice, balanced against a judgement about the potential for the development of side effects.

Extrapyramidal side effects are relatively common and consist of three types of symptoms: (1) akathesia or motor restlessness, which can be mistaken for the agitation of a psychotic individual and, compounding the problem, lead to increasing dosage of the medication causing the symptom, (2) dystonia, showing itself as abnormal movements of the face or body musculature, and (3) a Parkinsonian-like tremor and stiffness. There is some suggestion that young people may be particularly prone to the development of extrapyramidal side effects (Remington et al., 1998).

Use of antipsychotic medications can also lead to the unwanted development of tardive dyskinesia. The dyskinesia or movement disorder often takes the form of involuntary movement of the face – especially the mouth and tongue. This is a very worrying side effect, as it often appears irreversible even on stopping the drug treatment. While, in general, it is more common in the elderly and in those on long-term medication it can occasionally occur in the treatment of children and adolescents (Wolf and Wagner, 1993).

Neuroleptic malignant syndrome (Silva et al., 1999) is another uncommon, potentially fatal side effect that has been reported to occur with many of the antipsychotic medications. Its presentation is characterised by hyperthermia, muscular rigidity and autonomic dysfunction. It is a medical emergency that requires immediate cessation of drug therapy and often further active management in an acute hospital.

It is not surprising, given such side effect profiles, that the 'atypical' antipsychotic group has been developed. It is known that the presence of side effects is a commonly cited reason people give for stopping antipsychotic medication, a factor that has now been confirmed in an adolescent population (Lloyd et al., 1998). It is possible to attempt to manage any extrapyramidal side effects by reducing the dose of antipsychotic medication or, if this not clinically appropriate, through the addition of anti-Parkinsonian medication (e.g. procyclidine, orphenadrine). However, there is a compelling argument for using medication that has a reduced side effect profile as the first-line treatment.

Once the decision to use antipsychotic medication has been made then the prescription should be started at a low dose to check for sensitivities, given that this will, in many cases of adolescent-onset psychosis, be the first exposure to such treatment. It is essential that the dose of medication is raised to a therapeutic level, while recognising that the full benefits, on psychotic symptoms, will not be present for 2–3 weeks. Generally the therapeutic benefits will occur at the lower end of the dosing range and there is no need, during this period, to continue to increase the dose to the maximum indicated in the British National Formulary (1999). Once improvement has occurred, it is important to reduce the dose of antipsychotic medication to the lowest level that still maintains symptom control.

These early phases of treatment are often best managed in the controlled environment of an adolescent inpatient unit. Occasionally, in an acute situation, it may be necessary to contain the young person's behaviour and to require more sedation than is achieved with an antipsychotic alone. In such circumstances the addition of a benzodiazepine, such as lorazepam, is appropriate (Nottingham Healthcare NHS Trust, 1998). In such circumstances the medication may have to be administered intramuscularly. Such a senario is part of the information that should be discussed with the patient and family in considering both the immediate management and the longer-term treatment plan.

Taking the time to ensure that the patient and family are fully engaged with treatment is of particular importance in the first episode of a psychotic illness. It is essential, given the potential need for long-term contact with mental health services, that the opinion of both patient and carers is positively influenced in all aspects of the treatment. Continuing treatment with medication is important in the prevention of relapse of a psychosis (Hogarty and Ulrich, 1977). Reduced side effects, during the initial phase of treatment, could be expected to lead to greater compliance and argues strongly for the use of the newer compounds for first-onset psychosis. The use of the 'atypicals' is not uniform, often related to the economics, balancing the increased cost of the novel antipsychotics in comparison to conventional antipsychotics. However, this focus is too narrow and the issues are wider than a consideration of the drug costs alone. Cookson and Huybrechts (1998) studied the broader economics and found that the most important factor in overall cost–benefit analysis was a reduction of inpatient stay in long-term treatment with risperidone.

Another benefit of increased compliance with oral medication is a reduced need for depot formulations. Longer acting depot injections of antipsychotic medication are available. These are indicated when, with poor compliance, the response to oral medication leads to less than optimal treatment outcome. As with all medication there is a duty to gain fully informed consent before starting to use the preparation. The treatment protocol, using an initial small test dose, with subsequent careful monitoring of dosage and frequency of injection should, of course, be followed with young people as with all patients.

There are relatively few research studies to show the effectiveness of antipsychotic medication in the adolescent age group. The development of the group of new medications has provided an impetus and, in recent years, there has been a growth in the number of papers which have provided case reports or open studies of the atypical antipsychotics in the adolescent population. The clinical justification for the use of these medications, in the treatment of psychotic illnesses, is based on such studies as well as from extrapolation of the adult literature.

Risperidone was used to treat 10 young people who had a diagnosis of schizophrenia (Armenteros et al., 1997). After a withdrawal from previous medication, risperidone was given for 6 weeks. Rating scale scores showed a clinical improvement over the period of the trial. Olanzapine was used in the treatment of a group of eight young people with Schizophrenia for whom two different traditional neuroleptics had proved ineffective (Kumra *et al.*, 1998). By week 8 of the trial only three (of eight) patients were considered to have responded, but this is from a group who had already not responded to other classes of antipsychotic. It is hardly surprising that both these groups of authors suggest that the results from their studies identify the need for proper double-blind trials in this area.

Clozapine is of particular importance given its licence for schizophrenia unresponsive to other treatments. This illness, occurring with first onset in adolescence, has been found to be associated with a poor prognosis (Cawthron *et al.*, 1994). Case studies have described the successful use of clozapine in the treatment of two (Jacobsen *et al.*, 1994) and of three adolescents (Birmaher *et al.*, 1992). An open trial of clozapine in the treatment of 11 adolescents with schizophrenia reported that just over half of the young people were rated as improved in both positive and negative symptoms (Frazier *et al.*, 1994).

This latter group of authors, from the National Institute of Mental Health, Bethesda, has recruited a national sample of young people with a diagnosis of schizophrenia. The patients have taken part in a double-blind study comparing clozapine with haloperidol (Kumra *et al.*, 1996). Twenty-one patients were used in the 6-week comparison, the results of which revealed that clozapine was superior to haloperidol in the improvement of both positive and negative symptoms. However, the need to monitor blood cell count is integral to the use of clozapine and it must be noted that in this study half of the ten patients on clozapine had a drop in neutrophil count and for two this led to a cessation of the trial. A further two patients had to stop the treatment after developing seizures. Another side effect, that may be of particular concern to young people, was weight gain, a finding also reported in treatment with risperidone (Kelly *et al.*, 1998).

The variable response for any individual to antipsychotic medication, together with the relative infrequency of the presentation of psychotic disorder in this age group, means that a child and adolescent psychiatrist providing a district service will see very few new cases in any particular year. It is therefore not surprising that, in general, child and adolescent psychiatrists in Britain have continued to use traditional antipsychotic medication (Slaveska *et al.*, 1998).

Such is the importance of the early diagnostic and treatment interventions that there is an important role for the adolescent psychiatry inpatient multidisciplinary clinical teams. These consultant-led teams have the opportunity to assess all presentations of psychotic illness in their catchment area. As a specialist clinical team, dealing with a larger number of psychotic patients than seen by any one general outpatient service, it will be informed both about diagnosis (Werry *et al.*, 1991) and current treatment models. In such a service, best practice can be implemented, by enabling one clinical team to build up their expertise and knowledge, both of the newer antipsychotics together with the advances in other treatment approaches, to provide an early intervention treatment model (Birchwood *et al.*, 1998).

Clark and Lewis (1998) have recently proposed a treatment protocol for schizophrenia in young people. The authors suggest that a traditional anti-psychotic is used first, but with a change being made to an atypical if the side effects are not acceptable or if, after 6 weeks, there is no clinical improvement. If effective it is suggested that the medication be continued for a period of at least 12 months. This length of continuation of treatment is supported in the adult literature, where is demonstrated a higher risk of relapse if medication is stopped in the first year (Hirsch *et al.*, 1973). In this protocol, clozapine is reserved for those who have tried, with limited success, at least two other classes of antipsychotic. The developing research evidence of the effectiveness of the atypical antipsychotics in young people makes this seem a rather conservative protocol. There are now strong arguments for the newer antipsychotics being considered as a first line treatment.

CYCLICAL AFFECTIVE DISORDERS

The mood stabilisers are treatment options for the management of recurrent affective disorders occurring in adolescence. As with the long-term prescription of antipsychotics the prophylactic use of mood stabilizers, over many years, raises the issue of the appropriateness of their use in this age group. A balanced view has to be taken as to the recommendation for longer-term treatment and when this might be justified in the course of an evolving clinical presentation.

Although lithium salts can be used in the acute treatment of mania, they are generally considered for the longer term in the prevention of relapse. However, the medication may be introduced relatively early in the treatment of an episode of the disorder. This will reduce the need for prolonged use, with the associated risks, of antipsychotic medication necessary to control the acute presentation. The research basis, in young people, for lithium treatment is relatively well established. Fifty-seven studies were identified in a recent review of which nine (16%) were double-blind (Alessi *et al.*, 1994). The authors concluded that the evidence supports the use of lithium as being beneficial in the treatment of manic depressive disorder in adolescence. The indications also include the benefits in prophylaxis, as described by Strober *et al.* (1990), who identified a three-fold higher risk of relapse in those young people who did not finish an 18 month treatment trial as compared to the group who completed it. The evidence is available to support the use of lithium in the treatment of young people with an established diagnosis of cyclical affective disorder.

Lithium has also been used in the other recurrent disorders of adolescence. The rare Kleine–Levin syndrome, characterised by episodic hypersomnia with megaphagia and generally only occurring in males, has been reported to respond to lithium treatment (Cawthron, 1990). The periodic psychoses of puberty have been considered as having a distinct nosology. However, a case series of 11 young people, described by Abe and Ohta (1995), suggest that this is a presentation of a cyclical affective disorder which responds well to lithium therapy.

Lithium, when compared to the antipsychotics, has a different side effect profile. It is important for the young person and family to be aware of these side effects, which include the risk of weight gain, polyuria/polydypsia and a fine tremor. The need for caution in circumstances where there is significant loss of fluid such as gastrointestinal disturbance with vomiting or diarrhoea, the potential for thyroid dysfunction and the long-term risk of kidney damage have all to be considered. There is a need for repeated blood level monitoring of the lithium level together with continuing assessments for the development of such side effects. The frequency of the blood tests reduces over time if the lithium level is stable, making such a process slightly more acceptable to the young person.

Against this inconvenience has to be set the risk to the individual of a relapse of the manic-depressive illness. Disruption to the young person's development, noting in particular, the educational circumstances with the national examinations of the GCSE at 16 years and the A levels at 18 years. Of equal importance to young people embarking on the employment ladder is the need for stability to enable them to work towards fulfilling their potential.

The prediction of risk of recurrence for an individual patient after an initial episode cannot be known. Adopting a cautious attitude to reduce the risk of relapse, at such an important stage of development, lithium could be considered after a single episode of hypomania, on the basis that such a diagnosis implies the likelihood of a recurrent affective disorder. However, confirming that such a pattern is established before considering longer-term treatment is the more usual process. If lithium therapy has been used in the control of the acute phase of a manic illness, either with an antipsychotic or using benzodiazepines, these latter medications can be withdrawn first. The longer term management decision is then made whether to withdraw the lithium 3–6 months after the initial acute phase has resolved or whether to continue as prophylaxis against relapse for a further 2 years or more.

CLINICAL CASE

A 14-year-old girl is admitted to an adolescent unit with a presentation of hypomania. She is grandiose, has pressure of speech, is overactive and not sleeping. The symptoms respond to antipsychotic medication, which the young person reluctantly accepts. She needs even more support to maintain compliance when she develops side effects, notably sedation, increased salivation and rigidity. This is managed through a reduction of the dose of antipsychotic medication. The symptoms resolve and she returns to her pre-morbid state. On discharge from the inpatient unit the patient asks for a cessation of the medication. She acknowledges the clinical advice about risk of relapse but is determined and agrees a phased withdrawal while remaining in contact with the physician who is able to monitor her mental state. Five months later she has a further episode of her psychotic disorder, which again takes the form of hypomania. Treatment is instigated with antipsychotic medication but on this occasion the patient, and her parents, agreed to the additional use of lithium for prophylaxis. The psychotic symptoms again respond to the medication, the young person's mental state stabilises, the antipsychotic is withdrawn and she is discharged home on lithium mono-therapy. The patient missed a significant amount of education and dropped a year at school. She successfully passed her GCSEs 2 years later and then made a decision to stop the lithium before commencing her A level studies. Six months later she remained symptom free.

The case illustrates several issues: there is the general reluctance of the young person to take medication, which is reinforced by the initial side effects. She showed a preference, following the first episode, to come off medication. She reached an agreement, following relapse, to commence lithium and later, at a time when it fitted with her educational situation, to withdraw from lithium prophylaxis. Of importance is the need for the therapeutic relationship to remain positive, so that the reluctance to accept medication does not lead to a complete rejection of the contact with the healthcare professional.

Carbamazepine is also used as a mood stabiliser in young people. It is usually considered as the second line treatment if lithium is unsuccessful. However, the anticonvulsant has been identified as of particular use in rapid cycling affective disorder. Woolston (1999) describes the use of carbamazepine in the adolescent age group in a case study. Although it appears an effective treatment, as with many medications, there is clearly a need for proper trials using control groups of an appropriate age.

ATTENTION DEFICIT HYPERACTIVITY DISORDER (ADHD)

ADHD is one of the most investigated mental disorders of childhood. There remains, however, a lack of knowledge on the long-term history of the condition; in particular, the predictors for any individual child/adolescent (Richters et al., 1995). ADHD can be diagnosed in adolescents (Biederman et al., 1998). The place of medication, with psychostimulants, in the treatment of ADHD in childhood is well supported by the research evidence (Ottenbacher and Cooper, 1983). However, there remain a number of uncertainties, especially considering the place of medication in the treatment of ADHD in adolescents.

Some young people, not identified in childhood, will be diagnosed with ADHD for the first time in adolescence and will be likely to benefit from stimulant medication. Many other children, with diagnosed ADHD, will grow into adolescence and adulthood requiring continuing treatment and support. The place for medication will need individual evaluation, reconsidered over time, to ensure that the treatment benefits remain. This is usually assessed through the mechanism of having 'drug-free' holidays to monitor the differences 'on' compared to 'off' medication.

Psychostimulants are the first choice medication. If unsuccessful, other classes of drugs, including the TCAs, the SSRIs and clonidine, can be used as alternatives or adjuncts (AACAP Official Action, 1997a). When initiating treatment, with a psychostimulant, it is appropriate to start with a low dose increasing on a weekly basis, dependent on side effects and therapeutic benefits. One particular issue for the socially conscious teenager is the need to take three or four doses of medication a day. To increase the chances of compliance this regime will need careful consideration with the young person (Garland, 1998). Tactful discussion on the subject of compliance is also required if the medication appears to lose effectiveness rather than responding with an immediate increase in the dosage. Another specific concern, in the prescription of psychostimulants to young people, is the perceived risk of abuse. While the chances may be greater with increasing general levels of substance misuse, Hechtman (1985) found no evidence of abuse in a well-monitored treatment programme.

CONDUCT DISORDER

Conduct disorders are the commonest group of mental disorders seen in children and adolescents (Rutter et al., 1975). Medication is not generally countenanced for the treatment of this group of young people. From the American Academy of Child and Adolescent Psychiatry's (AACAP Official Action, 1997b) 'Summary of the practice parameters for the assessment and treatment of children and adolescents with conduct disorder' it is clear that medication alone cannot be the treatment for conduct disorder. However, there may be times, particularly when young people with this disorder are hospitalised, usually for associated self-harming behaviour, that medication is utilised to reduce the aggressive or the self-harming behaviour while trying to engage the young person in other therapeutic work. At the Hill End Adolescent Unit rationale for the use of antipsychotic medication, to contain the aggressive situation, was that it was indicated when staff anxieties were too great. The dilemmas of this approach are illustrated by Stuart-Smith (1994) who, in a follow-up of patients subject to this regime, revealed the young person's preference for alternative methods of trying to contain behaviour.

Some of the studies of the use of lithium in adolescence look at its role in the management of aggression. This is sometimes as an adjunct to prescription of the antipsychotics, but lithium can be used as an alternative. In general, reports in this area have investigated groups of young people who have a learning disability (DeLong and Aldershof, 1987) or a pervasive developmental disorder (Campbell *et al.*, 1972). In these situations it does appear that lithium has an effect in reducing aggressive or unmanageable behaviour. While the first line management, in these groups of patients, is to use behavioural techniques, medication can provide a useful back-up. In long-term treatment lithium does not have the same risks of tardive dyskinesia as the antipsychotics and is therefore the preferred option.

Managing conduct disorder, Schreier (1998), in an outpatient sample, report results of a positive response to risperidone in reducing aggressive behaviour. The dilemma, of this study, is the interpretation of the effects of medication on aggression in that the group of young people were co-morbid for a mood disorder. The importance of assessing co-morbidity in conduct disordered young people is highlighted in a survey of 'adolescents', with an age range of 13–28 years! (Arredondo and Butler, 1994). In this study, 41 out of 57 patients with conduct disorder were co-morbid for mood disorder, which included one-quarter of the group having bipolar disorder. Additionally, the conduct disorder patients were found to have associated ADHD and substance misuse.

Advances in our understanding of brain biochemistry and its relationship to aggression and other behavioural disorders (Zubieta and Alessi, 1993) will lead to further efforts to determine which medication acting on which system will be most beneficial. Equally important is to further clarify the subtypes or clinical co-morbid associations of conduct disorders.

COMBINED PHARMACOTHERAPY

While the debate on the clinical effectiveness of medication continues, concerns are being raised about a perceived trend towards polypharmacy or the prescription of more than one group of medicines. Behr (1998) describes a case report of a 13-year-old receiving four medications on a daily basis and questions the research evidence for such practice. Clinicians are faced with difficult situations in respect of individual patients, often where the adolescent has a pervasive developmental disorder, is aggressive and has symptoms of ADHD or a depressive disorder. Responding to the reports and concerns of parents and teachers, there is often a pressure to increase the dose or add another medication. The potential for causing the appearance of new symptoms, including the risks of toxicity, must be considered. Wakefield and Sagar (1997) make the point that it is necessary to review and to stop medication when the benefits are not apparent. Choice will generally need to be based on alternative classes of medication, as second-line treatment, rather than the addition of another compound.

There are some clinical situations in which polypharmacy is accepted practice. The alleviation of side effects caused by the antipsychotics or in the control of an acutely disturbed patient are two such scenarios. However, where combined pharmacotherapy (CPT) is used in an attempt to effect a change in a difficult clinical situation there is a limited research base to support such practice. If the decision is based on the supposed inefficiency of monotherapy then, as well as considering the general knowledge of efficacy and rate of non-response, consideration must also be given to individual circumstances and, in particular, the issue of compliance.

The clinical findings of substantial co-morbidity in the adolescent population may lead to targeting the treatment of the different disorders with individual medications. However, in these circumstances our knowledge of the relationship between such co-morbid disorders is limited. Further studies are needed to determine if one disorder can be considered 'primary' and for research to compare therapeutic interventions targeting one of the co-morbid disorders as opposed to treating all diagnosable disorders as separate entities.

It might be expected that the use of CPT is generally restricted to the more disturbed adolescent inpatient population. Connor et al. (1997), in a review of young people admitted to a residential treatment centre, identified 60% as having a history of CPT. However, in an outpatient service, Storch (1998) reports that almost half (48%) of those on medication were taking more than one treatment. Such results are not universal but indicate a need to carefully consider prescribing practices.

CONCLUSION

In recent years there have been genuine advances in the use of psychoactive medication in young people. The introduction of new generations of pharmacological agents, in the fields of antipsychotic medication and in antidepressant medication, has increased treatment options. Secondly, there has been an increase in the publication of more rigorous research findings in specific adolescent populations. There is now much stronger evidence to support the prescription of medication in a range of mental disorders. Psychiatrists who treat young people no longer have to rely on adult studies from which to extrapolate information on clinical effectiveness.

The depth of age relevant information is still limited and there is clearly a need for further studies. It would be beneficial to instigate several multicentre studies in Britain to give greater validity to psychopharmacological investigations. Such a development would be welcomed and, by placing this work firmly in the context of general clinical practice, make the findings more directly relevant to clinicians. At the same time the developments in non-pharmacological treatment interventions need to be considered. Drug treatments must not just be compared with other medication or placebo (Brown and Ievers, 1999). As examples, the place of cognitive-behavioural therapy in the treatment of depression, family therapy for the prevention of relapse in schizophrenia and psychological therapies in the management of hallucinations need to be evaluated alongside medication to establish the specific indications for, and the interactions between, the different therapeutic approaches for young people.

The aim of the CAMHS team is to provide an integrated approach to case management. It is important to determine, for any young person with a mental illness, the specific clinical diagnosis and co-morbid disorders, together with identifying the most effective combination of therapeutic interventions. As clinical knowledge expands, the range of skills in a multidisciplinary child and adolescent mental health team will need to develop. The national agenda of clinical governance (NHS Executive, 1999) will serve to increase emphasis on clinical effectiveness and provide a further impetus for the development of clinical guidelines. This will, in turn, lead to more rigour in general clinical practice with continuing refinements in the evaluation of treatment outcomes.

The general adoption of an organisational model of CAMHS into tiers (NHS Health Advisory Service, 1995) allows for the development of specialist services. While it is essential for every local service to determine its own organisation, continuing therapeutic developments will guide this process. Some areas will be able to develop teams targeting specific diagnostic groups, such as the psychoses, ADHD or major depressive disorder. Such teams will acquire substantial knowledge and significant expertise in psychopharmacology. However, all general, community-based CAMHSs will need to have adequate clinical input from consultant psychiatric staffing in order that medication can be properly considered alongside other therapeutic interventions.

There remain substantial challenges in considering the use of medication in young people. The gap between clinical practice and research evidence in the use of antidepressants is one such area. While there is now a more general acceptance, supported by research evidence, of the benefits of methylphenidate in the treatment of ADHD, the place for its continued prescription through adolescence and into adulthood needs further clarification. The slow acceptance, by many British child psychiatrists, of the benefits seems likely to be mirrored by those mental health professionals providing services to younger adults.

Young people suffering from a mental disorder have a range of treatment options available. Medication is an important and powerful intervention, but one that carries a clinical risk. Advances in psychopharmacology have diminished some of the risks but the increased choice available is not accompanied by clear research evidence to support its use. Future developments may bring additional concerns but also the potential of treatments for disorders for which there are currently no specific pharmacological interventions. Developments in non-pharmacological therapies will also lead to changes in the way medication is currently used, as will continuing exploration of the clinical indications for the use of existing drugs. Progress in further developing clinical practice can only be achieved by continuing and substantial research in the field.

REFERENCES

AACAP Official Action (1997a) Summary of the practice parameters for the assessment and treatment of children., adolescents and adults with ADHD. *Journal of the American Academy of Child and Adolescent Psychiatry*, 36, 1311–1317.

AACAP Official Action (1997b) Summary of the practice parameters for the assessment and treatment of children and adolescents with conduct disorder. *Journal of the American Academy of Child and Adolescent Psychiatry*, 36, 1482–1485.

Abe, K. and Ohta, M. (1995) Recurrent brief episodes with psychotic features in adolescence: periodic psychosis of puberty revisited. *British Journal of Psychiatry*, 167, 507–513.

Alderman, J., Wolkow, R., Chung, M. and Johnston, H. F. (1998) Sertraline treatment of children and adolescents with obsessive compulsive disorder or depression: Pharmacokinetics, tolerability, and efficacy. *Journal of the American Academy of Child and Adolescent Psychiatry*, 37, 386–394.

Alessi, N., Naylor, M. W., Ghaziuddin, M. and Zubieta, J. K. (1994) Update on lithium carbonate therapy in children and adolescents. *Journal of the American Academy of Child and Adolescent Psychiatry*, 33, 291–304.

Armenteros, J. L., Whitaker, A. H., Welikson, M., Stedge, D. J and Gorman, J. (1997) Risperidone in adolescents with schizophrenia: an open pilot study. *Journal of the American Academy of Child and Adolescent Psychiatry*, 36, 694–700.

Arredondo, D. and Butler, S. (1994) Affective co-morbidity in psychiatrically hospitilized adolescents with conduct disorder or oppositional defiant disorder: should conduct disorder be treated with mood stabilizers? *Journal of Child and Adolescent Psychopharmacology*, 4, 151–158.

Behr, R. (1998) Overzealous prescribing of medications (Letter). *Journal of the American Academy of Child and Adolescent Psychiatry*, 37, 900.

Biederman, J., Faraone, S., Taylor, A., Sienna, M., Williamson, S. and Fine, C. (1998) Diagnostic continuity between child and adolescent ADHD: findings from a longitudinal clinical sample. *Journal of the American Academy of Child and Adolescent Psychiatry*, 37, 305–313.

Birchwood, M., Todd, P. and Jackson, C. (1998) Early intervention in psychosis. The critical period hypothesis. *British Journal of Psychiatry*, 172 (Suppl. 33), 53–59.

Birmaher, B., Baker, R., Kapur, S., Quintana, H. and Ganguli, R. (1992) Clozapine for the treatment of adolescents with schizophrenia. *Journal of the American Academy of Child and Adolescent Psychiatry*, 31, 160–164.

Birmaher, B., Waterman, G., Ryan, N., Cully, M., Balach, L., Ingram, J. *et al.*

(1994) Fluoxetine for childhood anxiety disorders. *Journal of the American Academy of Child and Adolescent Psychiatry*, 33, 993–999.

Bramble, D. (1995) Antidepressant prescription by British child psychiatrists: practice and safety issues. *Journal of the American Academy of Child and Adolescent Psychiatry*, 34, 327–331.

British National Formulary (1999) London: British Medical Association and Royal Pharmaceutical Society of Great Britain.

Brown, R. T. and Ievers, C. E. (1999) Psychotherapy and pharmacotherapy treatment outcome research in pediatric populations. *Journal of Clinical Psychology in Medical Settings*, 6, 63–88.

Campbell, M., Fish, B., Shapiro, T., Collins, P. and Koh, C. (1972) Lithium and chlorpromazine: a controlled cross-over study of hyperactive severely disturbed children. *Journal of Autism and Childhood Schizophrenia*, 2, 234–263.

Cawthron, P. (1990) A disorder unique to adolescence? The Kleine–Levin syndrome. *Journal of Adolescence* 13., 401 – 406.

Cawthron, P., Dell, J., James, A. and Seagrott, V. (1994) Adolescent onset psychosis. A clinical and outcome study. *Journal of Child Psychology and Psychiatry*, 35, 1321–1332.

Clark, A. F and Lewis, S. W. (1998) Practitioner review: treatment of schizophrenia in childhood and adolescence. *Journal of Child Psychology and Psychiatry*, 39, 1071–1081.

Colle, L. M., Belair, J-F., DiFeo, M., Weiss, J. and LaRoche, C. (1994) Extended open-label Fluoxetine treatment of adolescents with major depression. *Journal of Child and Adolescent Psychopharmacology*, 4, 225–232.

Connor, D., Ozbayrak, K., Kusiak, K., Caponi, A. and Melloni, R. (1997) Combined pharmacotherapy in children and adolescents in a residential treatment center. *Journal of the American Academy of Child and Adolescent Psychiatry*, 36, 248–254.

Cookson, R. and Huybrechts, K. (1998) Risperidone: an assessment of its economic benefits in the treatment of schizophrenia. *Journal of Medical Economics*, 1, 103–1034.

DeLong, G. and Aldershof, A. (1987) Long term experience with lithium treatment in childhood: correlation with clinical diagnosis. *Journal of the American Academy of Child and Adolescent Psychiatry*, 26, 389–394.

DeVane, C. L. and Sallee, F. R. (1996) Serotonin selective reuptake inhibitors in child and adolescent psychopharmacology: a review of published experience. *Journal of Clinical Psychiatry*, 57, 55–66.

Eisenberg, L. (1996) Commentary: what should doctors do in the face of negative evidence? *Journal of Nervous and Mental Disease*, 184, 103–105.

Frazier, J. A., Gordon, C. T., McKenna, K., Lenane, M. C., Jih, D. and Rapoport, J. L. (1994) An open trial of clozapine in 11 adolescents with childhood-onset schizophrenia. *Journal of the American Academy of Child and Adolescent Psychiatry*, 33, 659–663.

Garland, E. (1998) Pharmacotherapy of adolescent attention deficit hyperactivity disorder: challenges, choices and caveats. *Journal of Psychopharmacology*, **12**, 385–395.

Hazell, P., O'Connell, D., Heathcote, D., Robertson, J. and Henry, D. (1995) Efficacy of tricyclic drugs in treating child and adolescent depression: a meta-analysis. *British Medical Journal*, **310**, 897–901.

Hechtman, L. (1985) Adolescent outcome of hyperactive children treated with stimulants in childhood: a review. *Psychopharmacology Bulletin*, **21**, 178–191.

Hill, P and Cameron, M. (undated) *Information for New Staff on Medication used in Attention Deficit Hyperactivity Disorder (DSM IV)/Hyperkinetic Disorder (ICD 10)*. St George's Hyperactivity and Attention Disorders Clinic, St George's Hospital.

Hirsch, S., Gaind, R., Rohde, P., Stevens, B. and Wing, J. (1973) Outpatient maintenance of chronic schizophrenic patients with long acting fluphenazine: double-blind placebo trial. *British Medical Journal*, **1**, 633–637.

Hogarty, C. and Ulrich, R. (1977) Temporal effects of drug and placebo in delaying relapse in schizophrenic outpatients. *Archives of General Psychiatry*, **34**, 297–301.

Jacobsen, L. K., Walker, M. C., Edwards, J. E., Chappell, P. B and Woolston, J. L. (1994) Clozapine in the treatment of a young adolescent with schizophrenia. *Journal of the American Academy of Child and Adolescent Psychiatry*, **33**, 645–650.

Jain, U., Birmaher, B., Garcia, M. and Al-Shabbout, M. (1992) Fluoxetine in children and adolescents with mood disorders: a chart review of efficacy and adverse effects. *Journal of Children and Adolescent Psychopharmacology*, **2**, 259–265.

Kashani, J and Orvaschel, H. (1988) Anxiety disorders in midadolescence: a community sample. *American Journal of Psychiatry*, **145**, 960–964.

Kelly, D. L., Conley, R. R., Love, R. C., Horn, D. S and Ushchak, C. M. (1998) Weight gain in adolescents treated with Risperidone and conventional antipsychotics over six months. *Journal of Child and Adolescent Psychopharmacology*, **8**, 151–159.

Klein, R., Koplewicz, H. and Kanner, A. (1992) Imipramine treatment of children with separation anxiety disorder. *Journal of the American Academy of Child and Adolescent Psychiatry*, **31**, 21–28.

Kumra, S., Frazier, J. A., Jacobsen, L. K., McKenna, K., Gordon, C. T., Lenane, M. C. *et al.* (1996) Childhood-onset schizophrenia: a double-blind clozapine–haloperidol comparison. *Archives of General Psychiatry*, **53**, 1090–1097.

Kumra, S., Jacobsen, L. K., Lenane, M., Karp, B. I., Frazier, J. A., Smith, A. K. *et al.* (1998) Childhood-onset schizophrenia: an open-label study of olanzapine in adolescents. *Journal of the American Academy of Child and Adolescent Psychiatry*, **37**, 377–385.

Kutcher, S. (1997) Practitioner review: the pharmacotherapy of adolescent depression. *Journal of Child Psychology and Psychiatry*, 38, 755–767.

Kutcher, S. and Mackenzie, S. (1988) Successful clonazepam treatment of adolescents with panic disorder. *Journal of Clinical Psychopharmacology*, 8, 299–301.

Kutcher, S. and Robertson, H. (1995) Electroconvulsive therapy in treatment resistant depression. *Journal of Child and Adolescent Psychopharmacology*, 5, 167–175.

Kutcher, S., Reiter, S., Gardner, D. and Klein, R. (1992) The pharmacotherapy of anxiety disorders in children and adolescents. *Psychiatric Clinics of North America*, 15, 41–67.

Leonard, H., Swedo, S., Lenane, M., Rettew, D., Cheslow, D., Hamburger, S. *et al.* (1989) Treatment of obsessive compulsive disorder with clomipramine and desipramine in children and adolescents: a double-blind crossover comparison. *Archives of General Psychiatry*, 46, 1088–1092.

Leonard, H., Swedo, S., Lenane, M., Rettew, D., Hamburger, S., Bartho, J. *et al.* (1993) A two to seven year follow up study of 54 obsessive-compulsive children and adolescents. *Archives of General Psychiatry*, 50, 429–439.

Leonard, H. L., March, J., Rickler, K. C. and Allen, A. J. (1997) Pharmacology of the selective serotonin reuptake inhibitors in children and adolescents. *Journal of the American Academy of Child and Adolescent Psychiatry*, 36, 725–736.

Lloyd, A., Horan, W., Borgaro, S. R., Stokes, J. M., Pogge, D. L and Harvey, P. D. (1998) Predictors of medication compliance after hospital discharge in adolescent psychiatric patients. *Journal of Child and Adolescent Psychopharmacology*, 8, 133–141.

March, J., Mulle, K. and Herbel, B. (1994) Behavioural psychotherapy for children and adolescents with obsessive-compulsive disorder: an open trial of a new protocol-driven treatment package. *Journal of the American Academy of Child and Adolescent Psychiatry*, 33, 333–341.

NHS Executive. (1999) *Clinical Governance: Quality in the New NHS*. London: Department of Health.

NHS Health Advisory Service (1995) *Child and Adolescent Mental Health Services: Together We Stand*. London: HMSO.

Nottingham Healthcare NHS Trust (1998) *Algorithm for the Control of a Seriously Disturbed Patient*. Nottingham: Nottingham Healthcare NHS Trust.

Ottenbacher, K and Cooper, H. (1983) Drug treatment of hyperactivity in children. *Developmental Medicine and Child Neurology*, 25, 358 – 366.

Pellegrino, E. D. (1996) Commentary: clinical judgement, scientific data, and ethics: antidepressant therapy in adolescents and children. *Journal of Nervous and Mental Disease*, 184, 106–108.

Power, P., Elkins, K., Adlard, S., Curry, C., McGorry, P. and Harrigan, S. (1998) Analysis of the initial treatment phase in first episode psychosis. *British Journal of Psychiatry*, **172** (Suppl. 33), 71–76.

Reineche, M., Ryan, N. and DuBois, D. (1998) Cognitive-behavioural therapy of depression and depressive symptoms during adolescence: a review and meta-analysis. *Journal of the American Academy of Child and Adolescent Psychiatry*, **37**, 26–34.

Remington, G., Kapur, S. and Zipursky, R. (1998) Pharmacotherapy of first-episode schizophrenia. *British Journal of Psychiatry*, **172** (Suppl. 33), 66–70.

Rey-Sanchez, F. and Gutierrez-Casares, J. R. (1997) Paroxetine in children with major depressive disorder: an open trial. *Journal of the American Academy of Child and Adolescent Psychiatry*, **36**, 1443–1447.

Richters, J., Arnold, L., Jensen, P., Abikoff, H., Conners, K., Greenhill, L. *et al.* (1995) NIMH Collaborative Multisite Multimodal Treatment Study of Children with ADHD: background and rationale. *Journal of the American Academy of Child and Adolescent Psychiatry*, **34**, 987–1000.

Riddle, M., Scahill, L., King, R., Hardin, M., Anderson, G., Ort, S. *et al.* (1992) Double-blind crossover trial of fluoxetine and placebo in children and adolescents with obsessive-compulsive disorder. *Journal of the American Academy of Child and Adolescent Psychiatry*, **31**, 1062–1069.

Rodriguez-Ramos, P., de Dios-Vega, J. L., San-Sebastian-Cabases, J., Sordo-Sordo, L. and Mardomingo-Sanz, M. J. (1996) Effects of paroxetine in depressed adolescents. *European Journal of Clinical Research*, **8**, 49–61.

Rosenberg, D., Stewart, C., Fitzgerald, K., Tawile, V. and Carroll, E. (1999) Paroxetine open-label treatment of pediatric outpatients with obsessive compulsive disorder. *Journal of the American Academy of Child and Adolescent Psychiatry*, **38**, 1180–1185.

Royal College of Psychiatrists (1998) *Higher Specialist Training Handbook. Occasional Paper OP43.* London: Royal College of Psychiatrists.

Rutter, M., Cox, A., Tupling, C., Berger, M. and Yule, B. (1975) Attainment and adjustment in two geographical areas. I: Prevalence of psychiatric disorder. *British Journal of Psychiatry*, **126**, 493–509.

Ryan, N., Puig-Antich, J., Ambrosini, P., Rabinovich, H., Robinson, D., Nelson, B. *et al.* (1987) The clinical picture of major depression in children and adolescents. *Archives of General Psychiatry*, **44**, 854–861.

Ryan, N., Meyer, U., Dachille, S., Mazzic, D. and Puig-Antich, J. (1988) Lithium augmentation in TCA-refractory depression in adolescents. *Journal of the American Academy of Child and Adolescent Psychiatry*, **27**, 371–376.

Safer, D. (1997) Changing patterns of psychotropic medications prescribed by Child Psychiatrists in the 1990s. *Journal of Child and Adolescent Psychopharmacology*, **7**, 267–274.

Schneier, F., Johnson, J., Horning, C., Leibowitz, M. and Weissman, M. (1992) Social phobia: comorbidity and morbidity in an epidemiological sample. *Archives of General Psychiatry*, **49**, 282–288.

Schreier, H. (1998) Risperidone for young children with mood disorders and aggressive behaviour. *Journal of Child and Adolescent Psychopharmacology*, **8**, 49–59.

Silva, R., Munoz, D., Alpert, M., Perlmutter, I. and Diaz, J. (1999) Neuroleptic malignant syndrome in children and adolescents. *Journal of the American Academy of Child and Adolescent Psychiatry*, **38**, 187–194.

Simeon, J. G., Dinicola, V. F., Ferguson, H. B. and Copping, W. (1990) Adolescent depression: a placebo-controlled Fluoxetine treatment study and follow-up. *Progress in Neuro-Psychopharmacology and Biological Psychiatry*, **14**, 791–795.

Slaveska, K., Hollis, C. and Bramble, D. (1998) Use of antipsychotics by child and adolescent psychiatrists. *Psychiatric Bulletin*, **22**, 685–687.

Storch, D. (1998) Outpatient pharmacotherapy in a community mental health center (Letter). *Journal of the American Academy of Child and Adolescent Psychiatry*, **37**, 249–250.

Strober, M., Morrell, W., Lampert, C. and Burroughs, J. (1990) Relapse following discontinuation of lithium maintenance therapy in adolescents with bipolar illness: a naturalistic study. *American Journal of Psychiatry*, **147**, 457–461.

Stuart-Smith, S. (1994) Reactions to Hill End Adolescent Unit: interviews with 20 ex-patients. *Journal of Adolescence*, **17**, 483–489.

Wakefield, T. and Sagar, P. (1997) Combined drug therapy debate (continued) (Letter) *Journal of the Academy of Child and Adolescent Psychiatry*, **36**, 2–3.

Walkup, J. T., Labellarte, M. J. and Riddle, M. A. (1998) Commentary: unmasked and uncontrolled medication trials in child and adolescent psychiatry. *Journal of the American Academy of Child and Adolescent Psychiatry*, **37**, 360–363.

Walter, G. and Rey, J. (1997) An epidemiological study of the use of ECT in adolescents. *Journal of the American Academy of Child and Adolescent Psychiatry*, **36**, 809–815.

Weinberg, N. Z., Rahdert, E., Colliver, J. D. and Glantz, M. D. (1998) Adolescent substance abuse: a review of the past ten years. *Journal of the American Academy of Child and Adolescent Psychiatry*, **37**, 252–261.

Werry, J., McClellan, J. and Chard, L. (1991) Childhood and adolescent schizophrenia., bipolar and schizoaffective disorders: a clinical and outcome study. *Journal of the American Academy of Child and Adolescent Psychiatry*, **30**, 457–465.

Wolf, D. and Wagner, K. (1993) Tardive dyskinesia, tardive dystonia and tardive Tourette's syndrome in children and adolescents. *Journal of Child and Adolescent Psychopharmacology*, **3**, 175–198.

Woolston, J. (1999) Carbamazepine treatment of juvenile-onset bipolar disorder. *Journal of the American Academy of Child and Adolescent Psychiatry* 38, 335 – 338.

World Health Organisation (1992) *ICD-10 Classification of Mental and Behavioural Disorders. Clinical Descriptions and Diagnostic Guidelines.* Geneva: World Health Organisation.

Zubieta, J. and Alessi, N. (1993) Is there a role of serotonin in the disruptive behaviour disorders? A literature review. *Journal of Child and Adolescent Psychopharmacology*, 3, 11–35.

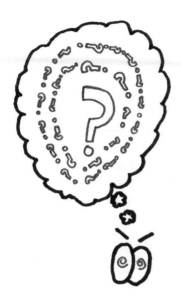

Chapter 19

COGNITIVE AND BEHAVIOURAL APPROACHES

Alison J. Wood

INTRODUCTION

Cognitive and behavioural approaches are being used increasingly with adolescents. There is a growing body of evidence for their efficacy in mood disorders and eating disorders. A cognitive approach is applicable to most adolescent psychiatric disorders and this may be one element of a multimodal treatment programme. This chapter aims to give an overview of applying cognitive and behavioural techniques in therapeutic work with adolescents. The theoretical background to cognitive-behavioural therapy (CBT) is outlined followed by a description of a comprehensive cognitive-behavioural assessment. Key components of a good cognitive-behavioural treatment programme are given. The final section of the chapter focuses on treatment planning and the application of these approaches to clinical problems.

THEORETICAL UNDERPINNINGS

Cognitive therapy is an active, problem-orientated treatment which can be conducted with individuals or groups and has a coherent theoretical foundation. Cognitive and behavioural approaches or procedures have the common distinguishing feature of simultaneous endorsement of the importance of the role of both cognitive and behavioural processes in shaping and maintaining psychological disorders. Cognitive therapy derives from the 'phenomenological' perspective that an individual's view of himself and the world is central, and that this personal conceptualisation or meaning is based on previous experiences. Behavioural therapies developed separately until the work of Meichenbaum (1975), Beck (1967), Beck et al. (1979) and Ellis (1962) promoted an integrated cognitive-behavioural approach. CBT has now been developed for most disorders encountered in psychiatric practice with adults (Hawton et al., 1992). Recent publications have described equivalent developments for children and adolescents (Graham, 1998; Reinecke et al., 1996; Zarb, 1992).

Theoretical underpinnings of CBT are transposed from work with adults. Cognitive therapy is founded upon the assumption that behaviour is adaptive and that there is an interaction between an individual's thoughts feelings and behaviours. The major focus of CBT is in understanding the nature and development of an individual's dysfunctional behaviours or emotions and the accompanying cognitive process. Cognitions are viewed as a body of knowledge or beliefs and a set of strategies for utilising this information in an adaptive manner. Cognitions include current thoughts or self-statements as well as perceptions, appraisals, schemas, attitudes, memories, goals, standards, expectations and attributions. The term 'cognition' also refers to the complex ways in which this information is processed, i.e. communication, problem-solving and interpersonal skills (Reinecke, 1996).

A large theoretical body of knowledge has grown up around the use of CBT in the treatment of depressive disorders. Beck's cognitive theory of depression (Beck, 1967; Beck et al., 1979) outlines three key concepts: negative automatic thoughts, cognitive distortions and dysfunctional beliefs. Although these relate specifically to the understanding of depressive disorders, the concepts are valuable when considering the wider use of CBT for child and adolescent psychiatric disorders. *Negative automatic thoughts* are superficial 'here and now' thoughts which can negatively influence mood states. Individuals with depressive disorders describe thoughts of personal failure and self-criticism, thoughts that their future is hopeless and not amenable to change, and misinterpretations of the world around them. The cognitive triad describes current automatic thoughts about the self, the future and the world. *Cognitive distortions or errors* are habitual errors in the logic of thinking that alter reality and lead to the types of automatic thoughts described above. A variety of slightly different classifications of these distortions exist (Beck et al., 1979; Burns, 1980). Wilkes et al. (1994) transposes this work into understandable material for adolescents. The most common are: all-or-nothing thinking, selective abstraction (mental filter), personalisation, fortune telling and emotional reasoning. These cognitive errors are thought to arise out of *dysfunctional core beliefs or schemas*. The deepest level of cognition is the core belief. Core beliefs are absolutistic statements about ourselves, others and the world (Greenberger and Padesky, 1995). These beliefs or schemas are relatively stable patterns of thinking that govern the ways in which external situations are interpreted. They are manifest as assumptions which are usually stated as 'If. . .then' sentences or 'should. . .' statements. Core beliefs provide rules for evaluating situations and are developed and shaped by life experiences. They may lie latent but are triggered by experiences which may be similar to those that led to the negative schema initially. Typical depressive assumptions might include 'if people find out how horrible I am as a person, they will hurt and reject me'. This reflects a core belief that 'I am unloveable'. It is therefore helpful to think of three layers of cognitive functioning and to work from a superficial level to a deeper level of understanding in therapy. Many adolescents will not reach the level of core beliefs and their modification in therapy.

Behaviour therapy comprises graded exposure to the feared or avoided stimulus with prevention of the typical response. This is based on the premise that anxiety is reduced by a process of habituation which is facilitated by both exposing patients to the problematic stimulus and by preventing or modifying their responses (Meyer, 1966). CBT encourages a wider understanding of symptoms to extend from behaviours and physical reactions to include thoughts, mood and environmental influences. When working with young people suffering from obsessive compulsive disorders, eating disorders and depressive disorders, this wider perspective is very helpful.

The final influence in the development of cognitive and behavioural approaches as used in adolescent psychiatry is social learning theory and the role of interpersonal relationships in the generation and maintenance of psychiatric disorders. A multitude of cognitive processes determine the actual behaviour of children in social situations. Social perception and social problem-solving skills are integral to the majority of CBT programmes (Spence and Donovan, 1998).

THE COGNITIVE–THERAPEUTIC RELATIONSHIP

Fundamental to CBT is the nature of the therapeutic relationship. 'Collaborative empiricism' refers to the therapist's stance as educator and facilitator, stimulating and empowering patients to solve problems and recover. This transposes particularly well to adolescents who often have a short attention span, dislike authority and need to be in control. The therapeutic intervention must take place within a social and educational context and it may be necessary to involve the family in treatment. The principles of working individually with adolescents are described in Chapter 20.

AN OVERVIEW OF COGNITIVE-BEHAVIOURAL THERAPY

A typical CBT programme is a short-term, time-limited therapeutic programme which is individual and problem-orientated, and planned to take place over an 8–12 week period. Initially, an in-depth assessment is completed of the adolescent's presenting problems within the context of their life situation. The treatment programme will usually begin with the identification of treatment goals together with further exploration and assessment of cognitive and behavioural phenomena. The central part of the programme will comprise cognitive, behavioural and interpersonal techniques, and the final part will aim to summarise progress and identify the need for further therapeutic work. It is important to involve parents/carers in this process. Each individual session should be 30–50 min duration, and start with setting an agenda and reviewing homework tasks. The therapist acts as a coordinator summarising each session at the end and planning the following week. CBT may be part of a multimodal treatment programme including medication, family and group therapies, and is therefore suited to being administered in a variety of inpatient, day patient or outpatient settings. CBT can be administered to individuals or groups. Young people with severe incapacitating symptoms, e.g. in acute depression or bulimia nervosa, may require twice-weekly therapy sessions in the early stages of treatment. However, it would be usual to plan 4–8-weekly sessions in the first instance followed by a review of progress. Towards the end of the treatment programme, sessions are held less frequently. Throughout the planning and the execution of the treatment programme, therapist and patient collaborate to use empirical methods to identify and resolve specific problems. CBT may be administered by any professional with therapeutic experience of working with adolescents who has had an appropriate training. Ongoing therapeutic supervision is essential.

COGNITIVE-BEHAVIOURAL ASSESSMENT

GOALS OF ASSESSMENT

The principal aim of a cognitive-behavioural assessment is to derive a formulation and treatment plan. The service context will also influence the assessment process and assessment will usually take place in stages. Following referral, the adolescent plus key members of their family or carers would be involved in a diagnostic assessment. This assessment would aim to develop a psychiatric formulation and an assessment of risk. This section aims to describe assessment methods that are useful in assessing suitability for CBT and starting to adopt a cognitive-behavioural approach with patients. Diagnostic interviewing and assessment of risk have been dealt with elsewhere.

PRINCIPLES OF ASSESSMENT

Assessment and intervention occur in parallel. Engagement in a therapeutic relationship begins at the first meeting with the therapist. It may be that the young person has been previously assessed and the first encounter with the therapist is for consideration of CBT or it may be that the CBT assessment is the first contact with the service. Key principles are to elicit the young person's views of the referral, identify broad areas which they perceive as a problem and to involve them from the outset in a collaborative exploration of their current difficulties. Who is present at the interview, the focus of the interview and the methods adopted will influence expectations and attitudes. Views about responsibility for the problem, the potential for change, and appreciation of the severity and extent of the difficulties may change during the initial assessment. The intervention begins with the assessment but the assessment continues throughout treatment. This will involve continuing assessment of key problem areas, ongoing assessment of risk, and continuing assessment and re-formulation of the adolescent's predicament. In practice CBT assessment will take place over a minimum of two sessions and will involve seeking corroborative information from other sources. Embarking on CBT is to begin a voyage of discovery!

ASSESSING SUITABILITY FOR COGNITIVE-BEHAVIOURAL THERAPY

A cognitive approach is applicable to most disorders in adolescent psychiatry. Assessing suitability and planning CBT involves identifying aspects of the presenting problems, the adolescent and their situation which best fit with this method of psychotherapeutic working. The remainder of this chapter concentrates on CBT administered by experienced professionals in an outpatient setting. An assumption is made that the adolescent is not receiving additional treatments.

The problem
Cognitive-behavioural approaches are suitable for young people presenting with clinical depression, eating disorders, obsessive compulsive disorder or any problem where cognitive distortions such as a negative self-appraisal are a key component. CBT is also indicated for the treatment of anxiety and panic, attention deficit hyperactivity disorder, conduct disorders, post-traumatic stress disorders, and the treatment of chronic pain and somatisation (Graham, 1998). CBT may have a place in the treatment of young people with psychotic disorders.

Characteristics of the adolescent
The young person must be able to identify a suitable focus for work and agree to 'give the treatment a try'. It is necessary that the young person has the ability of metacognition and is able to take responsibility for change. Clearly the approach is mainly verbal and a degree of insight and emotional literacy are necessary. The practicalities of treatment involve the ability to read and write, attending regularly for appointments and carrying out homework tasks. CBT is contra-indicated for adolescents with learning disabilities, those who externalise their

difficulties, those with immature verbal skills and young people with severe disorders affecting cognition. This last group of young people may benefit from CBT in combination with other therapies.

Characteristics of the context

Individual therapy with adolescents requires support from parents or carers. Practical assistance is required in facilitating attendance of appointments, and interest, support and feedback is necessary even if parents are not directly involved in therapy. It is necessary that the environment is safe and reasonably stable. Many young people presenting with psychiatric disorders have unstable and damaging home circumstances. These factors should be addressed prior to starting CBT. Young people may identify cognitions which are profoundly negative but founded in reality. CBT may still be a helpful approach; however, involvement and support of parents must be negotiated to a minimum acceptable level at the outset of treatment.

AREAS OF ASSESSMENT

Presenting problems

The nature of the key presenting problems is explored in detail. Descriptions and details of severity frequency and impact should be sought from informants. This will take up a significant proportion of the initial assessment interview.

Cognitive assessment

Important cognitive phenomena to focus on during a CBT assessment are self-statements, beliefs, attributions, self-efficacy expectations, perceptions and assumptions (Zarb, 1992). Important cognitive data are contained within reports of emotional responses, evaluations, plans and personal historical facts. Distorted information processing styles may be suggested by statements of both adolescents and their parents at interview:

Family assessment

Constructing a geneogram and obtaining details of family members, their relationship with the adolescent and descriptions of family functioning will identify predisposing and maintaining factors of the adolescent's difficulties.

Social relationships

Peer relationships are crucial in adolescence. Details of interpersonal and social skills deficits will need to be incorporated into the cognitive-behavioural formulation.

Intellectual and school functioning

The best assessment of whether a young person has the cognitive capacity to engage in verbal reflective therapy is their performance at a problem-focused interview. It may be important to assess intellectual ability for other purposes, e.g.

for examining reasons for school failure. A report from school of general academic and social functioning is very important.

Developmental history/general psychological adjustment
An understanding of pre-adolescent functioning is important and general adjustment and functioning. Some disorders arise *de novo* in adolescence and many are exacerbated by the developmental tasks of adolescence. An understanding of the young person's temperament and capacity for functioning will effect expectations of therapy outcome.

METHODS OF ASSESSMENT

Interview
The majority of the information can be obtained at clinical interview. It is important to interview the adolescent alone following a brief introduction involving all members of the family present. Baseline information should be recorded. Quantitative information should be obtained wherever possible. It is important to interview parents, although not essential that they are interviewed alone if the adolescent is unwilling for this to take place. Behavioural interviewing aims to develop a behavioural analysis of antecedents, behaviours and beliefs under assessment, and their consequences (Kirk, 1992).

Direct observation
Observations of family relationships are made throughout. Observations of the adolescent's reactions to the interviewer and their mental state over the course of the assessment are important.

Self-report measures
There are many self-report measures which can be incorporated into the CBT assessment. These may be standardised or devised informally to collect specific information. They provide a very useful method of quantifying symptoms and measuring change over the course of therapy.

Standardised interview measures
Similarly, there are many standardised methods of assessing functioning which are highly relevant to a CBT assessment. These are mainly used for research purposes in evaluating the efficacy of therapy. Often training is required and they are time-consuming to administer. For some disorders where the initial presentation may involve a high level of complexity such as young people with eating disorders or obsessive-compulsive disorders, a detailed analysis of the presenting problems are facilitated by such instruments.

Independent observation
Liaison with school, other professionals involved and other members of the adolescent's social network contributes to the development of cognitive-

behavioural formulation. It may be helpful for school to complete standardised behaviour ratings.

DEVELOPING A COGNITIVE-BEHAVIOURAL FORMULATION

The purpose of the cognitive-behavioural assessment is to be able to give the adolescent a preliminary formulation of their problem. This includes a brief description of the main areas of difficulty, an explanation of how the problem developed including predisposing factors and strengths as well as immediate precipitants and a summary of maintaining factors. As the CBT programme will be based on this formulation, it is important that it is shared with the adolescent and their parents in a helpful way so that a consensus can be reached.

COMPONENTS OF A COGNITIVE-BEHAVIOURAL THERAPY PROGRAMME

This section will describe cognitive, behavioural and social problem-solving components of a good CBT programme. The techniques used with adolescents with clinical depressive disorders are demonstrated in a training video (Wood *et al.*, 1997). The process of CBT involves regular reviews with the adolescent and parents, and if progress is not being made, further planning and changes in focus. The therapist must be fully conversant with a wide range of techniques and interventions, and be able to apply them flexibly according to the needs of the young person. In the final section of this chapter on applications of CBT, a clinical example will be developed to illustrate how such a programme would be implemented for adolescents presenting with clinical depression.

STARTING COGNITIVE-BEHAVIOURAL THERAPY

The initial phase of CBT is in many ways a continuation of the assessment. The following modules can usually be completed in two sessions following which the therapist should reappraise the overall goals and plan the central phase of treatment.

Rationale of cognitive-behavioural therapy

The introduction of the rationale and components of CBT to the adolescent and their parents is crucial in engaging them in a treatment programme. The adolescent should actively decide that they would like to give this treatment a try after hearing about it and actually commit themselves to an initial number of sessions. The importance of their participation should be emphasised; the necessity to complete tasks between sessions (any term other than 'homework' is helpful here) and the structure of the treatment programme should be outlined. Time must be taken to define the boundaries of confidentiality and involvement of parents. Finally, the therapist spends time focusing on educating the adolescent on the nature and rationale of CBT. The form and words of this will depend on the individual involved. Diagrams are helpful. Key concepts are: definition of 'cognitive', brief outline of techniques, importance of self-help and discovery, and team working. For each particular disorder the cognitive model will be different. Diagrams are very useful. For example (depressive disorders): *'Cognitive therapy is a particular form of talking treatment which focuses on the thoughts and beliefs that are circulating through our minds all of the time. These thoughts affect how we feel. Some people find that when they feel miserable or depressed they are having bad thoughts about themselves (I'm a failure); the future (nothing will ever change); and the people and things around them (everyone hates me). Treatment works by identifying these thoughts, understanding them and changing them. You will understand this better as we work through the treatment programme together'*. It is important to start to develop an understanding of the interconnection of physical reactions, thoughts, behaviours, moods and the young person's environment. The explanation for parents should outline their involvement and provide information regarding expectation of progress.

Identifying goals of therapy

Psychotherapy without goals is like a ship without a navigator, at the mercy of the prevailing elements (Wilkes *et al.*, 1994). CBT lays particular emphasis on agendas, goals and priorities. Goal identification will be based on information from the initial assessment of the patient's difficulties. The process of goal identification is to facilitate the adolescent in identifying problems, to translate these in to target symptoms, to agree on three or four initial goals of treatment and to rate each goal for severity at the outset. This is often difficult and can provide very helpful information about the young person. The focus of therapeutic intervention should be at a symptom level, e.g. 'to feel less depressed', 'to reduce my hand washing', 'to stop making myself sick'. Goals which are outside of the control of the adolescent or unrealistic should be avoided, e.g. 'to get on better with my parents' or 'to lose weight'. Rating the severity of problems on a Likert scale can help to set treatment priorities. It is essential that the adolescent 'owns' the treatment goals and often considerable therapist skill is needed to facilitate this.

Self-monitoring

Self-monitoring is a widely used technique both at the initial assessment stage and later in therapy. It is useful for monitoring change. There are two aspects involved in self-monitoring: (1) the individual has to note that the event (emotion, thought, behaviour) has occurred and (2) has to record that the event has happened. The accuracy of self-monitoring is increased if a few general rules are followed: only appropriate and meaningful information should be requested; the importance of the material in later sessions and how it will be used should be specified clearly by the therapist; and explicit agreement should be gained from the patient. The principles of self-monitoring and setting homework tasks should be described in the introductory phase of CBT. The first task is usually the completion of a diary task focusing on symptoms identified in goal setting.

MIDDLE PHASE OF COGNITIVE-BEHAVIOURAL THERAPY

Planning the middle phase of CBT will involve the use of a mixture of cognitive, behavioural and social problem-solving strategies as determined by the initial assessment and cognitive formulation. The middle phase would normally span over eight to 12 sessions. The following list of strategies is not exhaustive and it is beyond the scope of this chapter to describe any techniques in great detail.

Cognitive techniques

Emotional recognition
Affective education (teaching adolescents to recognise their emotions, to be able to distinguish between different emotions and to differentiate feelings from bodily sensations and thoughts) is a good starting point for CBT. There are two reasons for this: (1) one or more target problems are often concerned with emotional states and therefore focusing on this problem is relevant and logical to the young person, and (2) distinguishing emotions from thoughts provides an opportunity for the therapist to assess the ease with which the adolescent will grasp 'cognitive concepts'. The young person is asked to describe common mood states such as 'depressed', 'happy', ' angry', 'lonely', 'excited', etc. They are then asked to describe a recent personal experience of this mood state and to recount thoughts associated with it. This exercise can lead to linking emotional state with automatic thoughts and the concept of detecting negative automatic thoughts. An emotional recognition diary can be introduced in which the young person keeps a daily record of mood states by filling in three columns: 'What I was doing'; 'What I was thinking'; 'What I was feeling'.

Eliciting and recording automatic thoughts
Concrete and specific direct questions are the most straightforward means of eliciting automatic thoughts. Adolescents will not be familiar with registering the thoughts which are continuously passing through their minds and at the beginning may need significant prompting. If a young person is tearful or upset, simply asking *'What thoughts are going through your mind now?'* can be useful. Other helpful probing questions might include; *'What thoughts were going through your mind before you started to feel this way?'*, *'What does it say about you if the thoughts are true?'*, *'What are you afraid of?'*, *'What is the worst thing that could happen?'*, *'How do other people feel or think about you?'*, *'What images or memories do you have in this situation?'* (Greenberger

and Padesky, 1995). It may be that the thoughts and mental imagery are distressing and some young people have difficulty verbalising them. Simply stating thoughts and describing images can be highly arousing and upsetting for young people and the therapist must be aware of this. Other techniques include role play, video playback 'as if. . .' and the recall of pleasant and unpleasant events. Young people should be encouraged to record automatic thoughts as homework tasks using specially prepared charts. Having grasped the concepts of automatic thinking and self-monitoring, the next step is to identify the crucial most upsetting thought in generating the emotion or problem behaviour, the 'hot' thought.

Thought-stopping, distraction

Thought stopping aims to provide a strategy for dismissing unwanted thoughts and reducing their duration. The techniques are based on distraction and they cannot be learned in stressful situations. Techniques include focusing on an object, increased sensory awareness, engaging in mental exercises, remembering pleasant memories and fantasies, and counting thoughts. The immediate effect of counting thoughts may be to produce an apparent increase (Burns, 1980).

Identification of dysfunctional beliefs

Socratic questioning is the essence of cognitive therapy and forms the mainstay of a process of guided discovery which the therapist and patient embark upon together. The therapist asks a series of questions intended to lead the patient to examine his or her own beliefs and behaviours, and weaken their belief in them. It requires significant skill and experience to apply in a therapeutic relationship. This collaborative style of therapeutic communication will be liberating for some adolescents however requires a level of insight and creative or lateral thinking which may not be available to younger adolescents who may find it intimidating or threatening. Down arrow technique, innocent questioning, reflective empathy are variants of Socratic questioning. Useful references to the techniques are found in Wilkes *et al.* (1994), Burns (1980) and Blackburn and Davidson (1995). Effectively the therapist repeatedly asks 'Why?' or 'So what?' as a probe. For example: A 15–year-old boy was frightened of failing his maths exam. The therapist probes this fear in order to identify his belief that other people's approval are necessary in order for him to feel happy: '*What would it mean to you if you failed the exam?*'. . .'*So if you failed and everyone knew, why would that be so upsetting?. . .*', '*So why do you think it means so much to you what other people think. . .?*', and so on.

Identification of thinking errors

Cognitive errors have been described previously. It is often helpful from observation of the adolescent's responses and statements to reflect with them in the session on their thinking tendencies. A handout listing the thinking errors can be helpful in prompting adolescents to give personalised examples.

Cognitive restructuring

After identifying negative automatic thoughts and beliefs and cognitive errors, the next step is to use a series of techniques to replace dysfunctional cognitions with more accurate and adaptive thought patterns. The target symptoms of cognitive restructuring are automatic thoughts, self statements, interpretations, beliefs and distortions. Techniques used include pro/con evaluation, examining the evidence in support of the thought or belief, logical analysis and operationalising beliefs. These tasks lend themselves well to the use of charts and diaries. The aim is to replace dysfunctional thoughts with alternate more balanced thoughts or beliefs. Cognitive restructuring techniques are well developed for the treatment of depressive disorders. See Wilkes *et al.* (1994) and Greenberger and Padesky (1995).

Cognitive re-formulation

Following the preliminary formulation, it will now be possible to add to this and expand it to involve a shared understanding of the role of early experience in the formation of beliefs and how subsequent experience has reactivated these and produced symptoms and presenting problems.

Behavioural techniques

Activity scheduling

Activity scheduling is useful early on in treatment. Many adolescents with psychiatric disorders are socially avoidant and are not attending school. When an assessment of their daily activities is conducted it is clear that they spend a lot of time in bed, with day to night reversal and a loss of daily routine and a lack of rewarding activity. Modifying this can be quite a challenge, particularly when the adolescent perceives that this is the main aim of their parents! The result, however, is that they have little enjoyment or sense of mastery, they undervalue their abilities and they lack motivation. All of these factors reinforce their low self-esteem. The purpose of activity scheduling is to help the young person structure and plan activities. They are asked to keep a diary which involves recording activities during the day usually on an hour to hour basis. In addition they rate their enjoyment of activities on a Likert scale. The next step is to schedule pleasant and rewarding activities aimed at producing a sense of achievement. This usually requires support from parents or carers.

Self-reinforcement

Adolescents are asked to reward themselves when they complete an agreed task. The therapist and adolescent devise examples of rewards which are social, material and personal.

Behavioural analysis

The purpose of this intervention is to enable adolescents to analyse their dysfunctional behaviour patterns. It is a useful approach for anger or temper outbursts, panic attacks or a range of other behaviours identified by young people as a problem. Patients are taught to use a simple A (activating events), B (the behaviour in question) and C (consequences). Initially, examples are completed within the session; however, young people can them go on to complete dairies using this format for further discussion.

Relaxation training

Therapists usually have their own relaxation-training technique. Personal audiotapes are helpful, talking the patient through progressive muscular relaxation, and then mental imagery aimed at producing a peaceful and calm state of mind and body. This may be a helpful technique to accompany other behavioural and cognitive techniques for young people suffering from anxiety and panic, obsessive-compulsive disorder, and sleep problems accompanying clinical depression. It is not a helpful treatment alone. Therapeutic credibility can be lost if it is introduced as anything other than an experimental adjunct to other techniques.

Behavioural experiments

Behavioural experiments are designed for individual patients to help them to check out the validity of their negative cognitions. The behavioural experiment will depend on the particular beliefs it is designed to test. The treatment of anxiety and panic lend themselves well to the use of behavioural experiments. During panic attacks adolescents develop catastrophic interpretations of bodily experiences. Alternative hypotheses can be generated and discussed but testing these can be very helpful. For example, determining that voluntary hyperventilation reproduces the bodily symptoms of a panic attack can be very powerful.

De-sensitisation

Avoidance is a common symptom of many adolescent disorders. It may reach criteria for a phobia or it may be part of an obsessional phenomenon. The principle of treatment is in devising a graded hierarchy reflecting the full range of situations avoided by the patient from those which provide mild difficulty to those which provoke significant anxiety. The approach is used for school avoidance, and is usefully combined with the cognitive and behavioural techniques already described.

Exposure and response prevention

These are key behavioural techniques involved in the treatment of obsessive compulsive disorder (Salkovskis and Kirk, 1992). They should be combined with modelling and reassurance by the therapist.

Social problem-solving techniques

Communication and interpersonal skills

There is a large body of literature describing social skills intervention for young people (Spence and Donovan, 1998). Listening skills, conversation skills and self-presentation skills may form a part of a CBT programme. These can be conducted within the sessions using role play and modelling by the therapist together with examples from the adolescent's personal experience.

Social problem solving

Difficulties with problem solving are a common thread running through many adolescent mental health problems. Teaching the steps of problem solving (identifying problems, brainstorming solutions and examining the consequences of these) is effective and empowering for adolescents. The use of handouts and the application to real and fictitious social situations can form part of the central phase of a CBT package (Stark, 1990).

Interpersonal techniques

Many of the goals adolescents identify to work on in therapy are occurring in an interpersonal context. Examining interpersonal deficits, roles and the part these play in symptom formation and maintenance can be powerful (Mufson *et al.*, 1993).

ENDING COGNITIVE-BEHAVIOURAL THERAPY

The final phase of CBT will span over two to four sessions, but may include maintenance sessions spaced out to occur less frequently and facilitate a healthy separation from the therapist. The final sessions offer an opportunity for the adolescent to summarise what they have gained from the therapy and to re-rate their goals and identify continuing problems. The focus of this closure phase it to help the young person predict future problems and how to deal with them in the light of their therapeutic gains.

APPLICATION OF COGNITIVE-BEHAVIOURAL THERAPY TO CLINICAL PROBLEMS

OVERVIEW OF TREATMENT PROGRAMME

Figure 19.1 shows a typical CBT programme. There are no rigid rules and if improvement is occurring then the programme is assumed to be appropriately focused. The importance of assessment and goal definition can not be over-emphasised. Outcomes which are agreed at the initial phase can be monitored and treatment focus can be modified if improvements are not seen.

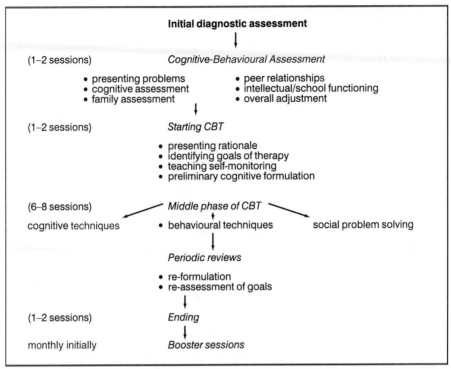

Figure 19.1 Overview of CBT programme.

COGNITIVE-BEHAVIOURAL THERAPY FOR CLINICAL DEPRESSION

There have been six randomised outcome studies of cognitive-behavioural interventions in childhood and adolescent depressive disorder (Brent *et al.*, 1997; Lewinsohn *et al.*, 1990; 1997; Reed, 1994; Vostanis *et al.*, 1996; Wood *et al.*, 1996) and a systematic review of these by Harrington *et al.* (1998) showed significant benefit of CBT over alternative inactive interventions. The following case illustration outlines a typical CBT intervention for a clinically depressed adolescent girl

SARAH

This case illustrates the use of cognitive techniques focused on symptoms of depression and suicidality in a 15-year-old girl with chronic individual and family problems. Prior to starting CBT, Sarah had been treated with antidepressants with little benefit. She was initially resistant to her mother being involved in her treatment.

Background

Sarah (aged 15) years lives with her mother, who works full-time as an administrator, and her four older sisters. Sarah's parents separated when she was 8 years of age and her father is now re-married with a 3-year-old daughter. Sarah was referred by her GP with symptoms of depression and school non-attendance leading to complete school refusal. She had been resistant to referral to an adolescent psychiatrist and had been treated with antidepressants by her GP. Sarah's mum had given up trying to get Sarah to go to school and had become increasingly concerned about Sarah's social withdrawal and mood swings at home. She acknowledged that it had been very difficult to bring up five girls relatively close in age after her husband had left, and that their father was inconsistent and 'not interested' in maintaining contact with them, particularly since his baby daughter had been born. Sarah's mum described a period of depression which responded to antidepressant medication following her separation but ongoing symptoms of dysphoria and anxiety and having to take increasing time off work. Both Sarah and her mum described difficulties in their relationship. Sarah has no past medical history of relevance, and her developmental and early educational history were unremarkable until the separation of her parents when she had a period of school refusal. At this time her mother moved her to another school and her attendance improved until the transition to secondary school. Sarah is bright academically and has always had a small number of close friends.

Assessment

The initial assessment consisted of meeting Sarah briefly with her mum to set an agenda but most of the session was spent interviewing her alone. This interview provided an in-depth assessment of Sarah's symptoms of depression and suicidality. Sarah revealed that she had taken a small overdose and cut her wrist recently, and had also experimented with cannabis and amphetamines. Sarah fulfilled diagnostic criteria for a depressive disorder. Other findings and observations included low self-esteem, a high level of introspection and personal attribution for her difficulties, but also an ability to engage in a collaborative style of working. It was clear that there was a significant level of conflict between Sarah and her mum, and Sarah was at times weepy and distressed at interview. Although she denied ongoing suicidal thoughts and impulses, the risk of further self-harm needed to be attended to. The parental interview revealed that Sarah's mum was also low in mood and demoralised. She was not aware of Sarah's suicidal thoughts and acknowledged a need for personal support.

Cognitive-behavioural formulation

Sarah presented with the following difficulties:

- **Affective**: depression moods, anger, anxiety
- **Motivational**: loss of interest and pleasure, social withdrawal
- **Behavioural**: avoidance of school and social situations
- **Cognitive**: hopelessness, suicidal thoughts, self-blame, low self-esteem, poor concentration, overconcern with appearance/body image
- **Somatic**: sleep disturbance, tiredness, disturbed eating patterns, headaches

Sarah is the youngest and was 8 when her father left home. She had always compared herself unfavourably with her older sisters who she felt had ongoing relationships with her father but that he 'never had any time for me'. For most of Sarah's childhood the marriage had been under stress and when he left Sarah had felt pleased. During these years Sarah's mum was intermittently depressed and Sarah had felt unwanted by both her parents. During her primary school years she had been supported by a close friend who had moved away at around the same time precipitating Sarah's difficulties in primary school.

- **Core beliefs**: *I'm worthless, I am inferior as a person, I am unloveable.*
- **Assumptions**: *If people get to know the real me, they will reject me. If I try to do anything I will fail.*
- **Critical incidents**: separation of parents aged 8 years, loss of close friend at the same time, father's re-marriage and birth of half sister. Difficulties with peer relationships and verbal bullying were the final triggers to the school non-attendance. Critical incidents for Sarah are likely to be around rejection and loss.
- **Negative automatic thoughts**: self: *I'm useless, a failure, I have no friends, I'm ugly*; future: *nothing can ever go right for me, I've wrecked my life, I will be alone for ever, nobody will ever understand me*; world: *everyone hates me, everything I try goes wrong, I hate school, I have no friends.*

Sarah is predisposed to becoming depressed by a family history of maternal depression and being temperamentally 'difficult' – demanding and stubborn and always clinging and close to her mum. She has a long history of school non-attendance and a conflicted relationship with her mother who has not been able to exert strong boundaries and acknowledges that Sarah 'got away with a lot' over the time of her divorce. Sarah was neglected by her dad who is inconsistent and does not make much effort to keep in touch. Sarah blamed her father for leaving and has had very little contact with him since. Maintaining factors are her isolation, her mum's unavailability and the many longstanding symptoms of her depressive disorder. Sarah had taken a trial of antidepressants which had caused side effects and she had abandoned them angry that they had not worked.

- **Strengths:** Sarah is very bright, imaginative and creative. She is thoughtful and insightful and has ambition. She can be assertive and hold strong opinions.

Cognitive-behavioural programme

Sarah agreed to a trial of four initial sessions of CBT. The initial two sessions aimed to engage Sarah in individual therapy, identify a list of goals and teach self-monitoring. It was important to outline the boundaries of confidentiality, and for Sarah to share with her mum the severity of her desperation and her wishes for change. Sarah came to sessions alone up to the review held with her mum after four sessions had been completed. Sarah identified the following goals of therapy: 'to feel less depressed', 'to go back to school' and 'to be less sensitive'. Emotional recognition was a helpful start to detecting negative automatic thoughts, assumptions and core beliefs. Sarah readily completed diary exercises and engaged well in collaborative working. There was an early improvement in her moods; however, Sarah resisted focusing on her inactivity and her relationship with her mother. At the review meeting, Sarah's mum was negative and critical of Sarah, and rather hostile to the therapist. It was important to reflect on the limitations of individual therapy in isolation for Sarah. Planning the next phase in treatment included building in joint meetings for Sarah and her mum at the end of Sarah's sessions and focus on activity scheduling and returning to school. The role of Sarah's father was discussed and the need for Sarah's mum to have psychological help independently. With renewed contact with school the next phase of treatment included social problem-solving and behavioural techniques focused on anxiety management as well as ongoing cognitive work. Sarah had found her individual time with the therapist very helpful and was clearly emotionally needy. Ending therapy was difficult and the sessions continued for sometime after her return to school. Sarah continued to experience mood swings and setbacks, however she seemed able to learn from experience and grew in confidence. She stopped attending sessions regularly when she 'fell in love'. Her acute treatment took place over approximately 12 weekly sessions.

OTHER CLINICAL APPLICATIONS

Obsessive-compulsive disorder

CBT is considered the treatment of choice for adults with obsessive-compulsive disorder (Salkovskis, 1996); however, work in adolescents has been hampered by the lack of clear cognitive theories for the maintenance and development of obsessive-compulsive disorder in the young, and there is no clear definition of the cognitive component of treatment (Shafran, 1998). There have been no systematically controlled treatment trials to date. March (1995) conducted a review of 32 articles describing treatment of obsessive-compulsive disorder. In conclusion, March states that CBT alone or in combination with pharmacotherapy is an effective treatment for obsessive-compulsive disorder in children and adolescents.

Post-traumatic stress disorders

Young people who have been exposed to extreme stressors manifest a range of reactions including anxiety, fears and depression as well as post-traumatic stress disorders. Cognitive approaches use imaginal and *in vivo* exposure techniques within a safe therapeutic environment to allow adequate emotional processing of traumatic memories (Smith *et al.*, 1998). The cognitive, behavioural and social problem-solving techniques described are applied according to a problem-oriented treatment plan.

Eating disorders

Cognitive models for both anorexia nervosa and bulimia nervosa have been described. The cognitive-behavioural model of bulimia nervosa has been translated into a CBT programme which has been the subject of much research in adults (Fairburn *et al.*, 1986, 1993). This has been shown to be highly effective. The treatment of eating disorders is fully discussed in Chapter 9.

Other disorders

Over the course of this chapter, I have emphasised the growing application of CBT for other adolescent mental health disorders and I have referred to several of the many text books describing these in more detail. The cognitive therapeutic relationship is effective in working with adolescents with a variety of problems, the reader is referred to these texts for further details.

SUMMARY AND CONCLUSIONS

- There is a wide diversity of techniques considered to be components of CBT. Core procedures aim to alter distorted thought processes.
- Cognitive models exist for many adolescent psychiatric disorders, the most coherent of which are those for depressive and anxiety disorders, bulimia nervosa, post-traumatic stress disorder, and obsessive compulsive disorder.
- As yet there is little evidence in favour of CBT in comparison with other interventions for most adolescent psychiatric disorders. The exception is clinical depression.

- CBT is most likely to be effective when it forms one component of multimodal therapy programme. The degree to which the therapist can work cooperatively within a multiprofessional team is likely to be an important predictor of positive outcome.
- The cognitive-behavioural assessment and formulation is a crucial part of the treatment process, and a key task in introducing CBT to a young person is engaging them in collaborative working.
- Designing a treatment programme should offer a flexible needs-oriented individual approach. Progress should be regularly reviewed and determine future treatment.
- Cognitive and behavioural approaches add significantly to the range of treatments available to mental health professionals working with adolescents. Clinical supervision and adequate training are essential.

REFERENCES

Beck, A. T. (1967) *Depression: Clinical, Experimental and Theoretical Aspects.* New York: Harper & Row.

Beck, A. T., Rush, A. J., Shaw, B. F. and Emery, G. (1979) *Cognitive Therapy of Depression.* New York: Guilford Press.

Blackburn, I. and Davidson, K. (1995) *Cognitive Therapy for Depression the Anxiety: A Practitioner's Guide.* Oxford: Blackwell.

Brent, D., Holder, D., Kolko, D., Birmaher, B., Baugher, M., Roth, C., *et al.* (1997) A clinical psychotherapy trial for adolescent depression comparing cognitive family and supportive treatments. *Archives of General Psychiatry,* **54**, 877–885.

Burns, D. (1980) *Feeling Good: The New Mood Therapy.* New York: Signet.

Ellis, A. (1962) *Reason the Emotion in Psychotherapy.* New York: Lyle Stuart.

Fairburn, C. G., Kirk, J., O'Connor, M. and Cooper, P. J. (1986) A comparison of two psychological treatments for bulimia nervosa. *Behaviour Research and Therapy,* **24**, 629–643.

Fairburn, C. G., Marcus, M. D. and Wilson, G. T. (1993) Cognitive behavioural therapy for binge eating and bulimia nervosa: a comprehensive treatment manual. In C. G. Fairburn and G. T. Wilson (eds), *Binge Eating: Nature Assessment the Treatment.* New York: Guilford Press.

Graham, P. (ed.) (1998) *Cognitive-Behaviour Therapy for Children and Families.* Cambridge: Cambridge University Press.

Greenberger, D. and Padesky, C. A. (1995) *Mind over Mood: A Cognitive Therapy Treatment Manual for Clients.* New York: Guilford Press.

Harrington, R. C., Whittaker, J., Shoebridge, P. and Campbell, F. (1998) Systematic review of efficacy of cognitive behaviour therapies in childhood and adolescent depressive disorder. *British Medical Journal,* **316**, 1559–1563

Hawton, K., Salkovskis, P. M., Kirk, J. and Clark, D. M. (eds) (1992) *Cognitive Behaviour Therapy for Psychiatric Problems: A Practical Guide.* Oxford: Oxford University Press.

Kirk, J. (1992) Cognitive-behavioural assessment. In K. Hawton, P. M. Salkovskis, J. Kirk and D. M. Clark (eds), *Cognitive Behaviour Therapy for Psychiatric Problems; A Practical Guide.* Oxford: Oxford University Press, pp. 13–51.

Lewinsohn, P., Clarke, G. N., Rowhde, P., Hops, H. and Seeley, J. (1997) A course in coping: a cognitive-behavioural approach to treatment of adolescent depression. In E. D. Hibbs and P. S. Jensen (eds), *Psychosocial Treatments for Child and Adolescent Disorders.* Washington, DC: American Psychiatric Association, pp. 109–135.

Lewinsohn, P. M., Clarke, G. N. and Andrews, J. (1990) Cognitive-behavioural treatment for depressed adolescents *Behaviour Therapy*, **21**, 385–401.

March, J. S. (1995) Cognitive-behavioural psychotherapy in children and adolescents with OCD: a review and recommendations for treatment. *Journal of the American Academy of Child and Adolescent Psychiatry*, **34**, 7–18.

Meichenbaum, D. H. (1975) Self-instructional methods. In F. H. Kanfer and A. P. Goldstein (eds), *Helping People Change: A Textbook of Methods.* New York: Pergamon, pp. 357–391.

Meyer, V. (1966) Modification of expectation of cases with obsessional rituals. *Behaviour Research and Therapy*, **4**, 273–280.

Mufson, L., Moreau, D., Weissman, M. M. and Klerman, G. L. (1993) *Interpersonal Psychotherapy for Depressed Adolescents.* New York: Guilford Press.

Reed, M. K. (1994) Social skills training to reduce depression in adolescence. *Adolescence*, **29**, 293– 302.

Reinecke, M. A., Dattilio, F. M. and Freeman, A. (1996) General issues. In M. A. Reinecke, F. M. Dattilio and A. Freeman (eds), *Cognitive Therapy with Children and Adolescents: A Casebook for Clinical Practice.* New York: Guilford Press, pp. 1–9.

Reinecke, M. A., Dattilio, F. M. and Freeman, A. (eds) (1996) *Cognitive Therapy with Children and Adolescents: A Casebook for Clinical Practice.* New York: Guilford Press.

Salkovskis, P. M. and Kirk, J. (1992) Obsessional disorders. In K. Hawton, P. M. Salkovskis, J. Kirk and D. M. Clark (eds), *Cognitive Behaviour Therapy for Psychiatric Problems: A Practical Guide.* Oxford: Oxford University Press, pp. 129–168.

Salkovskis, P. M. (1996) Cognitive behavioural approaches to the understanding of obsessional problems. In R. Rappee (ed.), *Current Controversies in Anxiety Disorders.* New York: Guilford Press.

Shafran, R. (1998) Childhood obsessive compulsive disorder. In P. Graham (ed.), *Cognitive-Behavioural Therapy for Children and Families.* Cambridge: Cambridge University Press, pp. 45–67.

Smith, P., Perrin, S. and Yule, W. (1998) Post-traumatic stress disorders. In P. Graham (ed.), *Cognitive-Behavioural Therapy for Children and Families.* Cambridge: Cambridge University Press, pp. 127–140.

Spence, S. H. and Donovan, C. (1998) Interpersonal problems. In P. Graham (ed.), *Cognitive-Behavioural Therapy for Children and Families.* Cambridge: Cambridge University Press, pp. 217–243.

Stark, K. D. (1990) *Childhood Depression: A School-based Intervention.* New York: Guilford Press.

Vostanis, P., Feehan, C., Grattan, E. and Bickerton, W. (1996) Treatment for children and adolescents with depression: lessons from a controlled trial. *Clinical Child Psychology and Psychiatry,* 1, 199–212.

Wilkes, T. C. R., Belsher, G., Rush, A. J. and Frank, E. (1994) *Cognitive Therapy for Depressed Adolescents.* New York: Guilford Press.

Wood, A. J., Harrington, R. C. and Verduyn, C. (1997) Cognitive behavioural therapy for depressed adolescents. *Training video.* University of Manchester.

Wood, A. J., Harrington, R. C. and Moore, A. (1996) A controlled trial of a brief cognitive-behavioural intervention in adolescent patients with depressive disorders. *Journal of Child Psychology and Psychiatry,* 37, 737–746.

Zarb, J. M. (1992) *Cognitive-behavioural Assessment and Therapy with Adolescents.* New York: Brunner/Mazel.

Chapter 20

INDIVIDUAL AND GROUP THERAPY

Andrew Weaver

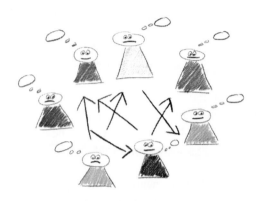

THERAPY WITH ADOLESCENTS – GENERAL ISSUES

In any interaction between a person seeking therapy and the professional providing that help there can be initial tensions, anxieties and discomfort until trust develops. In an adolescent these issues can be complicated by, for example, the fact that the youngster has probably not been the instigator of the help-seeking process. A teenager may have unspoken concerns about being seen by a psychiatrist, may have fears about being perceived as 'mad' or may view the therapist as representing aspects of authority figures from their daily life (Copley and Forryan, 1987).

A 15-year-old boy with behavioural problems was referred to a mental health service by his head teacher. During the initial session he remained sullen and withdrawn until it was explained that the psychiatrist seeing him was not working for the education department. Once he realised that the mental health team was not involved in discussions about excluding him from school he became much more spontaneous.

The process of engaging an adolescent in accepting individual help can therefore often take some time, perhaps a number of sessions, before sufficient trust is established. Professionals working with teenagers for the first time in their careers are often challenged by this process. It is natural to react by over zealous attempts to appear friendly and acceptable to the client, but teenagers usually have a knack of seeing through displays of false interest in teenage culture. In fact those aspects of therapist qualities such as genuineness and accurate empathy which underpin all successful approaches are more effective in promoting engagement.

Occasionally an adolescent may invest the potential therapist with an almost magical quality as if all their problems will be solved by the professional trying to help them or indeed the opposite process, denigration, can occur where the youngster's anger is projected onto the worker.

Silences during therapy sessions are not uncommon in adolescents. There is a natural tendency to fill such gaps by repeated questions but silences can be useful in giving clues about potential emotions, such as fear or anger, that the youngster may be feeling (Copley and Forryan, 1987).

One of the tasks of adolescence is to successfully negotiate the separation–individuation process, i.e. that of moving from a dependent to an independent, autonomous individual. The transition is unlikely to follow a smooth gradient, and progressions and regressions are par for the course. Equally, psychological development does not necessarily follow hand in hand with physical or social progress. An adolescent presenting for therapy is likely therefore to be something of a *pot-pourri* of various developmental stages. A therapist working with teenagers needs to hold this in mind. Flexibility is required. One youngster might respond to a verbal approach, whereas with another conversation may be unrewarding necessitating the use of art or drama.

'Control' is often a major factor related to psychiatric problems in adolescence. Disorders such as anorexia nervosa, bulimia, obsessive-compulsive disorder and oppositional defiance often have a fight for control as a central issue. In many of these cases it will be the parents, care givers or teachers who will be dictating the need for therapy. Tension can arise particularly where the therapist accepts that therapy is likely to be helpful but is faced with an adolescent who is unwilling to accept it as this would be akin to 'giving in' to the parents, thereby losing control. It is here that the process of engagement is particularly crucial. Successful therapy cannot be prescribed or 'done' to the person; in fact is likely that, whatever approach is utilised, a positive outcome will be directly related to effective engagement of the person in treatment. Green (1996) discusses this concept of the therapeutic alliance in a study of child psychiatry outpatients. He found that engagement in treatment explained more of the variance in outcome than any other variable. Crisp (1980) refers to a kindling process which enables a person with anorexia to take a risk about getting better. Indeed recovery from many emotional disorders involves taking a chance that giving up the symptom (and the comfort it somehow provides) is worth the risk. In engaging adolescents it is useful to assume that, whatever the symptom, the youngster is ambivalent about having that symptom or problem. A teenager with an eating disorder, whilst terrified of weight gain, is likely to be miserable about the effect the problem is having on daily life. Similarly an adolescent with a conduct disorder may be upset and angry about the negative consequences at home and school or fearful about what he sees as an inevitable progression to criminality and prison. An early discussion about the youngster's aspirations and expectations for the future may shed light on this. If the teenager agrees to come for sessions because it will please their parents or 'get the teachers off their back', it is unlikely to be very effective. Major progress often occurs when the adolescent, having been encouraged to recover for themselves and no-one else, actually begins to accept this notion.

Since the majority of teenagers receiving therapy will have parents or carers responsible for them it is important to ensure that the sessions are supported. In practice this means that one will have to check that the carers are in favour of the sessions, that they receive some feedback about important issues and that regular reviews are organised. Confidentiality issues are obviously relevant but it is equally important to be aware of the mechanism of 'splitting' which can sometimes occur; in this a therapist may find himself in competition with a parent due to processes relating to idealisation and denigration. Regular sessions for parents, or at least an opportunity for them to air their own views, will reduce the likelihood of the therapy being threatened by splitting.

The process of bringing therapy to an end is often an important one. It may be that the sessions reach a conclusion because of factors outside of the youngster's control, e.g. the therapist may leave or parents may decide that they are opposed to further work. However, if the ending of therapy can be predicted well in advance, and the adolescent and therapist can work towards it, then this in itself can be valuable therapeutically (Copley and Forryan, 1987).

INDIVIDUAL THERAPY – THE DEVELOPMENT OF 'TALKING TREATMENTS'

Individual therapy developed from the work of Freud (1909) with differing schools of psychotherapy evolving throughout the 20th century. Theories and treatments proposed by pioneers such as Klein (1932), Winnicott (1958) and Axline (1947, 1964) led to the adaptation of individual approaches for children. Child guidance clinics, originating in North America, were founded in the UK in the 1920s; the standard approach in such clinics became parenting work coupled with individual therapy for the child. Counselling, as originally described by Rogers (1951), was increasingly seen as relevant to the treatment of older children, particularly those with good verbal skills. Other influences such as cognitive-behavioural theory and solution-focused approaches have added to the plethora of influences on child mental health, and are described elsewhere in this book. In general, the indications for individual therapy are quite broad; most emotional disorders can benefit, e.g. depression, anxiety or phobias. In some cases of behavioural disorder, the emotional aspects can respond to individual interventions. Youngsters should be motivated enough, have relatively intact cognitions and be in a placement that is able to support the intervention.

INDIVIDUAL PSYCHODYNAMIC PSYCHOTHERAPY

The main focus of the psychodynamic therapist is on the client's internal experiences and their perception of reality. Although awareness of the external stresses, losses or life events are important factors in informing the therapist's thinking, the main concern once the therapy starts is how these external factors impinge on the internal reality of the client. There are a number of important principles which form the basis of effective psychodynamic work. The setting of the therapy is viewed as crucial. It is thought important to see the client at the same time each week, in the same place and, if relevant, with the same materials. By establishing such predictable, firm boundaries around the client a therapeutic space can develop for anxieties to be explored and expressed. In particular, the therapy aims to create a space within the mind of the therapist wherein the client's anxieties can be held (Daws and Boston, 1988). This process is referred to as containment and is crucial to the therapy. It is important that one of the goals of such work is to help teenagers begin to own both positive and negative feelings again for themselves i.e. to gradually take responsibility for them.

A 13-year-old girl recovering from anorexia nervosa would constantly complain about her parents, blaming them for any slip ups in her weight gain by their failure in providing suitable meals. She also tended to assign the cause of any other conflicts on to external agencies such as her parents, siblings or teachers. After a series of sessions in which she had had the experience of becoming irritable with the therapist but having this contained and explored, she began to take more responsibility for her own actions and recognised the part she often played in conflicts.

It is assumed that the client often lacks insight into his feelings and behaviour or in some cases may only have an intellectual understanding of them rather than an emotional one. The therapist endeavours to help the client with this 'block' by offering interpretations. These are spoken hypotheses about possible conflicts or defences. Two related issues of importance in such work are the 'transference' which explains how the client re-experiences the emotional aspects of his difficulties within the room and the 'counter-transference' which refers to feelings engendered within the therapist.

Brief therapy

Brief therapy (De Shazer, 1988) can often be useful for adolescents. In essence the approach aims to help the client by using a solution-focused interview. There is minimal discussion of problems, exceptions to the difficulties are sought and goals are set. 'Scaling' questions, in which clients are asked to evaluate their progress towards specified targets on a scale of 0–10, are fundamental to the approach.

Interpersonal psychotherapy

Interpersonal psychotherapy (IPT) was originally developed for use with depressed adults (Klerman *et al.*, 1984). Moreau *et al.* (1991) adapted it for adolescents whilst still proposing that its main use was in depression. The basis of the approach is on helping the person tackle the problem areas that are either a cause, or a consequence of, the current symptoms. Moreau argued that, as teenagers were often characterised by their tendency to drop out of therapy, they would find the brief nature of IPT attractive. Whereas psychodynamic therapy looks at the inner world, IPT addresses current problems such as disputes with parents, sexual relationships, peer problems and adolescent identity. It is not suitable for psychotic or suicidal adolescents or those with severe antisocial disorders. The therapy format is that an initial engagement is established during which the main problems are identified and the rationale for treatment explained. Following this the therapist endeavours to help the youngster learn to link their depressive symptoms with the problems listed. Techniques such as education and clarification are followed by approaches aimed at improving social skills (Scott, 1995).

COUNSELLING

The term 'counselling' can have a number of meanings. Rogers (1951) described client-centred counselling as a way of helping a person re-organise their subjective view of the world. The aim, he thought, was to encourage the person to become more spontaneous, independent and confident. The skills required from a counsellor included genuineness, empathic understanding and an unconditional positive regard for the client. Many child and adolescent mental health service (CAMHS) teams offer individual counselling to the adolescents who attend. Practice varies but most counselling in such services contains elements from a number of theoretical schools with a mix of cognitive, supportive and psychodynamic aspects. Supportive therapy is often an important component of successful interventions with adolescents in primary care. Professionals such as teachers, GPs or school nurses can be helpful in cases of milder severity by listening and offering advice. The primary care professional can also play a part in bridging the gap between services by, for example, continuing to support the youngster awaiting an appointment at a child psychiatry service.

There are several components of supportive therapy or counselling as often practised in mental health clinics. One aspect involves helping the youngster develop an understanding about the difficulties. If successful, this enables the adolescent to feel less helpless and ultimately more in control of their feelings, whereas previously they may have felt like the problems were controlling *them*. The therapist qualities referred to earlier, as originally described by Rogers, allow the development of a relationship which encourages the person to discover their own solutions. Sometimes it can be useful to incorporate psychodynamic theories into supportive work. In effect this means that the therapist, having an understanding about defence mechanisms and the relationship between past conflicts and current symptoms, uses this knowledge to understand his client more fully. However, interpretations or more in-depth analysis will not be offered. Equally, being aware of transference or counter-transference issues is important whatever form of therapy is used. Andrews (1993), writing about 'psycho-therapies' in adult mental health, refers to the importance of providing 'good clinical care'. Many of the aspects of this are equally relevant to adolescent therapy, and include establishing a relationship, being professional and enthu-siastic about the treatment offered, understanding the many elements under-pinning the therapeutic relationship and providing general care and support until the disorder resolves.

CREATIVE THERAPIES

The term creative therapy refers to the utilisation of media such as play, art or music to help people with psychological difficulties. At the forefront of the development of such therapies was the increasing interest in 'play' as a therapeutic tool.

Schiller, in 1875, wrote that play is the 'aimless expenditure of exuberant energy'.

However, the use of play as a form of therapy was developed by Axline (1947, 1964) whose books *Dibs in Search of Self* and *Play Therapy* are well known. Whereas psychoanalytical theorists such as Anna Freud (1926/27) and Melanie Klein (1932) tended to see the child's play as a way of accessing other parts of the person, in particular the unconscious conflicts, Axline thought that the play *itself* was a healing process. She proposed eight basic principles which she considered necessary in play therapy and they also apply to creative therapies in general:

• The development of good rapport
• Accepting the child as they are
• Allowing the child to express their feelings
• Being alert to the feelings that the child is expressing and reflecting them
• Believing that the child has the potential to solve their own problems

- Not directing the play
- Not hurrying the child
- Having safe limits around the therapy, thereby anchoring it to reality

Play therapy is one of the 'non-verbal' approaches often recommended for younger children but it can also be useful in certain circumstances with adolescents. Whilst a teenager would be unlikely to be over keen on a blunt offer of 'play therapy', it can sometimes be interesting to see how even older children enjoy the freedom of expression that sand or water play can give. In other situations of course, such as a child whose emotional development is impaired, the use of play therapy may be very appropriate.

A 13-year-old girl with a reactive attachment disorder following neglect, abuse and multiple care placements was referred to the child and adolescent mental health service. As she was now in a stable foster placement it was felt that individual sessions would be potentially helpful as she had a range of emotional symptoms which her carers were finding hard to understand and manage. Following the initial assessment it was evident that she found one to one conversation difficult but she showed great interest in the play room. Further sessions were arranged in the play room in which she gradually began to illustrate many of the conflicts in her life. Later, her play re-enacted themes of rejection, hurt and loss.

The aim of art therapy is to help the person deal with inner conflicts which are too difficult to express verbally. It particularly aims to foster the development of 'personal growth'. Harmony between the inner and outer worlds is a goal (Simon, 1992). It is an approach which can often be valuable in group settings such as on adolescent units.

Art therapy was offered to a 15-year-old boy, N, whose father had been imprisoned for the murder of the boy's mother. Although he engaged well in the sessions, N initially produced rather superficial paintings and denied feelings of anger towards his father. He also tended to project such feelings on to other relatives blaming them for his current situation. Eventually he produced a piece of work containing an image of his father behind bars which the therapist interpreted as analogous to N's experience of feeling trapped by his conflicts. This marked a turning point in the therapy and further sessions were used productively.

Music therapy is not widely available in child mental health clinics but can be a valuable tool in assisting youngsters. Teenagers generally enjoy music or at least have a view about it and there are benefits to be gained from adolescents creating music together. The group production of music, with the help of a therapist, is a powerful experience containing elements of creativity, socialising and working together.

GROUP THERAPY

Human beings are social animals and have always seen the value and strength of groups. The powerful effect of being part of a group which has an emotional issue in common is often described in the popular press. The term 'shared national experience' has recently been used in England as a recognition of this 'group effect' (e.g. following the death of Princess Diana). One of the first descriptions of a group process in the management of ill health was in the early part of this century when classes of patients with tuberculosis were seen for weekly meetings with the aim being to provide mutual support and instruction (Pratt, 1907). The term group therapy was first used by Moreno in 1920. In England, following World War II, two people were influential in the further development of group therapy. Bion (1961) wrote about experiential groups in military hospitals. He believed that the psychodynamic processes of projection and transference were just as relevant to group therapy as they were in individual analysis. He advocated a disciplined group but with an understanding leader. Foulkes (1964), who worked at the Institute of Group Analysis, considered that problems did not necessarily reside within individuals but in their network of relationships. He held that the group needed to be group-centred as opposed to leader-centred and was in favour of a focus on present difficulties.

Groups can be closed or open. In closed groups a set number of participants is established and the group remains intact from first session to the last. Open groups allow new members to join at later stages. When using a psychodynamic approach to group therapy with adolescents, a number of aims will be present. Evans (1998) suggests that the aims for the individual should be: the achievement of age-appropriate tasks (the development of an adult 'identity', acquiring a level of independence appropriate for their age and culture, coming to terms with sexual drives, and making effective use of their aggressive drives), improved object relations, improved defences and coping strategies, improved capacity to tolerate anxiety and frustration, improved reality testing, removal of fixations, and the recovery of repressed memories. The therapist should also have aims for the group. These include developing a group cohesion, ensuring that the group works on its problems, setting appropriate limits for behaviour and providing space for the development of individual identities (Evans 1998).

Educative groups are usually based on cognitive-behavioural principles. Examples include groups aimed at addressing problems such as social skills deficits or shared experiences (such as child sexual abuse survivor groups). These are described in more detail later.

PSYCHODRAMA

Psychodrama is a therapeutic approach which often lends itself to group work. For example, a lead group member or 'primary actor' might dramatise a particular conflict or difficulty in the group. This sets the scene and other group members might be co-opted to play subsidiary roles. The leader might encourage the main 'actor' to then take on another role. The therapist acts as a director and has the potential to influence the proceedings. Feelings are explored and shared and resolution is sought by acting out a different ending. The overall aim is for feelings and conflicts to be shared in a supportive forum, allowing the person (or persons) to experience alternative outcomes to their chosen conflict and ultimately to gain mastery over their difficulties (Johnson, 1982).

ISSUES RELEVANT TO ADOLESCENCE IN GROUP THERAPY

The use of group therapy can have particular advantages when considering the treatment of adolescents. Firstly, given that many teenagers will be initially reluctant to participate in therapy and may feel stigmatised by being in receipt of mental health input, taking part in a group may reduce some of their concerns. By meeting regularly with other youngsters who perhaps have the same disorder or problems a sense of 'belonging' can develop. It is often the case in clinical practice that an adolescent with a particular problem, e.g. obsessive-compulsive disorder, might think that they are the only one suffering from this ailment. Whilst mental health professionals can assure the youngster that this is not the case it may only be by actually meeting with similarly afflicted teenagers that the assertion is believed.

Secondly, groups can be a time efficient way of delivering health care to where it is needed. By developing and running a group in a school for instance a number of youngsters will be able to receive help whereas to see the same number of clients for individual work would take up a large proportion of a mental health service's time. However, it is also worth noting that planning, executing and reviewing therapy can also be a time consuming process. Thirdly, for teenagers who find the individual therapy approach too threatening, particularly if they are shy or anxious, a group setting can offer support and structure. Fourthly, the group process can often provide opportunities for clients to learn from each other. In an open group, for example, newer members can be supported by more experienced participants and, in time, develop the confidence to act in a similar fashion with future members. The environment also provides opportunities for modelling of social skills. Fifthly, the same mechanisms which occur in individual therapy such as projection can occur in the group setting; this can be useful in helping the participants not only understand the other members but also learn more about their own fears and conflicts.

These ideas are elaborated by Reid and Kolvin (1993) in an excellent review of the topic.

GROUPS FOR SURVIVORS OF DISASTERS

Yule and Williams (1992) have described their work with children and parents who survived a ferry sinking. A number of interventions were utilised, including groups for the children and adolescents involved. The groups met on a monthly basis and continued for up to 3 years. The authors comment that the therapeutic elements included helping the youngsters identify the problems they were struggling to understand and gradually assisting them in realising that most of their emotional reactions were normal, given the enormity of the stressor. In particular, the value for the children in sharing these feelings with others who had had the same experience was an important component. There was also a problem-solving aspect to the group process. Yule and Williams also stress the importance of parallel parents' groups which, amongst other strengths, had a role in helping the adults discuss how best they could assist their children.

There are differing views on the need for such interventions in the immediate aftermath of a disaster. Yule and Williams (1992) comment that such interventions need to be thought out carefully rather than applied indiscriminately. These and other approaches in primary care settings are discussed elsewhere in this book.

GROUPS FOR YOUNG PEOPLE WHO HAVE EXPERIENCED SEXUAL ABUSE

When children have experienced sexual abuse they may develop numerous fears as a consequence of that abuse. Anxieties about being 'different' from peers or feelings of being stigmatised in other ways can occur. One advantage of a group approach to survivors of abuse is that the youngsters encounter similarly affected peers and can be reassured that they appear 'normal' (Glaser 1992). Groups can be structured or unstructured, open or closed. Glaser (1992) suggests a number of important areas to consider when setting up sexual abuse survivor groups for young people. These include the importance of establishing a common language for the group when discussing aspects of anatomy, abuse and sexuality, and developing a way of discussing the experiences that the group feel comfortable with.

Evans (1998), writing about sexual abuse survivor groups, mentions the potential difficulty in recruiting youngsters. The issue of whether to accept only those where there is firm evidence of abuse or include those cases where there was less certainty is discussed. He points out that, as group therapists, his team were faced with three potential errors: non-selection of an abused case, automatically accepting memories of abuse as a reality and selecting case who were claiming abuse as a means of obtaining attention. Evans concludes that they decided to live with these uncertainties and youngsters were accepted into the group if they had claimed that they had been abused.

GROUPS FOR OFFENDERS

These may be set up for adolescents who commit major offences, e.g. sexual abuse. Key issues underling the use of such an intervention are that the adolescent is 'accountable' for what they did and the approach is specific to their particular offence (e.g. sexual abuse) rather than being more generalized. Work with a supportive peer group is carried out on stages of the cycle of offending. In abuse this will consist of identification, sharing and discussion of various stages from contemplation, committing the offence and subsequent feelings of guilt. Additional aspects such as education, raising awareness of victims' responses and strategies to help prevent re-offending are also incorporated (Bentovim et al., 1991).

SOCIAL SKILLS TRAINING GROUPS

Given that the acquisition of social skills necessarily involves the use of those skills in interactions with others, a group approach in helping youngsters with deficits in this area is intuitively appealing. There is an opportunity to develop confidence in relating with others by being in an environment which is supportive and non-threatening (as all the members of the group will be sharing similar anxieties). Schools or adolescent units are often suitable settings for such work.

Sessions usually take the from of an introductory activity which allows members to settle in. The group leaders will then outline the concept that the session will be focusing on, e.g. asking for an item in a shop. Role-plays are often then utilised to illustrate the skills required. Common topics which adolescents bring as themes include assertiveness, friendships, bullying and relationships with the opposite sex. The therapeutic components involve discussion of the topic, some didactic elements but, more importantly, role-play and modelling (Bulkeley and Cramer, 1994).

EVALUATION OF THERAPEUTIC APPROACHES

The critical evaluation of the effectiveness of therapies is bedevilled with stumbling blocks (Callias, 1992; Trowell, 1994). Some of these are worth discussing here. When a condition has an easily measurable outcome (such as a pathological test) evaluation is much easier. In mental health the measurement tools are more blunt and vague. A number of difficulties arise: firstly it is not always clear what a good outcome is. Weight gain in an anorexic would be generally deemed to be a sign of progress but the parents may consider the outcome unfavourable if the adolescent began to test limits more frequently as a result of her increased confidence. Measures of outcome are often needed from a variety of sources – adolescent, parents, referrers, etc. An equally difficult issue is when to measure the outcome. Many disorders in adolescent psychiatry have relapsing, remitting courses or may spontaneously improve. There are other factors complicating attempts to evaluate therapies in mental health such as ethical considerations (what should be offered to untreated controls?), the problem of co-morbidity (in that many disorders in childhood have associated problems) and the fact that drop-outs from treatment studies may receive help elsewhere.

Finally, there are added difficulties when evaluating approaches such as psychodynamic psychotherapy and non-verbal treatments. It is difficult to standardise such treatments so that there is uniformity of therapist style. The very nature of the approaches does not always lend itself to the use of treatment manuals as in cognitive therapy and the 'turning points' in the therapy are often hard to quantify, e.g. a 13-year-old boy with a mixture of depression, obsessive symptoms and anxiety made great progress after he had become very frustrated and irritable during the sessions. The cause of this frustration was that the therapist would not persuade his mother to buy him a new pet dog. During further sessions it was apparent that he had feared that this outburst would somehow 'destroy' the therapist but on realising that his feelings were not capable of causing such devastation began to feel confident in tackling his own fears. This moment would have been impossible to set up at the start of the treatment but was probably crucial in his progress.

Factors relating to the therapist who conducts the treatment are also relevant when considering outcomes. Patient attitudes, their belief in the approach, the level of skill of the therapist and their adherence to the treatment model are all thought to influence the outcome to some extent (Scott, 1995).

Weisz et al. (1995a), writing about the disparity between experimental study outcomes and those found in clinic studies, suggest that clinic procedures may well need to be altered so as to include more focused, structured approaches. Evaluation in practical terms may then be more easily achieved.

GENERAL REVIEWS AND OVERLAP WITH ADULT STUDIES

Early research was disappointing in its conclusions: in the late 1950s Levitt (1957, 1963) published two studies which cast doubt on the efficacy of treatment in child mental health. His results were that although 78% of youngsters receiving therapy improved, 72.5% got better without treatment. His conclusions filtered into the consciousness of professionals in this field such that new recruits to the speciality were often advised 'no matter what you do about two-thirds will improve'. A more critical appraisal of Levitt's work, however, reveals that his methodology was poor and many of the untreated group were in fact 'defectors' from therapy as opposed to controls. Nevertheless his work was relevant in that it emphasized the importance of always asking oneself 'what will happen if I do nothing?'. Another rule of thumb in the 1960s was that, whereas conduct disorders were expected to run a depressing course into adult delinquency and sociopathy, childhood emotional disorders were thought to have a benign prognosis (Robins, 1966). Recent research has shown this belief to be erroneous. We now know that emotional disorders in childhood and adolescence can run a relapsing course into adult life (Cantwell and Baker, 1989; Flament et al., 1990; Harrington 1993).

Tramontana (1980) reviewed 33 studies of therapies offered to adolescents, i.e. individual, family or group treatments. In only five of these articles did he decide that the methodology was sufficiently sound to allow robust conclusions to be drawn. The overall finding was that treatment produced a good outcome in about two-thirds, whereas only 40% of controls improved. Weisz et al. (1995b) conducted a meta-analysis of 150 studies looking at treatment in child and adolescent disorders. The overall mean effect of therapy was positive and significant. A broad definition of psychotherapy was employed such that the study included a heterogeneous sample of approaches. They found that more positive effects were found with behavioural approaches as opposed to non-behavioural, although improvements occurred generally with all forms of therapy. Professionals (as opposed to paraprofessionals or students) were more effective in treating problems such as anxiety or depression and, of relevance to this review, adolescent girls had better outcomes than other samples grouped by age or gender. Shirk and Russell (1992) offer one explanation as to why there have been fewer studies of psychodynamic approaches as compared to behavioural treatments. They discovered that, in many cases, the non-behavioural treatment had been carried out by a researcher who actually favoured the use of behavioural approaches in clinical practice! In addition, many studies had measured outcome at quite an early stage in treatment whilst many theorists of psychodynamic approaches emphasize the need for relatively lengthy treatment.

There have been some studies, which although aimed at addressing problems within adult mental health, have concerned disorders which overlap with adolescent psychiatry. In one such study, Crisp et al. (1991) compared several therapeutic approaches for 90 patients with anorexia nervosa. All the patients were female and, in most cases, the disorder had commenced in adolescence. Patients were randomly allocated to one of three treatment groups (inpatient treatment, outpatient individual and family psychotherapy or outpatient group psychotherapy). Dietary counselling was also offered to both outpatient groups. A fourth group was offered no treatment. One year after treatment all three treatment groups had been highly effective in promoting weight gain, return of menstruation and social adjustment as compared to the non-treatment (control) group. This study, whilst acknowledging some methodological difficulties, was well designed and evaluated. It is of relevance to the discussion of adolescent disorders as anorexia nervosa is a condition which usually starts in adolescence or, if occurring in adult life, is often related to the same developmental issues which teenagers encounter.

RESEARCH INTO INDIVIDUAL PSYCHOTHERAPY

PSYCHODYNAMIC APPROACHES

In 1991, Lush *et al.* compared 35 children and adolescents (aged 2–18) who received psychodynamic psychotherapy with 13 youngsters for whom the same treatment had been offered but 'didn't happen'. All the cases were either fostered or adopted. The clients were seen weekly for about 1 year in most cases. Twenty cases were available for evaluation at the end of the study. Ratings of outcome were derived from canvassing the views of parent, clinician and external professional. Their results were that of these 20 cases, 16 made good progress. Of seven cases who did not receive treatment, none improved. Perhaps the most important finding was that the improvement also reflected inner change within the child. Their encouraging results contrast with those of Weisz and Weiss (1989) who, comparing 93 youngsters receiving at least five sessions of individual therapy with 60 'drop outs' after an initial assessment, found no difference in outcome between the groups.

Target and Fonagy (1996) have conducted a series of chart reviews looking at therapy with over 700 children and adolescents at the Anna Freud Centre, England. In many cases the interventions were intensive, e.g. up to five times per week lasting up to 2 years. The findings of relevance to this review were that younger children generally responded more favourably than adolescents. However it is of interest to note that 69% of children with disruptive disorders responded to psychotherapy and that youngsters who had more frequent sessions (four to five times per week) did better than those who were seen once a week. There are problems with the research in that it is retrospective and, particularly in the case of emotional disorders, we do not know whether the same results would have occurred without treatment. One might reasonably assume that, as the average length of an episode of depression in an adolescent is 9 months (Kovacs, 1997), most of the depressed cases treated would have undergone spontaneous remission during the 2-year treatment programme. Despite these criticisms it is worth commending the study as being one of the few attempts to evaluate psychodynamic therapy in youngsters.

Tibbetts and Stone (1990) compared 10 'seriously emotionally disturbed' adolescents who received art therapy with 10 similar youngsters who were given weekly, non-therapeutic 'socialisation' sessions. Clients were randomly allocated to one of the two groups, sessions were weekly and lasted for 6 weeks. Ratings, before and after the input, were obtained from the youngsters' teacher and from a counsellor from another district. The authors found that the art therapy had a significant impact on the emotional growth and development of the youngsters who received it. However, the sample sizes were small and the authors also comment that the term 'seriously emotionally disturbed' was quite a broad one encompassing a wide range of potential symptomatology from school phobia through to schizophrenia! Valid conclusions are therefore difficult to make but, what is interesting, is that the art therapy was offered on a short-term basis and was still found to be effective.

Post-traumatic stress disorder is being increasingly described in children and adolescents. There are conflicting views about the usefulness of psychological debriefing. However, one study of interest is that of Goenjian *et al.* (1997) who looked at the efficacy of a brief trauma/grief-focused psychotherapy for adolescents who experienced an earthquake in Armenia. The authors report that the intervention was effective at reducing the severity of post-traumatic symptoms as compared to controls. Interestingly, they suggest that the approach lends itself to use in schools.

INTERPERSONAL PSYCHOTHERAPY

There have not been any controlled trials of IPT with young people although there is evidence of its effectiveness in the treatment of depressed adults (Elkin *et al.*, 1989; Weissman *et al.*, 1979). In an open trial of IPT in 38 adolescents with depressive disorders, Robbins *et al.* (1989) found that 47% improved. This rate of recovery was increased to 92% if IPT was used in conjunction with an antidepressant, Imipramine. In 1996, Mufson and Fairbanks reported on a 1-year naturalistic follow up of 14 adolescents treated with IPT. The therapy had lasted for 3 months in each case on average. Ten patients took part in the follow up study, only one of which was found to meet criteria for depression. This report suggests that IPT may be of benefit not only in treating depressed adolescents but also in preventing relapse. However, two caveats are required: the numbers in the study were very small and the adolescents may have recovered spontaneously.

RESEARCH INTO GROUP THERAPY

One of the most well-known and rigorously designed studies of the efficacy of group therapy (as well as other treatments) was that of Kolvin *et al.* (1981) at Newcastle. The study was comprehensive and detailed and only a brief overview can be given here. However, the key findings were as follows: 547 children and adolescents (up to age 14) were randomly allocated to one of four possible treatment options, i.e. behaviour modification, group therapy, parent counselling/ teacher consultation or nurture work. The results were that three treatments, i.e. nurture work, behaviour modification and group therapy, produced positive outcomes over and above what would have been expected by a natural improvement (what the authors referred to as a 'base rate' of recovery). Of the three treatments the most benefit was derived from group therapy which produced an improvement of over 30% above base rate. Kolvin *et al.*'s study produced results, which have been very heartening to clinicians, particularly those dismayed by Levitt's findings (1957). It is worth mentioning, however, that the Newcastle study was with non-referred children and utilised an approach which most clinics are not set up to provide.

Social skills training groups have been evaluated by some researchers. Jackson and Marzillier (1982) set up a youth club run on therapeutic lines for shy adolescents. Key elements in the sessions were modelling, role-play and feedback focusing on aspects of social skills such as eye contact, intonation, listening and dealing with teasing. The group was compared with similar youngsters who were introduced to the same topics but were not trained in using them. The authors found that the experimental group had an increased range of social activities by the end of the treatment. The use of social skills training has also been evaluated in the treatment of adolescents with depressive disorder. Fine *et al.* (1991) compared social skills training for 20 patients with 27 receiving therapeutic support. Both groups did well; however, interestingly, the adolescents who received 'therapeutic support' had a better outcome. There were many confounding variables including the fact that many of the adolescents received other treatments (such as antidepressants) in conjunction with the group work.

A meta-analytic study on the effectiveness of group therapy for sexually abused children was recently conducted (Reeker *et al.*, 1997). Fifteen studies met the researchers' criteria for inclusion in the analysis and effect sizes for each study calculated. An overall mean effect size was also obtained. The results were that the mean effect size across the studies was 0.79, with a trend for larger groups containing females to do better than other subgroups. The authors conclude that group treatments for sexually abused children and adolescents are effective, a finding supported by other published research in this area (Furniss *et al.*, 1988; Gomes-Schwartz *et al.*, 1990; Monck *et al.*, 1993).

FUTURE DIRECTIONS

In summary we still lack persuasive evidence as to which psychotherapeutic approaches work best for particular adolescent psychiatric disorders. The research findings are sometimes promising but, at this stage, inconclusive. It is often stated that 'further research is needed' and yet, although this statement is true (and it is hard to imagine when it would not be), it is not that helpful to clinicians. It may be more useful to consider the directions that further studies could take, e.g. there are numerous rating scales now available to assess both levels of psychopathology and outcomes (Achenbach and Edelbrock, 1983; Angold *et al.*, 1987; Berger *et al.*, 1993; Goodman, 1997; Gowers, 1999a,b; Schaffer *et al.*, 1983) and the use of such measures will be valuable in estimating degrees of change following therapy. The goals of treatment as described by Rutter (1985), including symptom reduction, the promotion of normal development and the generalisation of change (amongst others) are helpful for researchers to bear in mind when evaluating therapy. Good clinical care as referred to earlier may be a more acceptable control than the waiting list and more comparisons of differing treatments will help inform practice.

Ultimately, practitioners in this field have to deal with the ongoing conflict between empiricism and intuition. The former demands that we prove that what we do is efficacious and based on sound evidence; the latter is a key component of many successful therapeutic interventions. We need to learn to ask the right questions not only of published research but also of ourselves. Equally, case reports, conversations with colleagues and an enthusiasm for anything that increases our insight and empathy with young peoples' predicaments will facilitate the development of lasting therapeutic skills.

REFERENCES

Achenbach, T. M. and Edelbrock, C. S. (1983) *Manual for the Child Behavior Checklist and the Revised Child Behavior Profile*. Burlington, VT: University Associates in Psychiatry.

Andrews, G. (1993) The essential psychotherapies. *British Journal of Psychiatry*, **162**, 447–451.

Angold, A., Costello, E. J., Pickles, A. and Winder, F. (1987) *The Development of a Questionnaire for use in Epidemiological Studies of Depression in Children and Adolescents*. London: Medical Research Council Child Psychiatry Unit.

Axline, V. M. (1964) *Dibs in Search of Self*. London: Gollancz.

Axline, V. M. (1947) *Play Therapy: The Inner Dynamics of Childhood*. New York: Houghton Miffin.

Bentovim, A., Vizard, E. and Hollows, A. (1991) *Children and Young People as Abusers: An Agenda for Action*. London: National Children's Bureau.

Berger, M., Hill, P., Sen, E., Thompson, M. and Verduyn, C. (1993) *A Proposed Core Data Set for Child and Adolescent Psychology and Psychiatric Services*. London: Association for Child Psychology and Psychiatry.

Bion, W. R. (1961) *Experiences in Groups*. London: Tavistock.

Bulkeley, R. and Cramer, D. (1994) Social skills training with young adolescents: group and individual approaches in a school setting. *Journal of Adolescence*, **17**, 521–532

Callias, M. (1992) Evaluation of interventions with children and adolescents. In D. A. Lane and A. Miller (eds), *Child and Adolescent Therapy: A Handbook*. Milton Keynes: Open University Press, pp. 39–64.

Cantwell, D. P. and Baker, L. (1989) Stability and natural history of DSMIII childhood diagnoses. *Journal of the American Academy of Child and Adolescent Psychiatry*, **28**, 691–700.

Copley, B. and Forryan, B. (1987) *Therapeutic Work with Children and Young People*. London: Robert Royce.

Crisp, A. H. (1980) *Anorexia Nervosa: Let Me Be*. London: Academic Press.

Crisp, A. H., Norton, K., Gowers, S., Halek, C., Bowyer, C., Yeldham, D. *et al.* (1991) A controlled study of the effect of therapies aimed at adolescent and family psychopathology in anorexia nervosa. *British Journal of Psychiatry*, **159**, 325–333.

Daws, D. and Boston, M. (1988) *The Child Psychotherapist*. London: Karnac (Maresfield Library)

de Shazer, S. (1988) *Clues: Investigating Solutions in Brief Therapy*. New York: Norton.

Elkin, I., Shea, T., Watkins, J. T., Imber, S. D., Sotsky, S. M., Collins, J. F. *et al.* (1989) National Institute of Mental Health treatment of depression collaborative research programme: general effectiveness of treatments. *Archives of General Psychiatry*, **46**, 971–982.

Evans, J. (1998) *Active Analytic Group Therapy for Adolescents*. London: Jessica Kinglsey.

Fine, S., Forth, A., Gilbert, M., Haley, G. (1991) Group therapy for adolescent depressive disorder: a comparison of social skills training and therapeutic support. *Journal of the American Academy of Child and Adolescent Psychiatry*, **30**, 79–85.

Flament, M. F., Koby, E., Rapoport, J. L., Berg, C. J., Zahn, T., Cox, C. *et al.* (1990) Childhood obsessive-compulsive disorder: a prospective follow-up study. *Journal of Child Psychology and Psychiatry*, **31**, 363–380.

Foulkes, S. S. (1964) *Therapeutic Group Analysis*. London: George Allen & Unwin.

Freud, A. (1926/27) *Introduction to the Technique of Child Analysis*. Reprinted in: *The Psychoanalytic Treatment o Children*. London: Imago.

Freud, S. (1909) *Analysis of a Phobia in a Five Year Old Child*, standard edn 10. London: Hogarth Press.

Furniss, T., Bingley-Miller, L. and van Elburg, A. (1988) Goal-orientated group treatment for sexually abused adolescent girls. *British Journal of Psychiatry*, **152**, 97–106.

Glaser, D. (1992) Abuse of children. In D. A. Lane and A. Miller (eds), *Child and*

Adolescent Therapy: A Handbook. Milton Keynes: Open University Press, pp. 108–119.

Goenjian, A. K., Karayan, I., Pynoos, R. S., Minassian, D., Nejarian, L. M., Steinberg, A. M. *et al.* (1997) Outcome of psychotherapy among early adolescents after trauma. *American Journal of Psychiatry*, **154**, 536–542.

Gomes-Schwartz, B., Horowitz, J. M. and Cardarelli, A. (1990) *Child Sexual Abuse: The Initial Effects*. Beverley Hills, CA: Sage.

Goodman, R. (1997) The strengths and difficulties questionnaire: a research note. *Journal of Child Psychology and Psychiatry*, **38**, 581–586.

Gowers, S. G., Harrington, R. C., Whitton, A., Lelliott, P., Wing, J. and Beevor, A. (1999a) A Brief scale for measuring the outcomes of emotional and behavioural disorders in children (HoNOSCA). *British Journal of Psychiatry*, **174**, 413–416.

Gowers, S. G., Harrington, R. C., Whitton, A. , Beevor, A., Lelliott, P., Jezzard, R. and Wing, J. (1999b) Health of the Nation Outcome Scales for Children and Adolescents (HoNOSCA). Glossary for HoNOSCA score sheet. *British Journal of Psychiatry*, **174**, 428–431.

Green, J. M. (1996) Engagement and empathy: a pilot study of the therapeutic alliance in out-patient child psychiatry. *Child Psychology and Psychiatry Review*, **1**, 130–138.

Harrington, R. C. (1993) *Depressive Disorder in Childhood and Adolescence*. Chichester: Wiley.

Johnson, E. (1982) Principles and techniques in drama therapy. *International Journal of Arts and Psychotherapy*, **9**, 83–90.

Jackson, M. F. and Marzillier, J. S. (1982) The Youth Club Project: a community-based intervention for shy adolescents, *Behavioural Psychotherapy*, **10**, 87–100.

Klein, M. (1932) *The Psychoanalysis of Children*. London: Hogarth Press.

Klerman, G., Weissman, M. Rounsoville, B. and Chevron, E. (1984) *Interpersonal Psychotherapy of Depression*. New York: Basic Books.

Kolvin, I., Garside, R. F., Nicol, A. R., Macmillan, A., Wolstenholme, F. and Leitch, I. M. (1981) *Help Starts Here: The Maladjusted Child in the Ordinary School*. London: Tavistock.

Kovacs, M. (1997) The Emanuel Miller Memorial Lecture 1994 – Depressive disorders in childhood: an impressionistic landscape. *Journal of Child Psychology and Psychiatry*, **38**, 287–298.

Levitt, E. E. (1957) The results of psychotherapy with children: an evaluation. *Journal of Consulting Psychology*, **21**, 189–196.

Levitt, E. E. (1963) Psychotherapy with children: a further evaluation. *Behaviour Research and Psychotherapy*, **60**, 326–329.

Lush, D., Boston, M. and Grainger, E. (1991) Evaluation of psychoanalytic psychotherapy with adoptive or in-care children. *Psychoanalytic Psychotherapy*, **5**(3), 191–234.

Monck, E., Bentovim, A., Goodall, G., et al. (1993) Child Sexual Abuse: A Descriptive and Treatment Study. London: HMSO.

Moreau, D., Mufson, L., Weissman, M. M. and Klerman, G. L. (1991) Interpersonal psychotherapy for adolescent depression: description of modification and preliminary application. Journal of the American Academy of Child Psychology, 30 642–651.

Mufson, L. and Fairbanks, J. (1996) Interpersonal psychotherapy for depressed adolescents: a one-year naturalistic follow up study. Journal of the American Academy of Child and Adolescent Psychiatry, 35, 1145–1155.

Pratt, J. H. (1907) The class method of treating consumption in the homes of the poor. Journal of the American Medical Association, 49, 755–759.

Reeker, J., Ensing, D. and Elliott, R. (1997) A meta-analytic investigation of group treatment outcomes foe sexually abused children. Child Abuse and Neglect, 21, 669–680.

Reid, S. and Kolvin, I. (1993) Group psychotherapy for children and adolescents. Archives of Diseases of Childhood, 69, 244–250.

Robbins, D. R., Allessi, N. E. and Colfer, M. V. (1989) Treatment of adolescents with major depression: implications of the Dexamethasone suppression test and the melancholic clinical subtype. Journal of Affective Disorders, 17, 99–104.

Robins, L. N. (1966) Deviant Children grown up. Baltimore, MD: Williams & Wilkins

Rogers, C. (1951) Client Centred Therapy in Current Practice: Implications and Theory. New York: Houghton Miffin.

Rutter, M. (1985) Psychological therapies in child psychiatry: issues and prospects. In M. Rutter and L. Hersov (eds), Child and Adolescent Psychiatry: Modern Approaches, 2nd edn. Oxford: Blackwell Science.

Schaffer, D., Gould, M. S., Brasic, J., Ambrosine, P., Fisler, B., Bird, H. et al. (1983) A children's global assessment scale. Archives of General Psychiatry, 40, 1228–1231.

Scott, J. (1995) Psychological treatments for depression, an update. British Journal of Psychiatry, 167, 289–292.

Shirk, S. R. and Russell, R. L. (1992) A re-evaluation of estimates of child therapy effectiveness. Journal of the American Academy of Child and Adolescent Psychiatry, 31, 703–709.

Simon, M. R. (1992) The Symbolism of style: Art as Therapy. London: Tavistock/ Routledge.

Target, M. and Fonagy, P. (1996) Predictors of outcome in child psychoanalysis: a retrospective study of 763 cases as the Anna Freud Centre. Journal of the American Psychoanalysis Association, 44, 27–77.

Tibbetts, T. and Stone, B. (1990) Short term art therapy with seriously emotionally disturbed adolescents. The Arts in Psychotherapy, 17, 139–146.

Tramontana, M. G. (1980) Critical review of research on psychotherapy outcome with adolescents 1976–1977. Psychology Bulletin, 2, 29–450.

Trowell, J. (1994) Individual and group psychotherapy. In M. Rutter, E. Taylor and L. Hersov (eds), *Child and Adolescent Psychiatry: Modern Approaches*. Oxford: Blackwell Scientific Publications, pp. 936–945.

Weissman, M. M., Prusoff, B. A., Di Mascio, A., Nev, C., Goklaney, M. and Klerman, G. L. (1979) The efficacy of drugs and psychotherapy in the treatment of acute depressive episodes. *American Journal of Psychiatry*, **136**, 555–558.

Weisz, J. R., Donenberg, G. R., Han, S. S. and Kauneckis, D. (1995a) Child and adolescent psychotherapy outcomes in experiments versus clinics: why the disparity? *Journal of Abnormal Child Psychology*, **23**, 83–106.

Weisz, J. R., Weiss, B., Han, S. S., Granger, D. A. and Morton, T. (1995b) Effects of psychotherapy with children and adolescents revisited: a meta-analysis of treatment outcome studies. *Psychology Bulletin*, **117**, 450–468.

Weisz, J. R. and Weiss, B. (1989) Assessing the effects of clinic based psychotherapy with children and adolescents. *Journal of Clinical and Consulting Psychology*, **57**(6), 741–746.

Winnicott, D. W. (1958) *Collected Papers: Through Paediatrics to Psychoanalysis*. London: Tavistock.

Yule, W. and Williams, R. M. (1992) The management of trauma following disasters. In D. A. Lane and A. Miller (eds), *Child and Adolescent Therapy: A Handbook*. Milton Keynes: Open University Press, pp. 157–176.

Chapter 21

FAMILY THERAPY

Julia Nelki and Michael Göpfert

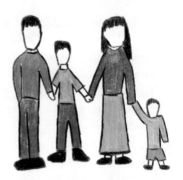

'Curiouser and curiouser', said Alice 'now I'm opening out like the largest telescope there ever was.'

Alice in Wonderland
(Carroll, 1867)

'She used to be such a good girl.' (*Dad*)
'If you'd all get off my back, I'd be fine.' (*Nicola*)

This is a familiar exchange between a parent and an adolescent. It easily escalates to a full-blown argument and if this happens in a family session the new family therapist may be longing to retreat to the safety of individual work. This chapter tries to give some alternative options.

ADOLESCENCE FROM A FAMILY SYSTEMS PERSPECTIVE

The task of adolescence in western European cultures is to move from functioning within a context determined by parental values to learning to define and determine ones own. Peer groups become the major reference point as adolescents develop a sense of identity, emerge into sexual beings, and begin the process of emotional and physical separation from their parents. Parental authority becomes relative with rules needing to be negotiated and openness to new ideas being important. How a young person manages these transitions will depend on their position in the family, what has happened before, how the family has managed other stages of development, and how the parents and grandparents managed their own adolescence.

Families are seen as groups of individuals in many possible constellations, living together in an intimate way over time, developing unique patterns of relating. Vertical connections over generations pass down beliefs, family stories and patterns which affect the present.

Work with adolescent patients can take many different forms, but family issues will always be of relevance. Working with the family does not imply an aetiological connection. Once a problem has arisen, for whatever reason, it may be possible to alter what maintains and sustains it, and this may be through family work.

Nicola, age 15, was the eldest of three and the first to approach the age of leaving home. Her mother had left home at 16 and a close family was very important to her. She had Nicola at 18 and described their relationship as a sisterly one. Nicola's father was a lot older than her mother and had always been a loner. He worked long hours, often away from home. The younger two, aged 7 and 5, argued with each other but little with their older, somewhat aloof sister.

Adolescence may be particularly difficult in families where there are unresolved issues for the parents. The competitiveness and challenges of adolescence may threaten the close relationship between Nicola and her mother.

HISTORY

The idea of the family as a unit, to be seen as a whole and understood in terms of a complex functioning system, developed after World War II. It was a revolutionary idea that brought ideological conviction with it. It was elaborated on by clinicians such as Bowlby (1949), Bell (1962), Ackerman (1959) and Skynner (1969), who found that working with families brought about more change than work with individuals alone.

EARLY PERIOD: 1945–1970

In the UK, a developing National Health Service and system of Social Services with a strong commitment to caring for children led to family therapy being developed mostly by practitioners in child and family services. The predominant therapeutic influences of the time were individual psychoanalysis and group analysis (Skynner, 1976). The main idea was that seeing families as units and people in context created different ways of understanding families, and opened up new, powerful ways of intervention and change.

Family therapy borrowed concepts from hard science such as systems theory (von Bertalanffy, 1968), cybernetics (Bateson, 1973; Wiener, 1961) and communications theory (Watzlawick *et al.*, 1967).

Some early applications of these ideas led to parents feeling blamed for their offspring's problems. However, in other families, changes were rapid and dramatic.

MIDDLE PERIOD: THE 1970s AND 1980s

Practitioners consolidated family therapy by developing different methods and theoretical frameworks for working with families. Separate schools were set up with areas of difference though also overlap and mutual influence. An important divide occurred during this time: Psycho-educational and other symptom-oriented approaches mainly aimed at supporting families dealing with a sick or disturbed member. This was contrasted by 'systemic' therapies including structural, strategic and the Milan systemic therapies, which aim to change the way that problems are perceived by looking at family functioning.

CONTEMPORARY FAMILY THERAPY

Family therapy is now an established approach within medicine and mental health. There has been a bridging of differences both across family therapy models and across disciplines, supported by research evidence and clinical trends. Central to this new tolerance of, and interest in, different approaches, has been the coming together of the philosophical idea of 'constructivism' (von Glaserfeld, 1984); the development of cybernetic thinking to the level of 'second-order cybernetics' (von Foerster, 1981), i.e. that there is no such thing as objectivity; the influence of the women's movement, and an increasing awareness of cultural relativity and the fundamentally ethnocentric nature of most Western schools of psychological therapies (Goldner, 1991; Gorell Barnes, 1990; Jones, 1993; Krause and Miller, 1995; Waldegrave, 1990). The idea of social constructionism, i.e. that meaning or knowledge is constructed through social interaction (Gergen, 1985), leads to the idea of there being no single 'truth'. Each individual therapist and family member actively 'constructs' their view of the world according to their own beliefs, experience and social context (Neimeyer and Ruskin, 2000). All perspectives have validity. The focus shifts from the systemic perspective of changing family interactions to creating different meanings and stories in therapeutic conversations (Worden, 1999). The emphasis is less on schools of thought, and more on understanding different viewpoints and crossing boundaries. The individual has now found their place within the system (McFadyen, 1997; Wilson, 1998) and the therapeutic relationship between the family and the therapist has greater focus than it had (Falaskas, 1997; Sprenkle *et al.*, 1999).

Training in family therapy is now part of psychiatric training, and Schmidt and Bonjean (1995) found that learning family therapy made psychiatric trainees more thoughtful and clinically competent.

FAMILY THERAPY FRAMEWORKS AND MODALITIES

THE FAMILY LIFE CYCLE AND TRANSGENERATIONAL FAMILY THERAPY

The concept of the family life cycle (Carter and McGoldrick, 1980) and its application in transgenerational family therapy (Bowen, 1978; Lieberman, 1980; Wetchler and Piercy, 1996) became very influential. Family issues can be formulated in terms of life cycle transition problems and families often present at times of transitions. Adolescence is such a transition period.

The family life cycle begins with the unattached adult; finding a partner; a couple becoming parents; birth of the first baby; moving through the pre-school years until the start of school; the middle years until adolescence; adolescence and leaving home; the time for all children to leave home and set up independent lives; the parents together without the children; death of the parents. Each stage is seen as having its own characteristics and tasks, and the move to the next stage as involving both losses and gains.

Nicola is anorexic. The effect was to freeze the family into a pre-adolescent phase. The difficulty of moving into the adolescent stage seemed linked to a feared loss of the family closeness. For Nicola, this was associated with a fear of becoming a woman and the sacrifices this had meant for her mother and grandmother. For her mother, her own adolescence had been stormy and explosive. She had run away from home and had no contact with her parents until recently. Nicola's father had children by a first marriage that he lost contact with when they were teenagers. His own father had died when he was 16. Death of a parent disrupts the normal family life cycle and expectations for a growing child. It was understandable that adolescence should be a difficult time for the family.

Although fundamentally useful, the model has limits. It is important to find out what the critical stages for particular family groupings are. Ethnic and cultural groups emphasise different life cycle transitions.

Transgenerational family therapy was born out of the psychoanalytic pre-occupation with the past, and conceptualizes the family as an ever unfolding process of patterns over the generations which is best communicated and understood as family stories or family myths (Byng Hall, 1995). Most people will be able to remember significant stories which in some way are characteristic for the particular family they come from.

In Nicola's case, a pattern was revealed over three generations of women sacrificing their own wishes and desires for their families, and, in particular, in relation to men. It became possible to talk about the meaning of becoming a woman and Nicola could express her concerns because there seemed no way out of living for, and through, someone else.

BEHAVIOURAL FAMILY THERAPY

Behavioural family therapy follows the principle of behavioural analysis of problem behaviours, looking at antecedents and consequences. It is now well supported by evidence (see below). Change techniques include role-play practice of possible alternatives to a problematic sequence of family interaction, role substitution (where the therapist plays the role of a family member), role reversal (where a parent plays the role of a youngster and the young person plays the parent) and modelling. The focus is on problem solving, communication and behaviour training (Falloon *et al.*, 1984). Cognitive techniques have recently been integrated into this work. 'Problem-solving family therapy', 'directive family therapy', 'functional family therapy', 'behavioural-systemic family therapy' and the McMaster model of family therapy could be considered here. There are also attempts at establishing more cognitively oriented models of family therapy. One of the more promising approaches is that of Procter (1996) who has developed a method of formulating 'family construct systems' based on Kelly's personal construct psychology. This blends in well with narrative approaches as described below, as well as with individual frameworks of psychological understanding and therapy such as cognitive-analytic therapy (Ryle, 1989).

The arguments around mealtimes were very distressing to all in Nicola's family. Nicola's mother would start to feel anxious before the meal, plead with Nicola to eat, and very quickly become tearful and upset when Nicola picked at the food. Nicola would shout to be left alone and storm out; her dad would get cross with her mum for 'nagging' at her. Often no one would eat. Through discussion and role play, the family agreed that dad would support mum through the meal; that both parents would be firm and clear that the food needed to be eaten but after 30 min whatever was left would be cleared away without comment. If mum got upset, dad was to support her away from Nicola.

PSYCHO-EDUCATIONAL MODELS OF FAMILY WORK

These are based on the evidence-based discovery that information itself can be helpful and make a substantial difference to how families interact and use services (McGill and Lee, 1986). There are many different and diverse frameworks, and considerable overlap with behavioural methods (Anderson *et al.*, 1986; Hogarty *et al.*, 1991; Miklowitz, 1995). Parent training is an educational approach just as much as the systematic provision of information about schizophrenia to a multi-family group of families with newly diagnosed schizophrenics (Webster-Stratton and Herbert, 1994).

Nicola's parents felt responsible for Nicola's anorexia and assumed the therapist felt the same. A lot of support was needed to help them grasp the idea that anorexia was a complicated issue. Especially important for the parent was the information that once it had taken a hold of their daughter it had self-perpetuating properties. The therapists' interest in examining some of their behaviour patterns was not based on causal explanatory models and finding a cause was ultimately less important than finding ways to move Nicola on. The family could accept their role in helping Nicola find a way out of anorexia.

STRUCTURAL FAMILY THERAPY

Structural family therapy is based on the notion that not all family members are equal. Family members have different roles and responsibilities, and problems result when these are unbalanced or unclear. Minuchin (1967) developed this approach in his work with delinquent boys from poor and chaotic Puerto Rican families. It offers both ways of looking at families and of working with them. It is highly structured using action and immediate techniques. The approach works on clarifying boundaries, building appropriate hierarchies and safe structures (Minuchin and Fishman, 1981). The therapist is active and interventionist, focusing on the minute details of transactions in the room, disrupting dysfunctional patterns and trying out more functional ones.

It is useful in adolescence where hierarchies may have become skewed and the young person appears to be in control of the parents rather than the other way round. The parents can feel very supported by this approach and the young person may be relieved to have safer limits set (Micucci, 1998). Some early studies of family therapy support its efficacy (see below).

> With Nicola, it became apparent that the parents had different ways of trying to get Nicola to eat, which resulted in tension between them and Nicola eating less. Nicola's father was calmer than her mother but was around less. Nicola would eat more with her father but wanted her mum to be around. It was agreed that the parents would make a unified approach and talk each evening about difficulties and plans for the next day.

STRATEGIC MODELS

There are many different models of family therapy that can be characterised as strategic. The basic assumption underlying any strategic family therapy is that the family has not brought about change with their attempts at problem solving. Otherwise they would not ask for help. This implies that their attempts at solving the presenting problem have become an integral part of the problem that needs addressing by therapy. Because the family cannot devise their own solution, the therapist takes responsibility for the therapy and develops a strategy for dealing with the problem in the patient's social context which is usually the family. Strategic family therapists have made a strong case that therapy in the first instance should dispel any notion of blame that by implication can be put on the parents (Price, 1996).

Brief therapy

The aim of therapy is to understand how the family sees the problem within its context and to understand the detail of their repeated attempts to solve it. The assumption is that the family is putting more and more energy into attempting to solve the problem, leading to a feeling of failure and despair (Weakland *et al.*, 1974). The therapist prescribes an 'uncommon' solution, one that they would not normally try and that prevents them from repeating their failed attempts (Procter and Walker, 1988).

Solution-focused therapy

De Shazer (1985) developed a model of brief solution focused therapy (BSFT). It is a behavioural model, but unlike the classical behavioural analysis works from the radical premise that the therapist does not need to know what the problem is in order to bring about change. Talking about problems is seen as reinforcing them. The therapist is only interested in when it does not occur or what possible solutions there might be. Therapists only need to know about the 'problem' to evaluate outcomes and because people would find it difficult to engage with a therapist who does not want to know what is wrong and painful.

> Nicola's family could only focus on the times Nicola would not eat and the resulting arguments. With help, they could remember and expand on the rare occasions that Nicola ate without being pressurised. She ate more after family meetings. The family linked this to everybody being able to express feelings such as anger that had previously been taboo. The family decided to make a regular time each day when they would talk together. They would talk in a non-critical way. The focus was to be on the difference in the family at times when Nicola could eat more from those times when she found eating difficult.

Strategic family therapy

Haley (1976) developed the original strategic family therapy. Symptoms are seen as crucially linked to the system, supporting the family as it is, holding things together or masking another area of difficulty. Families are not challenged directly, although recently parents have been encouraged to take more assertive actions when their youngsters are aggressive and abusive (Price, 1996). The importance of the symptom is acknowledged and strategies for dealing with the underlying problem without the need for the symptom are devised. It can be very creative and playful, using metaphor, drama, reframing and positive connotation (Madanes, 1974).

> The therapist likened Nicola's not eating to her being on strike. Her demands were not clear but he wondered whether she was angry with her parents but scared to show it because she was not sure whether they could cope with her being angry. The family was asked to have an argument at home that was not around food. An incident was found where there had been a mild disagreement. Her mum was encouraged to develop the argument rather than avoid it and the siblings were asked to set an example, as they were so good at it. This exercise highlighted their difficulty in having open arguments and allowed the fears and patterns around arguments to be explored with the family. Nicola's anger with her family was given a voice and could be expressed more directly than by refusing food.

MILAN SYSTEMIC FAMILY THERAPY

The 'Milan approach' is regarded by some as a strategic therapy too. It developed out of the work of four Italian psychoanalysts Selvini-Palazzoli, Prata, Boscolo and Cecchin (Selvini-Palazzoli *et al.*, 1978) who began working with families where there was a schizophrenic or anorexic member. The underlying assumption is that all family members equally influence each other. They recognised the power of the family as a cohesive group ('system') and believed that this needed to be countered by an at least equally powerful counter-system of the family therapy team, with one-way screens and messages going backward and forward between the team and the family (Selvini-Palazzoli *et al.*, 1980).

A new form of questioning was devised, based on feedback from information from the family about relationships and difference (Penn, 1982). Triadic questioning, whereby a person is asked to comment on the thoughts, behaviour or relationships of others, underlies many of these circular questions. Different types of circular questions include (Penn, 1985):

- Ranking: 'Who is closest to whom?'
- Change over time: 'Whose relationship has changed the most since Nicola became anorexic?'
- Hypothetical: 'How would your grandmother describe Nicola's relationship with her mother if she were here?'
- Feed-forward: 'What do you think everyone in the family will be doing in 10 years time?'

The questions were seen as very powerful and have developed as a major intervention themselves (Tomm, 1988). The fundamental premise is that the system of questioning helps the family question itself, which enables them to find their own solutions, without prescription from therapists.

NARRATIVE APPROACHES

The way we describe our lives is a narrative from a particular perspective. Usually one story becomes 'dominant'. Families in therapy often present with dominant stories that are problem-saturated and without hope. Different conversations and an understanding of the 'restraints' that prevent us seeing other possibilities can allow less dominant stories to have a voice, change the family's behaviour around a problem and restore hope (Jenkins, 1990). White (1984) combined aspects of BSFT (de Shazer, 1985) with the use of play and metaphor, and a focus on power and control. He developed externalisation and 'externalising conversations', which by separating the problem from the person can help this process. This approach 'enhances a view of self that centres on experiences of competence, avoiding failure, hopelessness and pathology' (White and Epston, 1990). It involves a shift in attitude of the therapist to 'a stance which suggests that the client's views about what is helpful are more salient than the therapist's belief about what is therapeutic' (Durrant and Kowalski, 1990). The solution cannot be predetermined and is more of an evolutionary process between the therapist and family (Hoffman, 1988).

Hoffman says that this approach means that psychiatric problems can be viewed as 'spells – collective illusions that must be dispelled rather than biological or social units that must be healed' (Hoffman, 1993).

Bringing the self in to the work means becoming aware of how, who you are, in terms of gender, ethnic origin, discipline, age, class, experience and family tradition, affects how you work and also the 'fit' between you and the family. It also makes one question how certain value systems, power relationships, theories and assumptions became such 'dominant stories' in Western society (Jones, 1996; Walters, 1990; Perelberg and Miller, 1990)

This approach makes it easier to accommodate seemingly contradictory frameworks, both within families and between professionals (Fishel, 1999).

An exercise to try this out is to imagine being with a family that you have recently seen.

Now imagine that you are a different gender, age and colour and imagine how the interaction between you and the family would be different.

What would your assumptions be about them and what would theirs be about you? What difference would this make?

For example, if Nicola is from a white middle-class family and sees me, a white female psychiatrist, assumptions may be different than if, for example, Nicola were from an Asian family or than if, for example, I were an Afro-Caribbean man.

IMPORTANT PRINCIPLES UNDERLYING FAMILY THERAPY

- Bringing the family together is a very powerful intervention in itself as it is for everyone to hear everyone else's point of view.
- The acknowledgement of each person's perspective particularly helps adolescents to feel taken seriously.
- There are many stories to be told and each has its validity – who the therapist is will determine what stories get told.
- The idea of working together collaboratively to find a useful solution rather than the therapist treating the family gives more scope for families to find their own solutions.
- Family therapy can be done with parts of the family.
- 'Facts' may not be as important as how they are perceived. Facts can be questioned, such as 'how did you make sense of that experience?', 'Is that how your dad/mum/sibling saw it too?', 'Is that how you saw it then or now when you look back?'.

- Criticism and other negative expressed emotion are associated with adolescent psychopathology (see below). Clinically this can be reinforced by a problem-focussed approach. Building on a family's strength may be more likely to facilitate therapeutic change.
- Family therapy cannot solve problems of poverty and deprivation (Knapp and Harris, 1998).

TECHNIQUES WHICH MAY BE USEFUL IN FAMILY THERAPY WITH ADOLESCENTS

THE USE OF METAPHOR

Metaphor can sometimes be a helpful way to get an idea across. Humour often engages people. With Nicola's family, the mother said at one point to father how she is sick of him never spending any time with the children or her. The therapist picked this up, made the link with Nicola's self-induced vomiting and eventually asked every family member what they were sick of in the family, thus 'normalising' to some degree Nicola's symptom.

BRING IN THE PEER GROUP

Ask questions that relate to their 'mates', such as 'how do your mates negotiate this with their parents?'; 'what advice would you give to a mate in the same predicament?'.

THE POWER OF QUESTIONS

'If you were spending more time with your mates and less time at home, and if your mum wasn't so worried about you, do you think your mum would spend more time with your dad or more time with your brother and sister?'

'I think she'd spend more time on her own and would feel lonely.'
'How would you know she was lonely?'
'She'd cry.'
'Would anyone else notice?'
'Dad wouldn't because she would not let him see, and the babies wouldn't because they just don't.'
'What would dad do if he knew?'
'He'd be worried and want to help.'
'Could you help your dad know?'

> The focus has shifted from Nicola's anorexia to her mum's loneliness and her parent's relationship. Nicola is given the role of helping rather than substituting for her father.

OFFER A DIFFERENT PERSPECTIVE

A family who arrives seeing their child as 'bad' might be surprised at the possibility that he is trying to distract them from their marital arguments.

THE USE OF GENEOGRAMS

Drawing a family tree with the family is a very good way of making contact with all family members, generating new ideas about the family by understanding patterns across generations, differing aspects of culture in father's and mother's family, father and mother as children, and how this compares with their parenting now (McGoldrick and Gerson, 1985). Geneograms enable unspoken dynamics related to the family of origin to become verbalised, and by way of putting it on a piece of paper or blackboard, they become 'externalised' and accessible.

FAMILY CIRCLES

Family circles give an indication of the perceived and desired strength of different current relationships and can be done quickly, in a setting such as general practice (Thrower et al. 1982; Tomson, 1998). An individual is asked to put themselves in the centre of a circle and mark other important individuals, family, friends and pets – in terms of their closeness and place within the circle or outside it. This can be done in terms of how the young person sees relationships currently and how they might desire them to be.

EXTERNALISING

> Seeing the anorexia as external to Nicola, a 'trickster' that made her not eat and dominated her life, could be used to unite the family together with Nicola to find ways of overcoming it. She could also express feelings of anger at her parents through her 'anorexic part' that she had not been able to express directly. Another story could be developed of a girl wanting to fulfil her parents expectations, desperate not to disappoint them but needing to do it in her own way.

AMBIVALENCE

The need to acknowledge and validate ambivalence in order to connect with the motivation of the family and identified patient.

> Nicola continued to lose weight while at the same time asserting that she wanted to gain weight. Eventually, the family could recognise and accept the valid and powerful reasons for Nicola's anorexia in conversation with the therapist and at home. Paradoxically, this enabled the family to negotiate eating patterns more constructively. Nicola's weight loss ceased until she eventually managed to put on more weight.

FAMILY THERAPY

INDICATIONS

Family therapy, as any other therapy, can only be considered if there is reasonable motivation. Working with the whole family should be considered in the following instances:

- Family life cycle events, such as death, family break-up or trauma experienced as a family
- Where family factors can be seen as relevant, e.g. in an adoptive family where the parent's know that the biological parent suffered from a mental illness, and disturbed behaviour is interpreted as the possible beginning of mental illness in the child
- Where family dynamics influence the course of a condition, e.g. anorexia nervosa, schizophrenia or diabetes
- When family patterns of relating and communication become difficult, e.g. where a parent or sibling has a life threatening illness
- When a disturbance only appears in one context but not in another – an out of control adolescent may appear 'mad' at home but normal in school when firm boundaries are in place
- Family-oriented, systemic therapy can be undertaken with any combination of family members, including individuals (Zawidowski, 1999)

CONTRAINDICATIONS

There are no absolute contraindications.

Sometimes family work can destabilise a precariously balanced equilibrium, e.g. in the case of a schizophrenic adolescent with an alcoholic father, where the anxiety triggered by the request for a family session led to an acute exacerbation of her symptoms and to a drinking spree of her father with increased domestic violence. Other ways of doing the much-needed work with this family had to be found.

ASSESSMENT FOR FAMILY THERAPY

REFERRAL

Pre-referral work is often crucial in clarifying motivation, the level of involvement of the referrer and the type of intervention likely to be helpful.

SETTING

Consider where might be the most appropriate place to see a young person, whether school, home or clinic. Ensure that the clinic setting is relevant to adolescents, by posters, magazines and information about other services, such as counselling, contraception, drug and alcohol support.

ENGAGEMENT

A first family meeting is as much an assessment of the therapist by the family as the other way round. All who live at home are generally invited to the first meeting. This can give the therapist an idea of available support; factors that may compound or ameliorate the problem; an observation of family functioning and an idea of motivation for change. Whatever the problem, the family will be important for the individual even if they never attend.

It is important to link with all members of the family, even though they may be in major conflict with each other. Asking questions about whose decision it was to come, and how, whoever has arrived was invited or decided to come, can allow anxieties and negative feelings to be brought into the open. Children of all ages have views on this. The youngest or least likely may give the most useful answers. Letters to missing members inviting them to come sometimes stimulates curiosity and allows them to come at a later date.

With adolescents, it is important to acknowledge their 'adult' part, both by respecting their viewpoint but also by encouraging them to take responsibility for their part in any problem behaviour. Their 'child' part needs addressing too though with care that they feel looked after in a way they can tolerate without feeling infantilised.

Young people have their own privacy and may need individual time with a therapist to talk about concerns. They might only be able to engage with family discussions if they know that they can have individual time too.

AGREEING AIMS

Asking what each person wants from the meeting needs clarifying in detail and checking on in subsequent sessions. Sometimes, there are great misperceptions as to what can be done. The young person may have been told that s/he can be taken into care if s/he continues to be naughty! The family may think the therapist can expedite school or house changes.

It is important to make a link with each person and ensure that each contribution is heard. Establishing how each person sees the problem can sometimes highlight important differences, which can be expanded into an understanding of family relationships and changes since the problem started. Finding out who most wants change may give an idea of who to work with. A geneogram on a theme, such as anger and arguments in Nicola's case, can involve the whole family.

For deliberate self-harm and other emergency referrals, risk assessment and management dominate the agenda of a family meeting (Asen, 1998):

- Is the young person safe at home or to go home and what would be needed to make it safe?
- What needs to happen to ensure the crisis is not repeated?
- Is further work possible or necessary?

> Key issues in the first meeting with Nicola were to ensure that Nicola's weight was not dangerously low; that the family understood the diagnosis of anorexia and the seriousness of her condition and that they might come again to think about how things could be different.

FAMILY FUNCTIONING

Important questions to be answered include:

- What are the roles of individual family members in the family? For example, one family member may have the role of taking care of parental distress, someone else may have to be a go-between if there is conflict.
- What is the family structure. Who makes executive decisions about what? Where is this family in their life cycle?
- What are the emotional and communication patterns in the family? For example, a family might never have any open conflict. What is the level of expressed emotion? A high level of criticism limits the possibility for change.
- What are family members' different perceptions of the 'problem' and motivations?
- What are the family members' perceptions of the role of the therapist?

FORMULATION

A formulation is an attempt to bring the information together from the meeting and give back the therapist's understanding of the problem so far. It will include a description of the problem, the family situation, a perspective from the therapist's position that will depend on the theoretical model, an estimate of the family's strengths, and motivation for change and suggestions for the next step. This may be further assessment or a treatment plan when an idea of prognosis can also be helpful. It is most useful if this is discussed with the family, modified as appropriate, then written and a copy given to the family and referrer. This process will give an idea of whether family work is indicated and what form it should take.

HOW EFFECTIVE IS FAMILY THERAPY?

This section explores how the views of family therapy are backed by research evidence. Family therapy research is clearly at a relative beginning stage and cannot yet provide conclusive evidence. As shown in the text so far, clinical material such as the case of Nicola can be looked at from within many different frameworks, which can lead to an enriched and helpful understanding in a complementary way (Roy and Frankel, 1995). This is at odds with current research practice and the way evidence is being used, where modalities of therapy are compared in a competitive way. The effect of this may be that evidence favouring one modality of therapy over another narrows the field of vision so that vital information may be lost.

Randomised controlled clinical trials have been hailed as the 'gold standard' of scientific clinical research. Yet, controlled clinical trials while giving important information are of limited use, because they do not evaluate real clinical services and usually measure only selected aspects of particular problems (Seligman, 1995). Research therapies reliably produce better outcomes than clinic therapies (Weisz *et al.*, 1995a,b, 1992) and using a particular, proven method of intervention does not guarantee effective delivery of services. Also there is an increasing agreement among the reviewers of family therapy outcome studies, that many outcome measures used to date tend to be too narrow and fail to measure complex family changes (Roy and Frankel, 1995).

The basic assumption of systemic therapists is that all causality is 'circular', i.e. all interactions between people are construed as totally interdependent. As may have become clear to the reader in the previous text, such a view has considerable implications for how one may relate to a family. This view can be seen as being at odds with the 'linear', scientific view of cause and effect with dependent and independent variables. For the integration of clinical with research evidence it may be better to concentrate more on user feedback at all levels of service structures, along with recursive audit procedures, so that clinicians, service users and purchasers know whether what they do works and works well enough (Stoep *et al.*, 1999).

It is in this spirit that some of the available evidence is reviewed below. It comes with all the usual characteristics and limitations of such a review, e.g. it does reflect the bias toward the more easily researchable modalities of family therapy, and it is less coherent and comprehensive in its coverage of the whole field. In its presentation a shift towards more 'factual' descriptions is noticeable. This does not, however, reflect a belief of the authors in any particular 'truth'.

GENERAL EVALUATION OF FAMILY THERAPY

Grawe *et al.* (1994) undertook a major meta-analytic study of all psychological therapies and assert that family therapy has a clearly different range of applicability in comparison with other modalities. Alexander *et al.* (1994, p. 623), in their review of family therapy research, conclude that attempts at bridging the gap 'between scientific demands for rigor and clinical demands for responsiveness and immediacy' are still at their beginning. Roy and Frankel (1995) note an increase in the numbers of research projects in the last two decades without an equivalent improvement of the quality of family research. Sprenkle *et al.* (1999) reviewed family therapy process research. They came to very similar conclusions in that family therapy research had not yet addressed the important issues. In particular, they criticise the 'bombast and hubris' (Sprenkle *et al.* 1999; p. 351) of much family therapy theory which they feel has prevented family therapy research from developing in line with other psychotherapy research with which it shares much common ground. A review of the *Cochrane Database of Systematic Reviews* yielded six reviews with materials about family therapy but no conclusive evidence.

Some textbook chapters review the evidence for family therapy and come to similar conclusions (e.g. Ravenscroft, 1996). Overall, the case of family therapy in general, and more particularly for adolescent psychiatric disorders is promising but there is no solid evidence base for it as yet.

SPECIFIC APPLICATIONS OF FAMILY THERAPY IN ADOLESCENT MENTAL HEALTH

Eating disorders

Eating disorders are prominent in family therapy research since Minuchin's well-known treatment project of anorectic families (Minuchin *et al.*, 1978) with its rather forceful family lunches, which aim at dealing with 'enmeshment' (lack of differentiation of family members) as a core dynamic. This has since been challenged (Hodes *et al.*, 1999). Family factors seem to contribute to eating disorders in young women (Hodes and Le Grange, 1993; Horesh *et al.*, 1996; Wichstrom, 1995) and especially 'expressed negative emotion' may be amenable to therapeutic intervention (Le Grange *et al.*, 1992; Hodes and Le Grange, 1993; Gowers and North, 1999).

Family interventions can make a significant difference, especially for patients under the age of 18, if anorexia is part of the presentation. In complex cases, family treatment is recommended as part of a wider package (Eisler *et al.*, 1997; Robin *et al.*, 1994; Roth and Fonagy, 1996). Some controlled studies confirm that family therapy is a good intervention for families with younger eating-disordered patients (Eisler *et al.*, 1997; Le Grange *et al.*, 1992; Robin *et al.*, 1994; Russell *et al.*, 1987). This seems to hold for naturalistic clinical settings (Gowers *et al.*, 1993). Family work in less serious cases of bulimia is useful (Dare and Eisler, 1995). There are common methodological problems, especially with often wide-ranging age spreads of samples (Steiner and Lock, 1998).

Schizophrenia

Family work can have a massive impact on relapse rates by reducing the level of negative expressed emotions such as criticism and hostility in the family (Falloon *et al.*, 1984; Goldstein *et al.*, 1978; Leff and Vaughn, 1985; Leff *et al.*, 1982). Falloon *et al.* (1998) found that family interventions over 2 years are more effective than shorter interventions. Reducing carer's stress alone reduces the likelihood of psychotic exacerbation by 10–25% and, overall, treatment reduced the incidence of schizophrenia from 7.4 to 0.75/100 000 over a 4-year period (Falloon, 1992). Leff *et al.* (1982) have demonstrated that the combination of family therapy and pharmacotherapy is particularly effective for a large proportion of sufferers.

Major affective disorder

Family therapy studies in adolescents with affective disorders are rare. York and Hill (1999) concluded that there is no evidence that family therapy is effective. Brent and collaborators (Brent *et al.*, 1996, 1997, 1998) report a randomised treatment trial of cognitive-behavioural therapy (CBT), systemic behavioural family therapy and supportive therapy for adolescent depression. On follow-up (Renaud *et al.*, 1998) patients with more severe depressions did better with specialized forms of treatment. There was no difference between the CBT modality and family intervention. It is premature to conclude that family therapy is not effective in depressed adolescents (Harrington *et al.*, 1998a).

Anxiety disorders

A controlled study of family treatment was reported by Barrett *et al.* (1996) with children age 7–14 who had anxiety disorders. A combined package of cognitive-behavioural psychotherapy and family management intervention was shown to be superior over CBT alone which in turn was better than a waiting list control. A controlled school-based 10-week group intervention focusing on the parent–child relationship showed maintained improvement at 6 months follow-up. There is evidence that family therapy may have something to contribute to the management of adolescent anxiety disorders.

Obsessive-compulsive disorder

March and Leonhard (1996) reviewed obsessive-compulsive disorder in childhood and adolescents. High negative expressed emotion is associated with exacerbations of the condition. The 'Practice parameters for the assessment and treatment of children and adolescents with obsessive-compulsive disorder' (AACAP Official Action, 1998b) are based on a combination of evidence and professional consensus. They recommend family therapy if the obsessive-compulsive disorder is accompanied by substantial family problems. March and Mulle (1996) make a similar recommendation.

Post-traumatic stress disorder

There are no controlled studies of family therapy. The 'Practice parameters for the assessment and treatment of children and adolescents with post-traumatic stress disorder' (AACAP Official Action, 1998a) recommend trauma-focused parental therapy. For families with high levels of conflict, harsh discipline or when post-traumatic stress disorder symptoms are present in more than one family member, family therapy is recommended.

Child sexual abuse

Bentovim et al. (1987) concluded that family consensus that abuse has occurred is an important factor in determining which children can be rehabilitated with one or both parents and whether families are capable of positive changes. Furniss et al. (1984) evaluated a family-oriented treatment service – 14% of victims could be rehabilitated with both parents and 33% with mothers only. The remainders were cared for in some other way.

Adolescent suicide and deliberate self-harm

Harrington et al. (1998b) conducted a controlled trial of a home-based family intervention for adolescents who had taken an overdose. There were no significant differences between the treatment and control group and the conclusion was that family therapy only made a difference to suicidal ideation for patients without major depression. Hawton et al. (1998), in a review of deliberate self-harm, compared the efficacy of psychosocial and pharmacological treatments and found no evidence in support of family therapy.

Substance abuse

Different modalities of family therapy have been tried in controlled studies with good effect (Weinberg et al., 1998). A meta-analytic study of family therapy in drug use which involved 1571 cases found in favour of structural and strategic family therapy over any form of individual therapy, peer group therapy and family education (Stanton and Shadish, 1997). Family therapy in cases of alcoholism has also been shown to be effective (Edwards and Steinglass, 1995), although no controlled studies of adolescent alcoholism could be found.

Conduct disorder and juvenile delinquency

Working systemically with schools can prevent emotional and behavioural problems (Nichol, 1998; Roth and Fonagy, 1996). Multi-systemic therapy (Brown *et al.*, 1997; Henggeler *et al.*, 1986, 1991, 1992, 1997) and functional family therapy (Alexander *et al.*, 1994, 1976; Alexander and Parsons, 1973, 1982) have been tried under controlled conditions with positive results. However, at the more severe end of the spectrum, therapeutic input may actually result in a deterioration in psychopathic disorders (Herpertz and Sass, 1997; Rice *et al.*, 1992).

Roy and Frankel (1995) in their review designate functional family therapy as the treatment of choice for conduct disordered and moderately delinquent juveniles. Target and Fonagy (1996) also support the use of family therapy. Kazdin (1996) includes functional family therapy or a combination of functional family therapy and CBT in the treatment modalities he recommends for conduct disorders.

Attention deficit hyperactivity disorder

A comparison of parent training, family-based problem-solving and communication training, and of structural family therapy in adolescents with attention deficit hyperactivity disorder resulted in improvement of up to 30% and a full recovery in up to 20% of all subjects on follow-up at 3 months. Family therapy did not differ in outcome from other treatment conditions (Barkley *et al.*, 1992). The relatively low rate of improvement may be due to the brevity of the interventions offered, in the face of the chronicity of this sample group (Anastopoulos *et al.*, 1996).

The '*Practice parameters for the assessment and treatment of children, adolescents and adults with ADHD*' recommend family therapy among 'other' treatment modalities for those symptoms that do not improve with medication (Dulcan and Benson, 1997).

Gender identity disorders

Cohen-Kettenis and van Goozen (1997) recommend consideration of gender reassignment in adolescence. However, a detailed case study reported by Reiner (1996) illustrates the risks associated with failing to work with the whole family. The parents, lacking support, disowned their only adolescent daughter after gender reassignment. Landen *et al.* (1998) conclude that lack of support from the patient's family for gender reassignment is associated with regret in the procedure. It may be that gender reassignment cannot ethically be carried out without family intervention, as part of the package, yet there are no controlled evaluations of family work in gender dysphoria.

Psychosomatic disorders and physical illness

Campbell and Patterson (1995) reviewed family interventions in the treatment of physical illness. Family intervention studies are inconclusive but encouraging yet very few interventions are actually directed toward the whole family or based on a family systems perspective. Panton and White (1996/99) conclude that some support has been demonstrated for the use of family therapy as an adjunct to medication in the treatment of childhood asthma, based on evidence from two random-controlled treatment studies.

Roy and Frankel (1995) have carried out a comprehensive review of family therapy in psychosomatic and medical disorders. They conclude that family therapy outcome studies with medical illnesses remain a 'novelty' in spite of suggestive evidence for beneficial effects of family interventions with abdominal pain, trauma (including terminal illness in a parent), diabetes, asthma and some other conditions. However, the evidence base is inconclusive.

Adolescent mothers

These are a vulnerable group for mental health problems because of the disruption to normal developmental processes due to the early transition to parenthood. Family factors clearly play a major part in this (Black and Nitz, 1996; Cassidy et al., 1996; McCullough and Sherman, 1998; Musick, 1993; Panzarine et al., 1995; Trad, 1995; Ward and Carlson, 1995). Yet, no controlled intervention studies of any treatment were available.

INTEGRATING FAMILY WORK AND MENTAL HEALTH PRACTICE

An overview of family therapy can only give pointers to different directions. Many ideas and techniques are mentioned in the hope that each reader will find something they wish to try out or explore further. We hope that the beginning psychiatrist will not be discouraged by the difficulties inherent in moving from one role (that of the psychiatrist) to another (that of the family therapist). While professional roles can reinforce and re-create professional divisions, the areas of overlap in the perceptions of mental health professionals are objectively much bigger than what may divide them (Tooth, 1996). Training practices may need to be reviewed in order to address this issue more widely (Tooth, 1996). However, training and working together where possible can help integrate practice. Appropriate blurring of professional boundaries is not only useful in the practice of family therapy but also in community mental health work generally (McKay and Pollard, 1996). Families do want help as families and this help may need to be delivered by the person who can identify the need for it, if it is to be made available at all. We hope that this chapter contributes to making that help more accessible.

CONCLUSIONS

After many decades of a separate journey for family therapy and child and adolescent psychiatry, they have begun to re-converge because of new research and clinical trends in both areas. This growing overlap is likely to give us a clearer understanding of what works in practice and what may lead to more effective interventions to help our youths cope with the adversity of their lives. Research may become a more integral and relevant part of clinical work and false dichotomies in adolescent mental health may be reconstructed as complementary viewpoints. In the meantime, clinical work can continue to improve on the basis of audit, user feedback and clinical impressions. Because some families will need help as families, and because sometimes family work can address issues that are more difficult to deal with in other ways, working with families will have to become an increasingly integral part of generic adolescent mental health service provision.

Nicola and her family made many changes during 18 months of therapy. Her weight increased and her periods returned, although arguments at home increased and were very painful for all. They culminated in her moving out but family sessions enabled good contact to be maintained and an ability to tolerate separation and change without relationship breakdown. Family and therapist acknowledged that the work had been difficult but the family also felt they could now move on.

ACKNOWLEDGEMENTS

Many thanks to Brenda Cox for moving us on and to Simon Gowers for his unwavering support.

RECOMMENDED FURTHER READING

Worden, M. (1999) *Family Therapy Basics*. Pacific Grove, CA: Brooks/Cole.

REFERENCES

AACAP Official Action (1998a) Practice parameters for the assessment and treatment of children and adolescents with post-traumatic stress disorder. *Journal of the American Academy of Child and Adolescent Psychiatry*, 37 (10 Suppl.), 4S–26S.

AACAP Official Action (1998b) Practice parameters for the assessment and treatment of children and adolescents with obsessive-compulsive disorder. *Journal of the American Academy of Child and Adolescent Psychiatry*, 37 (10 Suppl.), 27S–45S.

Ackerman, N. W. (1959) *The Psychodynamics of Family Life*. New York: Basic Books.

Alexander, J. F. and Parsons, B. V. (1973) Short-term behavioural intervention with delinquent families: impact on family process and recidivism. *Journal of Abnormal Psychology*, **81**, 219–225.

Alexander, J. F, and Parsons, B. V. (1982) *Functional Family Therapy: Principles and procedures*. Carmel, CA: Brooks/Cole.

Alexander, J. F., Barton, C., Schiavvo, R. S. and Parsons, B. V. (1976) Systems-behavioural intervention with families of delinquents: therapist characteristics, family behaviour and outcome. *Journal of Consulting and Clinical Psychology*, **44**, 656–664.

Alexander, J. F., Holtzworth-Munroe, A. and Jameson, P. (1994) The process and outcome of marital and family therapy: Research review and evaluation. In A. E. Bergin and S. L. Garfield (eds), *Handbook of Psychotherapy and Behaviour Change*. New York: Wiley, pp. 543–594.

Anastopoulos, A. D., Barkley, R. A. and Sheldon, T. L. (1996) Family based treatment: Psychosocial intervention for children and adolescents with attention deficit hyperactivity disorder. In E. D. Hibbs and P. S. Jensen (eds), *Psychosocial Treatments for Child and Adolescent Disorders: Empirically Based Strategies for Clinical Practice*. Washington, DC: American Psychological Association.

Anderson, C. M., Hogarty, G. E. and Reiss, D. J. (1986) *Schizophrenia and the Family*. New York: Guilford Press.

Asen, E. (1998) On the brink – managing suicidal teenagers. In P. Sutcliffe, G. Tufnell and U. Cornish (eds), *Working with the Dying and Bereaved*. London: Macmillan, pp 129–151

Barkley, R. A., Guevremont, D. C., Anasopoulos, A. d. and Fletcher, K. E. (1992) A comparison of three family therapy programs for treating family conflicts in adolescents with attention-deficit hyperactivity disorder. *Journal of Consulting and Clinical Psychology*, **60**, 450–462.

Barrett, P. M., Dadds, M. M., Rapee, R. M. (1996) Family treatment of childhood anxiety: a controlled trial. *Journal of Consulting and Clinical Psychology*, **64**, 333–342.

Bateson, G. (1973) *Steps to an Ecology of Mind*. St Albans: Paladin.

Bell, J. (1962) Recent Advances in family group therapy. *Journal of Child Psychology and Psychiatry*, **3**, 1–15.

Bentovim, A., Boston, P. and van Elburg, A. (1987) Child sexual abuse – children and families referred to a treatment project and effects of intervention. *British Medical Journal*, **295**, 1453–1457.

Black, M. M. and Nitz, K. (1996) Grandmother co-residence, parenting, and child development among low-income, urban teen mothers. *Journal of Adolescent Health*, **18**, 218–226.

Bowen, M. (1978) *Family Therapy in Clinical Practice*. Northvale, NJ: Jason Aronson

Bowlby, J. (1949) The study and reduction of group tension in the family. *Human Relations*, **2**, 123–128.

Brent, D. A., Holder, D., Kolko, D., Birmaher, B., Baugher, M., Roth, C. *et al.* (1997) A clinical psychotherapy trial for adolescent depression comparing cognitive, family, and supportive therapy. *Archives of General Psychiatry*, 54 (9), 877–885.

Brent, D. A., Roth, C. M., Holder, D. P., Kolko, D. J., Birhamer, B., Johnson, B. A. *et al.* (1996) Psychosocial interventions for treating adolescent suicidal depression: a comparison of three psychosocial interventions. In E. D. Hibbs and P. S. Jensen (eds), *Child and Adolescent Disorders: Empirically based Strategies for Clinical Practice*. Washington, DC: American Psychological Association, pp. 187–206.

Brent, D. A., Kolko, D. J., Birhamer, B., Baugher, M., Bridge, J., Roth, C. *et al.* (1998) Predictors of treatment efficacy in a clinical trial of three psychosocial treatments for adolescent depression. *Journal of the American Academy of Child and Adolescent Psychiatry*, **37**, 906–914.

Brown, T. L., Swenson, C. C., Cunningham, P. B., Henggeler, S. W., Schoenwald, S. K. and Rowland, M. D. (1997) Multisystemic treatment of violent and chronic juvenile offenders: bridging the gap between research and practice. *Administration and Policy in Mental Health*, **25**, 221–238.

Byng Hall, J. (1995) *Rewriting Family Scripts*. New York: Guilford Press.

Campbell, T. L. and Patterson, J. M. (1995) The effectiveness of family interventions in the treatment of physical illness. *Journal of Marital and Family Therapy*, **21**, 545–583.

Carroll, L. (1867) *Alice's Adventures in Wonderland*. London: Dean & Son, chap. 2, p. 18.

Carter, E, and McGoldrick, M. (1980) *The Family Life Cycle*. New York: Gardner Press.

Cassidy, B., Zoccolillo, M. and Hughes, S. (1996) Psychopathology in adolescent mothers and its effect on mother–infant interactions: a pilot study. *Canadian Journal of Psychiatry/Revue Canadienne de Psychiatrie*, **41**, 379–3384.

Cohen-Kettenis, P. T, and van Goozen, S. H. M. (1997) Sex reassignment of adolescent transsexuals: a follow-up study. *Journal of the American Academy of Child and Adolescent Psychiatry*, **36**, 263–271.

Dare, C. and Eisler, I. (1995) Family therapy. In G. Szmukler and J. Dare (eds), *Treasure: Handbook of Eating Disorders. Theory, Treatment and Research*. Chichester: Wiley, pp. 333–349.

De Shazer, S. (1985) *Keys to Solutions in Brief Therapy*. New York: Norton.

Dulcan, M. K., Benson, R. S. (1997) AACAP Official Action. Summary of the practice parameters for the assessment and treatment of children adolescents and adults with ADHD. *Journal of the American Academy of Child and Adolescent Psychiatry*, 36, 1311–1317.

Durrant, M. and Kowalski, K. (1990) Overcoming effects of sexual abuse: developing a self perception of competence. In M. Durrant and C. White (eds), *Ideas for Therapy with Sexual Abuse*. Adelaide: Dulwich Centre, p. 69.

Edwards, M. E. and Steinglass, P. (1995) Family therapy treatment outcomes for alcoholism. *Journal of Marital and Family Therapy*, 21, 475–509.

Eisler, I., Dare, C., Russell, G., Szmukler, G. le Grange, D. and Dodge, E. (1997) Family and individual therapy in anorexia nervosa: a five-year follow-up of a controlled trial of family therapy in severe eating disorders. *Archives of General Psychiatry*, 54, 1025–1030.

Falaskas, C. (1997) Engagement and the therapeutic relationship in systemic therapy. *Journal of Family Therapy*, 19, 263–283.

Falloon, I. R. H. (1992) Early intervention for first episodes of schizophrenia: a preliminary exploration. *Psychiatry*, 55, 4–15.

Falloon, I. R. H., Boyd, J. L. and McGill, C. W. (1984) *Family Care of Schizophrenia: A Problem-solving Approach to the Treatment of Mental Illness*. New York, Guilford Press.

Falloon, I. R. H., Coverdale, J. H., Laidlaw, T. M., Merry, S. and Kydd, R. R. (1998) Early intervention for schizophrenic disorders: implementing optimal treatment strategies in routine clinical services. *British Journal of Psychiatry*, 172 (33S), 33–38.

Fishel, A. K. (1999) *Treating the Adolescent in Family Therapy: A Developmental and Narrative Approach*. Northvale: Jason Aronson.

Furniss, T., Bingley-Miller, L. and Bentovim, A. (1984) Therapeutic approach to sexual abuse. *Archives of Disease in Childhood*, 59, 865–870.

Gergen, K. J. (1985) The social constructionist movement in modern psychology. *American Psychologist*, 40, 266–275.

Goldner, V. (1991) Feminism and systemic practice: Two critical traditions in transition. *Journal of Family Therapy*, 13, 95–104.

Goldstein, M. J., Rodnick, E. H., Evans, J. R., May, P. R. A. and Steinberg, M. R. (1978) Drug and family therapy in the aftercare of acute schizophrenia. *Archives of General, Psychiatry*, 35, 1169–1177.

Gorell Barnes, G. (1990) The 'little woman' and the world of work. In R. J. Perelberg and A. C. Miller (eds), *Gender and Power in Families*. London: Tavistock/Routledge, pp. 221–244.

Gowers, S. and North, C. (1999) Difficulties in family functioning and adolescent anorexia nervosa. *British Journal of Psychiatry*, 174, 63–66.

Gowers, S., Norton, K., Halek, C. and Crisp, A. H. (1993) Outcome of outpatient psychotherapy in a random allocation treatment study of anorexia nervosa. *International Journal of Eating Disorders*, **15**, 165–177.

Grawe, K., Donati, R. and Bernauer, F. (1994) *Psychotherapie im Wandel – Von der Konfession zur Profession.* Göttingen: Hogrefe-Verlag für Psychologie.

Haley, J. (1976) *Problem-solving Therapy.* San Francisco, CA: Jossey-Bass.

Harrington, R., Kerfoot, M., Dyer, E., McNiven, F., Gill, J., Harrington, V. *et al.* (1998a) Randomized trial of a home-based family intervention for children who have deliberately poisoned themselves. *Journal of the American Academy of Child and Adolescent Psychiatry*, **37**, 512–518.

Harrington, R., Whittaker, J. and Shoebridge, P. (1998b) Psychological treatment of depression in children and adolescents. A review of treatment research. *The British Journal of Psychiatry*, **173**, 291–298.

Hawton, K., Arensman, E. and Townsend, E. (1998) *Cochrane Depression, Anxiety and Neurosis Group, The Cochrane Database of Systematic Reviews* 4. Oxford: Update Software.

Henggeler, S. W., Rodick, J. D., Borduin, C. M., Hanson, C. L., Watson, S. M. and Urey, J. R. (1986) Multisystemic treatment of juvenile offenders: effects on adolescent behaviour and family interaction.. *Developmental Psychology*, **22**, 132–141.

Henggeler, S. W. Borduin, C. M., Melton, G. B., Mann, B. J., Smith, L. A., Hall, J. A. *et al.* (1991) Effects of multisystemic therapy on drug use and abuse in serious juvenile offenders: a progress report from two outcome studies. *Family Dynamics of Addiction Quarterly*, **1**, 40–51.

Henggeler, S. W., Melton, G. B. and Smith, L. A. (1992) Family preservation using multisystemic therapy: an effective alternative to incarcerating serious juvenile offenders. *Journal of Consulting and Clinical Psychology*, **60**, 953–961.

Henggeler, S. W., Melton, G. B., Brondino, M. J., Scherer, D. G. and Hanley, J. H. (1997) Multisystemic therapy with violent and chronic offenders and their families: the role of treatment fidelity in successful dissemination. *Journal of Consulting and Clinical Psychology*, **65**, 821–833.

Herpertz, S. and Sass, H. (1997) Psychopathy and antisocial syndromes. *Current Opinion in Psychiatry*, **10**, 436–330.

Hodes, M. and Le Grange, D. (1993) Expressed Emotion in the investigation of eating disorders: a review. *International Journal of Eating Disorders*, **13**, 279–288.

Hodes, M., Dare, C., Dodge, E. and Eisler, I. (1999) The assessment of expressed emotion in a standardised family interview. *Journal of Child Psychology and Psychiatry*, **40**, 617–625.

Hoffman, L. (1988) A constructivist position for family therapy. *British Journal of Psychology*, **9**, 110–129.

Hoffman, L. (1993) *Exchanging Voices.* London: Karnac, p. 31.

Hogarty, G. E., Anderson, C. M., Reiss, D. J., Kornblith, S. J., Greenwald, D. P., Ulrich, R. F. *et al.* (1991) Family psycho-education, social skills training, and the maintenance chemotherapy in the aftercare treatment of schizophrenia: II. Two-year effects of a controlled study on relapse and adjustment. *Archives of General Psychiatry*, **48**, 340–347.

Horesh, N., Apter, A., Ishai, J., Danziger, Y., Miculincer, M., Stein, D. *et al.* (1996) Abnormal psychosocial situations and eating disorders in adolescence. *Journal of the American Academy of Child and Adolescent Psychiatry*, **35**, 921–927.

Jenkins, A. (1990) *Invitations to Responsibility: The Therapeutic Engagement of Men who are Violent and Abusive*. Adelaide: Dulwich Centre.

Jones, E. (1993) *Family Systems Therapy*. Chichester: Wiley.

Jones, E. (1996) The gender of the therapist as contribution to meaning in therapy. *Human Systems: The Journal of Systemic Consultation and Management*, **7**, 237–245.

Kazdin, A. E. (1996) *Conduct Disorder in Childhood and Adolescence*. Thousand Oaks, CA: Sage.

Knapp, E. K. and Harris, E. S. (1998) Consultation-liaison in child psychiatry – a review of the past 10 years. Part II: Research on treatment approaches and outcomes. *Journal of American Academy of Child and Adolescent Psychiatry*, **37**, 139–146.

Krause, I. B and Miller, A. (1995) Culture and family therapy. In S. Fernando (ed.), *Mental Health in a Multiethnic Society*. London: Routledge, pp. 149–171.

Landen, M., Walinder, J., Hambert, G. and Lundstrom, B. (1998) Factors predictive of regret in sex reassignment. *Acta Psychiatric Scandinavica*, **97**, 284–289.

Leff, J. P. and Vaughn, C. (1985) *Expressed Emotion in Families*. New York: Guilford Press.

Leff, J. P., Kuipers, L., Berkowitz, R., Eberlein-Vries, R. and Sturgeon, D. (1982) A controlled trial of social intervention in the families of schizophrenic patients. *British Journal of Psychiatry*, **141**, 121–134.

Le Grange, D., Eisler, I., Dare, C. and Hodes, M. (1992) Family criticism and self starvation: a study of expressed emotion. *Journal of Family Therapy*, **14**, 177–192.

Lieberman, S. (1980) *Transgenerational Family Therapy*. London: Croom Helm.

Madanes, C. (1974) *Strategic Family Therapy*. San Francisco, CA: Jossey Bass.

March, J. S. and Leonhard, H. L. (1996) Obsessive-compulsive disorder in children and adolescents: a review of the past 10 years. *Journal of the American Academy of Child and Adolescent Psychiatry*, **35**, 1265–1273.

March, J. S. and Mulle, K. (1996) Banishing OCD: cognitive-behavioural psychotherapy for obsessive-compulsive disorders. In E. D. Hibbs and P. S. Jensen (eds), *Child and Adolescent Disorders: Empirically based Strategies for*

Clinical Practice. Washington, DC: American Psychological Association, pp. 83–102.

McCullough, M. and Sherman, A. (1998) Family-of-origin interaction and adolescent mother's potential for child abuse. *Adolescence*, **33**, 375–384.

McFadyen, A. (1997) Rapprochement in sight? Postmodern family therapy and psychoanalysis. *Journal of Family Therapy*, **19**, 233–240.

McGill, C. W. and Lee, E. (1986) Family psychoeducational intervention in the treatment of schizophrenia. *Bulletin of the Menninger Clinic*, **50**, 269–285.

McGoldrick, M. and Gerson, R. (1985) *Geneograms in Family Assessment.* New York: Guilford Press.

McKay, D. and Pollard, J. (1996) Community support networks in education and care settings. In M. Göpfert, J. Webster and M. V. Seeman (eds), *Parental Psychiatric Disorder: Distressed Parents and their Families.* Cambridge: Cambridge University Press.

Micucci, J. A. (1998) *The Adolescent in Family Therapy. Breaking the Cycle of Conflict and Control.* New York: Guilford.

Miklowitz, D. J. (1995) The evolution of family-based psychopathology. In R. H. Mikesell, D. D. Lusterman and S. H. McDaniel (eds), *Integrating Family Therapy: Handbook of Family Psychology and Systems Theory.* Washington, DC: American Psychological Association, pp. 183–197.

Minuchin, S. (1967) *Families of the Slums.* New York: Basic Books.

Minuchin, S. and Fishman H. C. (1981) *Family Therapy Techniques.* Cambridge, MA: Harvard University Press.

Minuchin, S., Rosman, B. L. Baker, L. (1978) *Psychosomatic Families: Anorexia Nervosa in Context.* Cambridge, MA: Harvard University Press.

Musick, J. S. (1993) *Young, Poor and Pregnant: The Psychology of Teenage Motherhood.* New Haven, CT: Yale University Press.

Neimeyer, R. A. and Ruskin, J. D. (2000) *Constructions of Disorder: Meaning-making Frameworks for Psychotherapy.* Washington D.C.: American Psychology Association.

Panton, J. and White, E. A. (1999; last substantive update 1996) Family therapy for asthma in children (Cochrane Review). *The Cochrane Library 1.* Oxford: Update Software.

Panzarine, S., Slater, E. and Sharps, P. (1995) Coping, social support, and depressive symptoms in adolescent mothers. *Journal of Adolescent Health*, **17**, 113–119.

Penn, P. (1982) Circular questioning. *Family Process*, **21**, 267–280.

Penn, P. (1985) Feed-forward: future questions, future maps. *Family Process*, **24**, 299–310.

Perelberg, R. and Miller, A. (1990) *Gender and Power in Families.* London: Routledge.

Price, J. A. (1996) *Power and Compassion: Working with Difficult Adolescents and Abused Parents.* New York: Guilford.

Procter, H. G. (1996) The family construct system. In D. Kalekin-Fishman and B. M. Walker (eds), *The Construction of Group Realities: Culture, Society and Personal Construct Theory*. Malaba, FL: Krieger, pp. 161–180.

Procter, H. G. and Walker, G. (1988) Brief therapy. In E. Street and W. Dryden (eds), *Family Therapy in Britain*. Milton Keynes: Open University Press, pp. 127–149.

Ravenscroft, K. (1996) Family therapy. In M. Lewis (ed.), *Child and Adolescent Psychiatry: A Comprehensive Textbook*. Baltimore, MD: Williams & Wilkins, pp. 848–862.

Reiner, G. W. (1996) Case study: sex-reassignment in a teenage girl. *Journal of the American Academy of Child and Adolescent Psychiatry*, 35, 799–803.

Renaud, J., Brent, D. A., Baugher, M., Birmaher, B., Kolko, D. J. and Bridge, J. (1998) Rapid response to psychosocial treatment for adolescent depression: a two-year follow-up. *Journal of the American Academy of Child and Adolescent Psychiatry*, 37, 1184–1190.

Rice, M., Harris, G. and Cormier, C. (1992) An evaluation of a maximum security therapeutic community for psychopaths and other mentally disordered offenders. *Law and Human Behaviour*, 16, 399–412.

Robin, A. L., Siegel, P. T., Koepke, T. Moye, A. W. and Tice, S. (1994) Family therapy versus individual therapy for adolescent females with anorexia nervosa. *Journal of Developmental and Behavioural Paediatrics*, 15, 111–116.

Roth, A. and Fonagy, P. (1996) *What Works for Whom? A Critical Review of Psychotherapy Research*. New York: Guilford Press.

Roy, R. and Frankel, H. (1995) *How Good is Family Therapy? A Reassessment*. Toronto: Toronto University Press.

Russell, G. F. M., Szmukler, G., Dare, C. and Eisler, I. (1987) An evaluation of family therapy in anorexia nervosa and bulimia nervosa. *Archives of General Psychiatry*, 44, 1047–1056.

Ryle, A. (1989) *Cognitive-Analytic Therapy: Active Participation in Change*. Chichester: Wiley.

Schmidt, G. L. and Bonjean, M. J. (1995) Family therapy education for psychiatry residents: a pilot study of efficacy. *Academic Psychiatry*, 19, 74–80.

Seligman, M. E. P. (1995) The effectiveness of psychotherapy: The Consumer Report Study. *American Psychologist*, 50, 965–974. Also: http://www.apa.org/journals/seligman.html

Selvini-Palazzoli M., Boscolo L., Cecchin G. and Prata G. (1978) *Paradox and Counterparadox*. New York: Aronson.

Selvini-Palazzoli, M., Boscolo, L., Cecchin G. and Prata G (1980) Hypothesising–circularity–neutrality: three guidelines for the conductor of the session. *Family Process*, 19, 3–12.

Skynner, A. C. R. (1969) A group-analytic approach to conjoint family therapy. *Journal of Child Psychology and Psychiatry*, 10, 81– 106.

Skynner, A. C. R. (1976) *One Flesh: Separate Persons*. London: Constable.

Sprenkle, D. H., Blow, H. A. and Dickey, M. H. (1999) Common factors and other non-technique variables in marital and family therapy. In M. A. Hubble, B. L. Duncan, S. D. Miller (eds) *The Heart and Soul of Change: What Works in Therapy?* Washington D.C.: American Psychological Association.

Stanton, M. D. and Shadish, W. R. (1997) Outcome, attrition, and family-couples treatment for drug use: a meta-analysis and review of controlled, comparative studies. *Psychological Bulletin*, **122**, 170–191.

Steiner, H. and Lock, J. (1998) Anorexia nervosa and bulimia nervosa in children and adolescents: a review of the past 10 years. *Journal of the American Academy of Child and Adolescent Psychiatry*, 37, 352–359.

Stoep, A. V., Williams, M., Jones, R., Green, L. and Trupin, E. (1999) Families as full research partners: what is in it for us? *Journal of Behavioural Health Sciences and Research*, **216**, 329–344.

Target, M. and Fonagy, P. (1996) The psychological treatment of child and adolescent psychiatric disorders. In A. Roth and P. Fonagy (eds), *What Works for Whom? A Critical Review of Psychotherapy Research*. New York: Guilford Press, pp. 263–320.

Thrower S. M., Bruce W. E. and Walters R. F. (1982) The family circle method for integrating family systems concepts in family medicine. *Journal of Family Practice*, 15, 451–457

Tomm, K. (1988) Interventive interviewing: part III. Intending to ask lineal, circular, strategic and reflexive questions. *Family Process*, 27, 1–15.

Tomson, M. (1998) Basic Guide 9. *Family Circles*. In Thinking Families Newsletter, October.

Tooth, B. (1996) Group construing: the impact of professional training. In D. Kalekin-Fishman and B. M. Walker (eds), *The Construction of Group Realities: Culture, Society and Personal Construct Theory*. Malaba, FL: Krieger, pp. 243–266

Trad, P. (1995) Mental health of adolescent mothers. *Journal of the American Academy of Child and Adolescent Psychiatry*, 34, 130–142.

von Bertalanffy, L. (1968) *General System Theory: Foundations, Development, Applications*. Harmondswoth: Penguin.

von Foerster, H. (1981) *Observing Systems*. Seaside, CA: Intersystems.

von Glaserfeld, E. (1984) An introduction to radical constructivism. In P. Watzlawick (ed.), *The Invented Reality*. New York: Norton, pp. 17–40.

Waldegrave, C. (1990) *Social Justice and Family Therapy. Dulwich Centre Newsletter*. Adelaide: Dulwich Centre.

Walters, M. (1990) A feminist perspective in family therapy. In R. Perelberg and A. Miller (eds), *Gender and Power in Families*. London: Routledge, pp. 13–33.

Ward, M. J. and Carlson, E. A. (1995) Associations among adult attachment representations, maternal sensitivity, and infant–mother attachment in a sample of adolescent mothers. *Child Development*, **66**, 69–79.

Watzlawick, P., Beavin J. and Jackson, D. (1967) *Pragmatics of Human Communication: A Study of Interactional Patterns, Pathologies and Paradoxes*. New York: W. W. Norton.

Weakland, J., Fisch, R., Watzlawick, P. and Bodin, A. (1974) Brief therapy: focused problem resolution. *Family Process*, **13**, 141–168.

Webster-Stratton, C. and Herbert, M. (1994) *Troubled Families. Problem Children*. Chichester: Wiley.

Weinberg, N. Z., Rahdert, E., Colliver, J. D. and Glantz, M. D. (1998) Adolescent substance abuse: A review of the last 10 years. *Journal of the American Academy of Child and Adolescent Psychiatry*, **37**, 252–261.

Weisz, J. R., Weiss, B. and Donenberg, G. R. (1992) The lab versus the clinic: effects of child and adolescent psychotherapy. *The American Psychologist*, **47**, 1578–1585.

Weisz, J. R., Donenberg, G. R., Han, S. S. and Weiss, B. (1995a) Bridging the gap between laboratory and clinic in child and adolescent psychotherapy. *Journal of Consulting and Clinical Psychology*, **65**, 688–701.

Weisz, J. R., Donenberg, G. R., Han, S. S. and Kauneckis, D. (1995b) Child and adolescent psychotherapy outcomes in experiments versus clinics: why the disparity. *Journal of Abnormal Child Psychology*, **23**(1), 83–106.

Wetchler, J. L. and Piercy, F. P. (1996) Transgenerational family therapies. In F. P. Piercy, D. H. Sprenkle, J. L. Wetchler and Associates (eds), *Family Therapy Sourcebook*. New York: Guilford Press, pp. 25–49.

White, M. and Epston, D. (1990) *Narrative Means to Therapeutic Ends*. New York: Norton.

White M (1984) Pseudo encopresis: from avalanche to victory, from vicious to virtuous cycles. *Family Systems Medicine*, **2**, 150–160.

Wichstrom, L. (1995) Social, psychological and physical correlates of eating problems. A study of the general adolescent population in Norway. *Psychological Medicine*, **25**, 567–580.

Wiener, N. (1961) *Cybernetics*. Cambridge, MA: MIT Press.

Wilson, J. (1998) *Child-Focused Practice*. London: Karnac.

Worden, M. (1999) *Family Therapy Basics*. Pacific Grove, CA: Brooks/Cole.

York, A. and Hill, P. (1999) Treating depression in children and adolescents. *Current Opinion in Psychiatry*, **12**, 77–80.

Zawidowki, E. (1999) *Single Session Family Staging: Breaking Family Spells*. London: Free Association Books.

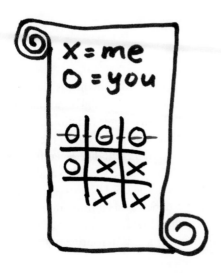

Chapter 22

OUTCOMES IN ADOLESCENT PSYCHIATRY

Simon G. Gowers

INTRODUCTION

There are a number of challenging issues in the assessment of outcomes in adolescent psychiatry. Some of these are generic problems of outcome assessment, but there are some unique challenges for our speciality. Eyberg *et al.* (1998), for example, have drawn attention to the need to take a developmental perspective in adolescent outcome research. Such an approach considers the range of normal development, the natural history of adolescent disorder and the age of maximum risk for its development. How many depressed adolescents, for example, go on to be depressed adults? What are the links between juvenile delinquency and adult criminality or other antisocial behaviours? What is the incidence of schizophrenia in each of the teenage years? Although the evidence base in our speciality has grown in the last 10 years, with a concomitant expansion in Britain of academic posts, research remains behind that in adult mental health. Hartmann (1998), in a useful editorial, argues that those involved in adolescent psychiatric research face particular difficulties of funding and of recruitment of clinical series due to the complexity of issues in the epidemiology of adolescent disorders, the organisation of services, and issues of consent and ethics.

This chapter will start by examining some of the issues in outcome evaluation, particularly with respect to adolescent mental health and the natural history of adolescent disorder. Secondly, and drawing on the earlier chapters, it will examine the effectiveness of interventions for these disorders. Finally, in a climate that increasingly stresses the importance of audit and evaluation, it will examine the demonstrable outcomes of adolescent mental health services.

GENERAL ISSUES IN OUTCOME ASSESSMENT

RELIABILITY

Although reliability data are published for standardised instruments as they are developed, the fact remains that different raters may not agree about an adolescent's level of functioning at a given time, whilst his or her functioning may vary to some extent from day to day. Much attention has been given to the inter-rater reliability of psychiatric diagnoses (e.g. Rey *et al.*, 1989). The reliability of most major diagnostic categories is said to be high (κ values between 0.6 and 0.8), whilst that for the subcategories is considerably lower. The US–UK cross- national study of diagnostic reliability of conduct, attention deficit and emotional disorder (Prendergast *et al.*, 1988) suggested, however, that highly trained researchers demonstrate much greater levels of agreement than clinicians in routine practice.

VALIDITY

This is concerned with whether a given test or assessment measures what it is designed to, whether it predicts outcome or whether its findings are generalisable, e.g. across cultures. The Eating Disorders Inventory is an example of a self-rated questionnaire, which has a subscale of 'Body Dissatisfaction'. Its value depends on whether it does indeed measure dissatisfaction with one's body and whether the scores it produces discriminate those for whom the test is likely to be used (i.e. those with eating disorders) from controls. Does it have predictive power in the sense that high scorers have a different course or respond to different intervention than low scorers? If this predictive power applies for white American teenagers, is it valid for black African subjects?

TIMING OF 'OUTCOME'

A distinction needs to be made between short-term symptom remission, behavioural change masking ongoing symptoms and longer-term outcome. Has the outcome been assessed during treatment, at the end of treatment or at follow-up some time later? When evaluating the effectiveness of an inpatient admission, for example, should outcome be assessed on discharge or later? On those occasions when there is a deterioration in functioning in the weeks following discharge, it is important to consider whether this represents a failure of the intervention, a relapse or possibly an unwanted effect of the admission (such as disruption of school attendance or peer relationships).

SENSITIVITY TO CHANGE

An outcome measure should ideally be sensitive enough to change that brief interventions can be evaluated. If the 'time-frame' under consideration at outcome review is too great (e.g. the previous 3 months), it may include the period of time before the intervention. A related issue concerns the difficulty in evaluating the outcome of episodic behaviours. If a teenager has committed three very violent assaults at 6-monthly intervals, how long a follow-up is required to assess whether this behaviour has been reduced or extinguished?

SPECIFIC ISSUES FOR ADOLESCENT PSYCHIATRY

Other branches of medicine often use very reliable, 'black and white' variables such as death rates as an outcome measure (either for a disorder, such as lung cancer, or for an intervention, such as a specific form of surgery). Alternatively they assess 'quality of life', which generally considers the current state against a steady and optimal pre-morbid level of functioning. An example might include the ability to wash and dress oneself or walk up a flight of stairs. Fortunately death is a rare outcome in our speciality, but quality of life is difficult to measure against a background of changing development and where limitations on quality of life tend to be subjective.

Some case examples may illustrate some of the points that need to be taken into account in considering outcomes.

- The first example concerns a 15-year-old girl who was very underweight at 35 kg before treatment. After 3 months treatment in an adolescent service, her weight had risen to an average 50 kg.
- A second 15-year-old girl also presented at 35 kg. A year later her weight was again 35 kg.
- A third 15 year old presented with mild depression. After 3 months she was more severely depressed.
- The parents of another girl were at their wits end with worry. Six months later they felt much better informed and able to cope.
- Another girl was attending school reliably. Four months later, she refused to attend.

Which of these cases have a good and which have a poor outcome?

The point here is that all the above descriptions concern the same patient. One gets a different view, depending on which symptom or behaviour is examined, whose view one takes, or when the outcome is measured. How then does one rate the relative merits of symptom change against social adjustment or clinical outcome against consumer satisfaction?

A review by Osher (1998) considers further the choice of appropriate target for outcome measurement and the perspective to measure outcomes from, i.e. that of the child, family, referrer or treating therapist. This article also points to the importance of taking context into account when evaluating outcome. Eddy *et al.* (1998) agree that the main issues in outcome measurement are the decision concerning which changes to measure, when and how. They also point to the need to consider mediating variables, when reporting outcomes.

WHAT IS THE GENERAL OUTCOME OF ADOLESCENT DISORDERS?

The chapters on individual disorders review this in detail. A few selected examples are highlighted in the following sections.

SCHIZOPHRENIA

Schultz *et al.* (1998) note that brain imaging studies suggest a continuity between adolescent and adult forms of the disorder in which the early-onset form can be considered to be more severe. Thus the adolescent form of schizophrenia may require especially energetic early intervention. These authors suggest that the newer atypical drugs might be especially indicated for this age group, due to relatively greater intolerance to the older preparations and consequent difficulties with compliance. McGorry (1998) shares this view of the importance of early intervention, in an argument for early preventive strategies from a psychosocial perspective.

SUBSTANCE MISUSE

The outcome of adolescent substance misuse appears poor. Myers *et al.* (1998) followed up 137 adolescents treated for substance misuse after four years. Sixty-one percent achieved DSM-III-R criteria for 'Antisocial personality disorder' and demonstrated poor functioning over a range of life domains. Poor outcome was associated with previous conduct disorder, particularly before the age of 10, diversity of deviancy and extensive pre-treatment drug use.

EMOTIONAL DISORDERS

The prognosis for an episode of depression appears to be good (see Chapter 4), though the risk of relapse is high. Those with an adult form of the disorder, i.e. with biological features and those without co-morbid conduct disorder, appear most at risk of a chronic course (Harrington, 1992).

Obsessive-compulsive disorder appears to follow a variable course with one-third remitting spontaneously and possibly 50% going on to have the disorder into adulthood (see Chapter 4).

Psychosomatic disorders appear to often have a good outcome though early adverse experience, with disorder of attachment, particularly where physical ill health is part of the picture, may predispose to chronic somatoform disorder extending into adulthood (see Chapter 10).

CONDUCT DISORDER

There is evidence that rates of minor conduct disorder reduce through adolescence. Cohen *et al.* (1993) give prevalence rates for boys of 16% at 10–13 years, dropping to 9.5% at 17–20%, whilst rates for girls are reported to peak at 14–16 years (9.2%) before dropping to 7.1% at 17–20 years.

Although the frequency of aggressive acts reduces with age, the potential to cause harm and the severity of attacks tends to increase. Whilst law-breaking gradually reduces in early adulthood, social and personality dysfunction continues (Farrington *et al.*, 1990)

EATING DISORDERS

The outcome of adolescent eating disorder does appear to be better than for those arising in adulthood. Predictors of good outcome include healthy family functioning by patient rating or clinician assessment and a severe negative life event precipitant (North *et al.*, 1997). Achievement of a weight below 65% of expected weight seems to be a negative prognostic feature. Admission to hospital, particularly for extensive psychiatric treatment is often associated with a poor outcome (Gowers *et al.*, 2000). Clearly cases with a number of adverse physical and psychological features are likely to be selected for admission, but it is probable that the negative effects of loss of schooling, on peer relationships and on self-esteem are underestimated.

WHAT IS THE EVIDENCE FOR THE EFFECTIVENESS OF TREATMENT?

GENERAL

A cautionary note has been sounded by Patton (1998) in an Editorial assessing the impact of adolescent psychiatry to reduce the burden of mental disorder over the past 25 years. He found little evidence that adolescent psychiatry was able to reduce psychopathology and disability from common disorders such as depression and substance misuse, in the long term. Kazdin and Weisz (1998) have considered the challenges in interpreting outcome research and report the most recent broad-based meta-analyses of treatment studies in child and adolescent research. These are said to show an effect size of 0.71, indicating that after treatment the average child is less symptomatic on various outcome measures than 76% of non-treated controls. They point also to the chief deficiencies in outcome research, i.e. focus on brief interventions designed for research, rather than typically used therapies, short follow-up and focus on symptom change rather than impairment or adaptation. They also claim that research publications rarely give adequate attention to mediators of change. Difficulties evaluating outcome research in child mental health abound, including failure to report basic data (Chorpita *et al.*, 1998). Such omissions include poorly defined patient groups, presence or absence of co-morbidity, poorly defined (non-manualised) interventions and lack of explanation of their presumed mechanisms of action.

A review of 10 years of consultation-liaison services (Knapp and Harris, 1998) demonstrated a shift over this time from descriptive articles to those describing interventions and measuring outcomes. These authors conclude that child psychiatrists are significantly better equipped than 10 years ago to use their growing skills in innovative ways.

PSYCHOTHERAPIES

A number of reviews have been critical of reports of the therapeutic outcome of child psychotherapy. Hibbs (1998), collating the views of a workshop convened by the National Institute of Mental Health, The MacArthur Foundation and The Child and Adolescent Psychosocial Interventions Consortium, highlighted a number of issues. These included the need to define psychotherapeutic interventions, their mechanisms of action, intensity and duration, and the effects of co-morbidity on outcomes.

Cognitive-behaviour therapy has yielded encouraging findings in depression in particular (Harrington, 1992), whilst its positive value as part of the psychosocial package for psychoses and in eating disorders in adults suggests that trials on younger patient samples are required.

Family therapy has been found to be more effective than individual therapy in the treatment of adolescent eating disorders after discharge from inpatient weight restoration (Eisler *et al.*, 1997). A family-based intervention, however, was found to be no more effective than 'routine care' in the treatment of adolescent self harm (Byford *et al.*, 1999).

Kibby *et al.* (1998) reviewed the effectiveness of psychological interventions in children and adolescents with chronic medical conditions using a meta-analysis of 42 outcome studies. They concluded that these interventions generally produced positive effects on disease management, emotional and behavioural problems, health promotion, and prevention. Furthermore, these gains were still evident at 12-month follow-up.

PHARMACOTHERAPY

The evaluation of newer atypical antipsychotic drugs in adolescent schizophrenia continues (Shultz *et al.*, 1998), with some promising results. The impact of antidepressant medication on depressive disorder remains uncertain (Hazell *et al.*, 1995), though early trials of selective serotonin reuptake inhibitors (SSRIs) are promising (Emslie *et al.*, 1997).

The effectiveness of methylphenydate in attention deficit hyperactivity disorder (ADHD) appears beyond doubt. Whilst 10 years ago, children were often withdrawn from this medication in adolescence, there is a growing case for continuation, if not commencement, in adolescence. Research into the long-term outcome of cases treated into adulthood is awaited.

PREVENTION PROGRAMMES

Harrington and Clark (1998) have reviewed the possibilities for primary and secondary prevention in reducing levels of depression in a population, and concluded that treatment and rehabilitation programmes will be more effective than primary prevention programmes, for the foreseeable future.

Durlak (1998) has considered the role of risk and protective factors in successful prevention programmes, based on a review of 1200 outcome studies. Many social and family risk and protective factors appeared to inter-relate, thus their possible causal relationship to outcome is unclear.

THE EVALUATION OF ADOLESCENT MENTAL HEALTH SERVICES

The systematic literature review and conceptual model of Hoagwood and colleagues (Hoagwood *et al.*, 1996; Jensen *et al.*, 1996) has offered a salutary lesson in research methodology in service outcome measurement. They defined five outcome domains, i.e. symptoms/diagnosis, functioning, consumer perspectives, environments and systems, and predicted that with the expansion of managed care, research into the efficacy of specific interventions or services will require credible evidence of their impact on all salient outcome domains.

In their review, only 38 studies met their required scientific criteria The same group have discussed the tensions in outcome research between clinical flexibility and scientific standardisation. They argue that standardised scientific protocols can undermine patient compliance if they do not involve them in goal setting and treatment planning. Hernandez *et al.* (1998) provide a conceptual and practical framework to the evaluation of outcomes through an emphasis on involving key stakeholders in the identification of outcomes to be measured and integrating outcome information in the service's decision making process.

Beck *et al.* (1998) have drawn attention to the value of outcome measurement to both service providers and purchasers. They describe the evolution of an outcome evaluation and monitoring system (SumOne for Kids) over 4 years and argue for functional rather than clinical outcomes. The project is presented in a way which is designed for replication. Glisson and Hemmelgarn (1998), in an interesting study of organisational 'climate' in Tennessee, drew attention to staff factors such as burnout, stress, job satisfaction and conflict as predictors of service quality and outcomes, arguing that more attention should be given to these factors rather than service configuration alone. Rosenblatt et al. (1998), meanwhile, described a model of continuing monitoring of outcomes and costs of service delivery employed in a Californian Youth Service. Key components include constant feedback at child, family and system level and selection of outcomes offering maximum value for all stakeholders.

Bickman et al. (1997) have used routine outcome measurement to cast doubts on the benefits of the American 'systems of care'. They compared two different types of service in a randomised trial of severely emotionally disturbed children and adolescents. There were no differences in 6-month follow up of symptoms and functioning for 350 families allocated to either traditional care or an 'exemplary' system of care. This finding appeared to replicate a similar result from the earlier Fort Bragg study (Bickman et al., 1996).

A British study (Leff and Bennett, 1998) examined referral pathways and outcomes in the care of emotionally and behaviourally disturbed children. The aim was to establish the necessity for referral guidelines for community child health staff, in ensuring that child and adolescent mental health services (CAMHS) focus on the most needy children with emotional and behavioural difficulties. They concluded that although the 9% of cases referred to CAMHS were generally appropriate, guidelines could be useful in assisting decision making. They suggested that early intervention by CAMHS could be very effective in reducing behavioural problems but that interventions needed to span 6 months or more to cover the possibility of relapse.

In 1998 and 1999, a number of UK policy initiatives focussed on proposals to improve the outcomes of CAMHS. The Quality Protects Initiative (Department of Health, 1998), for example, stressed the importance of early intervention in bringing about desired long-term outcomes.

Then the Audit Commission's review of CAMHS (Audit Commission, 1999) highlighted major inequalities around the country in staffing and budgeting of services. It also drew attention to the severity and complexity of cases presenting to most services.

Until recently, the evaluation of adolescent mental health services tended to be concerned with audit and process outcomes. More recently the routine measurement of clinical outcomes has begun to be addressed, not just by research groups, but by generic services.

AUDIT IN ADOLESCENT PSYCHIATRY

The NHS White Paper *Working for Patients* (1989) defines audit as the systematic, critical analysis of the quality of care. This includes the procedures used for diagnosis and treatment, the use of resources and the resulting outcome and quality of life for patients. Audit involves the setting and review of standards in the expectation of improvement of the quality of care, with an emphasis on the cyclical process of measurement and changing practice.

The components of audit include resources, process and outcome. Resources include the personnel, buildings and facilities available within the adolescent service, whilst it is also generally appropriate to include here consideration of such variables as the sociodemographic characteristics of the population under consideration, such as the Jarman index of deprivation (Jarman, 1983). The importance of taking such factors into account in assessing outcomes has been highlighted in education. Here consideration of school performance in published league tables clearly needs to take account of such factors as parental attitudes to education and baseline levels of attainment. The concept of 'added value' concerns the effect of an intervention over and above the predicted natural history.

Process involves the procedures of diagnosis and treatment. Until recently, given a number of theoretical difficulties in outcome measurement in psychiatry, much outcome measurement concerned process outcomes. These included throughput of patients, length of stay and waiting times both for first appointments and also in the waiting room, before being seen. Although there must be some relationship between efficiency and outcome, waiting time and customer satisfaction, the measurement of process outcomes often appears to put quantity above quality (Blackman, 1997). This may lead to such spurious conclusions as that an adolescent unit admission of 4 weeks is twice as good as one of 8 weeks whatever the clinical outcome.

The Scottish Child and Adolescent Audit Group (Hoare *et al.*, 1996) have, however, demonstrated how a large audit study can usefully elucidate aspects of such services, and have demonstrated a number of relationships between child, family and treatment variables.

Computer packages available for clinical audit in adolescent psychiatry are rapidly being developed. Features of an ideal system for adolescent psychiatry should include the following: affordability, user-friendliness, time-saving ability, and an ability to meet the needs of clinicians and managers simultaneously, whilst providing data for research (Sein, 1991). In addition it should be appropriately maintained and supported, and be flexible enough to support the individual needs of a particular service. To save duplication of effort it should link with other systems, to enable comparison with other similar services.

CONSUMER PERSPECTIVES AND SATISFACTION

Several recent publications have drawn attention to the importance of incorporating consumer perspectives into comprehensive service evaluations (Jensen *et al.*, 1996; Osher, 1998), although this is a relatively neglected area in practice.

Satisfaction does itself cover a number of areas, such as the comfort of surroundings and how service users feel they have been treated. In Britain, recent attention has focussed on such quality issues as the provision of information in a range of languages and the availability of interpreters. It seems reasonable to assume that levels of satisfaction are going to depend to some extent on expectation. One satisfaction study (Gowers and Kushlick, 1992) demonstrated that in general parents were more satisfied than adolescents with assessment in an adolescent service, but that the most crucial factor in determining their satisfaction was whether they agreed with the referral or otherwise. Those who had been referred by a third party without their full agreement were rarely satisfied with the opinion received. Interestingly, there was also an inverse association between satisfaction and complexity of treatment offered. That is to say, those receiving just an opinion or advice were generally happier than those offered ongoing outpatient management, whilst those recommended inpatient admission were least satisfied! One interesting study drawing attention to the need for multiple measures from multiple perspectives (Lambert et al., 1998) compared consumer satisfaction with outcome of psychopathology by different raters. It showed few associations.

REFERRERS' VIEWS

Many adolescent services, particularly where they incorporate an inpatient facility, are tertiary services drawing referrals from other professionals either in community mental health services or elsewhere in the community. Referrers are therefore also customers of such services. It may seem difficult in developing a service to balance the needs of different disciplines who bring a range of different perspectives to bear on adolescent problems. One survey (Gowers et al., 1991), however, suggested there is a great deal of agreement across disciplines about what is most required from an adolescent service. In this case it included urgent response to requests for assessment, good communication and provision of inpatient beds.

CLINICAL OUTCOME MEASUREMENT

The systematic literature review of Hunter et al. (1996) remains an important starting point from which to consider the merits of existing symptom questionnaires, interview schedules and general outcome measures. This review anticipated the results of the field trials of the Department of Health's general outcome measure for CAMHS, the Health of the Nation Outcome Scales for Child and Adolescent Mental Health (HoNOSCA). These scales measure a range of problem areas in the domains of symptoms, behaviours, impairments and social adjustment. They are designed to be used as a measure of severity at first assessment or as an outcome or change measure when rated at two or more time-points. Each rating takes 5–10 min. The field trials demonstrated HoNOSCA's satisfactory psychometric properties and suggested that the scales are acceptable to clinicians from a range of disciplines (Gowers *et al.*, 1999a,b).

The UK Audit Commission incorporated HoNOSCA into their recent review of CAMHS (Audit Commission, 1999). Although this exercise was conducted without the recommended training (Gowers *et al.*, 1998), it did help add to the growing belief in the importance of routine outcome measurement for generic CAMHS.

Yates *et al.* (1999) reported a comparison between HoNOSCA and the Paddington Complexity Scale (PCS) in three CAMHS. Both were found to be useful in describing clinical intakes to CAMHS and were sensitive to differences in patient populations in the three services. They correlated only weakly with parent and child measures of behaviour and quality of life. Subsequently, its sensitivity to change, reliability and validity have been confirmed (Garralda *et al.*, 2000). Clinician-rated outcome measures need to be balanced by the perspectives of young people and their families. The user version of HoNOSCA currently being piloted may be a useful contributor to this need for balance. The associations between clinician and family views of childrens' problem behaviour is often low (Yates *et al.*, 1999).

CONCLUSIONS

The last few years have seen a considerable growth in outcome research in three areas: the outcome of specific disorders, the impact of therapies and service evaluation. The importance of considering methodological issues in outcome measurement has implications for those in routine generic services as well as those involved in formal research. The critical reviews highlighting deficiencies in much child and adolescent outcome research ought to lead to improvements in future research design. It is encouraging that measures are increasingly becoming available for routine service use and that clinicians from the range of disciplines represented in CAMHS appear to be embracing them with some enthusiasm. The important contribution of users into outcome assessment is likely to continue to grow.

REFERENCES

Audit Commission (1999) *Children in Mind: Child and Adolescent Mental Health Services*. Abingdon: Audit Commission Publications.

Beck, S. A., Meadowcroft, P., Mason, M. and Kiely, E. S. (1998) Multiagency outcome evaluation of children's services: a case study. *Journal of Behavioural Health Services and Research*, **25**, 163–175.

Bickman, L., Heflinger, C. A, Lambert, E. W. and Summerfelt, W. T. (1996) The Fort Bragg Managed Care Experiment: short term impact on psychopathology. *Journal of Child and Family Studies*, 5, 137–160.

Bickman, L., Summerfelt, W. T. and Noser, K. (1997) Comparative outcomes of emotionally disturbed children and adolescents in a system of services and usual care. *Psychiatric Services*, 48, 1543–1548.

Blackman, C. (1997) Auditing CAMHS. *Young Minds Magazine*, 33, 4–5.

Byford, S., Harrington R. C., Torgerson, D., Kerfoot, M., Dyer, E., Harrington, V. et al. (1999) Cost effective analysis of a home based social work intervention for children and adolescents who have deliberately poisoned themselves. *British Journal of Psychiatry*, 174, 56–62.

Chorpita, B. F., Barlow, D. H., Albano, A. M. and Daleiden, E. L. (1998) Methodological strategies in child clinical trials: advancing the efficacy and effectiveness of psychosocial treatments. *Journal of Abnormal Child Psychology*, 26, 7–16.

Cohen, P., Cohen, J., Kasen, S. and Velez, C. N. (1993) An epidemiological study of disorders in late childhood and adolescence. I Age and gender specific prevalence. *Journal of Child Psychology and Psychiatry*, 34, 851–867.

Department of Health (1998) *Quality Protects: Transforming Children's Services*. London: Department of Health.

Durlak, J. A. (1998) Common risk and protective factors in successful prevention programs. *American Journal of Orthopsychiatry*, 68, 512–520.

Eddy, J. M., Dishion, T. J. and Stoolmiller, M. (1998) The analysis of intervention change in children and families: methodological and conceptual issues embedded in intervention studies. *Journal of Abnormal Child Psychology*, 26, 53–69.

Eisler, I., Dare, C., Russell, G. F. M., Szmukler, G. I and Le Grange, D. (1997) Family and individual therapy in anorexia nervosa. A 5 year follow up. *Archives of General Psychiatry*, 54, 1025–1030.

Emslie, G., Rush, A., Weinberger, W. A., Kowatch, A., Hughes, C., Carmody, T. et al. (1997) A double-blind, randomised placebo-controlled trial of fluoxetine in depressed children and adolescents. *Archives of General Psychiatry*, 54, 1031–1037.

Eyberg, S. M., Schuhmann, E. M. and Rey, J. (1998) Child and adolescent psychotherapy research: developmental issues. *Journal of Abnormal Clinical Psychology*, 26, 71–82.

Farrington, D. P., Loeber, R. and van Kammen, W. B. (1990) Long term criminal outcomes of hyperactivity impulsivity attention deficit and conduct problems in childhood. In L. Robins and M. Rutter (eds), *Straight and Devious Pathways from Childhood to Adulthood*. Cambridge: Cambridge University Press, pp. 62–81.

Garralda, M. E., Yates, P. and Higginson, I. (2000) Child and adolescent Mental Health Service use; HoNOSCA as an outcome measure. *British Journal of Psychiatry*, 177, 52–58.

Glisson, C. and Hemmelgarn, A. (1998) The effects of organizational climate and interorganizational coordination on the quality and outcomes of children's service systems. *Child Abuse and Neglect*, **22**, 401–421.

Gowers, S. G. and Kushlick, A. (1992) Customer satisfaction in adolescent psychiatry. *Journal of Mental Health*, **1**, 353–362.

Gowers, S. G., Symington, R. E. and Entwistle, K. (1991) Who needs an Adolescent Unit ? A referrer satisfaction study. *Psychiatric Bulletin*, **15**, 537–540.

Gowers, S. G., Harrington, R., Whitton, A., Beevor, A., Lelliott, P., Jezzard, R. *et al.* (1998) *Trainers Guide on Health of the Nation Outcome Scales Child and Adolescent Mental Health (HoNOSCA)*. London: CRU.

Gowers, S. G., Harrington, R. C., Whitton, A., Lelliott, P., Wing, J. and Beevor, A. (1999a) A brief scale for measuring the outcomes of emotional and behavioural disorders in children: HoNOSCA. *British Journal of Psychiatry*, **174**, 413–416.

Gowers, S. G., Harrington, R. C., Whitton, A., Beevor, A., Lelliott, P., Jezzard, R. and Wing, J. (1999b) Health of the Nation Outcome Scales for Child and Adolescents (HoNOSCA). Glossary for HoNOSCA Score Sheet. *British Journal of Psychiatry*, **174**, 428–431.

Gowers, S. G., Weetman, J., Shore, A., Hossain, F. and Elvins, R. (2000) The impact of hospitalisation on the outcome of adolescent anorexia nervosa. *British Journal of Psychiatry*, **176**, 138–141.

Harrington, R. C. (1992) Annotation: the natural history and treatment of child and adolescent affective disorders. *Journal of Child Psychology and Psychiatry*, **33**, 1287–1302.

Harrington, R. C. and Clark, A. (1998) Prevention and early intervention for depression in adolescence and early adult life. *European Archives of Psychiatry and Clinical Neuroscience*, **248**, 32–45.

Hartman, L. (1998) Child and adolescent psychiatry research remains a challenge. *American Journal of Psychiatry*, **155**, 453–454.

Hazell, P. and O'Connell, D. (1995) Efficacy of tricyclic drugs in treating child and adolescent depression. *British Medical Journal*, **310**, 897–890.

Hernandez, M., Hodges, S. and Cascardi, M. (1998) The ecology of outcomes: system accountability in children's mental health. *Journal of Behavioural Health Services and Research*, **25**, 136–150.

Hibbs, E. D. (1998) Improving methodologies for the treatment of child and adolescent disorders: introduction. *Journal of Abnormal Child Psychology*, **26**, 1–6.

Hoagwood, K., Jensen, P. S., Petti, T. and Burns, B. (1996) Outcomes of mental health care for children and adolescents: I. A comprehensive conceptual model. *Journal of the American Academy of Child and Adolescent Psychiatry*, **35**(8), 1064–1077.

Hoare, H., Norton, B., Chisholm, D. and Parry-Jones, W. L. (1996) An audit of

7000 successive child and adolescent psychiatry referrals in Scotland. *Clinical Child Psychology and Psychiatry*, **1**, 229–249.

Hunter, J., Higginson, I. and Garralda, E. (1996) Systematic literature review: outcome measures for child and adolescent mental health services. *Journal of Public Health Medicine*, **18**, 197–206.

Jarman, B. (1983) Identification of underprivileged areas. *British Medical Journal*, **286**, 1705–1709.

Jensen, P. S., Hoagwood, K. and Petti, T. (1996) Outcomes of mental health care for children and adolescents: II. Literature review and application of a comprehensive model. *Journal of the American Academy of Child and Adolescent Psychiatry*, **35**, 1064–107.

Kazdin, A. E. and Weisz, J. R. (1998) Identifying and developing empirically supported child and adolescent treatments. *Journal of Consulting and Clinical Psychology*, **66**, 19–36.

Kibby, M. Y., Tyc, Vl. and Mulhern, R. K. (1998) Effectiveness for psychosocial intervention for children and adolescents with chronic medical illness: a meta analysis. *Clinical Psychology Review*, **18**, 103–117.

Knapp, P. K, and Harris, E. S. (1998) Consultation-liaison in child psychiatry: a review of the past 10 years. Part II: Research on treatment approaches and outcomes. *Journal of the American Academy of Child and Adolescent Psychiatry*, **37**, 139–146.

Lambert, W., Salzer, M. S. and Bickman, L. (1998) Clinical outcome, consumer satisfaction, and *ad hoc* ratings of improvement in children's mental health. *Journal of Consulting and Clinical Psychology*, **66**, 270–279.

Leff, S. and Bennett, J. (1998) Developing guidelines for community child health staff and examining the referral pathways and outcomes of care in support of emotionally and behaviourally disturbed children. *Public Health*, **112**, 237–241.

McGorry, P. D. (1998) 'A stitch in time'. The scope for preventive strategies in early psychosis. *European Archives of Psychiatry and Clinical Neuroscience*, **248**, 22–31.

Myers, M. G., Stewart, D. G. and Brown, S. A. (1998) Progression from conduct disorder to antisocial personality disorder following treatment for adolescent substance abuse. *American Journal of Psychiatry*, **155**, 479–485.

North, C. D., Gowers, S. G. and Byram, V. (1997) Family functioning and life events in the outcome of adolescent anorexia nervosa. *British Journal of Psychiatry*, **171**, 545–549

Osher, T. W. (1998) Commentaries: outcomes in accountability from a family perspective. *The Journal of Behavioural Health Services and Research*, **25**, 230–232.

Patton, G. (1998) Editorial: adolescent psychiatry: its potential to reduce the burden of mental disorder. *European Archives of Psychiatry and Clinical Neuroscience*, **248**, 1–3.

Prendergast, M., Taylor, E., Rapoport, J. L., Bartko, J., Donnelly, M., Zametkin, A. *et al.* (1988) The diagnosis of childhood hyperactivity. A US–UK cross-national study of DSM III and ICD 9. *Journal of Child Psychology and Psychiatry*, **29**, 289–300.

Rey, J. M., Plapp, J. M. and Stewart, G. W. (1989) Reliability of psychiatric diagnoses in referred adolescents. *Journal of Child Psychology and Psychiatry*, **30**, 879–888.

Rosenblatt, A., Wyman, N., Kingdon, D. and Ichinose, B. (1998) Managing what you measure: creating outcome-driven systems of care for youth with serious emotional disturbances. *The Journal of Behavioural Health Services and Research*, **25**, 177–193.

Schulz, S. C., Findling, R. L., Friedman, L., Kenny, J. T. and Wise, A. L. (1998) Discussion: treatment and outcomes in adolescents with schizophrenia. *Journal of Clinical Psychiatry*, **59**, 55–56.

Sein, E. (1991) The information needs of clinicians and managers. In M. Berger (ed.), *Aspects of Audit: Collecting and Using Clinical Information. ACPP Occasional Paper 4*. London: Association for Child Psychology and Psychiatry, pp. 5–9.

Yates, P., Garralda, M. E. and Higginson, I. (1999) The PCS and HoNOSCA as measures of child mental health service intakes. *British Journal of Psychiatry*, **174**, 417–423.

INDEX

Note: page numbers in **bold** refer to figures, those in *italics* to tables. Abbreviations used in the index are: ADHD = attention deficit hyperactivity disorder; CAMHS = child and adolescent mental health services; CBT = cognitive-behavioural therapy; HEA = Health Education Authority; MDMA = Ecstasy; OCD = obsessive-compulsive disorder; PTSD = post-traumatic stress disorder.